Editors:
A. L. Baert, Leuven
K. Sartor, Heidelberg

Springer
Berlin
Heidelberg
New York
Barcelona
Hong Kong
London
Milan
Paris
Tokyo

F. Terrier · M. Grossholz · C. D. Becker (Eds.)

Spiral CT of the Abdomen

With Contributions by

C. Ala Edine · C. Bartolozzi · C. D. Becker · M. Bezzi · L. Bidaut · E. Biscaldi · D. A. Bluemke
V. M. Bonaldi · H.-J. Brambs · L. Broglia · R. Brooke Jeffrey Jr. · J. M. Bruel · C. Catalano
O. Cay · D. Cioni · L. Crocetti · J. F. Debatin · F. Donati · F. Dubrulle · J. H. D. Fasel · X. Fouillet
F. Fraioli · P. C. Freeny · B. Gallix · G. Georgakopoulos · G. Granai · N. Grenier · M. Grossholz
B. Hamm · P. R. Hilfiker · H.-M. Hoogewoud · N. Howarth · H. Hricak · W. A. Kalender
H.G. Khan · R. Kubale · A. Laghi · M. J. Lane · L. Lemaître · R. Lencioni · G. Marchal · J. Mareceaux
B. Marincek · L. Masquillier · J.-Y. Meuwly · W. Okuno · J. Palussiere · V. Panebianco
R. Passariello · P. Pavone · J.-P. Pelage · J. H. Pringot · M. Prokop · V.-D. Raptopoulos
G. A. Rollandi · L. Rubbia Brandt · S. G. Rühm · P. Soyer · L. Spadola · A. Spinazzi · P. Taourel
M. Taupiz · F. Terrier · H. Trillaud · H. Tschäppeler · D. Vanbeckevoort · B. E. Van Beers
L. Van Hoe · G. Verswijvel · V. Vilgrain · P. Vock

Series Editor's Foreword by
A.L. Baert

With 455 Figures in 818 Separate Illustrations, 51 in Color and 29 Tables

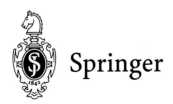

Springer

FRANÇOIS TERRIER, MD
Professor, Department of Radiology
Division of Diagnostic and Interventional Radiology
Geneva University Hospital
24, Rue Micheli-du-Crest
CH-1211 Genève 14
Switzerland

MARIANNE GROSSHOLZ, MD
Hôpital de la Tour
CH-1217 Meyrin
Switzerland

CHRISTOPH D. BECKER, MD
Department of Radiology
Division of Diagnostic and Interventional Radiology
Geneva University Hospital
24, Rue Micheli-du-Crest
CH-1211 Genève 14
Switzerland

MEDICAL RADIOLOGY · Diagnostic Imaging and Radiation Oncology

Continuation of
Handbuch der medizinischen Radiologie
Encyclopedia of Medical Radiology

ISBN 3-540-42291-9 Springer-Verlag Berlin Heidelberg New York

Library of Congress Cataloging-in-Publication Data. Spiral CT of the abdomen / F. Terrier, M. Grossholz, C. D. Becker, (eds.)
p.   cm. – (Medical radiology) Includes bibliographical references. ISBN 3-540-63463-0 (hard cover; alk. paper)
ISBN 3-540-42291-9 (soft cover; alk. paper) 1. Abdomen–Tomography. 2. Spiral computed tomography. I. Terrier, F. II.
Grossholz, M. (Marianne), 1952– . IV. Series. RC944.S678 1999 617.5'50757--dc21 98-52822 CIP

Springer-Verlag Berlin Heidelberg New York
a member of BertelsmannSpringer Science+Business Media GmbH

http://www.springer.de

© Springer-Verlag Berlin Heidelberg 2000, 2002
Printed in Germany

Cover Design and Typesetting: Verlagsservice Teichmann, Mauer

SPIN: 10905043   21/3111 – 5 4 3 2 1 – Printed on acid-free paper

Foreword

I am delighted to introduce a new volume in our series "Medical Radiology" devoted to the clinical applications of spiral CT for study of diseases of the abdomen.

Since the introduction of Spiral CT by W. Kalender a few years ago the technique has matured rapidly and has already found widespread applications in all areas of the body. Spiral CT has now attained a high level of sophistication, which requires from radiologists appropriate knowledge and skills in order optimally to exploit the numerous diagnostic potentials of this modality.

Notwithstanding the considerable progress achieved in abdominal MR due to the recent sucessful introduction of fast sequences and specific contrast media, CT still plays a major role in daily management of many abdominal conditions and many radiologists devote a considerable amount of their clinical time to this technique.

I would like to congratulate the editors for their excellent efforts in producing this comprehensive and up-to-date overview of abdominal spiral CT applications. They have been very sucessfull in securing the collaboration of so many leading experts in the field, from both Europe and the USA.

This splendid volume will be of benefit to all radiologists eager to remain on the cutting edge of abdominal CT as well as to gastroenterologists and to abdominal surgeons who are interested to learn more about the fascinating possibilities for better diagnostic and therapeutic management of their patients.

As responsible series editor I sincerely hope that this volume – like earlier volumes – will be well received by our colleagues in the different fields of medicine involved.

Leuven

ALBERT L. BAERT

Preface

Until the mid-1990s, the impressive, relentless progress of MRI had led many of us to believe that the days of abdominal CT were numbered. This feeling was made even stronger by the emerging concept of "interventional MRI", which gave the impression that one of the major achievements of CT, namely the guidance of diagnostic and therapeutic interventions, could soon be challenged.

Such pessimism about CT was a big mistake!

Indeed, the future of CT now appears brighter than ever. The advent of the slip-ring technology and the accelerating progress of information technology have laid the foundations for spiral data acquisition, which has allowed the move from slow, step-by-step scanning to fast, volumetric scanning. Highly optimised CT imaging protocols, based on a better understanding of the pharmacodynamics of iodinated contrast media, have resulted in greatly improved imaging of organs such as the liver, kidney and pancreas.

For the study of the aorta and its branches, the inferior vena cava and the portal circulation, powerful workstations can now calculate within a short time two- and three-dimensional reformatted images of exquisite quality from data acquired in the phase of maximal vessel enhancement and during a single breath-hold, a guarantee for high contrast and absence of respiratory misregistration artefacts. In many applications CT angiography has the advantage over MR angiography, and the respective roles of the two techniques still need to be clarified.

Virtual endoscopy provides completely new perspectives for imaging of tubular structures, including the gastrointestinal tract, and could have a major socio-economic impact if its potential in the secondary prevention of colonic carcinoma can be established by clinical studies.

Despite strong competition from US and MRI, CT remains the most informative and comprehensive modality for abdominal imaging in many clinical situations, especially in acutely ill patients and trauma victims and in perioperative situations. Most probably, the privileged role of CT will remain unchanged in the future and will even be strengthened by the breakthrough of multi-array detectors and perhaps also the introduction of tissue-specific contrast media in clinical practice.

All the new achievements in CT technology have led to a revival of CT as a field of exciting research and academic interest, besides its task as the workhorse in daily radiological practice. This is reflected in the large number of highly original publications on spiral CT in the recent literature.

It takes a highly competent team of radiologists and technologists to master state-of-the-art CT. Being in charge of a CT examination no longer just involves deciding whether or not to inject intravenous contrast material. The imaging protocol has to be tailored very precisely to the clinical question one has to answer and to the patient's condition, by adequate selection of scanning and contrast injection parameters. Furthermore, the sophisticated techniques of image reformatting require both familiarity with dedicated workstations and profound knowledge of the clinicians' requirements.

The daily work of the CT team is in no way less complex or challenging than that of the MRI team and requires constant adaptation to the rapidly changing computer environment, very close contact with the referring clinicians and, last but not least, hard work.

In this book, contributions from many leading radiologists and scientists in Europe and the United States have been collected to give a clinically oriented overview of state-of-the-art spiral CT of the abdomen.

We would like to thank all of them for their enthusiasm and excellent work. This book will be a great help to radiologists and technicians involved in the daily use of spiral CT as the prime imaging modality for the abdomen. For clinicians who are interested in abdominal imaging it may serve as a reference work on the capabilities of state-of-the-art CT in this field.

A final word of gratitude to the series editors of Medical Radiology, and to Professor A.L. Baert in particular, for their trust and patience, and to Ursula N. Davis, Janet Dodsworth, and Kurt Teichmann for their great help and professional spirit.

Geneva   FRANÇOIS TERRIER
                                                                                        CHRISTOPH D. BECKER
                                                                                            M. GROSSHOLZ

Contents

Technique 1

1 Principles
P. VOCK and W.A. KALENDER 3

2 Data/Image Processing
L. BIDAUT 13

3 Reconstruction Techniques for CT Angiography
M. PROKOP 41

Liver 55

4 Tailoring the Imaging Protocol
P.R. HILFIKER and B. MARINCEK 57

5 Segmental Anatomy of the Liver in Spiral CT
J.H.D. FASEL 65

6 Metastases
P. SOYER, D.A. BLUEMKE, and J.-P. PELAGE 73

7 Hemangioma
F. TERRIER, L. RUBBIA-BRANDT, L. SPADOLA, and N. HOWARTH 85

8 Adenoma and Focal Nodular Hyperplasia
V. VILGRAIN 99

9 Hepatocellular Carcinoma
R. LENCIONI, D. CIONI, and C. BARTOLOZZI 111

10 Perfusion Disorders
G. VERSWIJVEL, L. VAN HOE, and G. MARCHAL 133

Focal Liver Lesions: Role of Spiral CT and Controversies 149

11 The Case for Ultrasonography
R. LENCIONI, D. CIONI, L. CROCETTI, and C. BARTOLOZZI 151

12 The Case for Spiral CT
B. MARINCEK 157

13 Liver: Role of Helical CT and Controversies: the Case for MRI
     M. TAUPITZ AND B. HAMM 161

14 Synthesis
     F. TERRIER 165

Pancreas and Biliary Ducts 167

15 Tailoring the Imaging Protocol
     V.M. BONALDI 169

16 Benign and Malignant Biliary Stenoses
     M. BEZZI, L. BROGLIA 177

17 Choledocholithiasis and CT Cholangiography
     B.E. VAN BEERS AND J.H. PRINGOT 187

18 Spiral CT for the Diagnosis and Staging of Pancreatic Adenocarcinoma
     O. CAY AND V. RAPTOPOULOS 197

19 CT of Endocrine and Cystic Tumors of the Pancreas
     D.A. BLUEMKE and P. SOYER 215

20 Helical CT of Acute and Chronic Pancreatitis
     P.C. FREENY 227

Biliary and Pancreatic Diseases: Role of Spiral CT and Controversies 241

21 The Case for Ultrasonography
     R. LENCIONI, F. DONATI, G. GRANAI, and C. BARTOLOZZI 243

22 The Case for Spiral CT
     V. RAPTOPOULOS 247

23 The case for MRI
     P. PAVONE, A. LAGHI, V. PANEBIANCO, C. CATALANO, F. FRAIOLI,
     and R. PASSARIELLO 251

24 Synthesis
     C. D. BECKER 255

Urinary Tract 259

25 Tailoring the Imaging Protocol
     H.G. KHAN and F. TERRIER 261

26 Spiral CT of Renal Perfusion Abnormalities
     M.J. LANE and R. BROOKE JEFFREY JR. 269

27 Retroperitoneum and Ureters
    R. Lemaître, C. Ala Edine, F. Dubrulle, L. Masquillier, and J. Marecaux .. 277

28 Adrenals
    H.-M. Hoogewoud 319

29 Detection and Staging of Renal Neoplasms
    H. Trillaud, J. Palussiere, and N. Grenier 335

Renal Tumors: The Role of Spiral CT and Controversies 347

30 The Case for Ultrasonography
    J.-Y. Meuwly 349

31 The Case for Spiral CT
    H. Trillaud, J. Palussière, and N. Grenier 359

32 The Case for MRI
    W. Okuno and H. Hricak 361

33 Synthesis
    F. Terrier 365

Gastro-intestinal Tract 367

34 CT Enteroclysis
    G.A. Rollandi and E. Biscaldi 369

35 Virtual Colonoscopy
    H.-J. Brambs 385

36 Mesenteric Ischemia
    P. Taourel, B. Gallix, and J.M. Bruel 393

37 Synthesis: Impact of Spiral CT on Imaging of the GI Tract and Comparison
    with Other Imaging Modalities
    D. Vanbeckevoort, L. Van Hoe, and G. Verswijvel 407

Abdominal Aorta and its Branches 417

38 Aorta and Visceral Arteries
    M. Prokop 419

Abdominal Vessels: Role of CT Angiography and Controversies 441

39 The Case for Doppler Sonography
    R. Kubale 443

40 The Case for CT Angiography
    M. Prokop 451

41 The Case for MR Angiography
    S.G. Rühm and J.F. Debatin 459

42 Synthesis
    C. D. Becker 465

Special Topics 469

43 Helical CT in Patients with Abdominal Trauma
    H.G. Khan and C. D. Becker 471

44 Spiral CT of the Paediatric Abdomen: Technique and Applications
    H. Tschäppeler 481

45 Interventional Procedures
    M. Grossholz and N. Howarth 491

46 New Contrast Media for Liver CT
    A. Spinazzi and X. Fouillet 521

47 Spiral CT Imaging Protocols for Abdominal Studies
    G. Georgakopoulos, H. G. Kahn, N. Howarth, M. Grossholz, F. Terrier 531

Subject Index 547

List of contributors 551

Technique

1 Principles

P. VOCK, W.A. KALENDER

CONTENTS

1.1   Introduction: Spiral Versus Sequential CT   3
1.2   Hardware Modification for Spiral CT   5
1.3   Raw Data Interpolation in Spiral CT   5
1.4   Pitch, Slice Sensitivity Profile, and Slice
      Thickness   5
1.5   Reconstruction Interval and z-Axis
      Resolution   6
1.6   Image Noise and Artifacts   7
1.7   Radiation Exposure in Spiral Versus
      Sequential CT   7
1.7.1 Exposure During One Gantry Rotation   8
1.7.2 Exposure for Volume Coverage   8
1.7.3 Repeated Scanning of the Same Anatomical
       Area   9
1.8   Ongoing and Future Development of Spiral
      CT   10
      References   10

1.1
Introduction: Spiral Versus Sequential CT

X-ray computed tomography (CT), despite the great potential of ultrasound (US) and the astonishing ongoing improvement of magnetic resonance imaging (MRI), has a key role in imaging in abdominal disease. Its basic disadvantage in comparison with the other two techniques has long been the limitation to the transverse plane, with poor, hardly reproducible longitudinal resolution in the trunk. The transition from sequential to spiral (or helical) CT has significantly reduced the effects of this uniplanar approach and revolutionized clinical scanning. Although basically easy to understand as a simultaneous combination of table movement in the z-axis (as used for scout views) and continuous scanning (Fig. 1.1), the modification of spiral acqui-

P. VOCK, MD; Institut für Diagnostische Radiologie der Universität Bern, Inselspital, CH-3010 Bern, Switzerland
W. A. KALENDER, PhD; Institut für Medizinische Physik, Friedrich-Alexander-Universität Erlangen Nürnberg, Krankenhausstrasse 12, D-91054 Erlangen, Germany

sition means a philosophical switch from two-dimensional to three-dimensional acquisition of data, with the primary goal of improving z-axis resolution and the ultimate aim of isotropic imaging of a selected volume.

A number of obstacles had to be overcome before spiral CT was introduced into clinical imaging roughly 10 years ago (KALENDER et al. 1989, 1990; VOCK et al. 1989, 1990); several additional obstacles have been overcome in the meantime, and a couple still limit practical clinical work. This chapter will review these developmental steps, comparing sequential CT with spiral CT, and will try to estimate the potential achievement at the end of the ongoing improvement. It is primarily addressed to the clinical radiologist and will therefore not repeat the principles common to sequential and spiral CT, such as filtered backprojection for image calculation; nor will it cover the mathematical derivation of volumetric scanning.

Conventional sequential CT is a purely two-dimensional technique that measures one axial slice at a time and then moves the patient to the next longitudinal (z-axis) position before it can scan another slice of the body. Even with multiple scans taken during a single period of apnea, as used for dynamic imaging of the trunk, this principle is not modified, and the rhythm essentially remains discontinuous with repetition of the two phases involved: "planar scan – table motion – planar scan – table motion – ..." In contrast, spiral CT of the trunk uses one period of apnea to sample the complete information of a defined regional volume (Fig. 1.1). The raw data can be used to reconstruct scans at any z-axis position within the volume retrospectively without any new scanning (Fig. 1.2). This clearly means that spiral CT may be useful when continuous information of the entire volume is needed, whereas sequential CT will ordinarily be preferred whenever representative sampling can be obtained without complete gapless coverage. In other words, sequential CT is comparable to taking photos of the view from a mountain panorama by a camera (Fig. 1.3); the photo prints

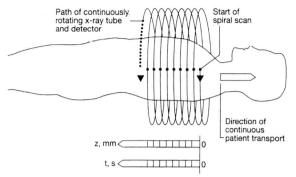

Fig. 1.1. The principle of spiral CT: during continuous tube and detector rotation, the patient is continuously transported along the z-axis; over the scanning time t (s), the z-axis is covered without a gap, and raw data are available for the entire volume (modified from Kalender et al. 1990)

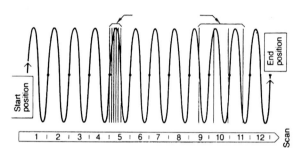

Fig. 1.2. z-Axis coverage and image reconstruction in spiral CT. Within the range of one spiral raw data acquisition (i.e., between the start position and the end position) positions of images to be reconstructed can be defined retrospectively at very short (*first arrow*) or at longer reconstruction intervals (*second arrow*), according to regional needs

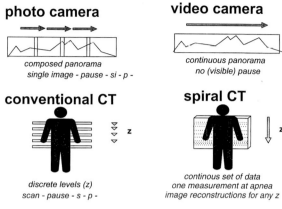

Fig. 1.3. The difference between conventional and spiral CT by analogy with photography. Like photography, conventional CT records single images (*si*) or scans (*s*) successively at discrete positions, whereas spiral CT, like a video camera, records a continuous set of data over the z-axis without interruption

show the beautiful landscape but even when they are placed together it is difficult to imagine the panorama. In contrast, spiral CT might be compared to a video camera, which captures the complete panoramic impression at once and still allows retrospective selection of a specific sector (Fig. 1.3). The main advantages of the volumetric measurement mode consist therefore first in a shorter acquisition to avoid any motion (typically 20–60 s, as opposed to many minutes in sequential scanning with inherent misregistration) and a better use of maximal contrast enhancement; and second, in the improved representation of the third dimension, which gives better z-axis resolution (reconstruction at arbitrarily fine increments), two-dimensional reformations and three-dimensional imaging.

Despite the basic difference between the two measuring techniques, spiral CT did not emerge as a new invention, but is rather an ongoing development of X-ray computed tomography that can now be ap-

plied as an alternative to sequential scanning and is increasingly replacing it. Most hardware and software features are common to both applications, such as X-ray generation, filtration, collimation, detector design, image calculation from planar raw data, and postprocessing to name but a few (Table 1.1), and both even offer the possibility of using either a rotating tube and a rotating detector array (3rd generation scanners) or a rotating tube and a stationary detector ring around the patient (4th generation scanners).

Table 1.1. Comparison of acquisition parameters in spiral CT and in conventional CT

Parameter	Prospective	Unique to spiral CT
Rotation time (t)	+	–
Collimation, section width (s)	+	–
Table feed per rotation (d)	+	+
Pitch $p=d/s$	+	+
Voltage (kVp)	+	–
mAs per rotation	+	–
Gantry angulation	+	–
Scanning direction	+	–
Scan duration	+	+
Multiple spiral scans	+	+
Patient position	+	–
Patient respiration	+	–
Contrast (i.v., etc.)	+	–
reconstruction increment (ri)	–[a]	+
Reconstruction center / size	–	–
Reconstruction algorithm	–	–

[a] Corresponding to scan increment in sequential CT (prospective)

In sequential CT, at the end of a – partial or complete – tube rotation of 360° around the stationary patient, all projection profiles can immediately be used for image reconstruction of the specific slice. In spiral CT, tube rotation and detector function remain identical but spiral raw data result, since the patient is continuously moved in the *z*-axis at the same time. This means that interpolation of planar raw data always precedes image calculation for any *z*-axis position specified.

1.2
Hardware Modification for Spiral CT

Traditional CT hardware was based on firmly attached connections between the high-voltage generator and the rotating tube and between the detectors and the computer; this design worked with alternating clockwise and anticlockwise rotations of the gantry. Independently of the spiral innovation, the need for dynamic studies of a single plane and for faster scanning of an entire region required continuous tube rotation, and the first scanners capable of multiple continuous rotations were produced in the late 1980s. Slip-ring technology – between the generator and the tube or between the source of current and the rotating generator – was an essential step in this achievement, being needed to guarantee a continuous power supply during many rotations; similarly, the increasing amount of data had to be brought back from the rotating detectors to the computer in 3rd generation scanners, by means of optical transfer, for example. Compared with this quantum leap, precise steering of table transportation simultaneous with tube rotation, as needed for spiral scanning, was a relatively small addition to the new hardware: this was probably the reason for the very fast and widespread introduction of the spiral scanning mode soon after presentation of the first clinical results in 1989 (KALENDER et al. 1989, 1990; VOCK et al. 1989, 1990). In the meantime, a number of additional improvements have been introduced, mainly to adapt the tube heat capacity and the computation capacity to the needs for increasing performance, but also to extend the spectrum of scanning options so that the protocols can be tailored to specific clinical needs. This is reflected by great flexibility in spiral acquisition times (mostly up to 60 s at maximum), repeated series of spiral scans with the same or different volumes, directions and acquisition parameters, as offered by most scanners on the market. Concerns about radiation exposure and tube heating led to the introduction of new, more dose-efficient solid-state detectors and of adaptive current (mA) modulation during scanning according to the patient's shape (see below). Indeed, spiral (or helical) CT has meanwhile become the standard examination mode in most conditions regarded as indications for investigation on modern scanners.

1.3
Raw Data Interpolation in Spiral CT

The longitudinal transportation of the patient during rotational scanning is responsible for spiral raw data, with only a single projection angle available immediately for any specific *z*-axis position; all other projection profiles have to be estimated by interpolating the many transmission signals obtained individually for the specific projection angle at *z*-axis positions of the table slightly above and below the specified position. This can be achieved in various ways; the simplest solution is linear interpolation from the values obtained at the identical tube position just above and just below the selected *z*-position, using the data from two consecutive 360° rotations for calculation of planar raw data. Modified interpolation may be nonlinear or differently weighted, or it may be obtained from little more than one rotation of 360°, based on 180° opposite projections. This popular method exploits the fact that the transmission signal in any projection angle at any angular tube position is available from a roughly opposite tube position (Fig. 1.4).

1.4
Pitch, Slice Sensitivity Profile, and Slice Thickness

When selecting a spiral CT protocol, the radiologist has the additional option of choosing the pitch (*p*), a factor defined as quotient between the table feed per rotation (*d*) and slice thickness (*s*): $p=d(\text{mm})/s\ (\text{mm})$ prospectively.

The higher the pitch, the larger the *z*-axis coverage and therefore the volume scanned during one period of apnea. Indeed, increasing the pitch from the theoretical value of 0 (dynamic scanning of one plane in conventional CT) to 1 (one slice thickness per rotation) and to the most frequently used range

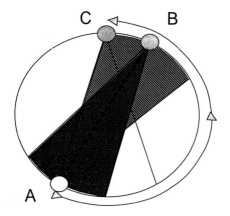

tube motion from A to C: 180° + 1/2 fan beam angle

Fig. 1.4. Raw data interpolation in spiral CT using opposite projections at 180° to each other. The absorption of the central ray, *AB*, is identical to the absorption of ray *BA* obtained from a tube position opposing the first at 180°. In the worst case of a peripheral ray, *AC*, the tube must rotate through 180° plus 1/2 the fan beam angle before it can produce ray *CA*. Compared with the original 360° interpolation, this technique provides interpolation of planar raw data from projections much closer to the image plane, improving the slice sensitivity profile

of 1.25–2.0 or even higher is very attractive and only limited by the fact that the slice profile is degraded.

Even with conventional CT, the longitudinal slice sensitivity profile (SSP) never has the ideal rectangular shape that would give an identical signal through the entire thickness in a homogeneous body. In spiral CT, the compulsory process of interpolating planar data from the original spiral raw data introduces information from outside the nominal slice. In consequence, the SSP is no longer rectangular but tends to become gaussian, with a small shoulder and a broad base, and the effective slice thickness clearly extends beyond the nominal limits of collimation (KALENDER et al. 1990; POLACIN et al. 1992; WANG et al. 1994; WANG and VANNIER 1996, 1997). This effect mainly depends on and is roughly proportional to the pitch; POLACIN et al. (1992) showed more than three-fold broadening from the nominal to the effective slice thickness [as defined by the full width at tenth-maximum value (FWTM)] in the worst case of a pitch of 2 and 360° raw data interpolation. In consequence, the contrast of structures and lesions will be slightly reduced for details smaller than the slice thickness (BRINK et al. 1992). When newer interpolation algorithms, such as those based on 180° opposite projections, are used, SSP blurring can be significantly reduced. However, it remains the main reason for not using a pitch of >2 in

routine protocols on current scanners with only one array of detectors. Therefore, in practice the slice thickness needed will largely determine the table feed per rotation allowed, and a reasonable pitch will often be in the order of 1.4, the square root of 2 (POLACIN et al. 1992; DAVROS et al. 1995; BRINK 1995; WANG and VANNIER 1996, 1997).

1.5
Reconstruction Interval and *z*-Axis Resolution

In-plane spatial resolution in spiral CT is very similar to that in conventional CT. Longitudinal (*z*-axis) resolution, however, is closely related to the effective slice thickness, i.e. the SSP, and to the reconstruction interval, a parameter chosen retrospectively during the process of image reconstruction from raw data. Therefore, *z*-axis resolution is basically different in conventional and spiral CT. The sequential mode, by taking overlapping scans (e.g. at scan distances of only one third of the slice thickness), might increase it significantly, but almost always at the cost of a nonrealistic examination time and radiation exposure (for the situation mentioned above: 300% of the value obtained with a scan distance of one slice thickness); this clearly eliminates the option of a major overlap in routine scanning. In spiral CT, for *z*-axis resolution, aside from the SSP discussed above, the reconstruction interval is the parameter analogous to scan distance in sequential CT; however, it comes without any cost in radiation exposure, examination time, and tube load. The raw data allow for image reconstruction at any minimal increment along the *z*-axis, and the cost is only the time needed for calculation and analysis of an increased number of images. Theoretical reasoning and phantom and practical experience all confirm that a reconstruction interval of less than one slice thickness is needed to reach the best *z*-axis resolution (URBAN et al. 1993; KALENDER et al. 1994; WANG et al. 1994; BRINK 1995; VANNIER and WANG 1996). As a rule of thumb, the reconstruction interval should be 1/2, 1/3 or 1/4 of slice thickness for a pitch of close to 2, around 1 or less than 1, respectively; smaller intervals do not improve the resolution significantly, whereas larger intervals clearly decrease it (VANNIER and WANG 1996).

1.6
Image Noise and Artifacts

Image noise in spiral CT, as in sequential CT, is critical and depends on many factors, such as the scanner hardware, dose (number of photons), patient geometry and density distribution, but also the reconstruction algorithm. Specifically, in spiral CT noise does not change when we increase the pitch (leaving all other parameters identical); but it increases when we use less than the raw data from two contiguous complete rotations for planar interpolation, i.e. as a function of z-interpolation (POLACIN et al. 1992). Most artifacts are similar to the ones encountered with sequential CT, mainly motion, metal and blurring artifacts (HERTS et al. 1993; VANNIER and WANG 1996). Motion artifacts – especially those caused by muscular contraction and by respiration – tend to be less disturbing owing to the shorter measurement period, whereas blurring caused by system imperfection is at least as important in spiral CT. Stair-step artifacts (WANG and VANNIER 1994; BRINK 1995) are associated with inclined surfaces in longitudinally reformatted images and increase with large reconstruction intervals and with asymmetric spiral interpolation; they can be minimized by using thin slice thickness and smaller pitch factors. A number of artifact-suppressing and deblurring postprocessing methods have been proposed; their use in clinical imaging, however, has been limited, and often it is more important just to be aware of the existence of artifacts in order to avoid misinterpretation.

1.7
Radiation Exposure in Spiral Versus Sequential CT

Awareness among the general population and concern about artificial exposure to ionizing radiation have grown during the last decade. During the same period, CT has become the single most important source of medical radiation exposure in industrialized countries (estimated at around 20–40%; JONES and SHRIMPTON 1991; SHRIMPTON and WALL 1995; MAYO and ALDRICH 1996; BUNDESMINISTERIUM FÜR UMWELT 1997; KAUL et al. 1997). This is explained by increasing numbers both of studies and of images per study, with an effective dose in abdominal CT of around 3–20 mSv (NISHIZAWA et al. 1991; POLACIN et al. 1992; LANGKOWSKI et al. 1994; CHANG et al. 1995; MINI et al. 1995; KALENDER 1998). Furthermore, in contrast to analogue roentgenography, where overexposure causes dark films, in all digital imaging techniques an increased dose is not easily detected, since it does not affect the gray scale of the monitor or the laser copy. It is therefore essential both to consider the risk of radiation exposure when choosing an imaging method and to minimize exposure once an X-ray method has been selected. For high-contrast organs, such as the lung or the skeleton, the tube current, which is proportional to the dose, can often be reduced without the loss of important information; unfortunately, in the abdomen contrast is mostly low and this option is of limited value. We will discuss the specific points of radiation exposure in spiral CT by pointing out three aspects (Table 1.2): exposure during one gan-

Table 1.2. Comparison of components of radiation exposure in spiral CT and in sequential CT

Principal contributions	Aspects	Comments
1. Per tube rotation	Tube output	kVp, mAs, tube age, filtration
	Scanner geometry	Generation, distances
	Detectors	Efficiency (geometric, quantum detection/conversion)
	Patient habitus (adaptation to)	Density/contrast/diameter (child, specific organ) dose modulation for noncircular cross-section
2. Type of volume coverage	Extra dose at top and bottom	Needed for interpolation (<2.5% with >10 and <1% with >25 tube rotations, 180° linear interpolation)
	Reconstruction interval (ri)	Dose reduction when ri < slice thickness
	Pitch	Dose reduction when pitch >1
3. Repeated scanning of same volume	Dynamic enhancement	Native, different phases of enhancement
	Functional CT	Respiratory, positional changes
	High resolution (thin slice)	Screening vs detailed imaging of subregion
	Intervention	CT guidance of biopsy, CT fluoroscopy

try rotation (one sequential scan/one subunit of a spiral scan), exposure for volume coverage, and exposure during repeated scanning of identical anatomical regions.

1.7.1
Exposure During One Gantry Rotation

A 360° rotation isolated from a spiral acquisition basically exposes the tissues to the same amount as a single sequential scan obtained on the same scanner and using identical parameters; differences are mostly limited to the local dose distribution caused by the different scanning geometry, with more homogeneously distributed values in spiral CT (HIDAJAT et al. 1998). Patient exposure mostly depends on the number and quality of photons entering the body (reflecting the voltage, mAs, tube performance, filtration, and the gantry geometry), and on their interaction with the patient. Newer detectors with increased overall dose efficiency [consisting of the geometric efficiency, the quantum detection efficiency (QDE), and the conversion efficiency] require less radiation: a QDE of >90% (as compared to 50–60% for Xe gas detectors) may result in a reduction of around 30% in the effective dose per study (VON DER HAAR et al. 1998). Similarly, a recent feature in some scanners enhances the potential of a patient-specific global dose reduction by modulating the tube current during rotation, that is to say by reducing mA specifically at tube angles with a smaller patient diameter. This is achieved either by estimating the diameter from two orthogonal projections (localizing scans; KOPKA et al. 1995; LEHMANN et al. 1997), or by interactively steering the output according to the number of photons exiting behind the patient (KALENDER et al. 1999; GREESS et al. 1998).

Exposure values are strongly hardware dependent, and there are important differences between different clinical scanners due to filtering, geometry, number of detectors and their efficiency, the number of readings per projection and other factors (SCHECK et al. 1998). The practical CT dose index (PCTDI, [mGy/100mAs]) was defined to help users estimate the exposure obtained in their scanner using a specific mAs setting.

1.7.2
Exposure for Volume Coverage

Volume coverage differs significantly between sequential and spiral scanning. In order to reconstruct the images at the top and the bottom of the volume scanned, the spiral mode has to extend exposure slightly beyond the top and bottom of the region of interest; this may be one rotation at worst for 360° interpolation or slightly more than half a rotation (twice the fan angle) for interpolation by 180° opposite projections (KALENDER 1998). Additional exposure is significant for short scans of only a few (≤5) rotations and for 360° interpolation; its proportional contribution soon decreases with longer scans such as are used in most clinical studies, and is <1% for ≥25 rotations (KALENDER 1998) and negligible for ≥30 rotations (HIDAJAT et al. 1998).

This detrimental aspect is, however, largely outweighed by two other options available with spiral CT: the possibility of using pitch values of >1 and the use of small reconstruction intervals of less than one slice thickness instead of overlapping scans (PITTON et al. 1995; VERDUN et al. 1996; HIDAJAT et al. 1998; PROKOP et al. 1998; SCHECK et al. 1998). As long as the effective SSP is adequate, increasing the pitch is appropriate and will bring an inverse, nearly proportional reduction in exposure (Tables 1.3, 1.4). For example, a spiral acquisition using a pitch of 1.5 instead of 1.0 over a length of 20 slices allows for an exposure reduction in the order of 32% (180° interpolation), and a reduction of 31% is realized compared with that resulting from 20 sequential scans. Sequential scanning mostly uses contiguous slices, with the scan distance equal to the slice thickness; however, when z-axis resolution is critical overlapping scans may be chosen, which means that the scan distance is lower than the slice thickness. The effect in radiation exposure is linearly related: 5-mm-thick slices spaced by 3 mm instead of 5 mm will increase exposure by 67% (Table 1.4). Owing to the complete volumetric set of data, spiral CT uses retrospective image reconstruction at reduced intervals instead of overlapping scans, with no additional exposure (Fig. 1.5). On the other hand, there is no reason to use complete volume coverage by spiral CT when only representative sampling of perhaps 10% of an organ is needed (such as for HRCT of diffuse lung disease, but also for the rather rare indication of hepatic densitometry); the sequential mode is clearly indicated in these situations.

Table 1.3. Influence of scan length and pitch on radiation exposure in spiral CT and in sequential CT. Values are indicated as percentages relative to sequential scanning, depending on the scan length expressed in number of contiguous sequential slices [same exposure parameters; 360° versus 180° opposite projections used for spiral interpolation (*intp.*)]

Scan length (no. of slices)	Pitch 1 360° intp.	180° intp.	Pitch 1.5 360° intp.	180° intp.	Pitch 2 360° intp.	180° intp.
10	110%	101%	80%	71%	65%	56%
15	107%	101%	76%	70%	60%	54%
20	105%	101%	73%	69%	58%	53%
25	104%	101%	72%	69%	56%	53%
30	103%	100%	71%	68%	55%	52%
35	103%	100%	70%	68%	54%	52%
40	103%	100%	70%	68%	54%	52%

Table 1.4. Influence of overlapping scan reconstruction (reduced reconstruction intervals) on radiation exposure in spiral CT and in sequential CT. Exemplary values for overlapping scanning using the conventional sequential technique at 5-mm slice thickness are indicated as percentages relative to contiguous scanning and to spiral CT, which stays at 100% no matter how small the reconstruction interval chosen

Slice thickness	Scan distance	Exposure Sequential	Spiral (pitch 1)
5 mm	5 mm	100%	100%
5 mm	4 mm	125%	100%
5 mm	3 mm	167%	100%
5 mm	2.5 mm	200%	100%

1.7.3
Repeated Scanning of the Same Anatomical Area

There are numerous reasons for repeated scanning of an identical area; many are inevitable, while others do not contribute to the diagnosis or do not have any implications for therapy. These reasons include: native and contrast-enhanced scans, contrast bolus tagging (with low-dose scans detecting bolus arrival), the need to obtain temporal information about early arterial, parenchymal, late venous or even urographic behavior, demonstration of functional changes in a different position or at a different level of inspiration, thinner slice collimation for more anatomical detail, and finally guidance of biopsy and intervention. Carrying out all the measurements needed at the specific anatomical area at the specific moment they are needed and using the specific correct conditions required while avoiding any excessive exposure is one of the most difficult parts of the radiologist's duty in prospectively planning

and supervising CT examinations. Modern fast scanners easily measure one or two additional volumetric scans and can therefore seduce the radiologist into adding delayed or slightly modified measurements of the same area. Unfortunately, the improvement to the study result may often be minimal or irrelevant, whereas additional radiation exposure may be significant. If the radiologist can draw on long years of varied experience and is continuously aware of exposure this will help him or her to resist (VAN HOE et al. 1998).

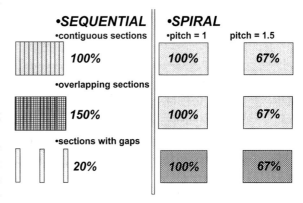

Fig. 1.5. Radiation exposure in spiral CT (simplified, excluding contribution at the top and the bottom of the volume outside the reconstructed volume). In conventional sequential CT, exposure increases in proportion to the degree of overlap; for example, with 3-mm-thick slices obtained every 2 mm, it is 150% of the value obtained with contiguous slices; conversely, it decreases with incomplete volume coverage, arriving at a relative value of 20% in the case of 3-mm-thick slices obtained every 15 mm. In spiral CT, the entire volume is always covered no matter what image reconstruction interval is chosen; this method is advantageous as soon as the reconstruction interval is below one slice thickness. In addition, it reduces exposure significantly whenever a pitch above 1 can be chosen

In conclusion, the total scanning period (which is closely related to the number of gantry rotations) becomes the single most important contributor to exposure that can be influenced by the operator during routine work. It can be reduced by decreasing the volume scanned, by avoiding repeated scanning of the same area, or – in the case of spiral CT – by increasing the pitch and using reconstruction at intervals far smaller than slice thickness instead of contiguous or overlapping sequential scans.

1.8
Ongoing and Future Development of Spiral CT

Currently, ceramic solid-state detectors with higher quantum detection efficiency are increasingly replacing gas detectors (VON DER HAAR et al. 1998); this is not only helping to limit radiation exposure, but also improving the flexibility of protocols and – with unchanged image quality – prolonging the lifetime of the tube. Interactive or scout-view-driven adaptation of the tube current to the shape of the body also reduces radiation exposure, based on the fact that a higher percentage of photons penetrates to the detector in children and at the shorter diameter of an oval body cross section (LEHMANN et al. 1997; KALENDER 1998; KALENDER et al. 1999; GREESS et al. 1998).

Faster acquisition may be achieved either by faster gantry rotation or by multiplying the row of detectors. The first approach of increasing the rotational speed, as long as the mechanical architecture is not replaced by an electron beam scanner, will run up against major technical obstacles; decreasing the time needed for one gantry rotation from the 0.7–2 s currently available to 0.5 s means mastering the enormous mechanical stress imposed by the rotating mass as well as the faster supply of power and the higher need for data reading and transfer. This significant challenge will be met by industry, but cost efficiency might be critical. The second approach of using two or multiple parallel rows of detectors seems to be much more attractive for the near future. Without increasing the heat load of the tube, just by opening the z-axis collimation, double or a multiple number of simultaneous readings can be obtained during the same scanning process, allowing for a higher pitch (e.g. 3) or a better z-axis resolution. One manufacturer, by using a double array of detectors, has realized the first product version of this innovation, while all major competitors are working hard on their own solution of multi-array detectors. Very probably, this will bring isotropic and three-dimensional imaging another step nearer (KALENDER 1995). At the end of the twentieth century, it seems to be clear that CT, despite its relative maturity, will continue to evolve for some years and will keep its primary imaging role in emergency situations and for many other indications. However, CT does not stand alone in the market, and the simultaneous development of other imaging methods, above all MRI and ultrasound, as well as other factors, such as cost efficiency, user friendliness and the political priority of radiation protection, will define the ultimate relative positions of imaging modalities.

References

Brink JA (1995) Technical aspects of helical (spiral) CT. Radiol Clin North Am 33:825–841
Brink JA, Heiken JP, Balfe DM, Sagel SS, Di Croce J, Vannier MW (1992) Spiral CT: decreased spatial resolution in vivo due to broadening of section-sensitivity profile. Radiology 185:469–474
Bundesministerium für Umwelt (1997) Umweltradioaktivität und Strahlenbelastung im Jahre 1996. Naturschutz und Reaktorsicherheit, Deutscher Bundestag 13. Wahlperiode. Drucksache 13/8630, 1.10.97
Chang LL, Chen FD, Chang PS, Liu CC, Lien HL (1995) Assessment of dose and risk to the body following conventional and spiral computed tomography. Chung Hua I Hsueh Tsa Chih 55:283–289
Davros WJ, Herts BR, Walmsley JJ, Obuchowski NA (1995) Determination of spiral CT slice sensitivity profiles using a point response phantom. J Comput Assist Tomogr 19:838–843
Greess H, Wolf H, Kalender WA, Bautz WA (1998) Dose reduction in CT by anatomically adapted tube current modulation: first patient studies. In: Krestin GP, Glazer GM (eds) Advances in CT IV. Springer, Berlin Heidelberg New York, pp 35–40
Herts BR, Einstein DM, Paushter DM (1993) Spiral CT of the abdomen: artifacts and potential pitfalls. AJR Am J Roentgenol 161:1185–1190
Hidajat N, Schröder R-J, Vogl T, Mäurer J, Steger W, Felix R (1998) Zur Dosisverteilung in konventioneller CT und Spiral-CT und zur Frage der Dosisreduktion mit Spiral-CT. Radiologe 38:438–443
Jones DG, Shrimpton PC (1991) Survey of CT practice in the UK. Part 3: normalized organ doses calculated using Monte Carlo techniques (NRPB-R 250). National Radiological Protection Board, Chilton, Didcot, UK
Kalender WA (1995) Thin-section three-dimensional spiral CT: is isotropic imaging possible? Radiology 197:578
Kalender WA (1998) Grundlagen der Spiral-CT. IV. Überlegungen zur Dosis. Z Med Phys 8:193–199

Kalender WA, Seissler W, Vock P (1989) Single-breath-hold spiral volumetric CT by continuous patient translation and scanner rotation. Radiology 173(P):414

Kalender WA, Seissler W, Klotz E, Vock P (1990) Spiral volumetric CT with single-breath-hold technique, continuous transport, and continuous scanner rotation. Radiology 176:181–183

Kalender W, Polacin A, Suess C (1994) A comparison of conventional and spiral CT with regard to contrast and spatial resolution: an experimental study on the detection of spherical lesions. J Comput Assist Tomogr 18:167–176

Kalender WA, Wolf H, Suess C, Gies M, Greess H, Bautz WA (1999) Dose reduction in CT by on-line tube current control: principles and validation on phantoms and cadavers. Eur Radiol 9:323–328

Kaul A, Bauer J, Bernhardt D, Nosske D, Veit R (1997) Effective doses to members of the public from the diagnostic application of the ionizing radiation in Germany. Eur Radiol 7:1127–1132

Kopka L, Funke M, Breiter N, Hermann KP, Vosshenrich R, Grabbe E (1995) Anatomisch adaptierte Variation des Röhrenstroms bei der CT. Untersuchungen zur Strahlendosisreduktion und Bildqualität. Fortschr Rontgenstr 163:383–387

Langkowski JH, Pogoda, Hess A (1994) Untersuchungen zur Strahlenexposition der CT-Diagnostik mit der Standard- und Spiraltechnik. Fortschr Rontgenstr 161:3–11

Lehmann KJ, Wild J, Georgi M (1997) Klinischer Einsatz der softwaregesteuerten Röhrenstrommodulation "Smart-Scan" in der Spiral-CT. Aktuel Radiol 7:156–158

Mayo JR, Aldrich JE (1996) Radiation Exposure. In: Rémy-Jardin M, Rémy J (eds) Spiral CT of the chest. Springer, Berlin Heidelberg New York, pp 33–40

Mini RL, Vock P, Mury R, Schneeberger PP (1995) Radiation exposure of patients who undergo CT of the trunk. Radiology 195:557–562

Nishizawa K, Maruyama T, Takayama M, Okada M, Hachiya J, Furuya Y (1991) Determinations of organ doses and effective dose equivalents from computed tomographic examination. Br J Radiol 64:20–28

Pitton MB, Harsini M, Mohr W, Schweden F, Duber C (1995) Strahlenexposition bei der CT-Diagnostik: Vergleich zwischen Spiral-CT und Standard-CT. Aktuel Radiol 5:289–292

Polacin A, Kalender WA, Marchal G (1992) Evaluation of section sensitivity profiles and image noise in spiral CT. Radiology 185:29–35

Prokop M, Schaefer-Prokop CM, Galanski M (1998) Dose reduction versus image quality in spiral CT: how far can we go in clinical practice? In: Krestin GP, Glazer GM (eds) Advances in CT IV. Springer, Berlin Heidelberg New York, pp 16–26

Scheck RJ, Coppenrath EM, Kellner MW, Lehmann KJ, Mayer M, Rock C, Rieger J, Rothmeier L, Schweden F, Sokiranski R, Bäuml A, Hahn K (1998) Dosismessung für Einzelschicht- und Spiralmodus bei 8 Spiral-CT-Scannern der neuesten Generation. Fortschr Rontgenstr 168:562–566

Shrimpton PC, Wall BF (1995) The increasing importance of X-ray computed tomography as a source of medical exposure. Radiat Prot Dosim 57:413–415

Urban BA, Fishman EK, Kuhlman JE, Kawashima A, Hennessey JG, Siegelman SS (1993) Detection of focal hepatic lesions with Spiral CT: comparison of 4- and 8-mm interscan spacing. AJR Am J Roentgenol 160:783–785

Van Hoe L, Van de Straete S, Bosmans H, Marchal G (1998) Relationships between time, dose, and quality in helical CT. In: Krestin GP, Glazer GM (eds) Advances in CT IV. Springer, Berlin Heidelberg New York, pp 3–8

Vannier MW, Wang G (1996) Principles of spiral CT. In: Rémy-Jardin M, Rémy J (eds) Spiral CT of the chest. Springer, Berlin Heidelberg New York, pp 1–32

Verdun FR, Meuli FO, Bochud FO, Imsand C, Raimondi S, Schnyder P, Valley JF (1996) Image quality and dose in spiral computed tomography. Eur Radiol 6:485–488

Vock P, Jung H, Kalender W (1989) Single-breathhold spiral volumetric CT of the hepato-biliary system. Radiology 173(P):377

Vock P, Jung H, Kalender WA (1990) Single-breathhold spiral volumetric CT of the lung. Radiology 176:864–876

Von der Haar T, Klingenbeck-Regn K, Hupke R (1998) Improvement of CT performance by UFC detector technology. In: Krestin GP, Glazer GM (eds) Advances in CT IV. Springer, Berlin Heidelberg New York, pp 9–15

Wang G, Vannier MW (1994) Stair-step artifacts in three-dimensional helical CT – an experimental study. Radiology 191:79–83

Wang G, Vannier MW (1996) Maximum volume coverage in spiral computed tomography scanning. Acad Radiol 3:423–428

Wang G, Vannier MW (1997) Optimal pitch in spiral computed tomography. Med Phys 24:1635–1639

Wang G, Brink JA, Vannier MW (1994) Theoretical FWTM values in helical CT. Med Phys 21:753–754

2 Data/Image Processing

L. BIDAUT

CONTENTS

2.1   Introduction *13*
2.2   Acquisition–Reconstruction *13*
2.3   Displaying CT Images *14*
2.3.1   Hounsfield Units *14*
2.3.2   Playing with Image Contrast *14*
2.3.3   Color Imaging *16*
2.3.4   2D Display of 3D Data *18*
2.4   Processing of Images for Enhancement
        or Restoration *21*
2.4.1   Value-based Enhancements *21*
2.4.2   Filters *22*
2.5   Advanced 3D Imaging *27*
2.5.1   Simple Measurements *27*
2.5.2   Segmentation/Extraction of Structures *28*
2.5.3   Creating Surfaces *29*
2.5.4   Volume Measurement *30*
2.5.5   Surface Visualization *30*
2.5.6   Manipulation *32*
2.5.7   Distribution of Digital Objects *32*
2.5.8   Volume Rendering *32*
2.6   Beyond "Simple" Imaging *34*
2.6.1   Navigation *34*
2.6.2   Use of Density Images for Calculation *34*
2.6.3   Parametric Imaging *36*
2.6.4   Computer-Assisted Manufacturing *36*
2.6.5   Finite Elements Modeling and Analysis *37*
2.6.6   Multimodality Imaging *37*
2.7   Picture Archiving and Communication Systems *38*
2.8   Conclusion *40*
        Suggested Further Reading *40*

2.1 Introduction

This chapter is intended to provide an insight into what is currently available to the medical imaging community for visualizing and processing digital images acquired with spiral CT. While even more sophisticated functions may also become available

L. BIDAUT, PhD; Division of Medical Informatics, Radiology Department, Geneva University Hospitals, 24 rue Micheli-du-Crest, CH-1211 Geneva 14, Switzerland

in the near future, most of these are still seldom implemented in current clinical practice.

As a general warning about processing images and data in a medical setting, it is worth mentioning that most display manipulation functions are provided on commercial equipment for enhancing their diagnostic capabilities. Obviously, the same functions can also significantly alter the content of the information, sometimes in a rather misleading way. For this reasons, caution should always be used in interaction with any display-related diagnostic equipment.

2.2 Acquisition–Reconstruction

Other chapters in this book describe the technique and technology of spiral CT in more detail.

In the classic CT approach, the X-ray generation/detection assembly describes a circle around the patient immobilized on the table at a specific location. This rotation generates a projection matrix, which encompasses a single planar disk across the patient. The projection matrix is often called a sinogram because of its appearance for a single off-centered object. From this sinogram, only one image plane – orthogonal to the rotation axis at the location of the table – can be reconstructed by the Radon back-projection transform.

In spiral CT, the table is moved at a known speed during the rotation of the X-ray generation/detection assembly. Thus, the projection sinogram describes a helix in space. This screw – with its main axis parallel to the motion of the table – cuts through a cylindrical portion of the patient's volume delimited by the starting and ending positions of the table. As the precise speeds of both rotation and translation are known, a classic planar sinogram at any location along the motion axis can be estimated by means of an interpolation of the sinogram data that have actually been acquired. Application of the standard Radon back-projection transform to this estimated sinogram then produces an estimated planar image of the cut through the patient's anatomy at the same location. Digital images are 2D (or 3D) arrays of picture (or volume) elements, respectively, which have been dubbed pixels (or voxels, respectively) for short.

Although mostly described for 2D images, all processing mentioned in this chapter can be extended to 3D data sets where 2D pixels expand into 3D voxels.

2.3
Displaying CT Images

2.3.1
Hounsfield Units

X-rays are photons produced by accelerated electrons hitting a metallic anode. X-rays travel through matter while being subjected to tissue absorption, which decreases their intensity. As a result, X-ray images are mainly an inverse representation of the tissues' density as measured by the attenuation of X-rays when they travel across the body. Classic 2D/planar X-ray images are film based, and the film is darkest where the most (i.e. the least attenuated) X-rays hit it. On this negative medium, "dense" tissues (e.g. the bones) appear white or opaque while "soft" tissues (e.g. the skin, fat and muscles) appear dark or transparent.

Because of the initial technical limitations of the analog/digital (AD) or digital/analog (DA) converters involved in the acquisition process, all reconstructed images from CT had values ranging over a 12-bit digital representation (from 0 to 4095=2^{12}-1). These limitations are now historical, but the useful range has stayed the same as its dynamics proved to be adequate to differentiate the density of all biological tissues. Other materials (e.g. metal from implants and prosthetic equipment) generally extend the density range upward. To normalize the density measurements across different types of equipment, Sir Godfrey Hounsfield came up with an absolute density scale (Table 2.1), which was defined as having air at its minimum and water at the value 0. The 12-bit reconstructed digital data (standard transform, ST) can be simply converted to Hounsfield units (HU) by means of a linear transformation:

HU = ST scale + offset (e.g. scale = 1.0, offset = –1000)

2.3.2
Playing with Image Contrast

2.3.2.1
Windowing

Historically, most digital displays had a single depth of 8 bits (also called a byte), producing luminance values from 0 to 255 (=2^8-1), which is enough dynamic range for the gray level resolution of the human eye. From this design came the immediate need to optimally convert 12-bit data (values from 0 to 4095) to an 8-bit representation, which was then fed to the display hardware. For this conversion, a simple proportional scaling ([0 to 4095]→[0 to 255]) would be the most obvious solution. Because of the undersampling it implies, however, (16 input values would produce only 1 output value), it becomes very difficult to assess the minute density variations actually contained within the initial 12-bit data range. For this reason – and because the full spectrum of densities is seldom of interest to radiologists – the concept of value windowing was introduced to expand the full contrast of the output/display range over the input density range actually of interest. Density (or Hounsfield units) windows are either defined by minimum and maximum values or by center and width in absolute units. Most often, such windows are defined to boost the contrast of specific tissue types as the examples in Fig. 2.1 show.

2.3.2.2
Look-up Tables

In modern systems, the conversion between a digital image and a display screen occurs through what is called a look-up table (LUT). A LUT is an addressing-based conversion scheme between an input value and an output one. This output value is then

Table 2.1. Hounsfield absolute units and ranges

Tissue	Hounsfield units	
	Lower limit	Upper limit
Air	–1000	–1000
Lung	–1000	–400
Fat	–150	–10
Water	–10	+10
Muscle	+10	+50
Bone	+250	+1000

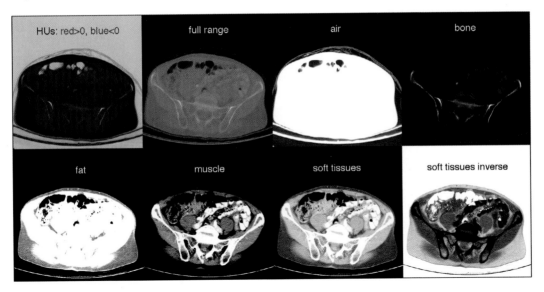

Fig. 2.1. Effect of applying various Hounsfield windows from the absolute values listed in Table 2.1

used to drive the luminance input on the display video tube through a digital-analog converter (DAC), which produces a point on the phosphor screen whose brightness will be proportional to the incoming signal at the corresponding image location (Fig. 2.2).

As a complement to the windowing approach, LUTs can also be used to enhance an image contrast by playing with the shape of what is called the transfer function between the stored image values and the corresponding index (or content) of the LUT component (Fig. 2.3). The transfer function is also called a sigma curve, by analogy with the S shape of the non-linear response of a photographic film to light (or X-ray) intensity. The standard way to use an LUT is to map incoming values linearly into the LUT indexing space. To simulate film response a sigmoid transfer can be applied, which will expand the contrast of the image in the intermediate values. If there is a need to expand the contrast in the low (or high) values a logarithmic (or exponential, respectively) transfer curve can be applied.

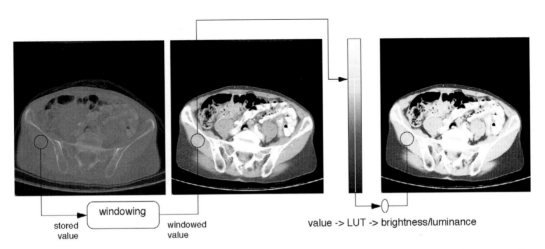

Fig. 2.2. Principle of the LUT approach: an incoming value is used as an index into a luminance array whose output is used to drive the display system

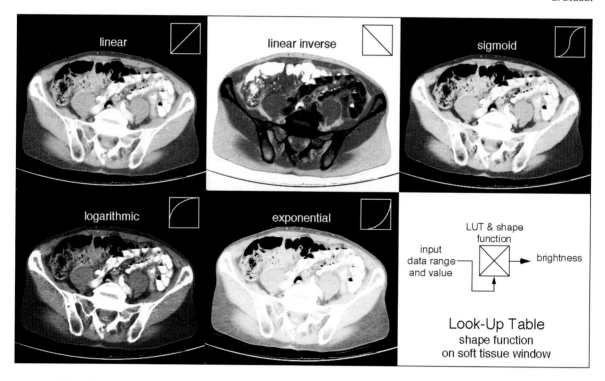

Fig. 2.3. Effect of changing the LUT shape function: besides correcting for distortions inherent to the display equipment, shape functions also provide a very effective way of enhancing the contrast of an image

2.3.3
Color Imaging

2.3.3.1
Creating Digital Colors

Any color of the spectrum can be represented as a linear combination of three fundamental colors, and this is how current display hardware has worked since the introduction of color video screens. The most common fundamental colors are red (R), green (G) and blue (B), but other colors can also be used, such as the RGB complements: cyan (C), magenta (M), and yellow (Y). The hardware-induced linear RGB paradigm is flexible enough to understand the additive color imaging concept and to interact with it. Other color reference domains have also been defined, such as hue-saturation-value (HSV), which closely matches the tint-shade-tone intuitive model of artists. Because of this intuitive foundation, the HSV model is more user oriented than the RGB, but its intrinsic nonlinearity makes it more difficult to use in the scope of digital imaging: while hue is the tint of the resulting color, saturation relates to the

amount of white in it, and value relates to the maximum intensity of the closest RGB fundamental color.

RGB and HSV spaces (Fig. 2.4) are reciprocal to each other and any color defined in one model can also be expressed in the other.

From any color image, a black-and-white (B&W) representation can be estimated based either on the magnitude (related to the modulus of the RGB vector) or on the luminance (actual equivalent luminosity of a specific RGB combination) of the individual colors:

$$magnitude = (R+G+B)/3$$
$$luminance = 0.3\,R + 0.59\,G + 0.11\,B$$

2.3.3.2
Pseudo-color Imaging

Traditionally in radiology, and by analogy with film, all displays have been – and still are for many – in B&W. Another reason for still using such displays today is that the color video screens use masks with a different phosphor point for each of the three fun-

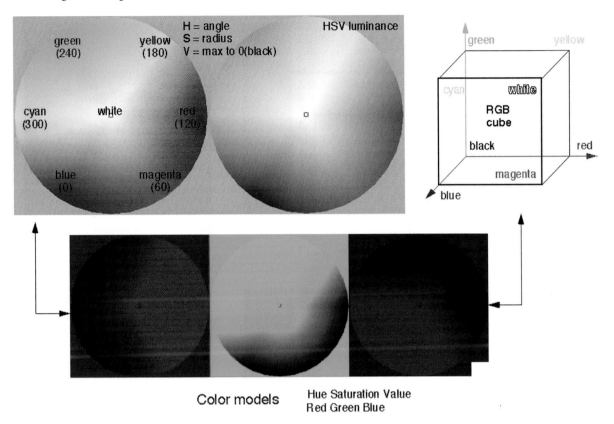

Fig. 2.4. Color models: HSV and RGB

damental colors. B&W video screens do not use such masks, and a point can – theoretically – be made as small as the impact of the electron beam itself. As a consequence, a single addressable point on a color screen is necessarily much bigger than a point on a B&W screen. For this reason, a color screen used for B&W imaging cannot be of the same intrinsic spatial resolution as its B&W counterpart. Nonetheless, when it is not just a matter of replacing standard radiological film, color can help by providing another contrast medium besides luminance, which can easily be distorted by hardware misalignment or even glare. With modern manufacturing processes and new technologies, computer color screens (including plasma or liquid crystal display devices) are getting much better in resolution, linearity and distortion. As new imaging techniques – such as parametric ones – also rely more on color for adding or enhancing information, and as the shortcomings can often be dealt with at the user level (i.e. through software features), color display systems should become even more popular in the very near future.

The LUT concept already described for B&W displays can easily be extended to color imaging, for which three separate video channels are driven by three independent signals, one for each of the fundamental colors (Fig. 2.5). In pseudo-color additive imaging, an LUT is a collection of as many color vectors as there are values in the incoming digital image. For any incoming image value, a three component vector (e.g. RGB or HSV) is created from the LUT content for this value. This color vector is then forwarded to the display system which translates it into a color on the screen at the corresponding image location.

2.3.3.3
True Color Imaging

"True color" imaging is the mode used for most photographic type color digital imaging. To best match the dynamic range of the human eye for colors, every fundamental color should be coded on at least 256 levels (8 bits). Considering three fundamental colors (e.g. through the RGB model) makes $256^3 = 16,777,216$ color nuances. Encoding that many different colors as a LUT is obviously not the most compact way of representing a true color image. For this reason, every RGB component of the composite

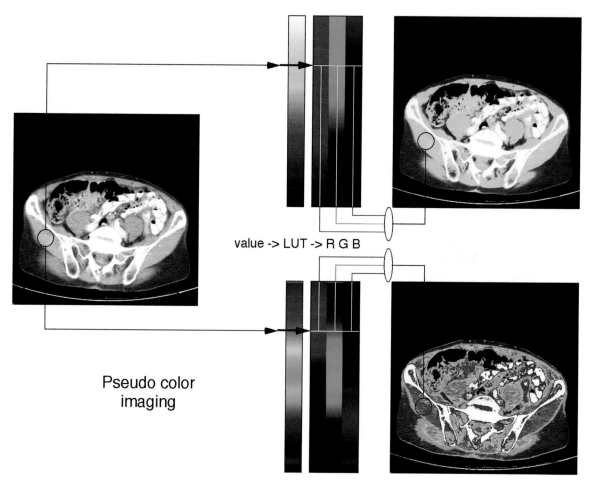

value -> LUT -> R G B

Pseudo color
imaging

Fig. 2.5. Principle of pseudo-color imaging: a color LUT is composed of RGB vectors which are fed to the display system

color image is actually stored as a separate image. To display such images, everything looks like three independent luminance channels with a single component (R, G or B) each, which are being used as the entry to the corresponding (R, G or B) DA converters and video channels (Fig. 2.6).

True color images are seldom used in radiology but they may for instance appear when a simulation or a real life scene (such as for histology, surgery, video-conference, etc.) needs to be displayed. As a common rule, and providing the display hardware permits it, true color mode is a more efficient approach than standard LUT whenever the combination of all colors results in a global LUT which contains far too many colors or entries for efficient handling (for example, see section 2.6.6.3).

2.3.4
2D Display of 3D Data

2.3.4.1
Slices and Multiplanar Reconstruction

Like all tomographic modalities, spiral CT produces slices (i.e. source images) across the patient's anatomy. Slices are 2D entities which can be displayed as such on any 2D screen (see pictures from this chapter and others). Window based display systems allow the screen space to be partitioned between various images which can either be from the same study or from different ones. Each data set can be displayed with its own parameters (value windowing, color scale, zoom, etc.). Compared to standard CT which produces single slices at significantly different times, spiral CT produces a collection of axial slices in a time (e.g. during a single breath-hold) when the body can be considered static

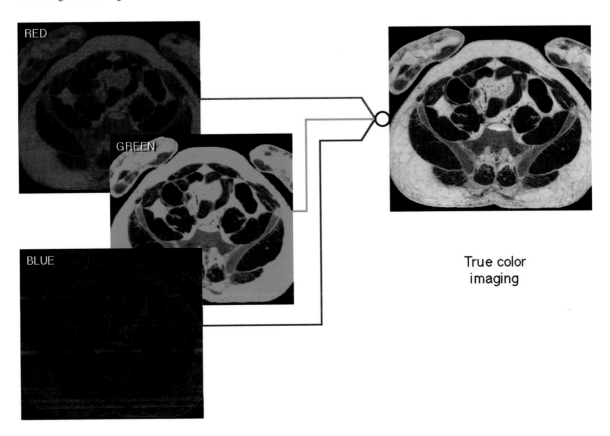

Fig. 2.6. Principle of true color imaging: an image is the combination of its three fundamental components

enough for 3D imaging purposes. Because of this capacity, the source slices can be stacked together to recreate the volume at the time of the acquisition. This volume can then be cut along orthogonal planes (standard multiplanar reconstruction, MPR) in order to produce images with other orientation than the originals (Fig. 2.7A). Such a tool, which is mostly based on an extended memory addressing scheme, can be very useful to display structures which are not "well oriented" in regard to the acquisition's main axis. A natural extension of the classical MPR approach is the oblique plane extraction and display which will show a cut of the reconstructed volume along any arbitrary plane (Fig. 2.7B). Another extension is the curved plane extraction and display which will show in 2D a nonplanar cut along a 3D curved path inside the reconstructed volume (Fig. 2.7 C).

2.3.4.2
Interpolation

Because of the way they are acquired and reconstructed, spiral CT volumes are very often anisotropic: the absolute size (e.g. in millimeters) of the elementary volume element (voxel) is different in all three axes. Generally, the source images (i.e. orthogonal to the table axis) have a pixel size smaller than 1 mm while there is less resolution in the third dimension (i.e. the one parallel to the table axis). Because of this anisotropy, data need to be interpolated in order to produce images which adequately represent real anatomical proportions and relationships, while also preserving an appearance which permits further exploitation (Fig. 2.7D). This interpolation – which is also needed when zooming the data – can be performed with several techniques which are more or less effective and/or computer or data intensive.

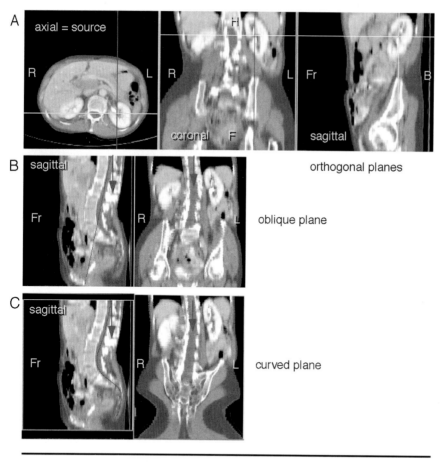

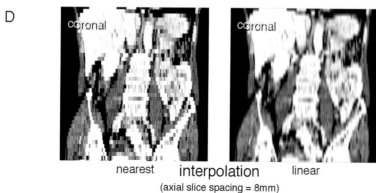

Fig. 2.7. Multiplanar reconstruction (MPR) on interpolated data for **A** orthogonal, **B** oblique, and **C** curved planes (from axial source images; some parts were generated with Analyze-AVW™). **D** Comparison of interpolation techniques; for anisotropic data sets, linear (or more complex) interpolation offers a dramatic improvement over the much simpler nearest mode

Let GT be a geometric transformation, i.e. any combination of rotations, scaling(zooms), translations, etc., and let the image G be the geometric transform of the image F (G = GT (F)). Resampling the bi-dimensional image/array F into the space of the bi-dimensional image/array G through GT means that for each pixel (u,v) (integer coordinates) of G, there will be a corresponding pixel location (x,y) in F's pixel space. The need for interpolation comes from the fact that (x,y) seldom are integers

which would point to a true pixel location in F. To best estimate the value of a pixel in G from the initial pixels in F several interpolation techniques can be used, including:

nearest voxel (or zero-order) interpolation:

(x,y)=inverse GT (u,v)

$i = $ floor$(x+0.5)$; $j = $ floor$(y+0.5)$
(where floor is the lower nearest integer)

$G(u,v) = F (i,j)$

bilinear (or first-order) interpolation:

(x,y) = inverse GT (u,v)

$i = \text{floor}(x)$; $j = \text{floor}(y)$
(where floor is the lower nearest integer)

$c = x-i$; $d = y-j$;

$t1 = bi(F(i,j), F(i+1,j), c)$

$t2 = bi(F(i,j+1), F(i+1,j+1), c)$

$G(u,v) = bi(t1, t2, d)$

where
$bi(y1,y2,a) = y1\,(1-a) + y2\,a$

2D interpolation techniques can be extended to 3D imaging. 3D interpolation is particularly relevant when creating or using image planes very "distant" from the source ones, such as in oblique or curved reslicing.

Other, more complex, interpolation techniques exist, which use polynomial or surface fitting, shape modeling, splines, etc. for a better estimate of missing data from that at hand. Such techniques are generally more computer intensive than the ones presented above. It is also important to bear in mind that interpolation techniques in fact always attempt to recreate missing data by making assumptions about the underlying data model. Except for very simple models, there is no ground truth to be found in their results, and their objective performances (i.e. their impact on diagnostic accuracy) will always vary depending on the actual features under scrutiny.

Another issue about image resampling arises when the size of the initial images is reduced (equivalent zoom factor <1.0). This type of processing should keep providing the most relevant information from the images (Fig. 2.8). Using the fast nearest pixel approach produces a rather crude representation of the initial image. Averaging or rank filtering (minimum, maximum or median value, see sections 2.4.2.2 and 2.4.2.4) can easily be used to keep an image aspect that is roughly comparable to the initial one. Other types of subsampling can also be implemented, which attempt to preserve the most significant information (edges, topology, etc.) concerning the structures of interest. Similar issues will be further detailed in section 2.4.2 (Fig. 2.8).

2.4
Processing of Images for Enhancement or Restoration

In the course of applying image processing techniques to CT images, it is interesting to note that these images are produced in an all digital world. As such, they do not suffer from the actual limitations of real life imaging (bad exposure, bad focusing, inhomogeneity, glare, etc.), but this does not prevent filter designs initially developed to cope with photographic issues from being successfully extended to the newer digital setting.

2.4.1
Value-based Enhancements

The contrast of images can be enhanced by other means than simply playing with the display window or the LUT transfer described before. For example, pixel values can be redistributed in such a way as to give optimal mapping of the complete display range available.

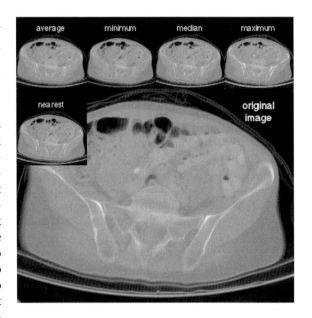

filtered sub-sampling for zoom<1.0
(example: zoom=0.25)

Fig. 2.8. Subsampling strategies; the small images are a sixteenth of the original one. Depending on the subsampling choice, the low, high or constant value areas are best exhibited in the small images; for simple consideration of the reduction of resolution actually underlying such processing, the average approach (similar to a sum) is the most obvious one

The most common processing of this type relies on the histogram of the initial image. Histogram equalization redistributes/spreads the initial image values so that its histogram becomes uniform or linear. This spreading – which can be confined to selected parts only – produces an optimal contrast for the image (Fig. 2.9).

2.4.2
Filters

As for standard photography, digital images can also be processed through filters to modify, suppress, or enhance some of their characteristics. As most digital filters are seldom truly problem oriented, their application is often empirical and is therefore always under the responsibility of the user who wants to ease diagnosis through improved – and hopefully not dangerously distorted – perception.

2.4.2.1
Space Versus Frequency

Any 2D image can be described both in the spatial domain – as a collection of picture elements or pixels – or in the frequency domain – as a collection (spectrum) of frequency components – after a bidimensional Fourier transform (FT):

Continuous forward FT (space to frequency)

$$F(\omega,v)=cFT(f)=\int\limits_{-\infty}^{+\infty}\int\limits_{-\infty}^{+\infty}f(x,y)e^{-j2\pi(\omega x+vy)}dxdy$$

Discrete forward FT (pixels to frequencies)

$$F(h,i)=dFT(f)=\frac{1}{n}\sum_{k=0}^{n-1}\sum_{l=0}^{n-1}f(k,l)e^{-j2\pi\frac{(kh+li)}{n}}$$

with $0\leq h,i\leq n-1$

Continuous inverse FT (frequency to space)

$$f(x,y)=ciFT(F)=\int\limits_{-\infty}^{+\infty}\int\limits_{-\infty}^{+\infty}F(\omega,v)e^{j2\pi(\omega x+vy)}d\omega dv$$

Discrete inverse FT (frequencies to pixels)

$$f(k,l)=diFT(F)=\frac{1}{n}\sum_{h=0}^{n-1}\sum_{i=0}^{n-1}F(h,i)e^{j2\pi\frac{(kh+li)}{n}}$$

with $0\leq k,l\leq n-1$

Because of the space/frequency duality of images through the FT (Fig. 2.10), frequency-based filters can generally be defined and applied in either of these two domains:

- On spatial images, a kernel (simple 2D array) is convoluted with the image: the original image array is multiplied and summed over the filter kernel at every pixel location to produce the new image.
- On frequency representations, a filter function (window, etc.) is convoluted (i.e., multiplied) with the 2D frequency spectrum representing the Fourier transform of the original image. The result is then transformed by the inverse Fourier transform to go back to the original 2D spatial domain where the image can be displayed.

The main interest of working in the Fourier (frequency) domain for digital filtering lies in the convolution theorem. In two dimensions, convolution is expressed by:

$$f*h(x,y)=\int\int f(t,u)h(x-t,y-u)dtdu$$

in the continuous form and by:

$$f*h(m,n)=\sum_i\sum_j f(i,j)h(m-i,n-j)$$

in the discrete form.

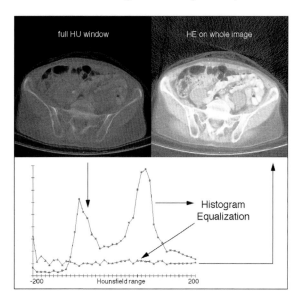

Fig. 2.9. Histogram equalization of an image; the spreading of values significantly enhances the aspect of the image which simultaneously exhibits contrast in the low and high values (see also Fig. 2.1)

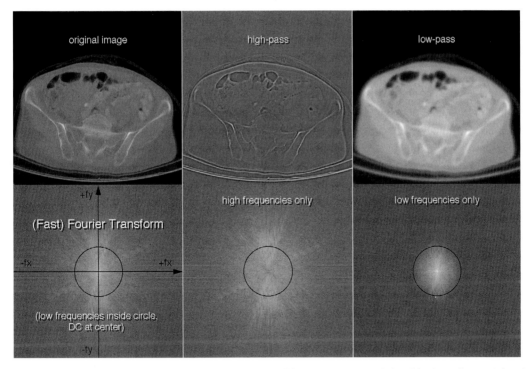

Fig. 2.10. (Fast) Fourier transform of an image with its high and low components exhibited both in the spatial and in the frequency domains (DC = Direct Current)

Based on convolution's definition, the convolution theorem is expressed as:

$$f * h = \text{iFT} [\text{FT}(f) \, \text{FT}(h)] = \text{iFT} (F \, H)$$

where FT is the Fourier transform, and iFT is the inverse FT.

Generally, because simple multiplications in the frequency domain take less time than matrix operations in the pixel domain, and despite the need for forward (FT) and reverse (iFT) Fourier transforms, there is a significant reduction in computing cost between spatial and frequency-based convolutions. For this reason, under suitable conditions, Fourier filtering is often used to speed up processing times. If the filtering to be applied is not physically and linearly based on suppressing or enhancing frequencies, or if the filters are on a small spatial kernel, Fourier filtering is generally not used. Because space is probably simpler to apprehend than frequencies, and because many filters use other pixel-based spatial information besides frequency, the following descriptions and examples will be provided in the "real life" spatial domain, where 2D filter masks/kernels are convoluted with a 2D image to produce the filtered image.

2.4.2.2
Smoothing Images

Images are smoothed to get rid of small details or some of the noise (i.e. high-frequency components). Such low-pass filtering (by analogy with frequencies) preserves larger structures while strongly attenuating smaller ones (Fig. 2.11).

The main parameter is the size of the kernel, which directly relates to the minimum size of the features to be preserved.

Smoothing at a specific location of an image is most commonly performed through direct averaging of neighbor pixels. Averaging over a 3 by 3 neighborhood will be a convolution of the original image with the following kernel:

	1	1	1
Average	1	1	1
	1	1	1

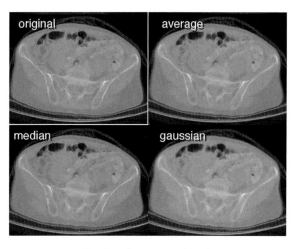

Fig. 2.11. Example of applying smoothing kernels (average, median and gaussian) to an image

If we weigh the values in the kernel by factors linked to the distance from the center location we can produce a weighted mean filter. A variation of such a filter is when the coefficients are assuming a gaussian shape centered on the middle of the kernel.

					1 1 2 1 1
Distance	1	2	1	Gaussian	1 2 4 2 1
Weighting	2	4	2	Mean	2 4 8 4 2
Mean	1	2	1		1 2 4 2 1
					1 1 2 1 1

Median filtering also uses neighbors, but it extracts and produces actual values from the image while preserving edges better than simple averaging. On a kernel of a specific size that selects which neighbors to consider, the output of the median filter is the value corresponding to the middle position when all values have been arranged in increasing (or decreasing) order. Median filtering is a type of rank filtering, which includes minimum and maximum filters (see section 2.4.2.4).

A variation of ordering the neighbors is called the mode filter, in which the output is the most common neighbor value over the kernel.

2.4.2.3
Enhancing Details and Edges

Several filters exist to enhance or extract small features (i.e. high-frequency components) from images

(Fig. 2.12). High-pass filters (by analogy with frequencies) are generally based on detecting and increasing differences and discontinuities within the images. The enhancements can also be based on simple combination of the original image with the output of the filters. The major problem with such filters is their sensitivity to digital noise, which generally lies in the high frequencies.

Gradient filters are based on a first-order derivative over a neighborhood of the pixel. Several variations exist with slightly different characteristics. Gradient filters always produce a vector, and this vector can be used through its components, its modulus, its orientation, or any combination of these.

Basic gradient: $G_x = \dfrac{\partial f}{\partial x}, G_y = \dfrac{\partial f}{\partial y}$

over a nonsymmetric 2 by 2 kernel:

$G_{x+1/2} = f(x+1,y)\text{-}f(x,y); G_{y+1/2} = f(x,y+1)\text{-}f(x,y)$

over a symmetric (i.e. centered) 3 by 3 kernel:

G_x
0	0	0
-1	0	1
0	0	0

G_y
0	-1	0
0	0	0
0	1	0

Prewitt operators are strict directional gradients on a larger kernel:

G_x
-1	0	1
-1	0	1
-1	0	1

G_y
-1	-1	-1
0	0	0
1	1	1

Sobel's operators are a combination of basic and Prewitt gradients, which reinforces the most local contribution:

G_x
-1	0	1
-2	0	2
-1	0	1

G_y
-1	-2	-1
0	0	0
1	2	1

Sometimes, the gradient is needed as a modulus

$$Gm(x,y) = \left| G(x,y) \right| = \sqrt{G_x^2 + G_y^2},$$

which is often considered as equivalent to $|G_x| + |G_y|$

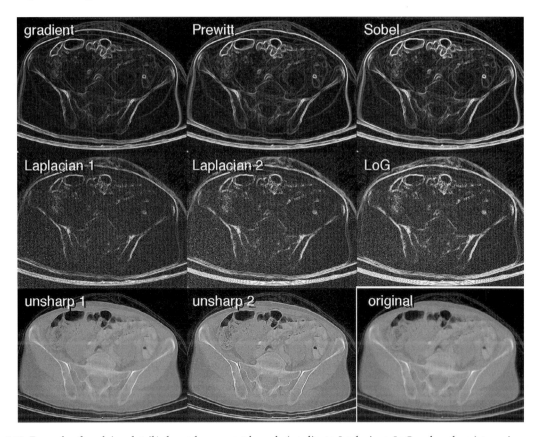

Fig. 2.12. Example of applying detail/edge enhancement kernels (gradients, Laplacians, LoG and unsharp) to an image

for imaging purposes. At other times, the gradient may be needed as an angle

$$Ga(x, y) = \tan^{-1}\left(\frac{G_y}{G_x}\right)$$

to provide an estimation of the orientation of an edge.

Laplacian filters are second-order derivatives. The masks for these filters can be calculated from the gradients. In 1D:

$$\frac{\partial f}{\partial x}(i) = f(i) - f(i-1)$$

$$\nabla^2 f(i) = \frac{\partial^2 f}{\partial x^2}(i) = \frac{\partial \left(\frac{\partial f}{\partial x}\right)}{\partial x}(i) = \frac{\partial f}{\partial x}(i) - \frac{\partial f}{\partial x}(i-1)$$

$$= [1 \;\; -2 \;\; 1] \; [f(i-2) \;\; f(i-1) \;\; f(i)]$$

After making the filter symmetric (centered on i) and after changing the sign of the coefficients, we get (–1 2 –1) as the basic mask for a Laplacian (or

rather its negative) in one direction. Current 2D 3 by 3 Laplacian masks then become:

$$
\begin{array}{ccc}
0 & -1 & 0 \\
-1 & 4 & -1 \\
0 & -1 & 0
\end{array}
\quad \text{or also} \quad
\begin{array}{ccc}
-1 & -1 & -1 \\
-1 & 8 & -1 \\
-1 & -1 & -1
\end{array}
$$

Laplacian filters are very sensitive to noise and they are often used in combination with smoothing filters. Laplacian-of-Gaussian filters (LoG; Mexican hats) are such filters where the image is first smoothed by a gaussian filter before enhancing edge detection with a Laplacian filter. These filters can be of any size in relation with the size of the edges to be detected but it is worth mentioning that the convolution of a gaussian kernel with a Laplacian kernel produces a resulting kernel which is much bigger than the initial ones. A small 5 by 5 mask for a LoG filter is:

$$
\text{LoG} \quad
\begin{array}{ccccc}
0 & 0 & -1 & 0 & 0 \\
0 & -1 & -2 & -1 & 0 \\
-1 & -2 & 16 & -2 & -1 \\
0 & -1 & -2 & -1 & 0 \\
0 & 0 & -1 & 0 & 0
\end{array}
$$

Unsharp masking (named by analogy with a similar photographic process) is another example of a filter combination which subtracts a blurred/smoothed image from the original, thereby enhancing the smaller details. In digital imaging, unsharp masking can also be produced through the addition of an image to its Laplacian:

$$uns(i,j) = f(i,j) + c\nabla^2 f(i,j)$$

where c is a scaling coefficient.

Various results can be achieved depending on the value of c and on the size of the Laplacian (respectively the smoothing) filter. With $c=1$, the previously defined 3 by 3 Laplacian masks give the following unsharp masks:

$$\begin{array}{ccc} 0 & -1 & 0 \\ -1 & 5 & -1 \\ 0 & -1 & 0 \end{array} \quad \text{and} \quad \begin{array}{ccc} -1 & -1 & -1 \\ -1 & 9 & -1 \\ -1 & -1 & -1 \end{array}$$

2.4.2.4
Morphological Filtering

Compared with other filters, morphological filtering does not have a duality in the frequency domain but is based solely on space. The spatial kernel of such filters represents the shape ("morphe" in Greek) of a structuring element, and their output is based on the convolution of this shape with the initial image or object.

All morphological filtering is based on combinations of two nonlinear operations: erosion and dilation. On binary data, erosion tends to shrink masks and open holes and gaps while dilation tends to expand masks and close holes and gaps (Fig. 2.13).

While morphology is best apprehended on binary masks (values 0 and 1) it can also be used on gray level images where erosion takes the minimum value of the image over the convoluted shape, and dilation the maximum one. With I the initial image, S the structuring element, S^s its symmetric (=S for an iso-

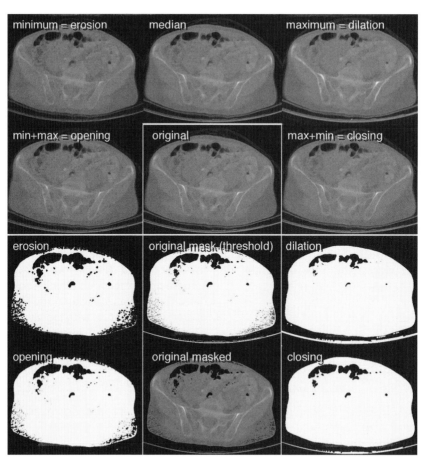

Fig. 2.13. Example of applying morphological filters (with a square 3 by 3 structuring element) over a gray level image (similar to rank filtering) and over a binary mask

tropic transformation), and $S_p = S$ translated to pixel p:

Erosion: $er[I(p)] = I \ominus S^s = \min\left[I(q)/q \in S_p^s\right]$

Dilation: $dil[I(p)] = I \oplus S^s = \max\left[I(q)/q \in S_p^s\right]$

From the two elementary operators, two more can be built: opening and closing. If the structuring element is symmetrical, opening is the combination of an erosion followed by a dilation and closing is the combination of a dilation followed by an erosion.

Opening: $op[I(p)] = (I \ominus S^s) \oplus S$

Closing: $cl[I(p)] = (I \oplus S^s) \ominus S$

By tuning the shape of the structuring element morphological filters can be fitted for many applications . In contrast to linear filters they are not reversible, but they can help in suppressing artifacts or unwanted features from images. They can be used for selecting objects with a specific shape from an image. They can also be used in combination with each other and with other processing to produce results that could not be reached through more standard approaches.

2.5
Advanced 3D Imaging

As mentioned before, spiral CT 3D data sets are stacks of 2D slices (source images) that have been acquired in a single breath-hold, i.e. which are representative enough of the same reality timewise. Under this assumption, such data can be used to extract and visualize information or objects directly relating to the patient's anatomy.

2.5.1
Simple Measurements

As well as being derivable from standard 2D imaging, distances and angles can be computed from 3D data sets providing the user specifies the points to be considered for these measurements (Fig. 2.14). Distances require two points and angles, three; calipers may use even more entries to provide extra information. In parallel with distances, linear (or even curved) profiles can also be computed inside the data sets, which may help in better assessing relative differences across an image.

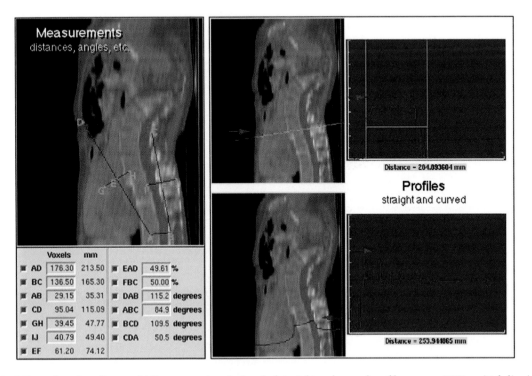

Fig. 2.14. Examples of a caliper tool (distances and angles) and of straight and curved profiles over an MPR sagittal slice (some parts were generated with Analyze-AVW^{TM})

2.5.2
Segmentation/Extraction of Structures

Besides the simple visualization of slices, the 3D spiral CT volume can also be used to extract (i.e. segment) structures and visualize or manipulate them in 3D.

A volume of interest (VOI) can be segmented from a volume of data using different means, depending on its characteristics and on the needs of the user. Con-

tours can be drawn around a structure of interest on each slice that shows part of it (Fig. 2.15A). At the end of the process, these contours can be displayed on a workstation and interactively manipulated (translations, rotations, zooms) in real time to provide a crude representation of the corresponding structure. Another way of extracting the structure would be to paint/tag it in every slice that contains part of it (Fig. 2.15B). The resulting mask can then be used to apply further processing on the data representing the struc-

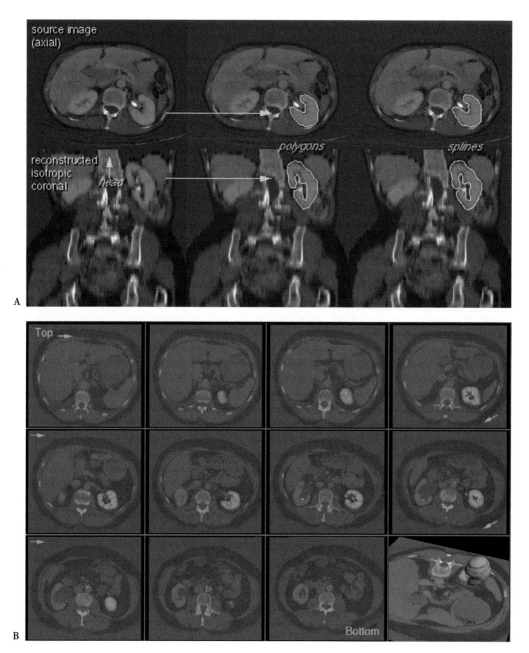

Fig. 2.15. Example of **A** contour-based and **B** paint/tag-based segmentation of a kidney on MPR slices

ture inside the full 3D data set. A semi-automated variation of the painting approach is the thresholding of data, which will extract only the voxels whose value falls within a user defined density range. Another variation of tagging is region growing, where all voxels falling into some kind of user-defined condition (e.g. a combination of value range, continuity, topology, etc.) are joined together iteratively from a user-specified seed until no more growing is possible. Providing that a good growing (and stopping) criterion can be defined, region growing is a very powerful semi-automated segmentation tool. The seed – which generally needs to be carefully selected – can either be any specific location inside the 3D volume, or an object which has previously been segmented out.

Tagging or growing produces a 3D mask over the structure of interest. Generation of such a mask is generally more comprehensive than contouring, as a mask may include finer details, which are not always easy to extract with contours. Other parameters can also be used to classify the voxels to be kept as part of a structure, such as texture analysis, topology, etc. While fully automatic techniques are seldom available for segmentation, even interactive (i.e. semi-automated) ones can benefit from preprocessing of the data through edge or contrast enhancement (see section 2.4.2.3 and Fig. 2.12), or from some other type of

filtering, which will attempt to make the relevant information more "visible" to subsequent processing. Very often, this preprocessing is a hidden component of the segmentation tools provided on clinical workstations.

2.5.3
Creating Surfaces

To further refine the representation of contours, their defining points can be joined together (tiled) by small triangular/polygonal surfaces, which will ultimately make up the outer shell of the structure of interest initially contoured.

A more direct way of creating surfaces is to use the 3D data set (or only a tagged part of it) directly through algorithms such as the widespread marching cubes (MCs). MCs are based on the classification of every cubic set of eight voxels from the volume (eight vertices/corners) into one of 15 possibilities as far as the inclusion of surfaces within this cube is concerned (Fig. 2.16).

Once surfaces have been created through MCs (or other algorithms), they may need to be processed further(Fig. 2.17). In order to correct for the artifacts brought in by working in a discrete (and often aniso-

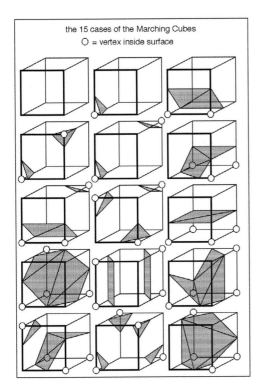

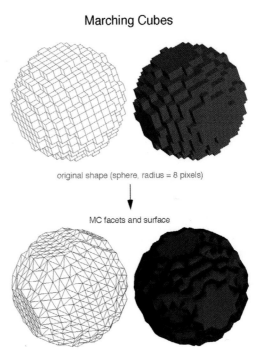

Fig. 2.16. The 15 possibilities of marching cubes (MCs), with an example of a discrete sphere (see also Fig. 2.18)

tropic) domain, surfaces can be smoothed by displacing their vertices to minimize the discontinuities between elementary patches. Also, for faster display or to decrease storage requirements, surfaces can be simplified by merging tiles/facets or suppressing redundant ones based on their orientation and on the local surface curvature.

Other surface extraction techniques exist, which attempt to correct for the intrinsic limitations of MCs or simply use parametric approximations of the surfaces (ellipsoids, superquadrics, etc.). The advantages of parametric surfaces is that they require only a few parameters to describe and manipulate them, and that their characteristics (local curvature, etc.) can be directly calculated from their equations. Parametric surfaces are often implemented in other types of software (computer-assisted design, computer-assisted manufacturing, finite elements, etc.), thereby making them generally easier to handle than real life arbitrary surfaces. The main disadvantage of parametric surfaces, though, is that they do not always fit anatomical structures well enough, and this is a limitation that may eventually lead to misrepresentation or misinterpretation in a true clinical setting.

2.5.4
Volume Measurement

Once a structure has been segmented out, it can be assessed in other ways than visually. For example, its contents can be analyzed to provide its density range or other relevant information, such as its total volume. The simplest way of calculating a segmented structure's volume is by multiplying the number of voxels that are believed to belong to the structure by the volume of a single voxel (Xsiz × Ysiz × Zsiz) calculated from the acquisition/reconstruction parameters (Fig. 2.18). While this calculation is the least disputable way of estimating a volume, using the shape of the structure – as provided by its polygonal or parametric surface estimate – may sometimes provide a more accurate approximation. This happens, for example, when the data set's sampling is poor but the surface model appropriate.

2.5.5
Surface Visualization

The easiest way to understand how a digital object can be represented to an observer is through the ray paradigm. Rays extend from infinity to the user (Fig. 2.19A). Some of the rays pass through empty space, while others intercept the object. Ray tracing implies

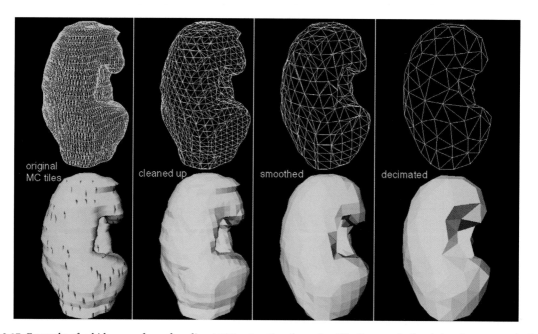

Fig. 2.17. Example of a kidney surface after direct MC extraction from the CT slices, and after it has been smoothed and decimated; the surfaces are shown both as their tile components and as constant (i.e. flat) rendering (see also section 2.5.5 and Fig. 2.20)

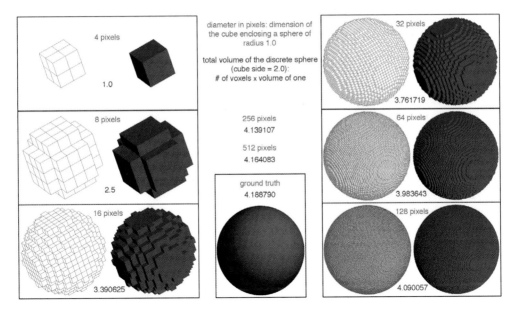

Fig. 2.18. Example of discrete volume calculation for a binary sphere as a function of the sampling resolution; obviously, the finer the resolution, the better the estimate. In real life, however, as resolution is limited for ionizing CT and as living objects are seldom binary, other (e.g. model-based) methods of volume calculation could sometimes provide better estimates than the discrete calculation

that all rays originate at infinity (beyond the object) and travel toward the observer. Ray casting goes the other way, from the observer to infinity (and beyond...). While the simplicity of the ray paradigm allows 3D imaging to be easily understood, its "brute force" application is far from being computationally optimal, and this is why it is always implemented through more efficient schemes.

Once a digital surface has been extracted, it can be given various properties regarding its representation, its color, its transparency (or opacity) and its response to external lighting. The visualization of the surface will then depend on the light model (Fig. 2.19B) used for the calculation and on the shading which is selected to render the surface in the most realistic or informative way (Fig. 2.20).

For example, depth shading shows the distance between the observer's virtual plane (i.e. the display screen) and the object surface on the corresponding ray; voxel shading displays the corresponding voxel value from the original 3D data set on the surface.

The constant light model places a single light source and the user/observer at infinity, while assuming that the surface is composed of flat polygonal (e.g. triangular) tiles. Every tile is then rendered as its polygonal projection in the direction of the observer, intensified by the light reflected to the user through the chosen model.

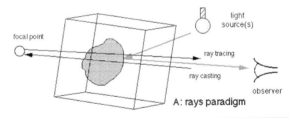

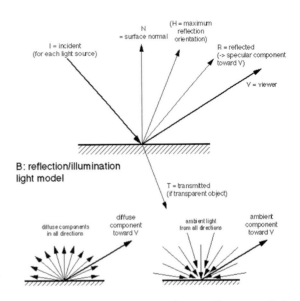

Fig. 2.19. A Rays paradigm and **B** reflection/illumination light model

In Gouraud shading (not shown), the intensity is calculated at each one of the elementary tile vertices by interpolating the normal vectors from the intersecting tiles. The projection of a tile to the observer is then interpolated from the values at the vertices, which makes the object appear smoother than in the constant model.

For a similar goal but a more realistic result, Phong shading actually uses normal vectors (not intensities) interpolated on the tiles' surface (not only at the vertices) for calculating the intensity to be projected toward the user.

Besides the intensity produced through the light shading model, the color of a surface can also be modified, either through interactive selection or by further use of the normals or of the values contained in the original data set. Interactive selection can include not only the base color of the surface (in the RGB or HSV model) but also all other characteristics that modify the surface response to any incoming light (e.g. specular, diffuse, ambient components). Finally, surfaces can be textured by projecting images or data onto the polygonal tiles. Such texturing can be used either to provide a more realistic look to the objects or to add other (e.g. parametric) information on the surface of the object. For example, the native 3D data set values can be used to calculate the 3D gradient on the surface.

2.5.6
Manipulation

To convey all its intrinsic information to an observer, a 3D object needs to be interactively manipulated and visualized on a screen. A successful concept for such manipulation is the virtual (or not so much so) trackball, which assumes that the object is at the center of a sphere. The user can then rotate and translate the object by simple manipulation of a standard input device.

The most standard input device is the mouse (or even a real trackball), which translates a 2D motion into the ones needed for manipulating the object (e.g. translations, rotations, zooms). Full 3D input devices also exist, which generally provide 6 degrees of freedom (3 translations and 3 rotations). These latter devices have generally been developed in the scope of virtual reality and are seldom used in combination with diagnostic workstations because the simultaneous manipulation of all six parameters is rarely required in such a setting. Most of the time, such devices are implemented on interventional

navigation systems (see section 2.6.1) which can use this type of interaction to simulate or accompany the free motion of the user.

2.5.7
Distribution of Digital Objects

On modern equipment, all surface rendering is generally taken care of by specialized hardware optimized for handling and rendering a large collection of polygonal surface tiles. Besides hardware itself – which continues to evolve at an ever-increasing pace – software standards have also been developed to allow 3D objects to be distributed and visualized on any platform available on the Internet. Virtual Reality Modeling Language (VRML) is such an achievement and – like images and movies at the beginning of the Internet – any 3/4D object can now be retrieved from a server on the worldwide web and manipulated in real time through standard plug-ins available on most workstations or PCs.

2.5.8
Volume Rendering

Compared with surface rendering, volume rendering does not intrinsically require the segmentation of structures but uses all voxels from the volume simultaneously. Voxels are assigned a color and an opacity/transparency, which can be linked to their value (though an LUT scheme) or to other characteristics (Fig. 2.21). The volume is then represented to the user/observer through the same ray tracing (or casting) paradigm as was described before for surfaces, and the opacity/transparency parameter can be selected to best tune the representation to the user's needs. A special (simplified) mode of volume rendering is maximum intensity projection (MIP) where only the highest value on a ray is projected to the user. This technique is mainly used when rendering isolated highly contrasted objects, such as bones or contrast-enhanced vascular structures. While considering all voxels along each ray is obviously the most comprehensive way of doing volume rendering, more effective multiresolution techniques – which also often limit the active length of the rays – are frequently implemented to shorten calculation times or to display only the information that is most relevant to a specific investigation.

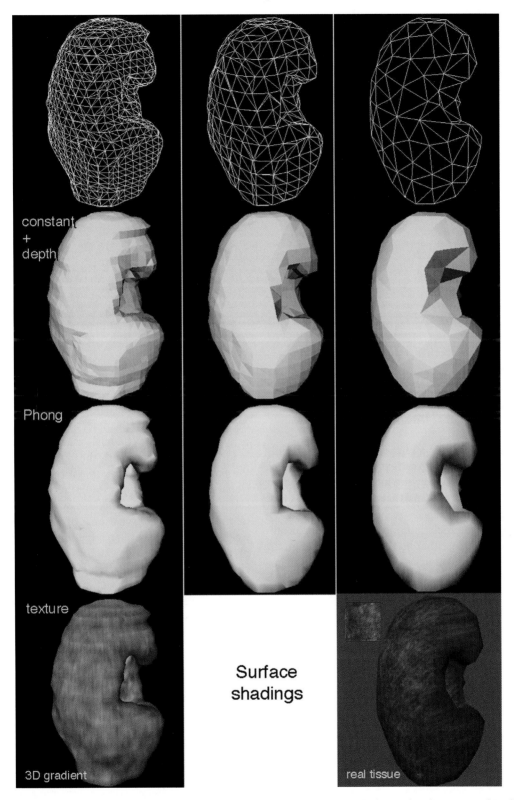

Fig. 2.20. Representations of the surface (with various resolutions) of a segmented kidney: tiles, distance combined with a constant shading, Phong shading, texture from a 3D gradient on the initial dataset, and texture from a real tissue sample

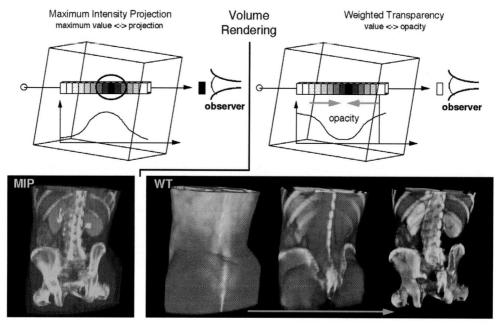

Fig. 2.21. Volume rendering paradigm with an example of maximum intensity projection and standard weighted transparency on a contrast enhanced abdominal data set

2.6
Beyond "Simple" Imaging

Most of this chapter attempts to provide a feeling about how digital images are produced, manipulated and displayed to convey the information needed for supporting diagnosis and therapy. While this is how most spiral CT images are being used nowadays, they can also be included into more complex protocols. For example, either on their own or through the fusion with other modalities at hand, spiral CT images can be used for actually planning and monitoring therapy.

2.6.1
Navigation

Most surgical suites now include a navigation system which allows image-based interventions (Fig. 2.22) to be carried out. Such a system mainly relies on a 3D pointer (Fig. 2.23) connected to a computer where all relevant objects can be extracted from the volumes and manipulated in relation with the motion of the pointer.

Most of the time, primary diagnosis selects a target for the intervention (biopsy, surgery or radiotherapy), which can be extracted on the navigation computer, along with other structures. At the time of the intervention, the patient is first aligned to the digital world through the detection and registration of paired features (fiducial markers, anatomical landmarks, etc.) from both the digital data set and the patient. After registration, all real-life interventional tools (or beams for radiotherapy) can be located inside the digital anatomy, which can be used to monitor the intervention. Although the major weakness of image based navigation is its reliance on presurgical data sets – which might not always be close enough to the ever-changing surgical reality – the increasing availability of interventional modalities (including US, CT and MR) should soon solve this issue by providing an accurate updating of the digital information during the intervention.

2.6.2
Use of Density Images for Calculation

Besides image-based targeting, CT density data can also be used as the base for calculating the optimal geometry of radiotherapy beams and the total dose to all structures irradiated (Fig. 2.24). Such capacity to use accurate digital data from the patient to fit the treatment to any individual anatomy and pathology insures both the best overlap at the tumor site and the least damage to other structures.

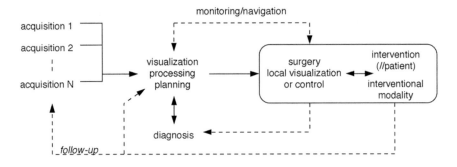

Image based navigation

Fig. 2.22. Flowchart of an image-driven interventional protocol; such a protocol relies on using diagnostic images to define a target and – possibly – on refreshing the target information through the use of interventional modalities or sensors

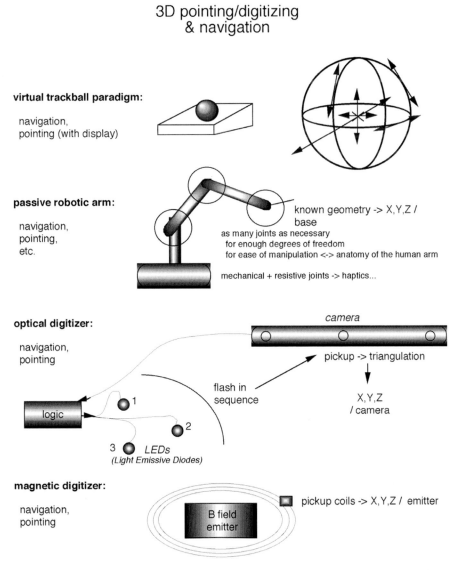

Fig. 2.23. Virtual trackball and other types of 3D pointer used in virtual reality but also for orienting objects or pointing at locations or directions in space

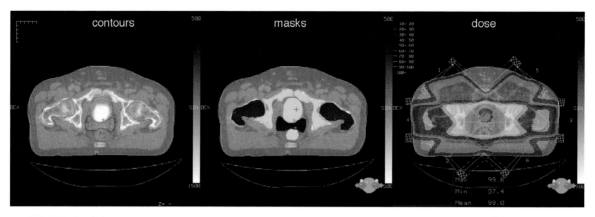

Fig. 2.24. Simulation and dose calculation from CT images for treating a prostate cancer (using a Varian™ system); relevant structures are segmented out and used to calculate the beam combination that will best overlap over the tumor while best preserving important areas

2.6.3
Parametric Imaging

Parameters may be any information associated with – or extracted from – images. Spiral CT is primarily intended to produce 3D volumetric data sets. The emphasis of this chapter has been put on such data. Using the same design, spiral CT can also provide fast dynamic data by leaving the table immobile and acquiring slices at the same location through time. Such data can – for example – show the spreading and washout of contrast agent during the time of the acquisition. From further calculation on this information [e.g. through compartmental analysis (Fig. 2.25)], parameters can be extracted which – for example – relate to the dynamic behavior of tissues or of blood flow. Such parameters can then be projected on the images and show computed values in regard to the actual anatomy.

2.6.4
Computer-Assisted Manufacturing

Segmented objects can be visualized on display screens. Still, sometimes, their assessment and clinical use might gain from constructing them with computer-assisted design/computer-assisted manufacturing (CAD/CAM) techniques and equipment. From the segmented objects, control points and models can be extracted, which can be fed to multi-dimensional digital manufacturing machines. Such machines can then mill rigid foam or any kind of material to reproduce the virtual object in the real world (Fig. 2.26). The most immediate application of such a technique was the making of models to build custom-made prostheses, but other applications can also be envisioned, even for soft tissues.

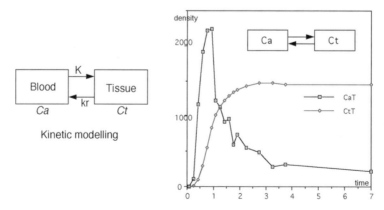

Fig. 2.25. Compartments and curves for a very simple model; the exchange parameters (K, kr) and the compartments' contents $[Ca(blood), Ct(tissue)]$ are fitted to the experimental data CaT (e.g. blood samples) and CtT (e.g. CT data) as a function of time

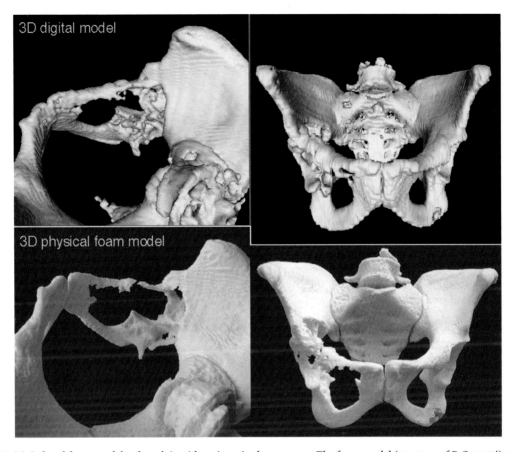

Fig. 2.26. Digital and foam models of a pelvis with an invasive bone tumor. The foam model (courtesy of P. Cerrutti) was built with a digital manufacturing milling machine driven by the shape of the pelvis structure as extracted from the CT data

2.6.5
Finite Elements Modeling and Analysis

Besides representing real-life objects, digital objects can also be used to provide more insight into the way real life ones behave through techniques such as finite element modeling (FEM). Digital objects are initially partitioned into elementary cells, which are set to represent the tissue at the same locations (Fig. 2.27). This setting occurs through the mixing of parameters and of constraints extracted from real life measurements and from physiological modeling of the tissues' behavior. Once completed and adequately validated, such models can be used to simulate whole organs or only some part of them. This "in vitro" digital simulation then permits analysis of normal or pathologic function, or estimation of the response to any external or internal variations in the environment.

2.6.6
Multimodality Imaging

2.6.6.1
Other Modalities

Spiral CT is providing information about the density of tissues as measured by the attenuation of X-rays. Other information can also be acquired for the same locations in the patient, either through other modalities (magnetic resonance, single photon emitted computed tomography, positron emission tomography, etc.) or through CT performed at different times (follow-up, etc.) or with different protocols (with and without contrast agent, etc.).

2.6.6.2
Registration

Although the data sets should all represent the same volume (or a reasonable overlap of it), they seldom

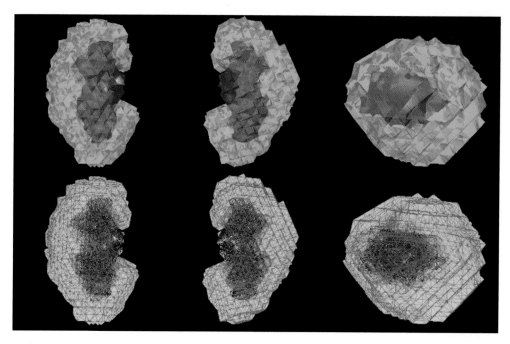

Fig. 2.27. 3D finite element (FE) mesh of a kidney and calix; physical, physiological, and other parameters can be attached to every FE cell so that the behavior of the model actually matches real life

do, and they therefore need to be registered together before direct comparison can take place. The simpler registration techniques align paired landmarks (either fiducial markers or anatomical landmarks) between two data sets. Other techniques rely on more robust 3D distance maps from the same object, identified in both data sets, or even on volumetric correlation when the information between the two data sets is considered to be sufficiently similar. Although there is a wealth of techniques now available to register two data sets, none of them is so comprehensive as to take care of all the registration situations. For this reason, and also to avoid putting all the burden on only one technique, it is often better to be able to use a selection of well-established techniques in such a way that the problem can actually be solved with the most efficiency and the least uncertainty. An important issue in the case of abdominal data sets is the wide variation of anatomical distribution between acquisitions simply due to vivid physiological motions. This variation often implies to use nonrigid registration techniques in which the geometric transformation between two data sets not only implements translations, rotations and scales, but also 3D warping and nonlinear motions. Extreme caution is always indicated when a registration between two data sets calls for such transformations, which are much more difficult to assess than rigid ones.

2.6.6.3
Visualizing Multimodality Data Sets

Once registered, two data sets can be represented as side-by-side 2D MPR images, with or without a coupled cursor. Another way is to blend both images – with different color scales and a varying blending ratio – into a single one (Fig. 2.28). When dealing with 3D objects, objects extracted from one data set can be visualized along objects extracted from the other one. Finally, information from one data set (e.g. the "functional" one) can be projected on the surface of objects from the other one (e.g. the "anatomical" one).

2.7
Picture Archiving and Communication System

In modern radiological imaging concepts, all equipment (though not its high-level functions) can now be considered as nodes of a picture archiving and communication system (PACS). Computed radiographs (CRs), ultrasounds (USs), CTs, MRs, SPECTs, PETs, workstations, archive servers, etc. are all connected together through a backbone/network, making up a PACS that is open to possible additions (Fig.

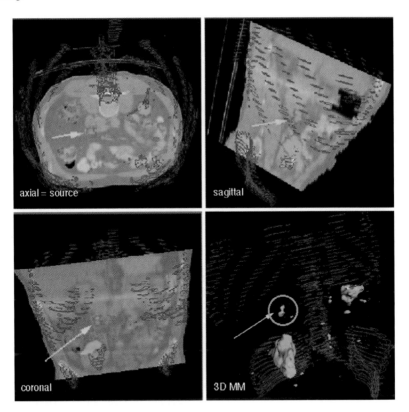

Fig. 2.28. Example of multimodality images: the tumor (insulinoma) was seen on the FDG-PET data set (courtesy of Geneva Hospitals' PET Center) though it remained invisible on the CT; after registration of PET and CT, the tumor could be accurately located inside the patient's anatomy

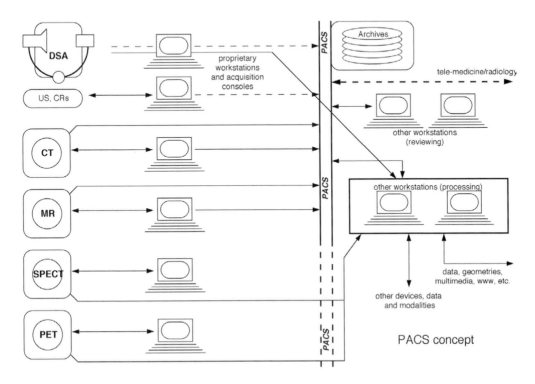

Fig. 2.29. Implementation of a picture archiving and communication system

2.29). Sometimes, the PACS concept also includes connections with the outside world, i.e. the tele-radiology and even the tele-medicine concepts. Though they initially suffered for a long time from the rather narrow-minded proprietary approach of most manufacturers, PACSs now benefit from the widespread acceptance and deployment of the DICOM (Digital Imaging & Communication in Medicine from the American College of Radiology-National Electrical Manufacturers Association) standard, which provides a realistic foundation for the exchange and storage of all medical imaging data over compatible equipment. DICOM has opened up access to most scanners' data and has provided the means for independent companies or universities to develop processing and workstations that can nicely complement the ones proposed by the major manufacturers.

2.8
Conclusion

Spiral CT provides a conceptually simple but still very efficient way to increase the dimension of traditional 2D CT data sets so that 3D volumes can be investigated as such. In parallel with the increasing functionality of workstations (through hardware and software developments) and of other clinical equipment, 3D CT now allows more complex protocols to take place and be used both in research and in clinic for the best interest of the patients. Also, based on 3D models that can be extracted from 3D CT, there is more knowledge to be gained from the morphology and behavior of structures that could not be adequately investigated in 2D. Although this chapter has attempted to provide an overview of what is presently available in clinical systems (and slightly beyond these), more is soon to come, which will add significantly to the current possibilities. More can be learned from the list of suggested fur-

ther reading and from the websites listed in Table 2.2. While this book is centered on spiral CT, development in image processing and analysis is obviously taking place in parallel and in combination with all other modalities available. This complex notion is currently extending the Sci-Fi concept of "X-ray vision" toward an ever-expanding horizon, which is not likely to be reached any time soon.

Table 2.2. Selected Internet sites

Grateful Med	http://igm.nlm.nih.gov/
Medical Imaging Center	http://www-sci.lib.uci.edu/HSG/ MedicalImage.html
LFMI	http://www.expasy.ch/LFMI/

Suggested Further Reading

American College of Radiology, National Electrical Manufacturers Association (1993) Digital imaging and communications in medicine (DICOM), vers 3.0 (draft standard VI). ACR-NEMA Committee Working Group, Washington, DC

Foley JD, Van Dam A (1982) Fundamentals of interactive computer graphics, Addison Wesley, Reading, Mass

Gonzalez RC, Wintz P (1987) Digital image processing. Addison Wesley, Reading, Mass

Niblack W (1986) An introduction to digital imaging. Prentice Hall International, London

Ratib O, Ligier Y, Scherrer JR (1994) Digital image management and communication in medicine. Comput Med Imaging Graph 18:73–84

Robb RA, Barillot C (1989) Interactive display and analysis of 3-D medical images. IEEE Trans Med Imaging 8:217–226

Russ JC (1994) The image processing handbook. CRC Press, Boca Raton

Todd-Pokropek AE, Viergever MA (eds) (1992) Medical images: formation, handling and evaluation. (NATO ASI series F: Computer and system sciences, vol 98) Springer, Berlin Heidelberg New York

Watt A, Watt M (1992) Advanced animation and rendering techniques. ACM Press/Addison Wesley, Reading, Mass

3 Reconstruction Techniques for CT Angiography

M. Prokop

CONTENTS

3.1   Introduction   *41*
3.2   Scan Parameters   *41*
3.3   Optimization of Scanning Techniques   *42*
3.3.1   Pre-contrast Scans   *42*
3.3.2   Scan Range   *42*
3.3.3   Scan Duration and Breath-holding   *42*
3.3.4   Slice Collimation   *43*
3.3.5   Pitch Factor   *45*
3.3.6   Rotation Time   *45*
3.3.7   Image Reconstruction   *45*
3.3.8   Multislice Detectors   *46*
3.3.9   Spatial Distortion Effects   *46*
3.4   Contrast Material Application   *47*
3.4.1   Flow Rate and Contrast Enhancement   *47*
3.4.2   Volume of Contrast Enhancement   *48*
3.4.3   Saline Flush   *48*
3.4.4   Start Delay/Test Bolus Injection   *48*
3.4.5   Bolus Triggering   *49*
3.5   CTA Evaluation and Image Presentation   *49*
3.5.1   Curved Reformats   *49*
3.5.2   Data Editing   *49*
3.5.3   Maximum Intensity Projections   *50*
3.5.4   Shaded Surface Displays   *51*
3.5.5   Volume Rendering Techniques   *52*
3.5.6   Thin Slab Rendering   *52*
        References   *53*

3.1
Introduction

CT angiography (CTA) is a minimally invasive technique for vascular imaging that is based on a rapid volume acquisition with spiral (or helical) CT and a properly timed intravenous contrast bolus injection. A contrast-enhanced three-dimensional data set from the examined vascular territory is obtained. This data set consists of overlapping transaxial CT images and can be interactively reviewed using arbitrary cut planes (multiplanar reformats) or transaxial CT images and can be interactively reviewed using arbitrary cut planes (multiplanar reformats) or trans-

M. PROKOP, MD; Allgemeines Krankenhaus der Stadt Wien, Universitätsklinik für Radiodiagnostik, Abteilung Radiologie für konservative Fächer, Währinger Gürtel 18–20, A-1090 Vienna, Austria

formed into angiographic displays using maximum intensity projections (MIP), 3D shaded surface displays (SSD) or new volume rendering techniques (VRT).

There is an absolute limit to spatial resolution in CTA, which so far precludes diagnostic assessment of abdominal vessels smaller than 1 mm. Otherwise, CTA has been shown to be an excellent tool for imaging of the abdominal aorta and its large side branches (BLUEMKE and CHAMBERS 1995). Advantages over arterial angiography include the intravenous approach, the direct information about vascular walls and perivascular structures, and the 3D visualization capabilities. However, CTA is only able to display anatomic information and lacks flow sensitivity.

While the basic idea of CTA is simple, a multitude of factors influence image quality and may cause artifacts. Attention has to be paid to scanning, contrast material application and reconstruction techniques in order to achieve images of optimum diagnostic quality.

3.2
Scan Parameters

In spiral (or helical) CT there is a trade-off between the scan range and the spatial resolution along the patient axis (z-axis). The reason for this is the limited number of times the X-ray tube can rotate around the patient during a single breath-hold phase. With larger scan ranges, the spiral acquisition has to be stretched, thus reducing the z-axis resolution.

There is a multitude of scanning parameters that can be influenced by the user. Manufacturers differ in how they name the various parameters (and how they define pitch when more than a single detector row is used). In the following section, all relevant parameters are defined to make it possible to correlate them with the specific names used by the various manufacturers.

For CT angiography it is important to know that the following three main parameters describe how a data set was acquired: slice collimation (SC), table feed (TF) per rotation, and reconstruction increment (RI). The three parameters determine the available scan range and spatial resolution along the z-axis.

3.3
Optimization of scanning techniques

Requirements in terms of spatial resolution and scan length vary substantially between the various imaging tasks for CT angiography. The aorta is most easily evaluated: it is large and runs almost perpendicular to the scan plane. Thus, the main diagnostic questions can be answered even with suboptimum z-axis resolution. On the other hand, the renal arteries pose a hard task for CT angiography: they run parallel or slightly oblique to the scan plane, and accessory renal arteries may be very small (<1 mm in diameter). Thus, the highest possible z-axis resolution should be used.

3.3.1
Pre-contrast Scans

The scan range is determined from a number of low-dose pre-contrast scans (7–10 mm collimation) with an interscan spacing that is tailored to the anatomic region, e.g. continuous scans for the renal arteries or 2- to 3-cm spacing for the abdominal aorta and iliac vessels. The scans also serve as an indicator of whether there is intraabdominal hemorrhage in acutely ill patients.

In aneurysmatic disease, these pre-contrast scans can detect involvement of the thoracic aorta or the iliac arteries. Involvement of the iliac arteries requires distal extension of the scan range in order to determine a proper site of anastomosis for surgery or to determine the correct type of endovascular graft. Involvement of the thoracic aorta rarely requires a proximal extension of the scan range, because simple measurements of the aortic diameter do not rely on contrast material and the only relevant side branches of the descending aorta (spinal supply) cannot be securely determined with present CTA techniques anyway.

For the renal arteries a few pre-contrast scans suffice, beginning at the level of T11/T12 and continuing until the origin of the SMA is identified. Unless renal calculi or a renal mass are suspected, pre-contrast scans of the kidneys are not required.

3.3.2
Scan Range

For CTA of the abdominal aorta, the scan range should start some 1–2 cm above the celiac artery and should at least include the common iliac arteries. If possible (fast scanners) or desirable (before bifurcated aortic graft), the scan range should be extended below the iliac bifurcation or, even better, down to the femoral bifurcation. Thus, the scan range may vary between 15 cm and 40 cm, depending on whether only the abdominal aorta or the whole aorto-iliac region is to be scanned. In patients with acute dissection it may be necessary to include the whole thorax and the abdomen down to the groins. This would increase the scan range to some 60 cm.

For the evaluation of the renal arteries, a scan range from above the superior mesenteric artery (SMA) to the common iliac arteries should be covered in order to avoid missing accessory renal arteries. Only a tiny fraction (<1%) of accessory arteries arise above the SMA or below the proximal portion of the common iliac arteries. Thus, some 10–12 cm have to be scanned.

3.3.3
Scan Duration and Breath-holding

The number of tube rotations increases with longer scan duration. In cooperative patients, a longer scan duration can be applied to make use of a narrower slice collimation and to improve z-axis resolution accordingly.

Patients are instructed to hold their breath for some 30 s and are then asked to breathe shallowly. The region of the liver and kidneys is covered during the breath-hold phase. The retroperitoneal arteries, which are subject only to negligible respiratory movement are then scanned during quiet breathing. The maximum available scan time depends on the scanner and on the vascular enhancement required. Arterial enhancement falls substantially after the plateau phase ends, but is usually sufficient for most diagnostic purposes in the pelvic and femoral arteries (Fig. 3.1). The end of the plateau phase varies between 40 s and more than 60 s, depending on individual circulatory factors in each patient.

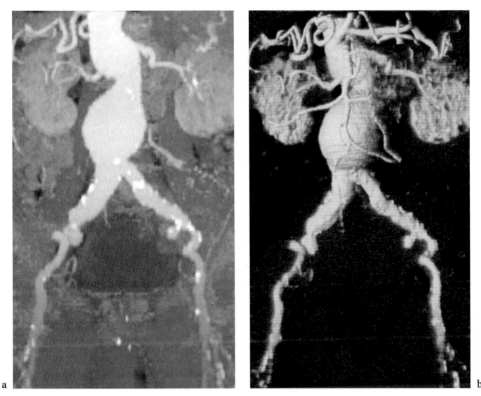

a b

Fig. 3.1a, b. CTA of a complex abdominal aortic aneurysm (SC/TF/RI = 3/5/2) with a large infrarenal portion and involvement of the right common iliac artery but also a second fusiform aneurysm in a perirenal location. Comparison of **a** maximum intensity projection (MIP) and **b** volume rendered image (VRT): the MIP displays the vascular calcifications excellently but suffers from the reduced contrast in the external iliac and femoral arteries (due to the end of the plateau phase in a 60-s scan) that almost lets these vessels blend into the background. The opacity curve for the VRT is set to yield a similar effect to a shaded surface display (SSD), but the display of small vessels is better than with a SSD and the distal portions of the pelvic arteries (low arterial enhancement) resemble that of a high-contrast MIP

All patients should be checked for their ability to hold their breath for the required time (usually 30 s). This can be done by instructing them to hyperventilate (i.e. take two to three deep breaths) and then hold their breath. By watching the abdomen of the patient, one can determine whether there are diaphragmatic movements during the breath-hold phase. If such movements occur the patient should be given further instruction. If sufficiently long breath-holding is not possible it is necessary to reduce the scan duration and increase the pitch or the collimation in order to take account of a shortened breath-hold phase. In the case of uncooperative patients, one should consider having them breathe shallowly (which is better than an uncontrolled deep inspiration during the scan) or even canceling the examination, since major distortion effects due to breathing may occur (cf. Fig. 3.4).

3.3.4
Slice Collimation

The slice collimation SC is defined as the width of a single slice (no spiral acquisition) measured at the center of the CT gantry as the full width at half maximum (FWHM) of the slice sensitivity profile (POLACIN et al. 1992).

Slice collimation should be chosen as small as reasonably possible (BRINK et al. 1995; GALANSKI et al. 1993; PROKOP et al. 1992). This optimizes spatial resolution along the z-axis and reduces partial volume effects (Fig. 3.2). Slice collimation depends on the required table speed using a pitch close to 2 (Tables 3.1, 3.2). It is important to note that a narrower slice collimation increases image noise. Therefore, a slice collimation of 3 mm may be the lower limit in adipose patients.

For the abdominal aorta, a slice collimation of 3–5 mm has been advocated (NAPEL et al. 1992; PROKOP et al. 1997a; RUBIN 1994). A larger collimation will

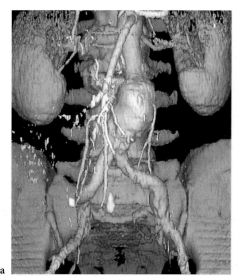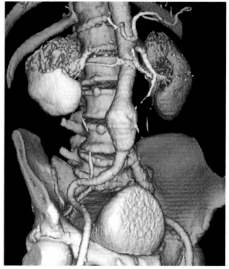

a b

Fig. 3.2a, b. Comparison of SSD images of infrarenal aortic aneurysms obtained with varying slice collimation: there is more longitudinal distortion of smaller arteries with **a** a SC/TF/RI = 5/8/2 protocol than with **b** a 3/5/2 protocol

Table 3.1. Suggested scanning techniques for CTA of the abdominal aorta (n detector rows (n=2: split detector, n=4: multirow detector), L scan length, TI scan time, SC slice collimation / single detector width, TF table feed per rotation, $Pitch$ TF/SC, RI reconstruction interval, V volume of contrast medium + saline flush, F flow rate; start delay is determined by test bolus or bolus triggering)

Scanner	n	L	TI	SC	TF	Pitch	RI	V	F
2-s scanner	1	25 cm	50 s	5	10	2	3	150+75 ml	3.5 ml/s
1-s scanner	1	36 cm	60 s	3	6	2	2	150+75 ml	3 ml/s
0.75-s scanner	1	40 cm	60 s	3	5	1.7	2	150+75 ml	3 ml/s
1-s scanner	2	40 cm	50 s	2	8	4	2	150+75 ml	3.5 ml/s
0.8-s scanner	4	40 cm	22 s	2.5	15	6	1.5	120+60 ml	5 ml/s
0.5-s scanner	4	40 cm	13 s	2.5	15	6	1.5	100+50 ml	5 ml/s

Table 3.2. Suggested scanning techniques for CTA of the renal and visceral arteries

Scanner	n	L	TI	SC	TF	Pitch	RI	V	F
2-s scanner	1	10 cm	40 s	3	5	1.7	2	150+75 ml	4 ml/s
1-s scanner	1	12 cm	40 s	2	3	1.5	1	150+75 ml	4 ml/s
0.75-s scanner	1	15 cm	38 s	2	3	1.7	1	150+75 ml	4 ml/s
1-s scanner	2	15 cm	25 s	2	6	3	1	120+60 ml	4 ml/s
0.8-s scanner	4	20 cm	21 s	1.25	7.5	6	0.8	120+60 ml	5 ml/s
0.5-s scanner	4	20 cm	13 s	1	6	6	0.7	100+50 ml	5 ml/s

severely impair the display of side branches (especially the celiac branches and the renal arteries) and should therefore be avoided. For large scan ranges, some authors suggest using a narrow collimation of 2–3 mm for the celiac axis and the renal arteries, and then adding a second scan of the lower aorta and iliac arteries (RAPTOPOULOS et al. 1996; VAN HOE et al. 1996a; ZEMAN et al. 1994). This is a feasible approach,

since arterial enhancement and z-axis resolution are less of a problem in the iliac arteries. However, superior results can be expected if the whole aorto-iliac region is covered with a single scan and a slice collimation of 3 mm (Fig. 3.1). As discussed above, this requires increasing the total scan time to some 55–65 s.

For the renal arteries, 2 mm collimation can be recommended for most scanners (BRINK et al. 1995).

Only if the scan range has to be particularly large, or if spatial resolution is less of a problem (such as in the evaluation of living renal donors), may slice collimation be increased to 3 mm (RUBIN et al. 1995a). An increase in slice collimation also becomes necessary if a slow scanner (>1 s time per 360° revolution of the X-ray tube) is employed.

3.3.5
Pitch Factor

The pitch factor P, is defined as the table feed TF, per rotation divided by the slice collimation SC:

$$P=TF/SC \qquad (1)$$

For multislice CT, the pitch is usually defined in an identical way. However, some manufacturers use the total collimation width (i.e. the number of active detector arrays n × the width of a single slice collimation) instead of the width of a single slice collimation SC:

$$P=TF/(n \cdot SC) \qquad (2)$$

For a multislice CT with four detector arrays, a pitch of 6 according to definition (1) corresponds to a pitch of 1.5 according to definition (2). Definition (1) has the advantage that it indicates the larger volume acquisition with multislice CT, while definition (2) indicates how much the radiation exposure to the patient is reduced when constant mAs are employed. Since the table feed per rotation is independent of either definition of pitch, it will be used instead of pitch in this article to define scan parameters.

For single-slice CT there is still some discussion about whether large or small pitch factors are more advisable. The discussion originates from the fact that the slice sensitivity profile is broadened with higher pitch factors, resulting in an increased effective slice thickness. This has led to the assumption that high pitch factors are generally bad for z-axis resolution.

With increasing pitch, however, volume coverage also increases. In fact, volume coverage (i.e. table feed) grows faster than the effective slice thickness: at any given collimation, increasing the pitch factor from 1 to 2 will increase the scan length by a factor of 2 but broaden the effective section thickness by only 30% (POLACIN et al. 1992). On the other hand, it is possible to calculate from these data that keeping the scan length constant and increasing the pitch factor by cutting the collimation in half will reduce the effective section thickness by 35%. Both arguments are strongly in favor of higher pitch factors but narrow collimation.

The question of how large a pitch factor is still acceptable depends mainly on the chosen slice collimation. For collimations of 3 mm or below, a pitch of 2 is acceptable. For 1 mm collimation, pitch factors up to 3 have been tested with sufficiently good results. In general, however, pitch factors of 2 or more will lead to undersampling artifacts in the periphery of the scan field. For the abdominal arteries, pitch factors between 1.5 and 2 are recommended.

3.3.6
Rotation Time

The maximum available speed is strongly dependent on the rotation time of the X-ray tube. While 0.75-s scanners can cover 33% more range than 1-s scanners, 2-s scanners can only cover half the scan range of standard 1-s scanners. This makes it necessary to increase the slice thickness with slow scanners. The resulting reduction in longitudinal resolution may impair the evaluation of side branch involvement in aortic disease or the visualization of small renal arteries.

3.3.7
Image Reconstruction

Once the scan is performed, images should be reconstructed using a 180° interpolation since this algorithm substantially reduces the effective section thickness by at least 30% (POLACIN et al. 1992). It is also the prerequisite for employing pitch factors larger than 1.

A smoothing filter kernel for CT image reconstruction (Fig. 3.3) suppresses image noise and improves the quality of 3D shaded surface displays (SSD) and maximum intensity projections (MIP) (RUBIN et al. 1993). However, it also slightly reduces the spatial resolution within the scan plane (xy-plane). The resolution in the xy-plane can be optimized using a field-of-view (FOV) between 15 and 25 cm (RUBIN et al. 1993).

Highly overlapping image reconstruction is mandatory for good results in those regions where the

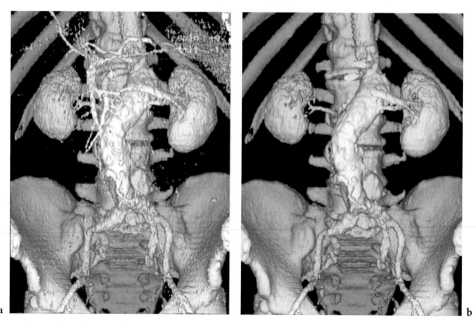

Fig. 3.3. Comparison of SSD images that were reconstructed from axial images obtained **a** with a standard reconstruction kernel and **b** with a smoothing kernel. Scan parameters were SC/TF/RI = 3/6/2

vessel course is parallel to the scan plane (KALENDER et al. 1994). This holds especially true for the renal arteries (GALANSKI et al. 1993; PROKOP et al. 1997b). In the upper abdomen, 1–1.5 mm reconstruction increments are advisable. Below the aortic bifurcation, an increment of 2–3 mm will suffice. However, changing the reconstruction increment is usually not considered worth the effort.

3.3.8
Multislice Detectors

The optimum scanning technique for CT angiography varies, depending heavily on the speed of the CT equipment. Excellent results are obtained with subsecond scanning. They can be further improved with split detectors and multislice detectors, which will dramatically improve the spatial resolution along the z-axis and allow for significantly shorter scan duration.

Split detectors consist of two parallel detector arrays. Two sections with equal width can be acquired simultaneously. For a given collimation SC of a single slice the maximum table feed TF per rotation can be double that with single slice detectors. This can be used either to improve z-axis resolution by a factor of two or to cut scan time in half (or a combination of both).

New multislice CT scanners employ multiple parallel detector arrays. At present, up to four sections can be acquired simultaneously. Wide slice collimations are obtained by combining two or more neighboring detector arrays (HU 1999). All systems use subsecond rotation of the X-ray tube (0.5–0.8 s). This increases performance by a factor of 4–8 over conventional 1-s single slice scanners.

As a consequence the region of the renal arteries can be scanned with some 1 mm slice collimation within 10–16 s given a table feed of 6 mm per rotation. The aorto-iliac region can either be scanned with 2.5-mm slice collimation within 10–20 s or with 1 mm slice collimation within 25–50 s.

With 1 mm collimation, near-isotropic imaging with a spatial resolution almost independent of the viewing plane is possible. A significant improvement of the display of small accessory renal arteries can be expected from these systems. In addition, the required scan time can be reduced. As a result, the contrast plateau can be shorter, thus allowing for a reduced amount of contrast material. In order to succeed, however, bolus triggering (see below) will become mandatory.

3.3.9
Spatial Distortion Effects

In CTA, spatial distortion of vascular structures is inevitable due to anisotropic voxel sizes with current scanners. Typically, the voxel dimensions in the *xy*-plane are some 0.5 mm, while the dimensions in the *z*-direction vary between 1.25 mm and 8 mm (effective slice thickness SL). Overlapping image reconstruction (RI < SL) does not reduce slice thickness but reduces step artifacts in CTA applications (PROKOP et al. 1997b).

The anisotropy of CTA data leads to a blurring of vessels along the *z*-axis together with a size-dependent contrast reduction due to partial volume effects (SCHAEFER et al. 1992). These effects are more pronounced for vessels that run parallel to the scan plane (e.g., renal arteries) than for those that run through the plane (e.g., aorta or mesenteric arteries). Due to voxel anisotropy, a viewing direction along the *z*-axis yields optimum results (*xy*-plane) while viewing directions perpendicular to the *z*-axis (such as ap or lateral views) suffer most from distortion effects (Fig. 3.4).

Contrast reduction plays a major part if small vessels cannot be visualized or if pseudo-stenoses or pseudo-occlusions occur when 3D display techniques such as MIP or SSD are used (HALPERN et al. 1995; PROKOP et al. 1997b). There is no single threshold level for 3D SSD or window setting for MIP that optimally displays vessels independently of a given size or orientation (HALPERN et al. 1995). Owing to the good *xy*-resolution, however, transaxial sections are able to display very small vessels (*d*<1 mm) even if the effective slice thickness is 5 mm (RUBIN 1994) or larger. The prerequisite is sufficient vascular contrast to compensate for the contrast reduction due to partial volume effects.

3.4
Contrast Material Application

CTA depends heavily on an optimized intravenous injection of contrast material. Optimum results are obtained if CTA is performed during the plateau phase of vascular enhancement. The start delay between the beginning of the contrast material injection and the start of the spiral scan should match the beginning of this phase as closely as possible. Thus, the individual transit time for the contrast material to flow from the injection site to the target volume has to be determined precisely (GALANSKI et al. 1993; RUBIN et al. 1993).

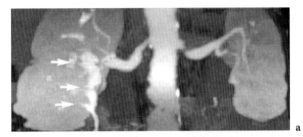

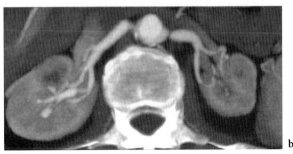

Fig. 3.4a, b. Bilateral renal artery stenoses (SC/TF/RI = 2/3/1): owing to the anisotropy of voxels, the MIP in antero-posterior direction (**a**) has a lower spatial resolution than the MIP in the caudo-cranial direction (**b**). Also note the irregular contours of the kidneys and the renal pelvis due to breathing artifacts (*arrows*)

3.4.1
Flow Rate and Contrast Enhancement

Maximum contrast enhancement is determined by the amount of iodine that is injected per second (PLATT et al. 1999). Thus, both flow rate and contrast material concentration influence arterial enhancement. In practice, a fixed concentration is used in most institutions. The suggestions for contrast material injection given in Tables 3.1 and 3.2 relate to a concentration of 300 mg iodine per ml.

A high contrast enhancement improves the visualization of small vessels such as accessory renal arteries. Thus, the highest possible flow rates should be employed while still providing a sufficiently long plateau phase of contrast enhancement. Most authors suggest flow rates between 3 and 5 ml/s (GALANSKI et al. 1993; RUBIN et al. 1995b; FARRES et al. 1996; KAATEE et al. 1998). With a flow rate of 4 ml/s the average peak aortic enhancement obtained with the injection of 150 ml contrast material was found to be 320 HU, while it was only 280 HU for a flow rate of 3 ml/s (PLATT et al. 1999).

With high injection rates, however, one has to keep in mind that the duration of contrast material injection and, thus, the length of the contrast plateau may be shortened. With a flow rate of 4 ml/s the aortic enhancement was found to be on average 15 s shorter than with a flow rate of 3 ml/s if 150 ml was injected (PLATT et al. 1999).

Even for a fixed flow rate, there are marked interindividual variations in maximum contrast enhancement, which can be explained by variations in cardiac parameters. In patients with high cardiac output (e.g. in young hypertensive patients with fibromuscular dysplasia), the contrast material is diluted substantially in the right heart, and maximum contrast enhancement is low. In patients with a low cardiac output (e.g., elderly patients with aortic aneurysms) the contrast is excellent, and the flow rate can be reduced.

3.4.2
Volume of Contrast Material

For a given volume of contrast material the duration of contrast injection depends on the flow rate. Since a sufficient amount of vascular opacification has to be obtained during the whole scan, higher flow rates also require higher volumes of contrast material. For CTA of the abdomen, 120–150 ml of contrast material is considered appropriate (GALANSKI et al. 1993; RUBIN et al. 1995b). An accurate estimation of the required volume of contrast material is not yet possible, since the individual circulatory parameters have a major influence on contrast enhancement.

3.4.3
Saline Flush

The injected contrast material can be utilized to better advantage if the injection is immediately followed by the injection of normal saline solution. The saline will push the contrast material forward and empty the injection veins. The approach is similar to that used in contrast-enhanced MRA or in intravenous DSA.

When normal CT injectors are used the syringe is kept in a strictly downward position. Some 50–90 ml of normal saline solution (0.9%) is loaded into the syringe, followed by the actual amount of contrast material (120–150 ml). When the injection begins, the intravenous contrast material is injected first, followed by the saline chaser bolus. This assures that the contrast material is pushed forward through the venous system, even past the end of the actual contrast material injection.

Alternatively, a double-headed CT injector can be used that immediately switches from contrast material to saline as soon as the required amount of contrast material has been injected.

With a 40-ml saline bolus and an injection rate of 4 ml/s, we found an average increase in plateau length of 8 s. Thus, a saline flush yields the effect of contrast material for the price of saline (PROKOP et al. 1995).

3.4.4
Start Delay / Test Bolus Injection

Patients with cardiovascular diseases are known to have wide variations in circulation times. Since scanning should only take place during the plateau phase of arterial enhancement, the optimum start delay between the beginning of contrast material injection and the start of the spiral scan is crucial for good results.

Test bolus injections have long been advocated for estimation of circulation time (GALANSKI et al. 1993). A test bolus of 10–20 ml contrast material is injected intravenously at a similar flow rate as the actual contrast material bolus (i.e. at 3–5 ml/s). Low-dose monitor scans are performed at the level of the renal arteries with a time delay of 1–3 s between successive scans. Enhancement in the aorta is measured using a circular region of interest, and the time to peak enhancement (TTP) is determined. Start delay is estimated from the time to peak. It is advisable to increase the start delay by up to 5 s over the TTP, especially in elderly patients, in order to compensate for the larger amount of contrast material injected during CT angiography (PROKOP et al. 1997a).

As a variant, a test bolus of 10 ml contrast material can be injected during the pre-contrast scan of the abdomen. The TTP is determined from the enhancement measured in the aorta as the scan progresses (SOKIRANSKI et al. 1997). This has the advantage that no additional test scans are necessary; however, most manufacturers do not support (semi-)automated evaluation of ROIs within different CT slice positions.

Test bolus injections improve the contrast enhancement during the beginning (in cases that otherwise would have started too late) and towards the end of a scan (in cases that otherwise would have started too early). Especially for high flow rates of 4 ml/s or more, they provide better results than a standardized scan delay (TELLO and HARTNELL 1994; VAN HOE et al. 1995).

However, the TTP measured during the test bolus and the actual time to peak aortic enhancement do not correlate well (KAATEE et al. 1998; PLATT et al. 1999). A better correlation is found between TTP and the time to reach a specific aortic enhancement, e.g. 200 HU (PLATT et al. 1999). The peak aortic enhancement is often reached much later during the scan, probably due to recirculation effects. When 140 ml is injected at 3 ml/s this peak occurs after 50–52 s (KAATEE et al. 1998). Since the renal arteries arise a few centimeters below the first sections of the scan, the proximal portion of the renal arteries was displayed in this study with maximum contrast when a start delay of 44 s was chosen. Such a technique, however, would result in a decreased contrast towards the end of the scan and therefore cannot be generally recommended.

If precise timing of contrast material injection is not possible or would take too much time, the flow rate has to be decreased to provide for a longer plateau to make up for suboptimum timing of the contrast material injection. With 150 ml contrast material and a flow rate of 3 ml/s, a plateau phase is maintained on average up to 60 s after the begin of contrast material injection (PLATT et al. 1999). Thus, a standardized start delay of 25–30 s may be employed with sufficiently good results (SHEIMAN et al. 1996).

3.4.5
Bolus Triggering

Bolus triggering is a technique that allows for an automated start of the CTA scan depending on the actual contrast enhancement in a target region. The starting level of the spiral scan is chosen as the reference level at which repeated low-dose scans are performed every 1–3 s. CT numbers in a circular ROI in the aorta are continuously measured and the actual spiral scan is initiated as soon as the aortic enhancement exceeds a preselected threshold level. It then takes another 4–7 s for the scanner to begin the spiral scan. Thus, a relatively low threshold of 50 HU should be selected in young patients in order to start as early as possible to optimally capture the plateau phase of contrast enhancement. In older patients the threshold may be raised to >100 HU, since the slope of the enhancement curve is flatter and optimum contrast levels are reached later.

With bolus triggering, contrast timing for CTA has become less cumbersome and can be generally performed in clinical routine.

3.5
CTA Evaluation and Image Presentation

Owing to the large number of axial CT sections (>100 images in most abdominal CTA studies), filming of all CT images is no longer feasible. For documentation purposes, filming of every 2nd to 4th image, but with digital archiving of the whole series, is recommended.

Axial CT images (source images) remain the basis for making the diagnosis, but the large data volume requires interactive viewing on a monitor display (GALANSKI et al. 1993; RUBIN et al. 1995a). In most situations, multiplanar reformats will be necessary to obtain a second orthogonal imaging plane. Both the longitudinal extent of disease and the vessel cross-section (e.g., in eccentric stenoses) can be evaluated to better advantage. If the available software allows, reformats should be performed interactively.

Further image processing of the 3D data set (curved MPR, MIP, SSD, VRT) is employed mainly for presentation purposes to make it possible to demonstrate the findings to referring physicians. For practical purposes, one may consider first looking at a rendered image (e.g., MIP), both in a coronal and in an axial viewing direction and then checking the findings by means of an interactive display of axial images and interactive multiplanar reformats. For the renal arteries it could be proven that a combination of axial images and MIP yields superior results over one modality alone (VAN HOE et al. 1996b).

3..5.1
Curved Reformats

Curved reformats along the course of the aorta and iliac arteries or along the renal arteries may be very accurate but depend heavily on precise definition of the center of the vessel (RUBIN 1994). Some manufacturers provide software that allows for an automated centering of curved cutlines parallel or perpendicular to the vessel course. This ensures an optimum longitudinal and cross-sectional display of aortic disease or renal artery stenoses in three perpendicular planes.

3.5.2
Data Editing

Bone structures are within the same range of CT numbers as the contrast-enhanced vessels. Thus, they have to be removed by editing prior to 3D image reconstruction (Prokop et al. 1997b). This can either be done by marking the structures to be included (i.e., vessels: positive editing) or by actively marking the structures to be excluded (i.e., bone: negative editing). Various computer programs are supplied to meet these tasks (Fishman et al. 1996).

These editing procedures used to be rather time consuming and tedious. Newer techniques such as watershed algorithms, require only very limited user interaction: the two structures to be separated have to be marked by a cursor (i.e., the aorta and the lumbar vertebrae) and the program determines a 3D cut plane that separates the two. Additional corrections can be preformed at multiple levels in an identical way but are required only in a very limited number of cases.

3.5.3
Maximum Intensity Projections

Maximum intensity projections (MIP) display the highest CT numbers encountered in a volume of interest (VOI) when this VOI is projected into a view plane. Contrast-enhanced vessels contain higher CT numbers than surrounding soft tissues and thus will be preferentially displayed using this technique. The results are angiography-like images. However, skeletal structures lie within the same range of CT numbers as the contrast-enhanced vessels. Thus, they have to be removed by editing prior to maximum intensity projection (Napel et al. 1992).

MIP images preserve CT attenuation values. Hence, they allow for differentiation of vascular wall calcification and contrast-filled vascular lumen. Problems arise because the maximum value (vessel) is preserved, while the background may change with the width of the VOI: the larger this width in the viewing direction, the higher the probability of large pixel values. This is most disturbing if parenchymal organs or veins are included in the VOI, and the background value may rise to an extent that obscures small vessels (Prokop et al. 1997b). Therefore, the width of the VOI has to be kept to a minimum (Fig. 3.5).

No depth information is encoded in MIPs; however, viewing of several MIPs from slightly different viewing angles in a cine loop enables the eye to integrate the information into a 3D image (Napel et al. 1992). Sliding thin-slab MIPs based on a few transaxial sections instead of the whole volume display small vessels better and allow for isolated dis-

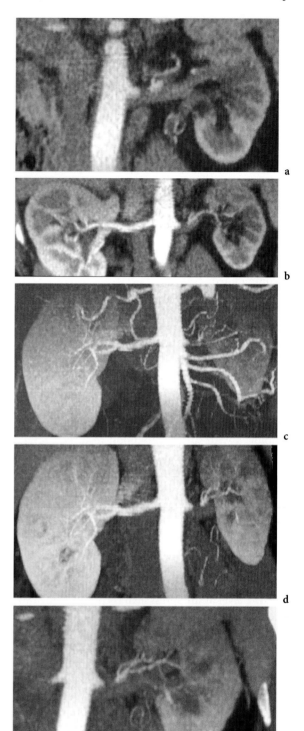

Fig. 3.5a–e. Left-sided occlusion of the renal artery (SC/TF/RI = 2/3/1): Comparison of **a** semicoronal multiplanar reformat, **b** curved multiplanar reformat, **c** MIP of the full data volume after editing of the bones, **d** MIP targeted only on the renal arteries, and **e** thin-slab MIP of the left renal artery. Note the display of the retroperitoneal collaterals with the different display modes

play of vessels of interest without overlying disturbing structures (NAPEL et al. 1993).

MIP images in antero-posterior direction require removal of all skeletal structures from the cross-sectional data set since they would superimpose over the aorta and the proximal portions of the aortic side branches. For MIP images in the lateral (Fig. 3.6) or caudo-cranial direction (Fig. 3.4b), however, editing is not generally necessary: it may be sufficient to use a narrow slab of 1–3 cm for projection and choose a projection angle that does not lead to superimposition problems (PROKOP et al. 1997b).

MIP images provide a comprehensive overview over the vascular lumen and are very sensitive for the display of vascular calcifications (Fig. 3.1). MIP are superior to axial images for the visualization of the string-of-pearls appearance of fibromuscular dysplasia (BEREGI et al. 1999). Quantification of the degree of arterial stenoses is not very reliable, however: overestimation is a frequent problem and requires a correlation with axial source images or MPR (VAN HOE et al. 1996b). Small arteries can often not be visualized with MIP. There is a multitude of potential artifacts and pitfalls that have been described elsewhere (PROKOP et al. 1997b).

3.5.4
Shaded Surface Displays

Surface shaded displays (SSD) require the definition of a binary object in the 3D data volume, e.g., by selecting a certain threshold range for CT numbers to be included in this object. A realistic '3D look' is obtained by casting rays onto the object surface and assigning gray-levels to each surface point according to the locally reflected or scattered light (voxel gradient shading) (HÖHNE and BERNSTEIN 1986).

SSD leads to a reduction of information from the primary data set, since no attenuation values are preserved and CT values outside the threshold range are not displayed. If the 3D object (vessel of interest) is properly chosen SSD is the superior display mode, because all irrelevant structures are excluded. However, if only one threshold is used, no discrimination of perfused lumen and calcifications is possible.

When a fixed threshold range is used, precise definition of all vessel borders is not possible due to partial volume effects that depend on vessel size and orientation. Lowering the threshold includes more small vessels in the 3D display but may also lead to obscuring effects of 'flying pixels due to image noise,' overlying enhancing parenchyma or venous struc-

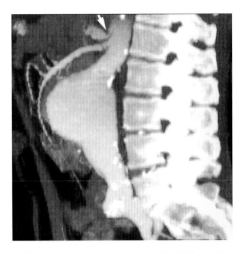

Fig. 3.6. Abdominal aortic aneurysm with high-grade stenosis (arrow) and poststenotic dilatation of the celiac artery due to compression by the median arcuate ligament of the diaphragm: lateral thin-slab MIP without prior editing of the vertebral column

tures. Although there is no ideal threshold, threshold values of some 40–50% of maximum vascular enhancement are useful in most instances.

SSD provide an excellent overview over the vascular situation, especially in complex anatomic situations (PROKOP et al. 1991). However, the results depend heavily on the chosen threshold: too low a threshold will lead to stenoses appearing as normal, while too high a threshold will simulate an occlusion (RUBIN et al. 1994). There is no single threshold that will correctly display all vascular structures. For a given stenosis, the optimum threshold that displays the degree of stenosis correctly depends upon the diameter of the vessel, the degree of stenosis, the scan parameters (mainly the effective section thickness) and the orientation of the vessel relative to the scan plane (SCHAEFER et al. 1992; HALPERN et al. 1995). Since SSD cannot differentiate between calcifications and vessel lumen (if only one threshold is used), evaluation of calcified stenoses is not reliable. Small or accessory (renal or hepatic) arteries pose an even bigger problem than with MIP.

For practical purposes, the following technique can be suggested for creating a realistic 3D display: first, one should find one section (axial or MPR) or MIP view that demonstrates the stenosis best. Then the window width should be reduced to 2 (binary = black-and-white image). Finally the level of the window setting has to be adjusted in such a way that the width of the stenosis is displayed correctly on the binary image. This level can then be used as the threshold for a shaded surface display and will result in a correct visualization of the degree of stenosis. This procedure requires that the degree of stenosis has already been determined using other display modes.

3.5.5
Volume Rendering Techniques

Volume rendering techniques (VRT) provide some of the advantages of both MIP and SSD (Fig. 3.7) (JOHNSON et al. 1996): since this technique does not rely on a single threshold but instead uses opacity curves to determine the influence of a single voxel on image display, a simultaneous display of calcified plaques and vessel lumen may be possible (SMITH and FISHMAN 1998). Still, the best results are obtained with prior editing of the data volume, excluding overlying vessels and skeletal structures. Given suitable opacity curves, the apparent degree of stenoses on these images is less dependent on vessel size and orientation.

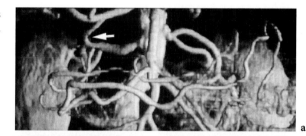

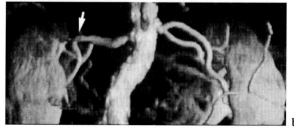

Fig. 3.8a, b. Volume rendering artifact. a For a wide VOI, volume rendering simulates an anastomosis (*arrow*) between the right renal artery and a mesenteric branch. b A slim VOI that excludes overlying vessels demonstrates the correct course (*arrow*) of the right renal artery and a right-sided renal artery stenosis

Artifacts may occur, however, and are still not too well understood: superimposing vessels may seem to merge and indicate a false anatomy (Fig. 3.8).

3.5.6
Thin Slab Rendering

Tools such as interactive thin-slab MIP (NAPEL et al. 1993) or multiplanar volume rendering techniques (MPVR) use various of the previously discussed display techniques for vessel visualization, but apply them only to a thin slab of some 5–20 mm in width. These tools have the advantage that, in the majority of cases, editing of overlying skeletal structures is not necessary if the slab can be appropriately placed excluding the vertebral bodies (Fig. 3.5e) (PROKOP et al. 1997b). At the same time the vessel course may be followed over a considerably longer range than in standard MPR.

In summary, CT angiography is an excellent imaging tool for the abdominal vasculature. For best results, the narrowest possible slice collimation and an individual timing of contrast application should be used. There is a multitude of 3D display techniques, of which MIP and SSD are presently the most important ones. In the future, however, it can be expected that these rendering techniques will be substituted by thin-slab rendering and volume rendering techniques that combine the advantages of both and require less editing time.

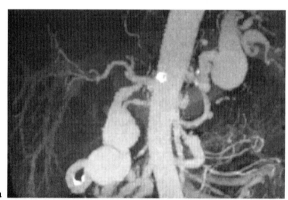

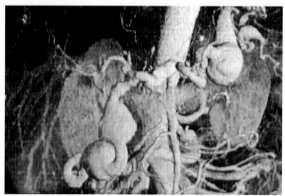

Fig. 3.7a, b. Multiple mycotic mesenteric aneurysms: comparison of a MIP and b VRT. Note the superimposition of various vessels on the MIP, which makes this modality unsuitable for this imaging task. VRT allows for demonstration of minute vascular detail while retaining three-dimensional foreground–background information

References

Beregi JP, Louvegny S, Gautier C, et al (1999) Fibromuscular dysplasia of the renal arteries: comparison of helical CT angiography and arteriography. AJR Am J Roentgenol 172:27–34

Bluemke DA, Chambers TP (1995) Spiral CT angiography: an alternative to conventional angiography. Radiology 195:317–319

Brink JA, Lim JT, Wang G, et al (1995) Technical optimization of spiral CT for depiction of renal artery stenosis: in vitro analysis. Radiology 194:157–163

Farres MT, Lammer J, Schima W, Wagner B, Wildling R, Winkelbauer F, Thurnher S (1996) Spiral computed tomographic angiography of the renal arteries: a prospective comparison with intravenous and intraarterial digital subtraction angiography. Cardiovasc Intervent Radiol 19:101–106

Fishman EK, Liang CC, Kuszyk BS, et al (1996) Automated bone editing algorithm for CT angiography: preliminary results. AJR Am J Roentgenol 166:669–672

Galanski M, Prokop M, Chavan A, et al (1993) Renal arterial stenoses: spiral CT angiography. Radiology 189:185–192

Halpern EJ, Wechsler RJ, DiCampli D (1995) Threshold selection for CT angiography shaded surface display of the renal arteries. J Digit Imaging 8:142–147

Hu H (1999) Multi-slice helical CT: scan and reconstruction. Med Phys 26:5–18

Höhne KH, Bernstein R (1986) Shading 3D-images from CT using grey-level gradients. IEEE Trans Med Imaging 1:45–47

Johnson PT, Heath DG, Kuszyk BS, Fishman EK (1996) CT angiography with volume rendering: advantages and applications in splanchnic vascular imaging. Radiology 200:564–568

Kaatee R, Van Leeuwen MS, De Lange EE, Wilting JE, Beek FJ, Beutler JJ, Mali WP (1998) Spiral CT angiography of the renal arteries: should a scan delay based on a test bolus injection or a fixed scan delay be used to obtain maximum enhancement of the vessels? J Comput Assist Tomogr 22:541–547

Kalender W A, Polacin A, Süss C (1994) A comparison of conventional and spiral CT: an experimental study on the detection of spherical lesions. J Comput Assist Tomogr 18:167–176

Napel S, Marks MP, Rubin GD, et al (1992) CT angiography with spiral CT and maximum intensity projection. Radiology 185:607–610

Napel S, Rubin GD, Marks MP, et al (1993) Sliding thin slab maximum intensity projection technique for improved visualization with CT scans and MR angiograms. Radiology 189(P):351

Platt JF, Reige KA, Ellis JH (1999) Aortic enhancement during abdominal CT angiography: correlation with test injections, flow rates, and patient demographics. AJR Am J Roentgenol 172:53–56

Polacin A, Kalender WA, Marchal G (1992) Evaluation of section sensitivity profiles and image noise in spiral CT. Radiology 185:29–35

Prokop M, Schaefer C, Doehring W, Laas J, Nischelsky, J, Galanski M (1991) Spiral CT for three-dimensional imaging of complex vascular anatomy. Radiology 181(P):293

Prokop M, Schaefer CM, Galanski M, et al (1992) 3D imaging with spiral CT: experimental evaluation of object distortion. Radiology 185(P):127

Prokop M, Engelke C, Schaefer-Prokop C, Jörgensen M (1995) Optimierung der Gefäßkontrastierung bei der Spiral CT Angiographie durch NaCl-Bolus. Radiologe 35:S167

Prokop M, Schaefer-Prokop C, Galanski M (1997a) Spiral CT angiography of the abdomen. Abdom Imaging 22:143–153

Prokop M, Shin HO, Schanz A, Schaefer-Prokop CM (1997b) Use of maximum intensity projections in CT angiography: a basic review. Radiographics 17:433–451

Raptopoulos V, Rosen MP, Kent KC, Kuestner LM, Sheiman RG, Pearlman JD (1996) Sequential helical CT angiography of aortoiliac disease. AJR Am J Roentgenol 166:1347–1354

Rubin GD (1994) Three-dimensional helical CT angiography. Radiographics 14:905–912

Rubin GD, Dake MD, Napel SA, et al (1993) Three-dimensional spiral CT angiography of the abdomen: initial clinical experience. Radiology 186:147–152

Rubin GD, Dake MD, Napel S, et al (1994) Spiral CT of renal artery stenosis: comparison of three-dimensional rendering techniques. Radiology 190:181–189

Rubin GD, Alfrey EJ, Dake MD, Semba CP, Sommer FG, Kuo PC, Dafoe DC, Waskerwitz JA, Bloch DA, Jeffrey RB (1995a) Assessment of living renal donors with spiral CT. Radiology 195:457–462

Rubin GD, Dake MD, Semba CP (1995b) Current status of three-dimensional spiral CT scanning for imaging the vasculature. Radiol Clin North Am 33:51–70

Schaefer C, Prokop M, Nischelsky J, Reimer P, Bonk K, Galanski M (1992) Vascular imaging with Spiral CT. In: Felix R, Langer M (eds) Advances in CT. II. 2nd European Scientific User Conference SOMATOM PLUS, Berlin 1992. Springer, Berlin Heidelberg New York, pp 109–115

Sheiman RG, Raptopoulos V, Caruso P, Vrachliotis T, Pearlman J (1996) Comparison of tailored and empiric scan delays for CT angiography of the abdomen. AJR Am J Roentgenol 167:725–729

Smith PA, Fishman EK (1998) Three-dimensional CT angiography: renal applications. Semin Ultrasound CT MR 19:413–424

Sokiranski R, Elsner K, Welke M, Gorich J, Rilinger N, Fleiter T (1997) Neues Verfahren zur Bestimmung der individuellen Verzögerungszeit fur die Bolusapplikation im Spiral-CT. Rofo Fortschr Geb Rontgenstr Neuen Bildgeb Verfahr 166:550–553

Tello R, Hartnell G (1994) Tailored timing as a critical factor in CT angiography. AJR Am J Roentgenol 162:997–999

Van Hoe L, Marchal G, Baert AL, Gryspeerdt S, Mertens L (1995) Determination of scan delay time in spiral CT-angiography: utility of a test bolus injection. J Comput Assist Tomogr 19: 216–220

Van Hoe L, Baert AL, Gryspeerdt S, Marchal G, Lacroix H, Wilms G, Mertens L (1996a) Supra- and juxtarenal aneurysms of the abdominal aorta: preoperative assessment with thin-section spiral CT. Radiology 198:443–448

Van Hoe L, Vandermeulen D, Gryspeerdt S, Mertens L, Baert AL, Suetens P, Marchal G, Stockx L (1996b) Assessment of accuracy of renal artery stenosis grading in helical CT angiography using maximum intensity projections. Eur Radiol 6:658–664

Zeman RK, Silverman PM, Berman PM, Weltman DI, Davros WJ, Gomes MN (1994) Abdominal aortic aneurysms: evaluation with variable-collimation helical CT and overlapping reconstruction. Radiology 193(2): 555–560

Liver

4 Tailoring the Imaging Protocol

P.R. Hilfiker, B. Marincek

CONTENTS

4.1   Introduction 57
4.2   Principles of Hepatic Contrast Enhancement 57
4.3   Imaging Technique (Spiral CT) 59
4.4   Imaging Applications 59
4.4.1 Non-Contrast-Enhancement CT Scan (NCECT) 59
4.4.2 Single-Phase CECT Scan 59
4.4.3 Dual-Phase (Biphasic) CECT Scan 60
4.4.4 Angiographically Assisted CT Scan 60
4.4.5 High-Dose Hepatic Helical CT 61
4.4.6 Delayed Contrast-Enhanced CT 61
4.4.7 3D Helical CT Angiography 62
4.5   Protocols 62
4.5.1 Liver (Abdomen) Survey Protocol 62
4.5.2 Dual-Phase Protocol 62
4.5.3 Triple-Phase Protocol 62
      References 62

4.1
Introduction

Despite extensive experience with CT for evaluating the liver, technological improvements accompanied by both experimental studies and widespread clinical experience have resulted in a gradual evolution of scanning protocols (FOLEY et al. 1994; HERTS et al. 1995; OLIVER and BARON 1996; SILVERMAN et al. 1998). Helical CT allows continual acquisition of data during a single patient breath-hold, profoundly affecting the relationship between contrast material administration and imaging. The short time required to image the entire liver using helical technique allows imaging to be performed with complete coverage of the liver during the optimal phase or phases of hepatic enhancement following intravenous administration of contrast (BERLAND 1995;

P.R. HILFIKER, MD; Institute of Diagnostic Radiology, University Hospital Zürich, Rämistrasse 100, CH-8091 Zürich, Switzerland
B. MARINCEK, MD; Institute of Diagnostic Radiology, University Hospital Zürich, Rämistrasse 100, CH-8091 Zürich, Switzerland

BLUEMKE et al. 1995b; BONALDI et al. 1995a; ZEMAN et al. 1993). Moreover, the fast data acquisition allows successive scanning of the entire liver at different moments after injection of contrast material, thus creating the possibility of multiphasic liver CT. In addition, advances in software are converting previously experimental concepts into feasible and clinically relevant applications.

4.2
Principles of Hepatic Contrast Enhancement

Intravenously administered contrast material is used to overcome a lack of inherent tissue contrast differences between certain liver tumours and liver parenchyma. The greater the differences in CT attenuation between the normal liver and tumours, the greater the tumour conspicuity. The liver receives a dual blood supply, with 25% of total liver blood flow being supplied from the hepatic artery and 75% from the portal vein (GREENWAY and STARK 1971). However, hepatic neoplasms receive their blood supply primarily from the hepatic artery, with relatively little supply from the portal vein (ACKERMAN et al. 1969; YOUNG et al. 1979). When administering exogenous contrast material, one should attempt to deliver the contrast material predominantly to the liver parenchyma or the liver tumour, but not both (OLIVER and BARON 1996).

Normal unenhanced liver parenchyma has an attenuation value of 40–70 HU (OLIVER et al. 1997). Hepatic neoplasms may have different attenuation values, depending on multiple factors, including vascularity, calcification, degeneration, necrosis and haemorrhage. Most hepatic tumours have a lower attenuation value than normal hepatic parenchyma. A neoplasm generally is indiscernible if its attenuation differs from that of the surrounding hepatic parenchyma by <10%.

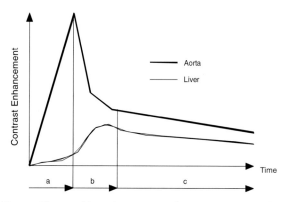

Fig. 4.1. Phases of hepatic contrast enhancement: _a_ vascular phase, _b_ redistribution phase, _c_ equilibrium phase

When a contrast agent is administered intravenously, it rapidly redistributes from the vascular to the extravascular space, while being continuously excreted by the kidneys. When it is administered by a power injector during helical CT scanning, three phases of hepatic contrast enhancement are produced: the arterial (vascular) phase (onset about 12–20 s after contrast initiation); the redistribution (arterio-portal) phase (onset about 30–60 s after contrast initiation); and finally the equilibrium phase (onset about 110–120 s after contrast) (Fig. 4.1). The vascular phase is characterised by a rapid rise in aortic enhancement, which reaches a peak shortly after the end of contrast medium injection (BONALDI et al. 1995b; KOPKA et al. 1996). During the hepatic arterial phase of enhancement, solid hepatic neoplasms are maximally enhanced due to their arterial supply. Simultaneously, hepatic enhancement increases gradually. Therefore, 'hypervascular' tumours appear as hyperattenuating masses against a minimally enhanced parenchymal background (BONALDI et al. 1995b). The arterio-portal phase occurs when sufficient portal venous contrast material is delivered to the liver, with resultant marked enhancement of liver parenchyma. Contrast material diffuses from the central blood compartment to the extravascular compartment of the liver, and it is only during this time that the liver parenchyma enhances substantially (OLIVER and BARON 1996). The arterio-portal phase is an excellent time to image hypovascular tumours, because such tumours receive minimal hepatic arterial or portal venous flow and therefore appear hypoattenuating compared with adjacent enhanced liver parenchyma. Hypovascular tumours optimally imaged during this phase include a minority of hypovascular HCCs and most metastases not considered hypervascular, such as metastases from the colon, the pancreas, and the

lung (OLIVER and BARON 1996). During the equilibrium phase, aortic and hepatic enhancement gradually decline as contrast medium from the liver slowly diffuses back into the central vascular compartment, which gradually loses contrast medium through glomerular filtration and diffusion into skeletal muscles and fat. Hepatic lesions may become obscured due to equal enhancement of hepatic lesions and liver parenchyma. With appropriate scan timing, the short scan duration used for liver spiral CT examinations technique largely eliminates the risk of imaging the liver during the equilibrium phase.

Multiple factors affect the magnitude of hepatic enhancement. It is well established that power injection of a monophasic bolus is superior to either drip infusion or a biphasic technique in which an initial bolus given at a higher injection rate is followed by drip infusion at a lower rate. Of greater interest are the contrast medium volume and concentration and the rate and type of injection (i.e. uniphasic versus biphasic). CHAMBERS et al. (1994a, b) demonstrated that an equal volume injected at the faster rate or a greater volume injected at the same rate results in greater liver enhancement; the effect on lesion conspicuity is not yet certain. The timing of peak hepatic contrast enhancement depends primarily on the injection duration (CHAMBERS et al. 1994a,b), rapid or low volume (shorter duration) injection producing earlier peak hepatic enhancement, whereas slow or high-volume (longer duration) injections result in later peak enhancement. It seems logical that an earlier maximal peak enhancement, as afforded by a faster injection rate, is desirable, because lesion conspicuity is greater prior to equilibrium. Decreased volume results in lower maximal peak enhancement, which may decrease the lesion conspicuity (CHAMBERS et al. 1994b). However, rapid injection rates do result in increased hepatic arterial enhancement and greater separation of the peaks of aortic and hepatic enhancement. These benefits of rapid contrast injection rate are helpful when dual-phase helical CT is used for detection of vascular hepatic neoplasms. Maximum hepatic enhancement decreases with increasing patient body weight (HEIKEN et al. 1995), which is the most important patient-related factor. Although diminished cardiac output causes delayed aortic and hepatic enhancement, it does not significantly alter the magnitude of hepatic contrast enhancement.

Recently, manufacturers have released an automated method of determining the adequacy of contrast enhancement during infusion of the contrast material intended for a diagnostic scan (bolus tracking). This is performed by acquiring a series of low-X-ray-dose transaxial images at a predetermined level representative of the scan volume (SILVERMAN et al. 1995). Once contrast enhancement is deemed adequate, the series of low-dose transaxial scans is interrupted and the diagnostic scan is commenced at the top of the imaging volume (KOPKA et al. 1995).

4.3
Imaging Technique (Spiral CT)

A study by BLUEMKE et al. demonstrated that 90% of outpatients are able to perform a 32-s breath-hold without significant respiratory motion (BLUEMKE et al. 1995a). The entire liver can be imaged during the plateau of peak hepatic enhancement without scanning during the equilibrium phase. Because a helical CT scan is completed within a very short scanning interval, a uniphasic injection using a relatively rapid flow rate (2.5–3.0 ml/s) is most advantageous, with a volume of 120–150 ml of contrast material (SILVERMAN et al. 1998). For helical CT of the liver, it is generally necessary to use a longer scan delay than is generally used for conventional CT. The scan delays normally used are 20 s for the arterial phase and 50–80 s for scanning during the portal venous phase (SILVERMAN et al. 1998).

Slice collimation for routine liver imaging is generally either 7 or 8 mm in most institutions, as demonstrated by SILVERMAN et al. (1998). Pitch is usually limited to 1.5:1 or less, with 1:1 pitch being ideal.

4.4
Imaging Applications

4.4.1
Non-Contrast-Enhancement CT Scan

Computed tomography scans of the liver without contrast medium administration are not routinely obtained, but may be useful in selected situations. These include identification of calcifications and haemorrhage and determination of the precontrast attenuation value of a lesion, which may be helpful in its characterisation. The evaluation of hypervascular liver tumours with non-contrast-enhancement CT scan (NCECT) is controversial. It is no longer considered an indication for the addition of NCECT to a contrast-enhanced scan (PATTEN et al. 1993), but one study demonstrated better results with the combination of NCECT plus portal venous phase (PVP) images than with HAP plus PVP images (OLIVER et al. 1997).

Indications for NCECT scans are diffuse liver diseases and primary liver neoplasms. Haemochromatosis shows on the NCECT images hyperattenuating liver parenchyma with HU greater than 70–80, compared to about 60 HU in normal livers (OLIVER et al. 1997). Other conditions that cause hyperattenuating livers on NCECT images are: glycogen storage disease (type 1); chemotherapy; amiodarone; gold therapy; and arsenic poisoning. Confluent fibrosis in cirrhotic livers is hypoattenuating on NCECT scans and iso- or minimally hypoattenuating on CECT (OHTOMO et al. 1993) and is frequently missed if only CECT is performed.

4.4.2
Single-Phase CECT Scan
(Liver/Abdominal Survey Helical CT)

The abdominal survey scan is used for screening patients with nonspecific abdominal pain or complaints (e.g. weight loss), and thus, while it is not focused on examination of the liver, it is an excellent and efficacious technique for screening of the upper abdomen and the liver (FREENY 1997). Other indications for the single-phase technique are nonhypervascular primaries or metastatic liver tumours, and trauma. Because the main hepatic parenchymal blood flow is supplied by the portal venous system, and lesion conspicuity is generally greatest during peak parenchymal enhancement, imaging during the portal venous phase of enhancement is desirable (BLUEMKE et al. 1995a). Thus, liver scanning begins about 60–70 s after the start of the injection (IRIE et al. 1995), and about 20 s is needed to scan completely through the liver using the spiral CT technique. This technique results in a consistent level of hepatic contrast enhancement, thus optimising the detection of focal lesions. If patients have problems with holding their breath during a CT scan using a standard pitch, then it is better to increase the pitch than to scan in two or more blocks.

4.4.3
Dual-Phase (Biphasic) CECT Scan

Helical CT provides the potential to image the entire liver twice, once during the arterial and once during the portal venous enhancement phase. Hepatic biphasic contrast-enhanced CT should be used in patients with known or suspected hypervascular neoplasms when documentation of the extent of liver disease may affect the choice of treatment (OLIVER and BARON 1996). The hypervascular neoplasms include (a) malignant neoplasms: HCC, renal cell carcinoma, breast carcinoma, neuroendocrine tumours (islet cell, carcinoid), sarcomas, thyroid carcinoma, and melanoma and (b) benign tumours: focal nodular hyperplasia (FNH) and hepatic adenoma. These tumours have an unusually rich arterial supply. They are often not seen on portal venous phase imaging because they enhance to a similar degree to the surrounding liver parenchyma. SILVERMAN et al. (1998) revealed that 83% of institutions relied on dual-phase scanning to improve the detection of hypervascular lesions, whereas 17% used triple-phase scanning including a baseline unenhanced CT scan. However, KANEMATSU et al. (1997) reported that a biphasic helical CT scan is still less sensitive than a CT arterial portography (CTAP) scan.

With the exception of patients with severe cardiovascular disease and altered circulation times, the optimal time to start imaging during the hepatic arterial phase depends most on the rate of delivery of intravenous contrast material. The faster rates of infusion (4.0–6.0 ml/s) require less scanning delay than the lower infusion rates (2.5–3.0 ml/s) (OLIVER and BARON 1996). A standard 20 s scanning delay is employed if the contrast material is being infused at 4.0–6.0 ml/s, and a 28-s scanning delay if the injection rate is less than 4.0 ml/s (OLIVER and BARON 1996). The portal venous scans are then acquired at a standard, fixed delay of 60–70 s after initiation of the contrast bolus.

4.4.4
Angiographically Assisted CT Scan

Determination of the exact number, extent and relation to vascular structures is essential in the preoperative setting of curative partial liver resection in patients with metastatic disease and occasionally primary malignant neoplasms, in order to decrease the false-positive rate of resectability (BLUEMKE and CHAMBERS 1995; BLUEMKE and FISHMAN 1993). CT hepatic angiography (CTHA) scan and CT arterial portography (CTAP) scan have improved detection rates of focal liver lesions. Indeed, with these techniques, an increase in lesion-to-liver contrast results from CT scanning following angiographically assisted administration of contrast agent into the hepatic arterial or portal venous system, respectively (BLUEMKE and CHAMBERS 1995). In several series the CTAP detection rate for tumour nodules was as high as 91% (OLIVER and BARON 1996; SOYER et al. 1993), while CTHA had detection rates of up to 94% (SITZMANN et al. 1990).

Lipiodol CT scan is a third method and is performed 1–4 weeks after injection of a small amount of iodised oil into the hepatic artery (NELSON 1991). This technique is helpful in the detection of small foci of HCC in cirrhotic liver, thanks to increased retention of this contrast agent in HCCs (NELSON 1991).

4.4.4.1
CT Hepatic Angiography

The liver receives a dual blood supply, with about 75% of total liver blood flow being supplied from the portal vein and 25% from the hepatic artery. All hepatic neoplasms (primaries and metastases) are largely supplied by the hepatic artery (ACKERMAN et al. 1969; YOUNG et al. 1979). CT hepatic angiography (CTHA) produces direct lesion contrast enhancement against a background of nonenhanced liver parenchyma. The degree of lesion enhancement depends on the vascularity of the lesion. CTHA scan has not become a commonly used preoperative examination in the staging of focal liver disease. Images are sometimes difficult to read owing to altered haemodynamics secondary to hepatic neoplasms or cirrhosis. Most institutions prefer CTAH for detection of hypervascular lesions (FREENY 1997), such as hepatocellular carcinoma or hypervascular metastasis, or in combination with CTAP scans for challenging cases (CHEZMAR et al. 1993; KANEMATSU et al. 1997). Although HCC tends to show homogeneous to heterogeneous enhancement on CTHA scan images, metastatic foci predominantly reveal a ring-enhancement pattern.

To perform CTHA, an angiographic catheter is placed into the hepatic artery using a modified Seldinger technique (CHEZMAR et al. 1993; IRIE et al. 1994). To avoid significant artefacts related to high contrast density, 70 ml of diluted iodinated contrast agent (15–30%) is injected at a flow rate of 3–5 ml/s.

Helical CT acquisition, which begins approximately 3–5 s after the initiation of contrast agent injection, is carried out with a single breath-hold of up to 30 s, with a 5- to 8-mm collimation and with the pitch adjusted (1:1 to 1:1.6) to cover the liver during the single breath-hold.

4.4.4.2
CT Arterial Portography

CT arterial portography (CTAP) produces contrast enhancement only of the normal liver parenchyma following selective administration of contrast material through either the superior mesenteric artery or the splenic artery (BLUEMKE and FISHMAN 1993; FREENY et al. 1995). Thus, on CTAP images hepatic neoplasms appear as hypoattenuating masses because they receive predominantly an arterial supply, whereas the normal hepatic parenchyma is supplied predominantly by the portal venous system. Metastases of colorectal carcinomas are a typical example of hypovascular hepatic tumours.

To perform CTAP, 150 ml of 30% contrast material is infused at a rate of 3 ml/s through a catheter placed into the superior mesenteric or splenic artery. CT scanning is initiated 30 s after the start of the infusion with helical CT (BLUEMKE et al. 1995b; GRAF et al. 1994). If scanning begins too early, suboptimal enhancement of the hepatic veins cause interpretation problems in differentiating venous structures from focal liver lesions. Helical CT acquisition is carried out with a single breath-hold of up to 30 s, using a 5- to 8-mm collimation and with the pitch adjusted (1:1 to 1:1.6) to cover the liver during the single breath-hold. Delayed CT scan at 4–6 h after the initial scan may be obtained (without additional i.v. contrast medium). Delayed CT scan following CTAP scan is the method suggested for differentiation of pseudolesions from true focal liver lesions (NELSON et al. 1992).

4.4.4.3
Iodised Oil CT Scan

Iodised oil (e.g. Lipiodol) CT scanning was introduced 1985, and it is still regarded as a sensitive method for diagnosing small HCC and additional small satellite intrahepatic metastatic nodules of HCC (ITAI 1997; LENCIONI et al. 1994, 1997; NGAN 1990; YUMOTO et al. 1985). The iodised oil is angiographically injected into the hepatic artery. It is rapidly cleared from the hepatic parenchyma by the reticuloendothelial system, but is retained in vascular hepatic neoplasms, especially HCC. This results in high-density foci on CT scans 7 or more days later. However, small avascular, necrotic, or fibrotic subtypes of HCC can be overlooked.

After complete angiographic study of the arterial supply, an amount of 5–20 ml of iodised oil is selectively administered in the proper hepatic artery, as well as in accessory hepatic arteries. The optimal timing for the liver CT scan is 7 days to 4 weeks after the intra-arterial injection.

4.4.5
High-Dose Hepatic Helical CT

CTAP has been the gold standard for determining the precise number and location of hypovascular hepatic tumours, particularly colorectal carcinoma (SOYER et al. 1993, 1994a, b). CHOI et al. (1996) reported that helical CT carried out using 200 ml of contrast (64 g iodine) injected at a rate of 5 ml/s can produced hepatic enhancement equal to 86% of that obtained with CTAP. Preliminary results in patients with potentially resectable hypovascular metastases, primarily colorectal carcinomas, are encouraging (IKEDA et al. 1996). High-dose hepatic helical CT can provide a level of accuracy similar to that of CTAP in the preoperative detection of hypovascular liver neoplasms.

4.4.6
Delayed Contrast-Enhanced CT

If a dynamic bolus contrast-enhanced CT or CTAP examination is equivocal, delayed hepatic scanning 4–6 h after administration of at least 60 mg iodine may be helpful (NELSON et al. 1992). This technique is based on the fact that 10–12% of intravenously or intra-arterially administered iodine is actively excreted by the hepatocytes into the biliary system within 4–6 h after contrast administration. This produces an increase of at least 20 HU in hepatic attenuation over baseline scans. An advantage of delayed CT is that it provides a more accurate assessment of tumour size than dynamic contrast-enhanced CT. However, small lesions are difficult to differentiate from hepatic vessels. Thus, the delayed images should always be evaluated in conjunction with the dynamic contrast-enhanced images.

4.4.7
3D Helical CT Arteriography

Three-dimensional CT scan arteriography is evaluated as a potential substitute for conventional angiography in the preoperative evaluation of the hepatic arterial anatomy (WINTER et al. 1995). A test injection of 20 ml of contrast and dynamic imaging at the T11–12 interspace is used to determine the optimal scan delay (average delay 12 s). Following the test bolus, 180 ml of contrast is injected at 5 ml/s, and the data are acquired using a 3-mm collimation with a pitch of 1:1 to 1:1.7 during a 30- to 35-s breath hold. Data are reconstructed at 1-mm intervals and used to reconstruct the 3D shaded surface or maximum intensity projection images on a computer workstation.

4.5
Protocols

4.5.1
Liver (Abdomen) Survey Protocol

Volume	120–150 ml
Flow rate	2.5–3.0 ml/s
Scan delay	60 s
Collimation	5–8 mm
Pitch	1:1–1.6:1
Scan range	Dome to caudal end of liver (single breath-hold); continue scanning to pelvic floor

4.5.2
Dual-Phase Protocol

Volume	150 ml
Flow rate	3.0–4.0 ml/s
Scan delay	
1. Arterial phase	20 s
2. Porto-venous phase	60 s
Collimation	
1. Arterial phase	3–5 mm
2. Porto-venous phase	5–8 mm
Pitch	1:1–1.6:1
Scan range	
1. Arterial phase	Dome to caudal end of liver (single breath-hold)
2. Porto-venous phase	Dome to caudal end of liver (single breath-hold); continue scanning to pelvic floor

4.5.3
Triple-Phase Protocol

Precontrast scan and dual-phase protocol

References

Ackerman NB, Lien WM, Kondi ES, Silverman NA (1969) The blood supply of experimental liver metastases. I. The distribution of hepatic artery and portal vein blood to "small" and "large" tumors. Surgery 66:1067–1072

Berland LL (1995) Slip-ring and conventional dynamic hepatic CT: contrast material and timing considerations. Radiology 195:1–8

Bluemke DA, Chambers TP (1995) Spiral CT angiography: an alternative to conventional angiography (editorial; comment). Radiology 195:317–319

Bluemke DA, Fishman EK (1993) Spiral CT arterial portography of the liver. Radiology 186:576–579

Bluemke DA, Soyer P, Fishman EK (1995a) Helical (spiral) CT of the liver. Radiol Clin North Am 33:863–886

Bluemke DA, Soyer PA, Chan BW, Bliss DF, Calhoun PS, Fishman EK (1995b) Spiral CT during arterial portography: technique and applications. Radiographics 15:623–637; discussion 638–639 [erratum: Radiographics 1995, 15:1190]

Bonaldi VM, Bret PM, Reinhold C, Atri M (1995a) Comparison of helical and conventional computed tomography of the liver. Can Assoc Radiol J 46:443–448

Bonaldi VM, Bret PM, Reinhold C, Atri M (1995b) Helical CT of the liver: value of an early hepatic arterial phase. Radiology 197:357–363

Chambers TP, Baron RL, Lush RM (1994a) Hepatic CT enhancement. I. Alterations in the volume of contrast material within the same patients. Radiology 193:513–517

Chambers TP, Baron RL, Lush RM (1994b) Hepatic CT enhancement. II. Alterations in contrast material volume and rate of injection within the same patients. Radiology 193:518–522

Chezmar JL, Bernardino ME, Kaufman SH, Nelson RC (1993) Combined CT arterial portography and CT hepatic angiography for evaluation of the hepatic resection candidate. Work in progress. Radiology 189:407–410

Choi CS, Freeny PC, Heyano BS (1996) High-dose helical CT of the liver with computer-automated scan technology: comparison with helical CT arterial portography and conventional helical CT. Radiology 201:P145

Foley WD, Hoffmann RG, Quiroz FA, Kahn CE Jr, Perret RS (1994) Hepatic helical CT: contrast material injection protocol. Radiology 192:367–371

Freeny PC (1997) Helical computed tomography of the liver: techniques, applications and pitfalls. Endoscopy 29:515–523

Freeny PC, Nghiem HV, Winter TC (1995) Helical CT during arterial portography: optimization of contrast enhancement and scanning parameters. Radiology 194:83–90

Graf O, Dock WI, Lammer J, Thurnher S, Eibenberger KL, Wildling R, Niederle B, Lang EK, Lechner G (1994) Determination of optimal time window for liver scanning with CT during arterial portography. Radiology 190:43–47

Greenway CV, Stark RD (1971) Hepatic vascular bed. Physiol Rev 51:23–65

Heiken JP, Brink JA, McClennan BL, Sagel SS, Crowe TM, Gaines MV (1995) Dynamic incremental CT: effect of volume and concentration of contrast material and patient weight on hepatic enhancement. Radiology 195:353–357

Herts BR, Paushter DM, Einstein DM, Zepp R, Friedman RA, Obuchowski N (1995) Use of contrast material for spiral CT of the abdomen: comparison of hepatic enhancement and vascular attenuation for three different contrast media at two different delay times. Am J Roentgenol 164:327–331

Ikeda AK, Freeny PC, Ryan JA, Crane RD, Nghiem HV, Winter III TC (1996) Preoperative high-dose helical CT of the liver: comparison with surgery, pathology, and intraoperative US in the detection of hypovascular hepatic neoplasms. Radiology 201:P420

Irie T, Takeshita K, Makita K, Yamauchi T, Kusano S (1994) A one-stage method for obtaining CT during arterial portography and hepatic arteriography. Acta Radiol 35:135–137

Irie T, Suzuki S, Yamauchi T, Kusano S (1995) Prediction of the time to peak hepatic enhancement to optimize contrast-enhanced spiral CT. Acta Radiol 36:154–158

Itai Y (1997) Lipiodol-CT for hepatocellular carcinoma (editorial; comment). Abdom Imaging 22:259–260

Kanematsu M, Hoshi H, Imaeda T, Murakami T, Inaba Y, Yokoyama R, Nakamura H (1997) Detection and characterization of hepatic tumors: value of combined helical CT hepatic arteriography and CT during arterial portography. Am J Roentgenol 168:1193–1198

Kopka L, Funke M, Fischer U, Vosshenrich R, Oestmann JW, Grabbe E (1995) Parenchymal liver enhancement with bolus-triggered helical CT: preliminary clinical results. Radiology 195:282–284

Kopka L, Rodenwaldt J, Fischer U, Mueller DW, Oestmann JW, Grabbe E (1996) Dual-phase helical CT of the liver: effects of bolus tracking and different volumes of contrast material. Radiology 201:321–326

Lencioni R, Caramella D, Vignali C, Russo R, Paolicchi A, Bartolozzi C (1994) Lipiodol-CT in the detection of tumor persistence in hepatocellular carcinoma treated with percutaneous ethanol injection. Acta Radiol 35:323–328

Lencioni R, Pinto F, Armillotta N, Di Giulio M, Gaeta P, Di Candio G, Marchi S, Bartolozzi C (1997) Intrahepatic metastatic nodules of hepatocellular carcinoma detected at lipiodol-CT: imaging-pathologic correlation (see comments). Abdom Imaging 22:253–258

Nelson RC (1991) Techniques for computed tomography of the liver. Radiol Clin North Am 2:1199–1212

Nelson RC, Thompson GH, Chezmar JL, Harned RK, Fernandez MP (1992) CT during arterial portography: diagnostic pitfalls. Radiographics 12:705–718; discussion 719

Ngan H (1990) Lipiodol computerized tomography: how sensitive and specific is the technique in the diagnosis of hepatocellular carcinoma? Br J Radiol 63:771–775

Ohtomo K, Baron RL, Dodd GD, Federle MP, Miller WJ, Campbell WL, Confer SR, Weber KM (1993) Confluent hepatic fibrosis in advanced cirrhosis: appearance at CT. Radiology 188:31–35

Oliver JH, Baron RL (1996) Helical biphasic contrast-enhanced CT of the liver: technique, indications, interpretation, and pitfalls. Radiology 201:1–14

Oliver JH, Baron RL, Federle MP, Jones BC, Sheng R (1997) Hypervascular liver metastases: do unenhanced and hepatic arterial phase CT images affect tumor detection? Radiology 205:709–715

Patten RM, Byun JY, Freeny PC (1993) CT of hypervascular hepatic tumors: are unenhanced scans necessary for diagnosis? (See comments.) Am J Roentgenol 161:979–984

Silverman PM, Roberts S, Tefft MC, Brown B, Fox SH, Cooper C, Zeman RK (1995) Helical CT of the liver: clinical application of an automated computer technique, SmartPrep, for obtaining images with optimal contrast enhancement. Am J Roentgenol 165:73–78

Silverman PM, Kohan L, Ducic I, Javadi S, Meyer C, Sharma N, Cooper C, Zeman RK (1998) Imaging of the liver with helical CT: a survey of scanning techniques. Am J Roentgenol 170:149–152

Sitzmann JV, Coleman J, Pitt HA, Zerhouni E, Fishman E, Kaufman SL, Order S, Grochow LB, Cameron JL (1990) Preoperative assessment of malignant hepatic tumors. Am J Surg 159:137–142; discussion 142–143

Soyer P, Lacheheb D, Levesque M (1993) CT arterial portography of the abdomen: effect of injecting papaverine into the mesenteric artery on hepatic contrast enhancement. Am J Roentgenol 160:1213–1215

Soyer P, Bluemke DA, Fishman EK (1994a) CT during arterial portography for the preoperative evaluation of hepatic tumors: how, when, and why? Am J Roentgenol 163:1325–1331

Soyer P, Bluemke DA, Hruban RH, Sitzmann JV, Fishman EK (1994b) Hepatic metastases from colorectal cancer: detection and false-positive findings with helical CT during arterial portography. Radiology 193:71–74

Winter TC, Freeny PC, Nghiem HV, Hommeyer SC, Barr D, Croghan AM, Coldwell DM, Althaus SJ, Mack LA (1995) Hepatic arterial anatomy in transplantation candidates: evaluation with three-dimensional CT arteriography. Radiology 195:363–370

Young SW, Hollenberg NK, Kazam E, Berkowitz DM, Hainen R, Sandor T, Abrams HL (1979) Resting host and tumor perfusion as determinants of tumor vascular responses to norepinephrine. Cancer Res 39:1898–1903

Yumoto Y, Jinno K, Tokuyama K, Araki Y, Ishimitsu T, Maeda H, Konno T, Iwamoto S, Ohnishi K, Okuda K (1985) Hepatocellular carcinoma detected by iodized oil. Radiology 154:19–24

Zeman RK, Fox SH, Silverman PM, Davros WJ, Carter LM, Griego D, Weltman DI, Ascher SM, Cooper CJ (1993) Helical (spiral) CT of the abdomen. Am J Roentgenol 160:719–725

5 Segmental Anatomy of the Liver in Spiral CT

J.H.D. FASEL

CONTENTS

5.1   Introduction   *65*
5.2   Materials and Methods   *65*
5.2.1   Materials   *65*
5.2.2   Methods   *65*
5.3   Results   *67*
5.4   Discussion   *69*
       References   *70*

5.1
Introduction

Delineation of the portal venous segments and subsegments in the human liver (GOLDSMITH and WOODBURNE 1957; COUINAUD 1957; BISMUTH 1982; FASEL et al. 1996a) has become a matter of increasing importance to radiologists during recent years, particularly because of the growing need for accurate preoperative localization of focal intrahepatic lesions. Indeed, for today's segment-oriented liver surgery, the planes of resection are considered to be determined largely on the basis of the precise position of the lesion relative to this vascular frame of reference (MUKAI et al. 1987; SUGARBAKER et al. 1990; SOYER et al. 1994).

Procedures for delineating segmental and subsegmental anatomy on CT and MR images have, therefore, been the subject of several studies during the past 10 years or so (MUKAI et al. 1987; SUGARBAKER et al. 1990; SEXTON and ZEMAN 1983; NELSON et al. 1990; LAFORTUNE et al. 1991; SOYER et al. 1991, 1995; GAZELLE and HAAGA 1992; DODD 1993; WAGGENSPACK et al. 1993; GORE et al. 1994; VAN LEEUWEN et al. 1994). Essentially, these procedures are based on the concept of three vertical planes that divide the liver into four segments and of

a transverse scissura that further subdivides each of these segments into two subsegments (SUGARBAKER et al. 1990; SOYER et al. 1994; NELSON et al. 1990; WAGGENSPACK et al. 1993). Although convenient for daily radiologic practice, use of this concept is highly questionable from an anatomical point of view (PLATZER and MAURER 1966; FASEL et al. 1996b). Radiologists have also recently expressed their skepticism and described observations that are incompatible with the concept (VAN LEEUWEN et al. 1994; DOWNEY 1994; OHASHI et al. 1996).

The purpose of this chapter is therefore to offer evidence for the unreliability of this concept and, hence, of the procedures presently used in daily radiologic practice.

5.2
Materials and Methods

5.2.1
Materials

Ten vascular corrosion casts of human livers were used. The specimens were obtained as follows. The portal vein and the inferior vena cava of 10 unembalmed cadavers (3 men and 7 women, age at death: range 70–95 years, mean 84 years, none with any history of liver disease) were injected in situ with acrylic resin of different colors. After the resin hardened, the injected livers were carefully removed en bloc and were corroded.

5.2.2
Methods

5.2.2.1
Radiologic Investigation

Helical CT scans of the 10 corrosion casts were acquired with a PQ 2000 scanner (Picker, Cleveland,

J.H.D. Fasel, MD; Division of Anatomy, Department of Morphology, University Medical Center, Rue M. Servet 1, CH-1211 Geneva 4, Switzerland

USA). To obtain optimal visualization of the vessels up to the periphery of the segments and subsegments, the following parameters were used: slice thickness 1.5 mm, pitch factor 1.0, reconstruction index 1 mm, 120 kV, 130 mA. On the sequential CT scans, the subsegments (after Couinaud and Bismuth) were delineated according to the guidelines currently used in radiologic practice (SOYER et al. 1994; DODD 1993): The right posterior, right anterior, left medial and left lateral segments were defined by three vertical planes traced from the inferior vena cava through the right, middle, and left hepatic veins, respectively. Each segment was then further divided into a superior and an inferior subsegment by a transverse plane drawn at the level of the right and left branch of the portal vein.

5.2.2.2
Anatomical Investigation

The intact surfaces of the corrosion casts were photographed (Fig. 5.1a) and the true anatomical borders between the portal venous subsegments of COUINAUD (1957) and BISMUTH (1982) were identified. For this, the peripheral branches for each subsegment were carefully removed, beginning at its center, until only a 1-cm band that contained the most distal branches at the intersubsegmental boundaries remained (Fig. 5.1b). Gentle moving of the dissected branches made precise determination of the boundaries of the territories between the most peripheral branches within these unchanged bands possible, and these were drawn on the photographs of the original casts. The intersubsegmental boundaries were transferred to the axial CT scans as follows. Each vessel depicted on each CT scan was identified on the corresponding anatomical cast. On the cast, the vessel could be attributed to the anatomically correct subsegment, which was determined by dissection as described in the previous paragraph. The intersubsegmental boundaries were then manually traced onto the CT scans between the next neighboring vessels that belonged to adjacent subsegments.

5.2.2.3
Radiologic–Anatomical Correlation

The radiologically determined subsegments were compared with the authentic anatomical subsegments obtained on direct investigation of the 10 corresponding casts. In addition to the qualitative comparison, the quantitative differences between

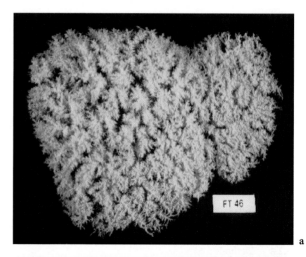

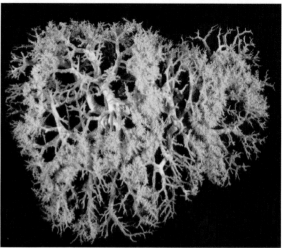

Fig. 5.1a, b. Anatomical determination of liver subsegments. **a** Native corrosion cast in a frontal view; **b** Cast after dissection, with a persisting band of peripheral branches along the intersubsegmental boundaries

the radiologic and anatomical subsegments were measured for five casts. These measurements were performed on the CT slices at four key levels, namely: at the level of the three hepatic vein trunks, at the left branch of the portal vein, at the right branch of the portal vein, and caudal to the bifurcation of the portal vein. The total area of the liver on the CT section was measured. For each subsegment, we then measured the area as delineated radiologically that did not correspond to the anatomical subsegment and, by dividing the sum of these areas by the total area of the liver, were able to calculate the percentage of the total liver area that would have been radiologically attributed to an incorrect subsegment. In addition to these percentage values, the maximum distances (in millimeters) of the radiologically determined subsegmental boundaries from the true anatomical boundaries were measured. To do this, it is first necessary to compute the minimum distance from each point on the radiologically delineated subsegment boundary to every point on the anatomical subsegment boundary, and vice versa. The largest of these minimum distances is then the maximum deviation of the radiologically determined boundary from the anatomically determined boundary.

5.3
Results

The radiologic–anatomical correlation between segments and subsegments was poor. An example is given in Fig. 5.2, in which subsegments obtained according to the current radiologic concept are compared with the authentic anatomical subsegments seen on a frontal view of the same liver. The ten livers investigated confirmed the wide anatomical variability of the portal venous territories. This variability was expressed in terms of the shape, size and number of subsegments. The boundaries between the subsegments proved to be complex, undulating scissurae rather than simple, flat planes. A uniform transverse plane, which is the assumption in the radiologic concept, could not be observed anatomically for either the right or the left hemiliver. The vertical scissurae were also observed not to be simple planes, but undulating boundaries.

These anatomical facts are depicted on axial CT scans in Fig. 5.3, in which the subsegments, delineated radiologically and anatomically at four key levels, are compared. In no case did the lines drawn from the inferior vena cava through the right, middle and left hepatic veins coincide with the real boundaries between the corresponding portal venous segments and subsegments. The most cranial level (Fig 3a, b) corresponds to the plane at which the trunks of the three hepatic veins can be recognized clearly. Contrary to the information obtained at routine radiologic examination, the presumably caudal subsegments 3, 4B and 5 can in fact be identified even at this cranial level. At the level of the left branch of the portal vein (Fig. 5.3c, d), subsegment 5 can also be recognized, and at the level of the right branch of the portal vein (Fig. 5.3e, f), parts of subsegment 2 can be seen. At the lowest key level – caudal to the bifurcation of the portal vein (Fig 3g, h) – not only the anticipated subsegments 3, 4B, 5 and 6

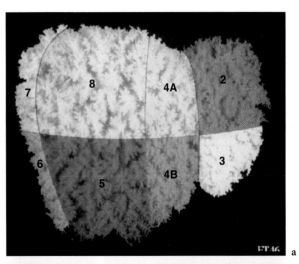

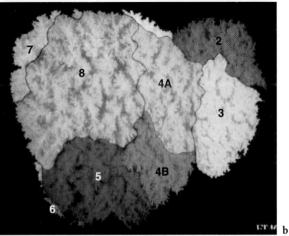

Fig. 5.2a, b. Comparison of radiologically and anatomically delineated subsegments in a frontal view of the corrosion cast shown in Fig. 5.1. a Subsegments according to the concept usually applied in daily radiologic practice; b Real anatomical subsegmentation in the liver under consideration. Comparison reveals the discrepancy between the rigid radiologic concept and the more complex anatomical reality. The *numbers* indicate the subsegment designations

are visible, but also parts of subsegments 7 and 8. Subsegment 8 extends caudally, like a wedge, between subsegments 5 and 6, and subsegment 7 extends caudally posterior to segment 6 in the liver illustrated. The observations on the CT scans thus confirm that the assumption of a flat, transverse scissura between the cranial and caudal subsegments is far from the anatomical reality.

Table 5.1 summarizes the quantitative results that support our observations. At the most cranial level, the average value ±1 standard deviation of the incorrectly determined subsegmental areas was

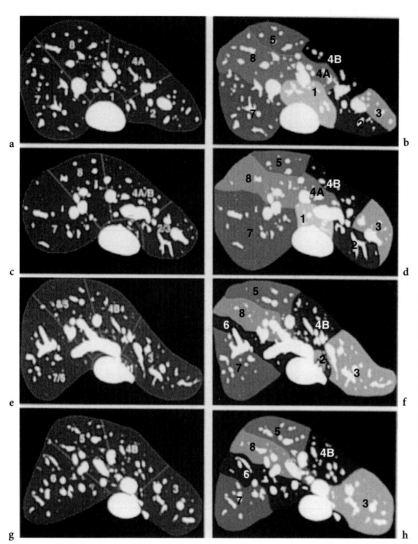

Fig. 5.3a–h. Sequential CT scans of a vascular liver cast with Couinaud's subsegments delineated at four key levels. Determination was performed according to the current procedure used in radiologic practice (*left column*: **a, c, e, g**) and compared with the true anatomical portal venous subsegmentation in the liver under consideration (*right column*: **b, d, f, h**). The radiologically assumed plane of division between the superior and inferior subsegments (the so-called transverse scissura) is noted with *dual subsegment numbers*. The synopsis confirms that it is not possible to determine the authentic subsegmental anatomy with the procedures currently used in radiologic practice

19.1±4.8% of the total liver area in the same plane. At the levels of the left and right branches of the portal vein, the corresponding values were 50.2±23.1% and 52.9±18.6%, respectively. Caudal to the portal vein bifurcation, the divergence averaged 15.4±7.7% of the liver area. In other words, the subsegmental determinations on axial CT scans made on the basis of the procedures presently used in daily radiologic practice were incorrect, on average, for 17.3±6.5% of the liver surface at the cranial and caudal regions of the liver, and for 51.6±19.9% at the central regions near the right and left branch of the portal vein. Expressed in absolute values (Table 5.2), the maximum deviation of the subsegmental boundaries, as determined radiologically on axial scans, was 40 mm (range: 10–40 mm, mean: 23±10 mm).

Table 5.1. Quantitative comparison between the subsegments as determined according to the procedures used in daily radiologic practice and the real anatomical subsegmentation, in five vascular casts. Data are percentages of the liver area per CT scan that would have been attributed to incorrect subsegments. The measurements were taken at four key levels for each cast. These levels correspond to the levels indicated in Fig. 5.3

Level	Cast 1	Cast 2	Cast 3	Cast 4	Cast 5	Average
I	12.7	20.5	25.7	17.1	19.7	19.1
II	44.1	40.3	55.7	24.4	86.4	50.2
III	39.6	44.4	41.9	84.8	53.7	52.9
IV	17.3	14.6	12.3	27.2	5.6	15.4

Table 5.2. Maximum distances (millimeters) between the boundaries of the subsegments as determined radiologically and the true anatomical boundaries on CT scans. The measurements were taken at the four key levels indicated in Fig. 5.3

Level	Specimen 1	Specimen 2	Specimen 3	Specimen 4	Specimen 5	Average
I	13	22	20	20	21	19.2
II	22	23	26	27	27	25.0
III	30	20	40	27	34	30.2
IV	12	18	16	31	10	17.4

5.4
Discussion

The first systematic investigations of the intrahepatic course of the portal and hepatic veins were undertaken by anatomists about 100 years ago (REX 1888; CANTLIE 1898; MELNIKOFF 1924). Fifty years later, in the middle of this century, the question was raised again, particularly by surgeons, and this time deliberations on it culminated in the fundamental work of HJORSTÖ (1951), ELIAS and PETTY (1952), HEALY and SCHROY (1953), GANS (1955), COUINAUD (1957), and GOLDSMITH and WOODBURNE (1957). Today, we are witnessing a third wave of interest, which has arisen during the past few years, spurred by the dramatic developments in medical imaging techniques. Brought about principally by radiologists and the need for accurate preoperative localization of focal hepatic lesions, this revival has ended up in publications reporting several studies concerned with the radiologic determination of segmental and subsegmental anatomy of the liver (MUKAI et al. 1987; SOYER et al. 1991, 1994; NELSON et al. 1994; GAZELLE and HAAGA 1992; WAGGENSPACK et al. 1993; VAN LEEUWEN et al. 1994).

The basic concept used by radiologists for this purpose is credited to COUINAUD (1957) and BISMUTH (1982) and is illustrated in Fig. 5.2a. The liver is divided into eight subsegments by means of three vertical scissurae and one transverse scissura. The vertical planes contain the inferior vena cava and the right, middle and left hepatic veins. The transverse plane passes through the right and left branches of the portal vein.

From a morphologic point of view, this concept is questionable. In particular, the anatomists PLATZER and MAURER (1966) pointed out that the variability of the segmental boundaries is too wide to render any scheme viable. FASEL et al. (1996b), who also used an anatomical approach, confirmed that the vertical planes that intersect the trunks of the hepatic veins do not correspond to the presumed intersegmental boundaries. Radiologists, too, have recently published observations that call into question the routine radiologic methods currently used for delineation of the segmental anatomy of the liver. NELSON et al. (1990) evaluated the preoperative subsegmental localization of focal hepatic lesions with the use of CT during arterial portography (CTAP) and concluded that the radiologic localization disagreed with the extent observed at surgical resection in 11 of 36 (31%) lesions. SOYER et al. (1991) reported a discrepancy in 8 of 36 (22%) cases in an analogous study with two-dimensional CTAP images. They concluded that indirect landmarks are not reliable for the correct delineation of the portal venous segments and subsegments. DOWNEY (1994), in a letter to the editor, called attention to the fact that the scissurae may curve, undulate, or even interdigitate within the liver. VAN LEEUWEN et al. (1994) used two- and three-dimensional MR imaging in healthy volunteers and concluded that localization of liver lesions and preoperative delineation of resection planes necessitate consideration of the variations in the segmental anatomy of the liver. Following a study in which three-dimensional spiral CT renderings were used, this same group reported (VAN LEEUWEN et al. 1994) that the right hepatic vein was an inaccurate indicator of the position of the right scissura and that no clear transverse scissura can be seen in the right hemiliver. OHASHI et al. (1996) observed discrepancies between the imaginary intersegmental boundaries and the margins of the areas actually enhanced on axial CT arteriograms obtained with selective injections, especially in the region under the right side of the diaphragm.

These radiologic observations accord well with the results obtained in the present study. The correlation of the subsegments as determined radiologically and anatomically was indeed poor, because the shape, size and number of portal venous territories varied greatly, and the territorial boundaries were not flat planes but were undulating. The pronounced discrepancy between the radiologically determined segmental and subsegmental anatomy and the real anatomical territories in the central regions of the liver (the second and third key levels in Table 5.1) – that is, in the region of the so-called transverse scissura – was also to be expected, because the portal venous territories show especially increased undulations in this transitional region (see Fig. 5.2b). The discrepancies between radiologically determined subsegmental anatomy and anatomical reality are less pronounced in the more cranial and caudal parts of the liver (the first and fourth key levels in Table 5.1), where the areas incorrectly determined on axial CT scans were, on average, 19.1%±4.8% and 15.4%±7.7%, respectively.

These divergences remain too high to permit reliable determination of segmental and subsegmental anatomy. Expressed in absolute numbers, the maximum distances measured on the axial CT scans between the subsegmental boundaries as determined radiologically and the true anatomical boundaries was as large as 40 mm (Table 5.2). In other words, focal hepatic lesions, such as metastases from colorectal cancer, with an axial diameter of up to 4 cm can be radiologically attributed to an incorrect subsegment. Thus, our results confirm that it is not possible, with current radiologic procedures based on indirect landmarks, to determine the authentic segmental and subsegmental anatomy of the liver. Every concept of flat planes that delimit the portal venous territories is an oversimplification that is not in agreement with the anatomical reality.

In view of these results, it seems to be necessary to develop more accurate radiologic means of determining the segmental and subsegmental portal venous anatomy. We believe that accurate segmental and subsegmental determination will be possible only with methods that take into account the actual anatomy of the portal vein tree, including the smallest peripheral branches in the liver under consideration. In principle, there seem to be two ways of achieving this goal. One is to produce a complete radiologic visualization and reconstruction of the portal vein tree, but even the most up-to-date imaging techniques, such as helical CT during arterial portography or MR imaging with gadolinium enhancement, do not provide the needed resolution. The other approach is to develop mathematical models that allow computation of the segmental and subsegmental boundaries on the basis of the radiologic data that can currently be obtained in vivo. At present, such computational models are undergoing development and preclinical validation (Evertsz et al. 1996).

Acknowledgement

This chapter is based essentially on the article of Fasel et al. (1998), with kind permission of the Radiological Society of North America, Baltimore.

References

Bismuth H (1982) Surgical anatomy and anatomical surgery of the liver. World J Surg 6:3–9

Cantlie J (1898) On a new arrangement of the right and left lobes of the liver. J Anat Physiol 32:IV–IX

Couinaud C (1957) Le foie: études anatomiques et chirurgicales. Masson, Paris, pp 9–12

Dodd GD III (1993) An American guide to Couinaud's numbering system. AJR Am J Roentgenol 161:574–575

Downey PR (1994) Radiologic identification of liver segments (letter). AJR Am J Roentgenol 163:1267

Elias II, Petty D (1952) Gross anatomy of the blood vessels and ducts within the human liver. Am J Anat 90:59–111

Evertsz CJG, Peitgen HO, Fasel JHD, Selle D, Klose KJ, Juergens H (1996) Laplacian approximation of the segmental anatomy of the liver and lung: a new method for the correct determination of subsegments. Paper presented at the 82nd scientific assembly and annual meeting of the RSNA, December 1996

Fasel JHD, Gailloud P, Terrier F, Mentha G, Sprumont P (1996a) Segmental anatomy of the liver: a review and proposal for an international working nomenclature. Eur Radiol 6:834–837

Fasel JHD, Gailloud P, Grossholz M, Bidaut L, Probst P, Terrier F (1996b) Relationship between intrahepatic vessels and computer-generated hepatic scissurae: an in vitro assay. Surg Radiol Anat 18:43–46

Fasel JHD, Selle D, Evertz CJG et al (1998) Segmental anatomy of the liver. Poor correlation with CT. Radiology 206:151–156

Gans H (1955) Introduction to hepatic surgery. Elsevier, Amsterdam

Gazelle GS, Haaga JR (1992) Hepatic neoplasms: surgically relevant segmental anatomy and imaging techniques. AJR Am J Roentgenol 158:1015–1018

Goldsmith NA, Woodburne RT (1957) The surgical anatomy pertaining to liver resection. Surg Gynecol Obstet 105:310–318

Gore RM, Levine MS, Laufer I (94) Textbook of gastrointestinal radiology. Saunders, Philadelphia, 1788–1795

Healy JE, Schroy P (1953) Anatomy of the biliary ducts within the human liver. Arch Surg 6:599–616

Hjortsö CH (1951) The topography of the intrahepatic duct systems. Acta Anat 599–615

Lafortune M, Madore F, Patriquin H, Breton G (1991) Segmental anatomy of the liver: a sonographic approach to the Couinaud nomenclature. Radiology 181:443–448

Melnikoff A (1924) Architektur der intrahepatischen Gefäße und der Gallenwege des Menschen. Z Anat Entw Gesch 70:411–465

Mukai JK, Stack CM, Turner DA et al (1987) Imaging of surgically relevant hepatic vascular and segmental anatomy. 1.

Normal anatomy. AJR Am J Roentgenol 149:287–292

Nelson RC, Chezmar JL, Sugarbaker PH, Murray DR, Bernardino ME (1990) Preoperative localisation of focal liver lesions to specific liver segments: utility of CT during arterial portography. Radiology 176:89–94

Ohashi I, Ina H, Okada Y (1996) Segmental anatomy of the liver under the right diaphragmatic dome: evaluation with axial CT. Radiology 200:779–783

Platzer W, Maurer H (1966) Zur Segmenteinteilung der Leber. Acta Anat 63:8–31

Rex H (1888) Beiträge zur Morphologie der Säugerleber. Morphol Jahrb 14:517–617

Sexton CC, Zeman RK (1983) Correlation of computed tomography, sonography, and gross anatomy of the liver. AJR Am J Roentgenol 141:711–718

Soyer P, Roche A, Gad M et al (1991) Preoperative segmental localization of hepatic metastases: utility of three-dimensional CT during arterial portography. Radiology 180:653–658

Soyer P, Bluemke DA, Bliss DF, Woodhouse CE, Fishman EK (1994) Surgical segmental anatomy of the liver: demonstration with spiral CT during arterial portography and multiplanar reconstruction. AJR Am J Roentgenol 163:99–103

Soyer P, Bluemke DA, Choti MA, Fishman EK (1995) Variations in the intrahepatic portions of the hepatic and portal veins: findings on helical CT scans during arterial portography. AJR Am J Roentgenol 164:103–108

Sugarbaker PH, Nelson RC, Murray DR, Chezmar JL, Bernardino ME (1990) A segmental approach to computerized tomographic portography for hepatic resection. Surg Gynecol Obstet 171:189–195

van Leeuwen MS, Noordzij J, Fernandez MA, Hennipman A, Feldberg MAM, Dillon EH (1994) Portal venous and segmental anatomy of the right hemiliver: observations based on three-dimensional spiral CT renderings. AJR Am J Roentgenol 163:1395–1404

Waggenspack GA, Tabb RD, Tiruchelvam V, Ziegler L, Waltersdorff K (1993) Three-dimensional localisation of hepatic neoplasms with computer-generated scissurae recreated from axial CT and MR images. AJR Am J Roentgenol 160:307–309

6 Metastases

P. Soyer, D. A. Bluemke, J.-P. Pelage

CONTENTS

6.1   Introduction   *73*
6.2   Clinical and Pathophysiological Background   *73*
6.3   Technique for Spiral CT of the Liver in Patients with Hepatic Metastases   *74*
6.3.1   Technical Considerations   *74*
6.3.2   Spiral CT with Intravenous Iodinated Contrast Material   *74*
6.3.3   Spiral CT During Arterial Portography   *75*
6.4   Clinical Performance of Spiral CT in Patients with Hepatic Metastases   *76*
6.4.1   Spiral CT with Intravenous Iodinated Contrast Material   *76*
6.4.2   Spiral CT During Arterial Portography   *77*
6.5   Clinical Benefits of Using Spiral CT Compared with Conventional CT   *78*
6.5.1   Detection of Hepatic Metastases   *78*
6.5.2   Multiplanar and 3-D Reformations   *80*
6.5.3   Volumetric Analysis   *82*
6.6   Future Research into Spiral CT of Hepatic Metastases   *82*
       References   *83*

6.1 Introduction

Hepatic resection is an accepted procedure in the management of hepatic metastases from colorectal cancer and, when feasible, improves the 5-year survival rate of the patients with this disease (Iwatsuki et al. 1986; Hughes et al. 1988). Unfortunately, less than 10% of patients with hepatic metastases from colorectal cancer may benefit from partial hepatic resection, because it is contraindicated by extrahepatic disease, bilateral hepatic involvement by me-

P. Soyer, MD, PhD; Department of Radiology, Hôpital Lariboisière, 2 rue Ambroise Paré, 75745 Paris cedex 10, France
D. A. Bluemke, MD, PhD; Department of Radiology, Johns Hopkins Hospital, 600 North Wolfe Street, Baltimore, MD 21287-6953, USA
J.-P. Pelage, MD; Department of Radiology, Hôpital Lariboisière, 2 rue Ambroise Paré, 75745 Paris cedex 10, France

tastases or the presence of too many metastases by the time the hepatic metastases are discovered. Also, new surgical techniques, including cryosurgery and radiofrequency ablation, have placed more demands on preoperative evaluation. Careful preoperative selection of the hepatic surgery candidate is therefore crucial to avoid needless laparotomy (Balfe 1992). A major factor in determining the success of surgery for hepatic metastases is the extent of hepatic resection. Besides the histological nature of hepatic metastases, preoperative evaluation of their number and location determines which patients' metastases are resectable and what type of surgical resection is necessary (right or left hemiliver, segmental or multisegmental).

The usefulness of computed tomography (CT) in the detection and characterization of hepatic metastases is well established. Requirements for high-quality examinations include rapid bolus administration of iodinated contrast material, rapid acquisition of data, and minimal respiratory motion from the patient being examined. These requirements are fully satisfied by spiral CT (Bluemke and Fishman 1993b, Heiken et al. 1993, Kalender et al. 1990, Zeman et al. 1993). Spiral scanning allows volumetric complete coverage of the liver in a single breath-hold (about 90% of patients are able to hold their breath during acquisition of the images), providing thin reconstruction of images. In addition, the images obtained can be manipulated in several ways (including cine mode, oblique reformation, and three-dimensional views).

6.2 Clinical and Pathophysiological Background

Evaluation of the liver for metastatic disease is a common indication for spiral CT examination. Metastatic disease is approximately 20 times as common as primary hepatic malignancies; about 30% of patients who die of malignancy have hepatic metastases (WILKES 1973). In autopsy series, the liver is the most common organ involved in colorectal carcinoma (65% of the cases) and rectal carcinoma (47% of the cases) (ABRAMS et al. 1950), and it is rare for metastases to be present in other sites if the liver and lung are free of tumor (WEISS et al. 1986). In addition, in many patients the presence of liver metastases is the main determinant of survival (GOSLIN et al. 1982). The primary mode of metastatic cell delivery in gastrointestinal cancer is the portal vein (CHAUDHURI and FINK 1991). The most common neoplasms that may give rise to hepatic metastases are colorectal, breast, lung, and pancreatic cancers, melanoma and sarcomas. Metastatic disease usually becomes manifest as focal hepatic masses, but infiltrative involvement is also found, particularly with lymphoma and breast carcinoma. Although metastases may be found anywhere in the liver, metastases are more frequently located in the right hemiliver than the left hemiliver (CHAUDHURI and FINK 1991).

Hepatic metastases receive most of their blood supply from the hepatic artery, although in some cases they may receive blood flow from the portal vein (KAN et al. 1993). Basically, hepatic metastases can be divided into two categories based on their enhancement relative to the adjacent hepatic parenchyma. Hypervascular lesions enhance rapidly during the arterial phase of the intravenous administration of the iodinated contrast material and become hyperattenuating compared with the liver. Metastases in this category include metastases from breast, islet cell, and renal cell carcinoma, sarcoma, and, to a lesser degree, metastases from melanoma and lymphoma (PATTEN et al. 1993, FREDERICK et al. 1996). Hypovascular metastases are relatively hypoattenuating compared with the liver during the arterial phase of intravenous administration of the iodinated contrast material. Most hepatic metastases from the gastrointestinal tract are hypovascular. Because of this variation in the apparent enhancement of hypervascular and hypovascular hepatic metastases, spiral CT should ideally be tailored to the specific metastases suspected (BLUEMKE et al. 1995c). However, it is difficult to predict the vascular status of a given metastasis before spiral CT examination is performed, because some "hypervascular" metastases may behave in a similar way to hypovascular metastases owing to the specific treatment given to the patient. For example, hepatic metastases from islet cell cancer may be necrotic after chemotherapy, so that they become hypovascular.

6.3
Technique for Spiral CT of the Liver in Patients with Hepatic Metastases

6.3.1
Technical Considerations

Although the distance to be covered may vary among patients, in general 20 cm is enough to cover the whole liver in patients with hepatic metastases. The distance to be covered depends on slice collimation, pitch, and total scan time. Collimation is the "section thickness" at which the imaging data are acquired (typically, from 4 to 6 mm). The pitch value is the distance of table advance per 360° rotation divided by the collimation thickness (KALENDER et al. 1990). The total scan time for hepatic spiral CT depends on the patient's ability to hold a breath and the heat load capacity of the X-ray tube. Reconstruction intervals are selected to create overlapping reconstructed images, which have been shown to improve the level of confidence for hepatic metastases detection (URBAN et al. 1993) and subsequent multiplanar and three-dimensional reconstruction.

6.3.2
Spiral CT with Intravenous Iodinated Contrast Material

Because spiral CT allows so much faster acquisition of images than conventional CT, administration of contrast agents has been extensively studied during the last 3 years to determine the optimal dose and rate of injection of iodine, and the best scan delay time for peak parenchymal enhancement. Although it is difficult to develop a single strategy that works for every case, it is generally admitted that a single-phase technique can be used in the majority of patients with hepatic metastases. For this single-phase technique, a scan delay time of 50-60 s is optimal following a single-phase administration of 100–120 ml of a 300-350 mg iodine/ml nonionic contrast medium delivered at a rate of 3-4 ml/s (the equilibrium occurring 100 s after the beginning of the injection) (SILVERMAN et al. 1995b). It is important to scan the liver before the equilibrium phase, because some metastases may become isoattenuating relative to the adjacent hepatic parenchyma. Portal venous phase imaging (also called single spiral scan) is most often used in clinical practice to investigate patients with hepatic metastases, because it is rapid and generally effective in the detection of hepatic metastases (KUSZYK et al. 1996).

For patients with suspected hypervascular hepatic metastases, or for patients scheduled to undergo partial hepatectomy, dual-phase spiral scanning is more appropriate. For a dual spiral scan, two consecutive back-to-back spiral acquisitions are performed during both the arterial and the venous phase of hepatic parenchymal enhancement. The first spiral acquisition is obtained during the arterial phase of the bolus (20 s after the start of the bolus), allowing arterial vascularity of the tumor to be assessed or subsequent three-dimensional reformation of the hepatic artery to be done (this may be useful for the surgeon to plan hepatic resection in selected cases) (WINTER et al. 1995). The second spiral acquisition is obtained 60-70 s after the start of the injection during the portal phase. The dual spiral scan technique potentially allows depiction of more tumors, some being seen during the arterial phase only and others, during the portal phase only (HOLLETT et al. 1995, BONALDI et al. 1995). However, a cost-efficiency assessment of this technique has to be done (dual spiral scan increases the acquisition time, double the numbers of films, and burns out the X-ray tube faster). For patients who are not able to hold their breath for 20 s, a cluster technique can be used to scan the liver in two or three acquisitions separated by one or two intervals during which the patients can breathe. Automated computer programs can be used to optimize the scan delay time after the start of the bolus (SILVERMAN et al. 1995a). Such software is now available on most scanners to optimize image acquisition during the best temporal window during which the highest degree of parenchymal enhancement is obtained. SILVERMAN et al. have shown that the use of an automated computer program allows a more consistent examination of the liver by automatically determining the best delay time to the beginning of spiral scanning after administration of iodinated contrast material.

The use of a triple-phase spiral CT technique has been advocated by several groups because it helps to better characterize focal liver lesions (VAN LEEUWEN et al. 1995). The triphasic spiral CT technique involves two different strategies. One of these consists in three consecutive spiral CT acquisitions after the injection of iodinated contrast material. Thus, the liver is scanned during the arterial (scanning delay, 22-27 s), portal (scanning delay, 49-73 s), and equilibrium (scanning delay, 8-10 min) phases. Although this technique has not yet been evaluated in terms of hepatic metastasis detection, it does convey a better level of confidence for lesion characterization (VAN LEEUWEN et al. 1995). This technique may be useful in patients with a known primary in whom hepatic lesions are discovered. Another triple-phase spiral scanning strategy consists in the combination of an unenhanced phase followed by an arterial and a portal phase acquisition (FREDERICK et al. 1996; PAULSON et al. 1998).

6.3.3
Spiral CT During Arterial Portography

Spiral CT during arterial portography has been widely embraced as the ultimate preoperative examination in patients with hepatic metastases. Although spiral CT during hepatic arteriography can be used to improve detection of hepatic metastases, this technique has not gained as much acceptance as spiral CT during arterial portography. VAN OOIJEN et al. found that spiral CT during hepatic arteriography has a sensitivity of 94%, but the high sensitivity is accompanied by a high false-positive rate, particularly because of variations in the perfusion of normal liver parenchyma (VAN OOIJEN et al. 1996). This accuracy of spiral CT during hepatic arteriography reaches only 74%, which hampers its routine application in patients with hepatic metastases. Conversely, in our experience spiral CT images obtained during arterial portography are associated with better degrees of accuracy (BLUEMKE et al. 1995a, b). This imaging technique consists of spiral CT images obtained during infusion of iodinated contrast material into the superior mesenteric or splenic artery (BLUEMKE and FISHMAN 1993a, BLUEMKE et al. 1995a). The tip of a 5-F angiographic catheter is placed in the superior mesenteric or splenic artery, and patency of the portal vein may then be determined by angiography using a limited amount of iodinated contrast material. In most cases angiography is not needed because the status of the portal vein can be determined by noninvasive imaging modalities. The patient is then transferred immediately to the CT suite. A noncontrast CT scan is obtained to define the lower and upper limits of the liver and for image centering on the scan monitor. Spiral CT during arterial portography is obtained with collimation of 4-6 mm and a table speed of 4-10 mm/s during transcatheter infusion of 100-120 ml of an iodinated contrast medium (iodine, 150-200 mg/ml). Before spiral CT during arterial portography, the patient is instructed to hold his breath during spiral scanning to eliminate motion artifact. Contrast material is injected via the catheter at a rate of 3 ml/s through a power injector. Spiral CT during arterial portography examination is obtained with craniocaudal table incrementation. With spiral CT, the use of a vasodilating agent is not mandatory prior to intraarterial administration of the iodinated contrast agent. Spiral scanning begins 30-35 s after the start of the contrast injection, as previously described (Bluemke and Fishman 1993a). Studies from the Johns Hopkins Hospital have showed that spiral CT during arterial portography allows high contrast between liver parenchyma and hepatic metastases, so that small metastases can be confidently depicted with an acceptable false-positive rate (Bluemke et al. 1995b, Soyer et al. 1994c). To enhance confidence in lesion characterization and decrease the false-positive findings rate, it is possible to combine spiral CT during hepatic arteriography and spiral CT during arterial portography in the same patient (Kanematsu et al. 1997).

6.4
Clinical Performances of Spiral CT in Patients with Hepatic Metastases

6.4.1
Spiral CT with Intravenous Iodinated Contrast Material

Using a single phase spiral technique, Kuszyk et al. (1996) were able to depict 84% of hepatic metastases in a series of 43 metastases. The 7 metastases not seen on spiral CT originated from colorectal cancer in 5 instances and from pancreatic neuroendocrine tumors in 2 others. Hollett et al. showed that dual-phase scanning improved the detection rate of hepatic neoplasms 1.5 cm or less in diameter over that yielded by a single spiral acquisition obtained during the portal phase of enhancement, which was used in the study by Kuszyk et al. (Hollett et al. 1995; Kuszyk et al. 1996) (Figs. 6.1, 6.2). As noted by Hollett et al. (1995), the added value of arterial phase scanning was more manifest in patients with hypervascular metastases, such as metastases from carcinoid of the small bowel (Fig. 6.3). However, in a few cases, hypovascular metastases such as metastases from colorectal carcinoma can be unexpectedly depicted during the arterial phase scanning only (Hollett et al. 1995). A study by Bonaldi et al. (1995) based on a series of 119 focal liver lesions found nine lesions (8%) that were seen on the arterial phase scanning only. To better address this concern, a study from the group at Durham (N.C., USA)

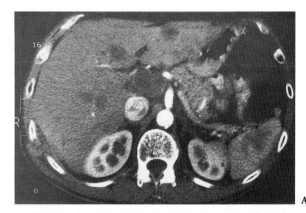

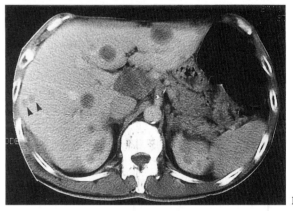

Fig. 6.1A, B. Hepatic metastases from colorectal carcinoma. Spiral CT scans obtained **A** during the arterial phase and **B** during the portal phase. Additional metastases are depicted during the portal phase scanning (*arrowheads*) compared with the arterial phase scanning

compared noncontrast CT, hepatic arterial phase, and portal venous phase spiral CT for the detection of hepatic metastases from breast carcinoma. Portal venous phase spiral CT showed more metastases than did the other two phases (85% vs 59% for arterial phase scanning and 61% for unenhanced scanning (Frederick et al. 1997). Two metastases were seen during the arterial phase only, three during the unenhanced phase only and 10 during the portal venous phase only. The remainder of the metastases were seen on more than one phase (Frederick et al. 1997). From a pragmatic point of view, in the study by Frederick et al. (1997) no spiral CT scan obtained during the portal venous phase was converted from negative to positive because of the addition of unenhanced or arterial phase scanning. Therefore, in cases of suspected hepatic metastases from breast carcinoma the routine use of these two phases has not been justified when the clinical concern is the presence or absence of metastases

Metastases

(FREDERICK et al. 1997). Another and more recent
study from the same group showed that unenhanced
scanning is helpful in showing calcified hepatic metastases from carcinoid tumors that may be partially
obscured after the administration of iodinated contrast material (PAULSON et al. 1998). In addition, in
the same study a significant number of metastases
were seen only during the arterial phase and 2 patients had all their carcinoid metastases visible during the arterial phase only (PAULSON et al. 1998). It is
reasonable to conclude that arterial phase scanning
is helpful in that it depicts more metastases in a subset of patients with hypervascular metastases. However, the impact of this dual-phase technique relative
to a single-phase technique in terms of patient outcome has not been fully evaluated to date (Fig. 6.4).

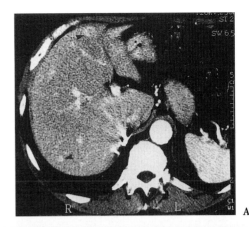

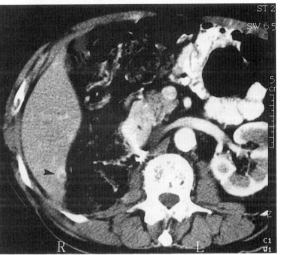

Fig. 6.3A, B. Hypervascular hepatic metastases from renal cell
carcinoma. Spiral CT scan obtained during the arterial phase
at two different levels of slice shows tiny hyperattenuating
metastases (*arrowheads*) that were not visible during the
portal venous phase scanning. Surgical clips are present because of prior nephrectomy

6.4.2
Spiral CT During Arterial Portography

Spiral CT during arterial portography is the ultimate
examination in patients scheduled to undergo curative partial hepatic resection. This technique is regarded as the most sensitive preoperative imaging
technique for the detection of hepatic metastases
(Figs. 6.5, 6.6). Also, this technique is used to exclude
the presence of metastases in the portion of the liver
that will be left in place after partial hepatectomy
(Fig. 6.7). In one of our studies that was based on the
comparison with pathological findings, a total of 35
hepatic metastases from colorectal cancer were
identified pathologically in the resected specimens
in 23 patients (SOYER et al. 1994c). The mean num-

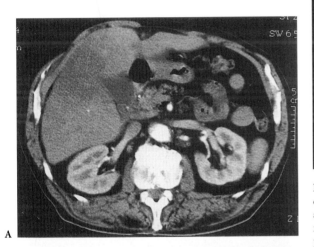

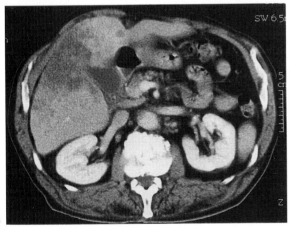

Fig. 6.2A, B. Hepatic metastases from colorectal carcinoma.
Spiral CT scans obtained A during the arterial phase and B
during the portal phase. The portal phase scanning shows a
more diffuse metastatic involvement than the arterial phase
scanning

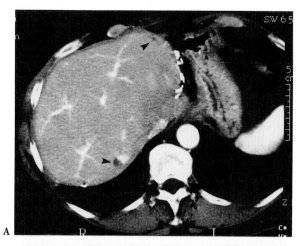

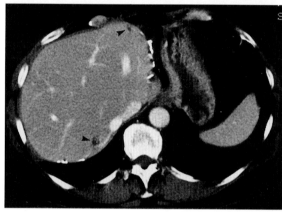

ber of hepatic metastases from colorectal cancer per patient was 1.5 (range, 1-4) and the mean diameter of the hepatic metastases was 37 mm (range, 4-95 mm). Thirty three of 35 hepatic metastases from colorectal cancer were correctly depicted by spiral CT during arterial portography, yielding a sensitivity of 94% (95% confidence interval, 0.83-0.99). The two hepatic metastases (6%) that were not detected on spiral CT during arterial portography were present in two different patients and had greatest diameters of 4 and 5 mm (SOYER et al. 1994c). The false-positive rate based on all lesions detected with spiral CT during arterial portography was 13% (95% confidence interval, 0.05-0.28). The false-positive percentage calculated on a per-patient basis was 17% (95% confidence interval, 0.00-0.29) (SOYER et al. 1994c).

6.5
Clinical Benefits of Using Spiral CT Rather than Conventional CT

6.5.1
Detection of Hepatic Metastases

Spiral CT improves detection of hepatic metastases, and this improvement, which is attributable in part to the use of thin collimation with overlapping reconstruction, is critical when small metastases are present (URBAN et al. 1993). The success of partial hepatic resection in patients with metastases de-

Fig. 6.4A, B. Intrahepatic recurrence of hepatic metastases from colorectal carcinoma after prior partial hepatectomy. Spiral CT scans obtained **A** during the arterial phase and **B** during the portal phase. Both phases allow comparable depiction of two tiny metastases (*arrowheads*)

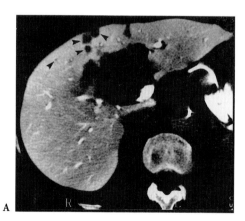
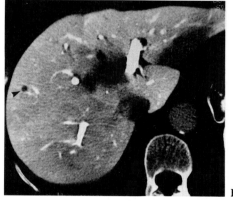

Fig. 6.5. A, B. Hepatic metastases from carcinoid tumor. Spiral CT scan obtained during arterial portography using a splenic artery injection of iodinated contrast material shows large central hepatic metastasis from carcinoid tumor. At both levels of slice (**A, B**), owing to increased density difference between metastases and the hepatic parenchyma, additional metastases (*arrowheads*) not seen with other imaging techniques are depicted on this examination only. In **A** portal involvement by tumor is clearly seen

pends on a careful preoperative selection of the hepatic resection candidate. Spiral CT during arterial portography is now established as an important method yielding results that can usefully be applied in the preoperative planning for patients with hepatic metastases (Fig. 6.8). Although no study directly compares spiral and conventional CT during arterial portography, the advantages of spiral technology over conventional CT for CT during arterial portography become self-evident on analysis of the explanations that have been suggested for the low

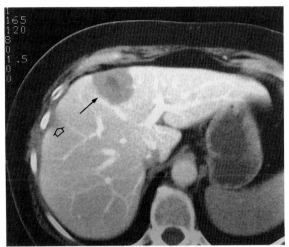

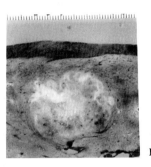

Fig. 6.6.8A, B. Hepatic metastasis from colonic carcinoma. A Spiral CT scan obtained during arterial portography using a superior mesenteric artery injection of iodinated contrast material shows a single metastasis (*arrow*) in segment 4 of the liver. Nontumorous subcapsular perfusion defect is seen (*open arrow*). B Resection of segment 4 only (segmentectomy) was successfully performed

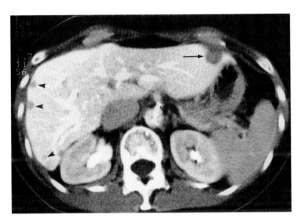

Fig. 6.6. Hepatic metastases from neuroendocrine tumor. Spiral CT scan obtained during arterial portography using a superior mesenteric artery injection of iodinated contrast material shows a metastasis in the left hemiliver (*arrow*). However, additional unsuspected metastases (*arrowheads*) are detected in the right hemiliver, changing the therapeutic strategy

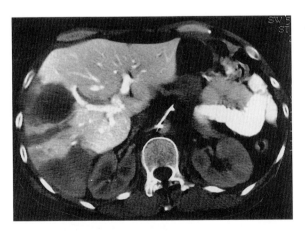

Fig. 6.7. Hepatic metastases from colonic carcinoma. Spiral CT scan obtained during arterial portography using a superior mesenteric artery injection of iodinated contrast material shows diffuse metastatic involvement of the right hemiliver. However, partial hepatectomy (resection of the right hemiliver) was considered and successfully performed owing to the exclusion of metastases in the left hemiliver by spiral CT during arterial portography

detection rate of small metastases with conventional CT during arterial portography. Respiratory motion and a partial volume phenomenon, which have been suggested as the cause of low sensitivity for small neoplastic nodule detection, are eliminated. In addition, the systemic recirculation of contrast to the hepatic artery that can occur with prolonged scanning times (this is likely to diminish contrast differences between metastases and disease-free hepatic parenchyma), potentially obscuring small metastases scanned late after the bolus), is eliminated by fast scanning (BLUEMKE et al. 1995a, SOYER et al. 1994b). In addition, 3- to 4-mm overlapping reconstruction intervals that increase detection of hepatic metastases with spiral CT may have a favorable effect on the sensitivity of spiral CT during arterial portography. Our experience at the Johns Hopkins Hospital confirms this assumption (SOYER et al. 1994c). The sensitivity of 94% (33 of 35 metastases) for spiral CT during arterial portography in the detection of hepatic metastases from colorectal cancer compares favorably with the upper limit of the range obtained using conventional CT technology (conventional CT during arterial portography has a reported sensitivity for detection of hepatic metastases from colorectal cancer ranging from 78% to 91%; SOYER et al. 1994b). The false-positive percentage (based on all lesions detected with spiral CT during arterial portography) of spiral CT during arterial portography is 13%, the false-positive percentage calculated on a per-patient basis being 17% in the same study (SOYER et al. 1994c).

6.5.2
Multiplanar and Three-Dimensional Reformations

Spiral technology has focused attention on the postprocessing of data, and most sites with spiral scanning units routinely use multiplanar reformation. One of the most exciting capabilities of spiral CT for the liver is its ability to give extremely high-quality two-dimensional multiplanar and three-dimensional images. This is due to the large number of overlapping thin slices (up to 80 for a complete study of the liver) that can be obtained with spiral technique. However, at this time, except for two-dimensional multiplanar reformation, which includes bone and abdominal structures, no automatic editing system for three-dimensional reformation is widely available and a large amount of time for manual or operator-defined editing is needed. However, as spiral CT has placed more demand on data postprocessing, postprocessing systems have improved in speed and quality and have become more user-friendly. Typically, spiral CT images are quickly transferred to a free-standing workstation for further analysis. Multiplanar reconstructions are then obtained in the oblique, coronal, and sagittal planes (Figs. 6.9, 6.10), SOYER et al. 1994a). Three-dimensional images of the hepatic vasculature can be obtained by using a surface rendering technique or a maximum intensity projection (MIP) technique; this latter technique is a two-dimensional image presentation of three-dimensional data (Fig. 6.11) (HEATH et al. 1995).

Two-dimensional multiplanar reformations are useful for defining anatomic structures and for determining segmental location and extent of tumors (Fig. 6.12) (SOYER et al. 1994a). Three-dimensional reformations are useful for analyzing the same criteria and for determining the exact volume of the liver

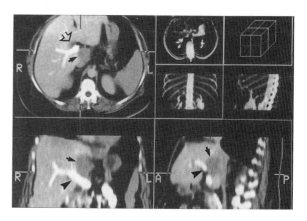

Fig. 6.9. Hepatic metastasis from colonic carcinoma. Spiral CT scan obtained during arterial portography using a superior mesenteric artery injection of iodinated contrast material in the axial, sagittal and coronal planes (clockwise) shows a single hepatic metastasis (*arrows*) in segment 1 of the liver. Reformatted images allow precise localization of tumor (*arrows*) and assessment of relationships to portal vessels (*arrowheads*). Nontumorous triangular perfusion defect (*open arrow*) is seen adjacent to right portal vein

and the estimated volume of the remaining liver volume when a partial hepatic resection is planned (Fig. 6.13). In addition, application of the segmental terminology to the imaging planes defined solely by axial CT slices may be difficult when anyone is attempting to define the transverse and vertical scissuras adequately. The transverse scissura, in particular, is nearly parallel to the axial imaging plane and may be difficult to depict. Reformatted images obtained with spiral CT are particularly useful for showing segmental anatomy of the liver. This technique provides vivid enhancement of both the hepatic veins and the portal branches, which are the landmarks of the subsegmental anatomy of the liver, so that three-dimensional displays can show the hepatic veins and fifth-order portal branches with the volume and MIP rendering techniques. In our experience, "stair-step" artifacts markedly degrade the three-dimensional displays obtained with the surface rendering technique, making this technique inappropriate for imaging the intrahepatic venous structures (HEATH et al. 1995). MIP reformatted images may be useful for the assessment of portal encasement by metastases, which are sometimes better seen on reformatted images than on axial images. However, it must be borne in mind that no study has yet elucidated the respective values of axial and MIP reformatted spiral CT images for the assessment of portal involvement by hepatic tumor.

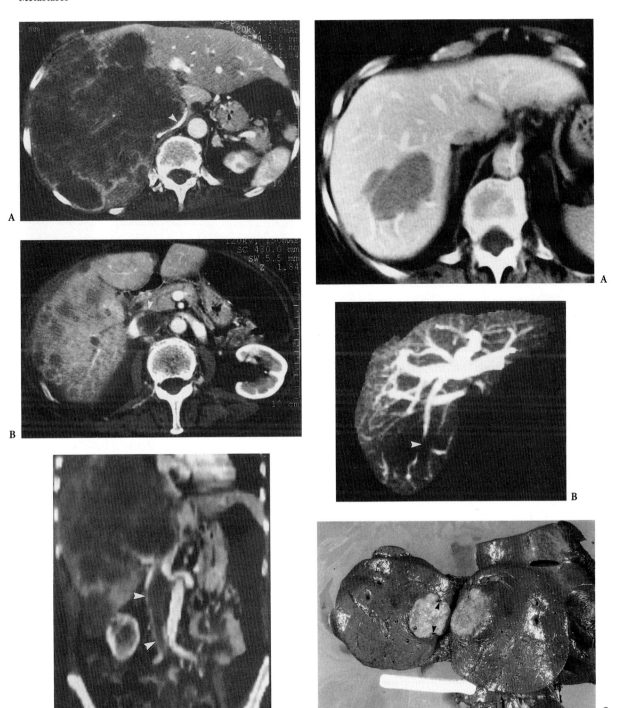

Fig. 6.10A-C. Hepatic metastasis from colonic carcinoma. Spiral CT scan obtained during the portal venous phase allows depiction of diffuse metastatic involvement of the liver and compression of the inferior vena cava. **A** At this level of slice, spiral CT shows protruding metastasis compressing the inferior vena cava (*arrowhead*). **B** At a lower level, a thrombus (*arrowhead*) is seen within the inferior vena cava. **C** Reformatted image obtained in the coronal plane confirms the presence of the thrombus (*arrowheads*) and helps to define its limits better

Fig. 6.11A-C. Hepatic metastasis from colonic carcinoma. **A** Spiral CT scan obtained during arterial portography using a superior mesenteric artery injection of iodinated contrast material shows a single metastasis in the right hemiliver. **B** Reformatted image using a maximum-intensity projection technique shows vessel encasement by the metastasis. **C** Vessels (*arrowheads*) within the metastasis are seen on the gross specimen

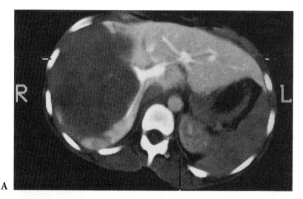

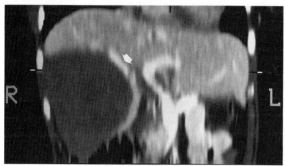

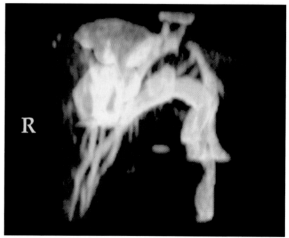

Fig. 6.13. Hepatic metastases from colonic carcinoma. Three-dimensional image obtained with a volume rendering technique from data obtained with spiral CT during arterial portography shows two metastases located at the hepatic dome in the right hemiliver. This technique allows definite tumor localization and estimation of the volume of the remaining liver after partial hepatectomy

Fig. 12A, B. Hepatic metastasis from colonic carcinoma. **A** Spiral CT scan obtained during arterial portography using a superior mesenteric artery injection of iodinated contrast material shows a large metastasis in the right hemiliver. **B** Reformatted coronal image shows that the metastasis is located mainly in inferior segments of the right hemiliver. Relationship of segmental portal branch for segment 8 (*arrow*) to metastasis is clearly seen

6.5.3
Volumetric Analysis

One role of spiral CT in the preoperative evaluation of patients with hepatic metastases is to estimate, preoperatively, the volume of the remaining liver that will be left in place after partial hepatic resection. One principle of hepatic resection is that sufficient liver volume must be left in place to support life (BISMUTH et al. 1982). Although survival after removal of up to 80% of the liver has been reported (MALT 1985), more than 30% of the functional liver should be left in place to avoid the risk of postoperative liver failure (SUGARBAKER 1990). Presently, 35% is accepted as the estimated postoperative liver volume needed for safe performance of hepatic resection (SOYER et al. 1992). In a prospective study, we demonstrated that the assessment of estimated postoperative liver volume using three-dimensional CT during arterial portography provides preoperative

data that are vital for reducing the risk of postoperative liver failure (SOYER et al. 1992). When the estimated postoperative liver volume is insufficient, it is possible to perform portal vein embolization preoperatively, which results in marked hypertrophy of the unembolized healthy part of the liver (SOYER et al. 1992). Such volumetric information can be obtained with a spiral CT study (STAPAKIS et al. 1995).

Also, another possible role of volumetric measurement obtained with spiral CT is to determine the volume of a given hepatic metastasis, which may be used to assess the response to therapy in patients with hepatic metastases treated by systemic chemotherapy or loco-regional treatment. VAN HOE et al. (1997) demonstrated that three-dimensional measurements obtained from spiral CT data are as reproducible as one- and two-dimensional measurements for the assessment of hepatic metastasis volume.

6.6
Future Research into Spiral CT of Hepatic Metastases

While some "academic" radiologists routinely prepare two-dimensional reformatted images or three-dimensional reconstructions from spiral CT data, extensive use of these postprocessing techniques is not common. Several reasons may be proposed for this: difficult cases are mostly examined in tertiary care and teaching hospitals (most surgical resections of the liver are performed in tertiary care hospitals), postprocessing is time consuming (requiring sometimes extensive editing on specialized workstations), and image reformatting needs additional workstations (which are expensive). Future developments of postprocessing software to make it more efficient and more user-friendly are needed. Currently, there is a need for automatic editing algorithms to obtain three-dimensional images of the liver. To our knowledge, except for bone removal, there is no system currently available that allows automatic editing to display the liver only.

Virtual reality is another trend in research on liver imaging, and especially when a surgical resection is planned. In the future, after three-dimensional images have been obtained with a volume rendering technique, it will be possible to simulate a surgical resection with a computer, with precise depiction of the remaining liver and the part of the liver that will be resected, and estimation of the volume of the remaining liver. However, it must be borne in mind that it is crucial to focus on the needs of physicians and not be tempted by the technology available to obtain images that are splendid and impressive (in terms of marketing) but expensive (in terms of time) and not clinically relevant (i. e. do not affect patient's care).

References

Abrams HL, Spiro R, Goldstein N (1950) Metastases in carcinoma. Cancer 3:74-85

Balfe DM (1992) Hepatic metastases from colorectal cancer: radiologic strategies for improved selection. Radiology 185:18-19

Bismuth H, Houssin D, Castaing D (1982) Major and minor segmentectomies « réglées »in liver surgery. World J Surg 6:10-24

Bluemke DA, Fishman EK (1993a) Spiral CT arterial portography of the liver. Radiology 186:576-579

Bluemke DA, Fishman EK (1993b) Spiral CT of the liver. AJR Am J Roentgenol 160:787-792

Bluemke DA, Soyer P, Chan BW, Bliss DF, Calhoun PS, Fishman EK (1995a) Spiral CT during arterial portography: techniques and applications. Radiographics 15:623-637

Bluemke DA, Soyer P, Fishman EK (1995b) Nontumorous low-attenuation defects in the liver on helical CT during arterial portography: frequency, location, and appearance. AJR Am J Roentgenol 164:1141-1145

Bluemke DA, Soyer P, Fishman EK (1995c) Helical (spiral) CT of the liver. Radiol Clin North Am 33:863-886

Bonaldi VM, Bret PM, Reinhold C, Atri M (1995) Helical CT of the liver: value of early hepatic arterial phase. Radiology 197:357-363

Chaudhuri K, Fink S (1991) Physiological considerations in imaging liver metastases from colorectal carcinoma. Am J Physiol Imaging 6:150-160

Frederick MG, Paulson EK, Nelson RC (1997) Helical CT for detecting focal liver lesions in patients with breast carcinoma: comparison of noncontrast phase, hepatic arterial phase, and portal venous phase. J Comput Assist Tomogr 21:229-235

Goslin R, Steele G Jr, Zamcheck N, et al. (1982) Factors influencing survival in patients with hepatic metastases from adenocarcinoma of the colon or rectum. Dis Colon Rectum 25:749-754

Heath DG, Soyer P, Kuszyk BS, et al. (1995) Three-dimensional spiral CT during arterial portography: comparison of three rendering techniques. Radiographics 15;1001-1011

Heiken JP, Brink JA, Vannier MW (1993) Spiral (helical) CT. Radiology 189:647-656

Hollett MD, Jeffrey RB Jr, Nino-Murcia M, Jorgensen MJ, Harris DP (1995) Dual-phase helical CT of the liver: value of arterial phase scans in the detection of small (<15 mm) malignant hepatic neoplasms. AJR Am J Roentgenol 164:879-884

Hughes KS, Rosenstein RB, Songhorabodi S, et al. (1988) Resection of the liver for colorectal carcinoma metastases: a multi-institutional study of long-term survivors. Dis Colon Rectum 31:1-4

Iwatsuki S, Esquivel CO, Gordon RD, Starzl TE (1986) Liver resection for metastatic colorectal cancer. Surgery 100:804-810

Kalender WA, Seissler W, Klotz E, Vock P (1990) Spiral volumetric CT with single breath-hold technique, continuous transport, and continuous scanner rotation. Radiology 176:181-183

Kan Z, Ivancev K, Lunderquist A, et al. (1993) In vivo microscopy of hepatic tumors in animal models: a dynamic investigation of blood supply to hepatic metastases. Radiology 187:621-626

Kanematsu M, Hoshi H, Imaeda T, et al. (1997) Detection and characterization of hepatic tumors: value of combined helical CT hepatic arteriography and CT during arterial portography. AJR Am J Roentgenol 168:1193-1198

Kuszyk BS, Bluemke DA, Urban BA, et al. (1996) Portal-phase contrast-enhanced helical CT for the detection of malignant hepatic tumors: sensitivity based on comparison with intraoperative and pathologic findings. AJR Am J Roentgenol 166:91-95

Malt RA (1985) Surgery for hepatic neoplasms. N Engl J Med 313:1591-1596

Patten RM, Byun JY, Freeny PC (1993) CT of hypervascular hepatic tumors: are unenhanced scans necessary for diagnosis? AJR Am J Roentgenol 161:979-984

Paulson EK, McDermott VG, Keogan MT, DeLong DM, Frederick MG, Nelson RC (1998) Carcinoid metastases to the liver: role of triple-phase helical CT. Radiology 206:143-150

Silverman PM, Brown B, Wray H, et al. (1995a) Optimal contrast enhancement of the liver using helical (spiral) CT: value of SmartPrep. AJR Am J Roentgenol 164:1169-1171

Silverman PM, O'Malley, Tefft MC, Cooper C, Zeman RK

(1995b) Conspicuity of hepatic metastases on helical CT: effect of different time delays between contrast administration and scanning. AJR Am J Roentgenol 164:619-623

Stapakis J, Stamm E, Townsend R, Thickman D (1995) Liver volume assessment by conventional vs helical CT. Abdom Imaging 20:209-210

Soyer P, Bluemke DA, Bliss DE, Woodhouse CE, Fishman EK (1994a). Surgical segmental anatomy of the liver: demonstration with spiral CT during arterial portography and multiplanar reconstruction. AJR 163:99-103

Soyer P, Bluemke DA, Fishman EK (1994b) CT during arterial portography for the preoperative evaluation of hepatic tumors: how, when, and why? AJR 163:1325-1331

Soyer P, Bluemke DA, Hruban RH, Sitzmann JV, Fishman EK (1994c) Hepatic metastases from colorectal cancer: detection and false-positive findings with helical CT during arterial portography. Radiology 193:71-74

Soyer P, Bluemke DA, Hruban RH, Sitzmann JV, Fishman EK (1994d) Primary malignant neoplasms of the liver: detection with helical CT during arterial portography. Radiology 192:389-392

Soyer P, Roche A, Elias D, Levesque M (1992) Hepatic metastases from colorectal cancer: influence of hepatic volumetric analysis on surgical decision making. Radiology 184:695-697

Sugarbaker PH (1990) Surgical decision making for large bowel cancer metastatic to the liver. Radiology 174:621-626

Urban BA, Fishman EK, Kuhlman JE, Kawashima A, Hennessey JG, Siegelman SS (1993) Detection of focal hepatic lesions with spiral CT: comparison of 4- and 8- mm interscan spacing. AJR Am J Roentgenol 160:783-785

Van Hoe L, Van Cutsem E, Vergote I, Baert AL, Bellon E, Dupont P, Marchal G (1997) Size quantification of liver metastases in patients undergoing cancer treatment: reproducibility of one-, two-, and three-dimensional measurements determined with spiral CT. Radiology 202:671-675

Van Leeuwen MS, Noordzij J, Feldberg MA, Hennipman AH, Doornewaard H (1996) Focal liver lesions: characterization with triphasic spiral CT. Radiology 201:327-336

Van Ooijen B, Oudkerk M, Schmitz PIM, Wiggers T (1996) Detection of liver metastases from colorectal carcinoma: is there a place for routine computed tomography arteriography? Surgery 119:511-516

Weiss L, Grundmann E, Torhorst J, et al. (1986) Haematogenous metastatic patterns in colonic carcinoma: an analysis of 1541 necropsies. J Pathol 150:195-203

Wilkes RA (1973) Secondary tumours of the liver, 3rd edn. Butterworths, London, pp 175-183

Winter TC III, Freeny PC, Nghiem HV, et al. (1995) Hepatic arterial anatomy in transplantation candidates: evaluation with three-dimensional CT arteriography. Radiology 195:363-370

Zeman RK, Fox SH, Silverman PM, et al. (1993) Helical (spiral) CT of the abdomen. AJR Am J Roentgenol 160:719-725

7 Hemangioma

F. Terrier, L. Rubbia-Brandt, L. Spadola, N. Howarth

CONTENTS

7.1   Introduction 85
7.2   Macroscopic and Microscopic Pathology 86
7.3   Double-phase CT 87
7.4   CT Features of Liver Hemangiomas 88
7.4.1   Atypical Hemangiomas 90
7.4.2   Why "Atypical Hemangioma" Is a Misnomer 93
7.5   Other Imaging Modalities 96
7.6   Conclusions 96
        References 96

7.1
Introduction

Hemangiomas are benign vascular tumors of the liver of unknown etiology. According to literature reports on autopsy series, their prevalence may be as high as 20% in adults (Karhunen 1986). They can be multiple in up to 10%. There is a female predominance (F-to-M ratio 5–6 :1).

Liver hemangiomas are usually asymptomatic and do not cause any morbidity. Only in a few patients (less than 1%) can so-called giant hemangiomas (larger than 4–6 cm) produce symptoms sufficiently severe to require treatment, usually surgical resection, although embolization may be an alternative (Choi et al. 1989; Graham et al. 1993; Soyer and Levesque 1995; Weimann et al. 1997). Symptoms are abdominal pain, nausea, or vomiting, a palpable mass, cardiac failure, coagulopathy, or hemoperitoneum due to rupture (Scribano et al. 1996; Iqbal

F. Terrier, MD; Department of Radiology, University Hospital of Geneva, CH-1211 Geneva 14, Switzerland
L. Rubbia-Brandt, MD; Department of Pathology, CMU, University Hospital of Geneva, CH-1211 Geneva 4, Switzerland – (Section 7.2)
L. Spadola, MD; Department of Radiology, University Hospital of Geneva, CH-1211 Geneva 14, Switzerland
N. Howarth; Department of Radiology, University Hospital of Geneva, CH-1211 Geneva 14, Switzerland

and Saleem 1997). Occasionally, liver hemangiomas enlarge considerably over time (Takayasu et al. 1990; Nghiem et al. 1997). In such cases, estrogen has been suggested as a possible factor, because growth has been observed in association with exogenous administration of estrogens (Morley et al. 1974) and during pregnancy (Fouchard et al. 1994). However, in other cases there is little supportive evidence for sex hormone involvement.

In the vast majority of patients, the clinical significance of liver hemangiomas arises not because of the symptoms they produce, but due to the diagnostic challenge they represent. As a very frequent incidental finding on routine imaging studies of the abdomen, they have to be distinguished from other benign and malignant liver tumors, especially metastases. Small hemangiomas are particularly troublesome. The high sensitivity achieved with spiral CT for detection of small liver nodules has created the new problem of characterizing lesions that are too small to exhibit distinctive morphologic features (Hollett et al. 1995; Jones et al. 1992; Schwartz et al. 1999). Ferrucci (1990) has referred to these tiny lesions as "nuisance nodules." In fact, with the advent of spiral CT of the liver, we now encounter the same problems as those we have been facing for some time already with chest CT. Thanks to the exquisite resolution obtained in CT imaging of the lung parenchyma, small peripheral nodules a few millimeters in size are frequently detected. In a given patient, it is often impossible to decide with certainty whether these are benign lesions, such as granulomas, or malignant lesions, such as metastases. This is of concern, particularly in a patient with a known malignancy, because the presence or absence of lung metastases may be crucial in the choice of appropriate therapy. In the liver, tiny cysts and small hemangiomas rather than granulomas most frequently cause differential diagnostic dilemmas. One further aspect to consider is that percutaneous biopsy of small lesions is difficult in both the lung and the liver, with a low yield for cytologic or histologic diagnosis.

Despite the fact that liver nodules of less than 1 cm, even in oncologic patients, are frequently benign on a statistical basis (in 51% and 80.2% according to JONES et al. 1992 and SCHWARTZ et al. 1999, respectively), in an individual patient management has to rely on a clear-cut diagnosis. In this chapter, we review the features of hemangiomas on spiral CT, emphasizing those that allow a definite diagnosis, and explain why small hemangiomas may lack these features in a relatively large proportion of cases. The further work-up of such small hemangiomas will also be briefly discussed.

7.2
Macroscopic and Microscopic Pathology

Hemangiomas are one of the most common soft tissue tumors (7% of all benign tumors). The majority are superficial lesions that have a predilection for the head and neck region, but they may also occur in organs, notably in the liver.

Hepatic hemangiomas occur in both sexes and at all ages. They range in size from a few millimeters to up to 20 cm. Most are solitary and visible from the external surface. A few are pedunculated or multiple (ELLIS et al. 1985). Multiple diffuse small hepatic hemangiomas are usually part of the involvement of multiple organs (such as bone, lung) occurring in diffuse systemic hemangiomatosis.

According to pathological criteria, hepatic hemangiomas in adults are usually of the cavernous type and most often occur on an otherwise normal liver.

Macroscopically, cavernous hemangiomas are bright red and have a spongy cut surface, which may partially collapse on sectioning. Their margins are usually well circumscribed but without evidence of a capsule. Occasionally, vascular extensions penetrate irregularly into the adjacent parenchyma. Large cavernous hemangiomas may have areas of dense fibrosis or calcification (Fig. 7.1).

Microscopically, cavernous hemangiomas are composed of vascular channels lined by a single layer of flat endothelial cells on thin, fibrous stroma (Fig. 7.2). The blood-filled spaces vary in size and may contain recent or old thrombi (Fig. 7.3). The stroma is poorly cellular and occasionally has a myxoid appearance. Major blood vessels, often corresponding to arterial branches, may be identified in larger septa.

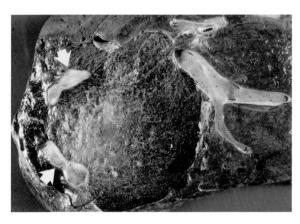

Fig. 7.1. In macroscopic appearance, this cavernous hemangioma of the right hepatic lobe corresponds to a red hemorrhagic mass approximately 8 cm in diameter on the undersurface of an otherwise normal liver. The margins are slightly irregular. Areas of fibrosis are present within the tumor (*arrows*)

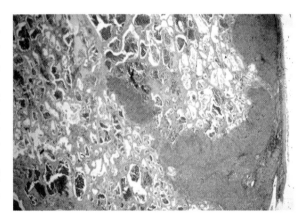

Fig. 7.2. Microscopically, cavernous spaces of this subcapsular hepatic hemangioma are of various sizes and filled with blood. Margins with the surrounding liver are irregular

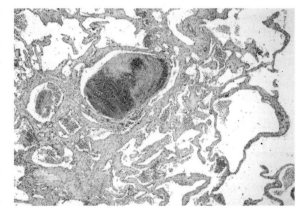

Fig. 7.3. A higher magnification of the hemangioma in Fig. 7.2 illustrates the vascular walls made of a single layer of flat endothelial cells underlined by fine, occasionally hyalinized, stroma. Two vascular spaces contain recent thrombi

The natural history of these lesions is variable. Cavernous hemangiomas essentially show no tendency to regress and may even be locally destructive by virtue of the pressure they exert on neighboring tissue. Nevertheless, they possess a limited growth potential and most hemangiomas remain stable. Moreover, there is no evidence that they undergo malignant transformation.

Occasionally they can undergo thrombosis and progressive fibrosis. Dystrophic calcifications may develop within organizing thrombi. Occasionally large cavernous hemangiomas may produce platelet sequestration with consumption coagulopathy (Kasabach-Meritt syndrome).

Focal involution occurs more often in large cavernous hemangiomas and may be accompanied by tissue necrosis. Entirely sclerosed cavernous hemangiomas are nevertheless rare, corresponding usually to small hemangiomas. They result from complete occlusion of the vascular space and appear as solitary fibrous nodules. Multiple sections and special stains are then necessary to identify vascular outlines within the fibrous stroma and to determine the vascular origin (Fig. 7.4).

From the pathological point of view, differential diagnosis of hemorrhagic vascular lesions may include angiosarcoma and Kaposi's sarcoma, peliosis hepatitis and, possibly, hereditary hemorrhagic telangiectasia. The presence of pleomorphic lining cells with large atypical nuclei, mitosis and imaging of parenchymal and large vein invasions indicate angiosarcoma. Kaposi's sarcoma with hepatic involvement usually occurs in patients with acquired immune deficiency syndrome (AIDS). The lesions are usually confined to portal areas and composed of atypical spindle cells and few vascular spaces.

Hereditary hemorrhagic telangiectasia, also called Osler-Weber-Rendu disease, is an inherited condition with multiple organ involvement by hemangiomatous lesions that also affect the liver. Hepatic involvement is rare and, if present, is diffuse; there are no isolated focal, vascular lesions as there usually are in cavernous hemangiomas. Nevertheless, lesions that are histologically similar to cavernous hemangiomas may be present. The dilated vascular channels lack the supporting stroma found in cavernous hemangiomas, however.

Finally, peliosis hepatitis is the presence of multiple, small (less than 5–10 mm in diameter) dilated blood-filled cavities that are not necessarily lined with endothelium, but occasionally directly with hepatocytes. There is no supporting stroma such as is noted in hemangiomas. Peliosis hepatitis occurs in

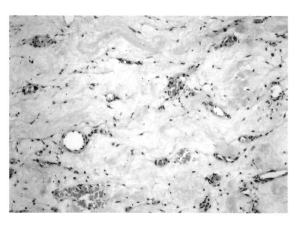

Fig. 7.4. A high magnification of this sclerosed cavernous hemangioma shows abundant fibrosis, containing a few scattered residues of small vascular channels

association with a wide variety of conditions, including drug-induced pathologies, malignancy, and chronic infections, and it is a reversible lesion.

7.3
Double-phase CT

The concept of double-phase CT is based on the following facts:

The liver has a double blood supply, 20–25% from the hepatic artery and 75–80% from the portal vein.

- On injection of contrast medium into a peripheral vein, enhancement of the hepatic artery (hepatic-arterial phase) occurs first, followed by enhancement of the portal vein (portal-venous phase) because blood has a longer circulation time in the splenic and superior mesenteric artery than in the hepatic artery before it reaches the liver.

- Liver tumors have an exclusively or predominantly arterial blood supply. Hypervascular tumors contain more arteries, hypovascular tumors, fewer arteries per unit volume than liver parenchyma.

Contrast medium injection directly into the hepatic artery allows selective enhancement of the liver in the hepatic-arterial phase (CT hepatic arteriography, CTHA). Contrast medium injection directly into the splenic or superior mesenteric artery allows selective enhancement of the liver in the portal-venous phase (CT arterial portography, CTAP). Using

CTHA, the conspicuity (i.e. the difference between tumor enhancement and liver parenchymal enhancement) of hypervascular tumors is increased. Using CTAP, the conspicuity of both hyper- and hypovascular tumors is increased. Hypervascular tumors appear as hyperattenuating nodules on CTHA, whereas hyper- and hypovascular tumors both appear as hypoattenuating nodules on CTAP. In order to achieve a similar result noninvasively, with contrast medium injected into a peripheral vein instead of selectively into a visceral artery, it is possible to take advantage of the lag time between the two phases, that is to say, to obtain a first set of images during the hepatic-arterial phase, when the hepatic-arterial perfusion predominates (within 44 s after initiation of contrast medium injection according to Frederick et al. (1996), followed by a second set of images during the portal-venous phase, when the portal-venous perfusion predominates. This is the rationale behind double-phase CT (Oliver and Baron 1996). However, there are several problems with this approach:

1. Scanning must be fast enough to ensure coverage of the entire liver volume within the hepatic-arterial phase.

2. The contrast medium bolus must be quite compact, so that a sufficient amount of contrast medium reaches the liver during the hepatic-arterial phase before the portal-venous phase.

3. As opposed to CTAP, in which no contrast medium reaches the liver via the hepatic artery, so that even hypervascular tumors appear hypoattenuating, on double-phase CT a hypervascular tumor enhances rapidly during the hepatic-arterial phase. As a consequence, it can still be sufficiently loaded with contrast medium in the following portal-venous phase to appear as hyperattenuating or, as would be more troublesome, as isoattenuating, thus becoming invisible.

4. For any given tumor in the liver, in each phase data are acquired at only one single time point, whereas contrast medium flow through the liver is a continuously changing and dynamic process.

The first two problems have been discussed in detail elsewhere in this book as well as in the literature (Frederick et al. 1996). In practical terms, double-phase CT has greatly benefited from spiral technology, which allows fast scanning. The solution to the third problem is also fast scanning, in order to be able to image the entire liver in the hepatic-arterial phase. Concerning the fourth problem, it must be appreciated that the definition of the two phases is arbitrary. They overlap, and of course there is no clear-cut transition in time from one to the other. This is reflected by the fact that the literature contains no definite rules on the optimal imaging protocol for double-phase spiral CT (Bonaldi et al. 1995). In addition, it is conceivable that for a particular tumor the enhancement pattern during one of the predefined phases is not necessarily constant and that it may matter whether the tumor is imaged at the beginning, the middle, or the end of a particular phase. Scanning of the entire liver is not instantaneous but has to proceed from the top to the bottom of the liver (or inversely). The appearance of a tumor on a double-phase CT may therefore depend on its location in the liver, which determines whether the tumor is imaged at the beginning, middle or the end of the hepatic-arterial phase (or portal-venous phase). As we will see, this remark is particularly pertinent to the imaging of hemangiomas.

In the very near future, multi-array detector CT could offer an ideal solution for some of the aforementioned problems.

7.4
CT Features of Liver Hemangiomas

On native CT images, hemangiomas present most commonly as a hypoattenuating mass, with density values similar to those measured in the lumen of the major abdominal blood vessels, such as the inferior vena cava or the aorta. They are less well defined and less hypodense than liver cysts (Fig. 7.5). In large hemangiomas the border is frequently lobulated, whereas small hemangiomas simply consist of rounded lesions. Rarely, dystrophic calcifications within areas of thrombosis and scarring or phleboliths are found, mostly in large hemangiomas (MITSUDO et al. 1995). Large cystic cavities have also been observed (HIHARA et al. 1990).

Double-phase spiral CT is helpful in distinguishing hemangiomas from other hepatic lesions (HANAFUSA et al. 1995). During the hepatic-arterial phase, strong peripheral enhancement is typically observed (Fig. 7.6). A finding of dense globular enhancement, which is isodense to that of the aorta, is a very specific and the most reliable sign of hemangiomas (GAA et al. 1991; QUINN and BENJAMIN 1992; LESLIE et al. 1995). Globular enhancement is defined when enhancing nodules less than 1 cm in diameter are seen within the lesion. In analysis of the latter it is particularly important to look at its border, which

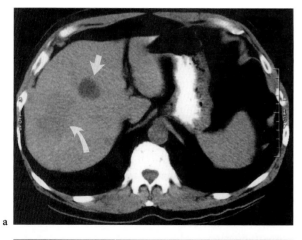

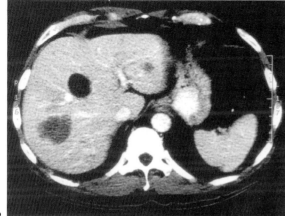

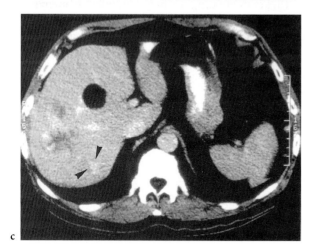

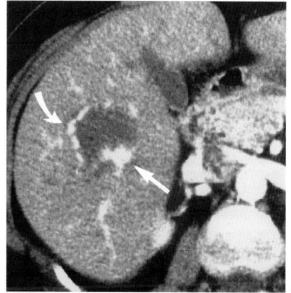

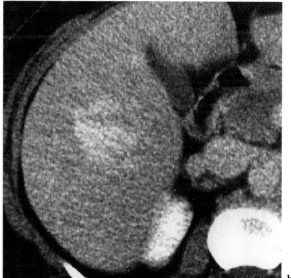

Fig. 7.6a, b. Typical enhancement pattern of an hemangioma. **a** Hepatic-arterial phase: globular enhancement (*arrow*). A feeding artery (*curved arrow*) is seen at the border of the hemangioma. Note that some portions of the lesion border are free from enhancement (no ring enhancement). **b** Late phase: the hemangioma is hyperattenuating

Fig. 7.5a–c. Liver hemangioma and cyst. **a** Native scan. The measured density of the cyst (*arrow*) was 7±12 HU, that of the hemangioma (*curved arrowheads*), 46±12 HU. Typically, the border of the hemangioma is less well defined than that of the cyst. **b** Scan in the portal-venous phase: globular enhancement is not yet obvious. **c** Scan performed 4 min after that shown in b: globular enhancement with almost complete filling-in is now seen. A second small hemangioma (*arrowheads*) is detected

should show areas without any enhancement in the early phase next to the globular areas of strong enhancement. This type of enhancement must be differentiated from ring (or rim) enhancement, which is continuous enhancement at the periphery of the lesion and is a strong argument against a hemangioma! (Fig. 7.7). In one study (LESLIE et al. 1995), globular enhancement was observed in 67% of a series of 54 hemangiomas and in none of the me-

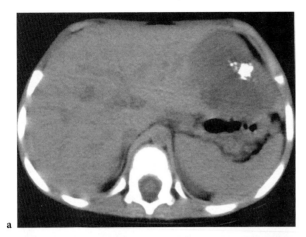

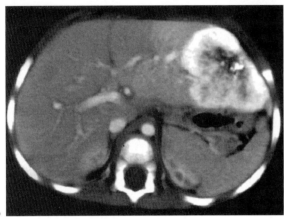

Fig. 7.7a, b. Malignant hemangio-endothelioma. **a** Native scan: mass in the left liver lobe with central calcification. **b** Postcontrast scan: ring enhancement

On delayed images, the contrast agent diffuses into the large blood-filled lakes, so that the enhancing globules coalesce centrally, yielding a centripetal pattern of enhancement. Finally, depending on the size of the hemangioma, the latter becomes isodense with the surrounding liver parenchyma (so called filling-in). The filling-in phenomenon is no longer considered a hallmark of hemangiomas, because it is also observed in the case of malignant neoplasms, owing to delayed interstitial diffusion of contrast medium from the well-vascularized periphery of the tumor into its hypovascularized center (ITO et al. 1992). In large hemangiomas, central areas of hemorrhage, thrombosis or scarring may remain hypoattenuating.

7.4.1
Atypical Hemangiomas

With the advent of spiral CT more small hemangiomas are detected, whose behavior often differs from the characteristic enhancing pattern described above. They are called atypical hemangiomas, and there are two main types, distinguished by the findings in the hepatic-arterial phase:

1. Hemangiomas with instantaneous and strong homogeneous rather than globular enhancement (hyperattenuating or "hypervascular" hemangiomas);
2. Hemangiomas with slow and faint enhancement (hypoattenuating hemangiomas).

7.4.1.1
Hyperattenuating or Hypervascular Hemangiomas

In a study performed on a series of 51 hemangiomas with two-phase dynamic incremental CT (30- to 71-s and 96- to 137-s phase), Hanafusa et al. (1997) found a considerable proportion of atypical hemangiomas (22%), which changed from hyper- to isoattenuation (14%) or showed persistent low attenuation during both phases (8%). Out of 15 hemangiomas that had homogeneous high attenuation in the early phase, 8 still had hyperattenuation, whereas 7 had isoattenuation in the late phase. None had low attenuation, a fact that it is important to stress, as we will see below.

Furthermore, early parenchymal enhancement adjacent and peripheral to the lesion (interpreted as indicating the presence of arterio-portal shunt) (Fig. 7.8), was observed in 12 hemangiomas, and early

tastases (n=47) imaged (sensitivity of 67% and specificity of 100%). In giant hemangiomas, enhancement may be nonperipheral and flame-shaped instead of globular.

The globular areas of strong enhancement consist of vascular spaces directly supplied by arteries; their attenuation should therefore theoretically be identical to that of the aorta, which was discussed and observed by LESLIE et al. (1995). Conversely, QUINN and BENJAMIN (1992) found that the qualitative attenuation of hemangiomas globules was similar to that of the adjacent hepatic and portal veins but lower than that of the aorta. This can be explained by too long a delay between contrast medium injection and imaging as a consequence of technical limitations (this study was performed before the advent of spiral CT). Thus, the hemangiomas were not imaged in the true hepatic-arterial phase but when the portal-venous phase was already starting.

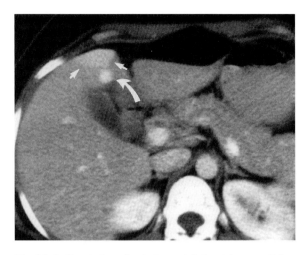

Fig. 7.8. Indirect sign of arterio-portal shunt in a small hemangioma. In the periphery of a homogeneously hyperattenuating nodule (*curved arrow*) of segment IV, there is a wedge-shaped area of increased attenuation (*small arrows*), reflecting early parenchymal enhancement as a consequence of arterio-portal shunt

opacification of portal branches, in 5 of the 12. At angiography, arterio-portal shunt was demonstrated in 10 of the 12.

The subset of hemangiomas, which demonstrate rapid diffuse enhancement during the hepatic-arterial phase of scanning, has also been identified on contrast-enhanced MR imaging (SEMELKA et al. 1994; OUTWATER et al. 1997).

The difference in enhancement pattern between hemangiomas with strong peripheral globular enhancement and those with instantaneous homogeneous enhancement reflects differences in the spread of contrast material within the lesion. It is not surprising that hemangiomas showing the latter pattern are small, because the smaller the lesion, the more rapid the spread of contrast material within the lesion (Fig. 7.9).

Hyperattenuating hemangiomas of this type, which show an homogeneous enhancement in the hepatic-arterial phase, have to be differentiated from other hypervascular liver tumors, such as hepatocellular adenoma or carcinoma, focal nodular hyperplasia and some metastases (VAN HOE et al. 1997) (Fig. 7.10). An important clue for the differential diagnosis is the fact that hypervascular liver tumors are frequently (but not always) hypoattenuating in the portal-venous phase, as a consequence of the rapid contrast medium wash-out, whereas hyperattenuating hemangiomas are either still hyperattenuating or isoattenuating, but not hypoattenuating, because of their sluggish blood circula-

tion (HANAFUSA et al. 1997). However, small hypervascular tumors (especially small hepatocellular carcinomas), which remain hyper- or isoattenuating in the portal-venous phase, may be very difficult to distinguish from hypervascular hemangiomas. Because immediate and persistent homogeneous enhancement is the most frequent pattern in small hemangiomas, persistent hyperattenuation in the portal-venous phase is fairly common in this type of hemangiomas, whereas larger hemangiomas with globular enhancement still show hypoattenuating regions in their center, owing to slow filling-in (Fig. 7.11). Arterio-portal shunts have generally been recognized as characteristic of malignant tumors. Whereas such shunts tend to occur in large hepatocellular carcinomas, the aforementioned study has shown that they also frequently occur in hemangiomas, in contrast to hepatocellular carcinomas, especially small ones (HANAFUSA et al. 1997). In larger hemangiomas arterio-portal shunts have also been observed, giving rise to a differential diagnostic problem with hepatocellular carcinomas (WINOGRAD and PALUBINSKA 1977; SHIMADA et al. 1994).

7.4.1.2
Hypoattenuating Hemangiomas

Small hemangiomas that show hypoattenuation during both the hepatic-arterial phase and the portal-venous phase represent another, less frequent, type of atypical hemangiomas. In a series of 377 hemangiomas (in 249 consecutive patients), JANG et al. (1998) found 30 (9%) hemangiomas with such a behavior. All these hemangiomas were less than 2 cm in diameter. These authors described a new useful sign for the diagnosis of atypical small hemangiomas, namely the appearance of a tiny enhancing dot within the hemangioma, which they called the "bright dot sign" (Fig. 7.12). In the aforementioned study, the tiny enhancing dots were as bright as the portal vein during the portal-venous phase in 77%. However, during the hepatic-arterial phase they were less bright than the hepatic arteries in 55%. A partial-volume averaging effect due to the small size of the dots might have affected the results. Nevertheless, most of the dots were relatively bright for their small size, a reliable indication of vascular spaces. Therefore, the "bright dot" most probably corresponds to the "miniature" form of the globular enhancement. It reflects the small size and the propensity for slow filling-in of this particular type of hemangioma.

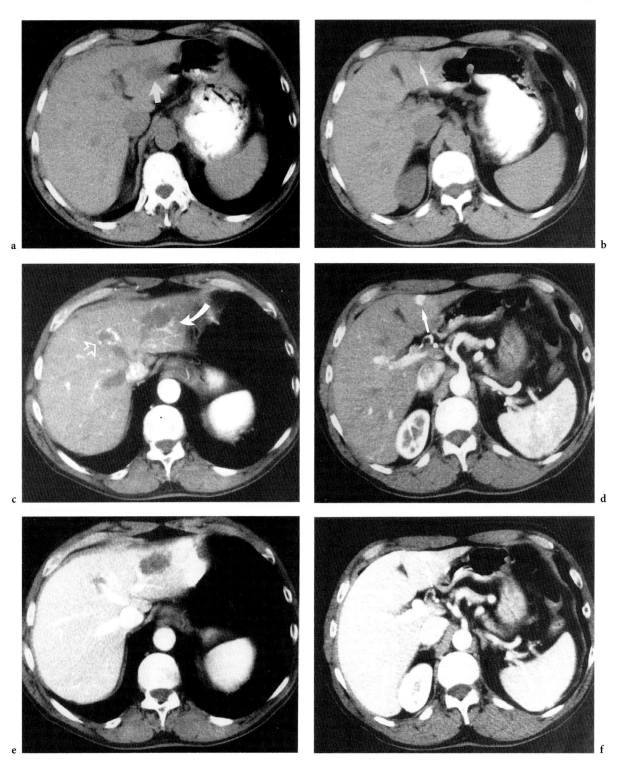

Fig. 7.9a–h. Different enhancement patterns of hemangiomas in the same patient depending on their size. **a, b** Native scans: two hypoattenuating lesions are seen in the left liver lobe, one measuring 2 cm (*large arrow*) and the other, 5 mm (*small arrow*). **c, d** In the hepatic arterial phase, the larger lesion shows faint globular enhancement (*curved arrow*), whereas the smaller one (*small arrow*) is homogeneously enhanced. There is a third typical hemangioma (*open arrow*) in segment 4, presenting globular enhancement. **e, f** In the portal-venous phase (1 min after c and d, the two larger hemangiomas are still hypoattenuating, whereas the smaller lesion is still hyperattenuating (*small arrow*). **g, h** On late images (10 min after **e** and **f**), all the hemangiomas are isoattenuating and no longer visible

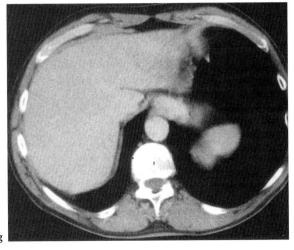
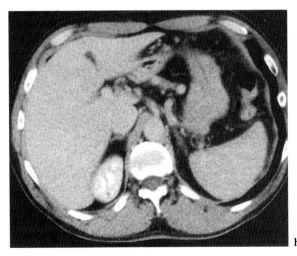

g   h

Fig. 7.9. Continued

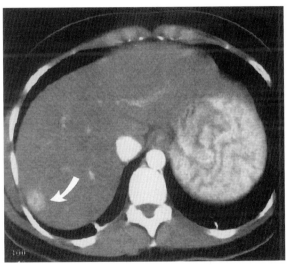
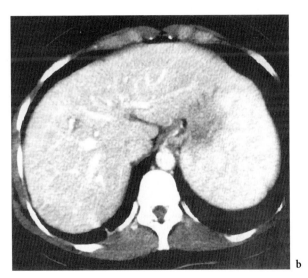

a   b

Fig. 7.10a, b. Small hepatocellular carcinoma in a patient with liver cirrhosis. **a** Hepatic arterial phase: homogeneously enhancing nodule (*curved arrow*) in segment VII. **b** Portal-venous phase: the lesion is isoattenuating and no longer visible

Sporadically, nonenhancing hemangiomas have been reported. At histology, hyalinization of the entire hemangioma has been described (TAKAYASU et al. 1986).

7.4.2
Why "Atypical Hemangioma" Is a Misnomer

The appearance of hemangiomas on spiral CT after intravenous bolus injection of contrast medium depends on several factors, including:
1. Factors related to the imaging protocol, the most important ones being the amount, iodine concentration and injection rate of the contrast medium and the delay after injection before the hemangioma is imaged.
2. Factors related to the angioarchitecture of the hemangioma.

The hemangioma is a vascular tumor consisting of interconnected vascular spaces supplied by arterial branches entering into some of the vascular spaces at the periphery of the hemangioma. During the hepatic-arterial phase, the spaces directly fed by the arterial branches enhance first and vividly. From there, the contrast medium diffuses into the remaining volume of the hemangioma from the periphery

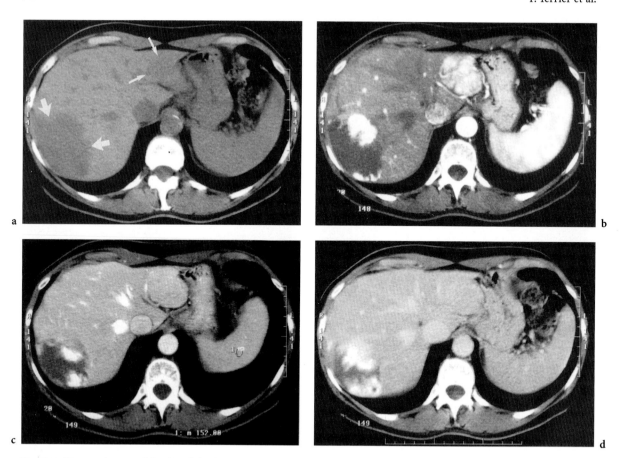

Fig. 7.11. Hemangioma and focal nodular hyperplasia (FNH). a Native scan: a large lobulated hypoattenuating lesion is seen in segment VII (*large arrows*). Another lesion (*small arrows*) bulging over the liver surface is scarcely recognized in the left liver lobe. b In the hepatic-arterial phase, the lesion in the right liver lobe show the typical globular enhancement (same density as the aorta) of an hemangioma. The lesion (FNH) in the left liver lobe shows immediate complete enhancement, albeit less dense than that of the aorta. A nodular pattern as well as feeding arteries penetrating into the nodule are recognized. c In the portal-venous phase (1 min after b), there is still globular enhancement of the hemangioma and incomplete filling-in, whereas the FNH is already almost isoattenuating compared with the liver. d In the late phase (3 min after c), the enhancement of the hemangioma has slowly progressed. The FNH is no longer recognizable

toward the center (filling-in phenomenon) (Fig. 7.13). The rate at which this occurs depends on the turnover of blood within the hemangioma. This turnover most probably varies greatly from one hemangioma to another, depending of course on the size of the hemangioma, but also and certainly more importantly, on the ratio between arterial supply and size of the hemangioma. In other words, if the total arterial flow to the hemangioma (depending on the number of arterial branches entering into the hemangioma and their diameter) is low in relation to the size of the hemangioma, the filling-in of the hemangioma with contrast medium will be sluggish. On the other hand, if the arterial flow is high, the filling-in will be rapid. To the best of our knowledge, this hypothesis of variation in relative arterial flow to the hemangiomas has not been verified. The size

of the individual spaces within the hemangioma should be of less importance on the rate at which the hemangioma is filled-in by contrast medium.

In fact, the term atypical hemangioma is a misnomer. In the past it has been used for large hemangiomas lacking complete filling-in by contrast medium on delayed images, because of central thrombosis or scarring (TAKAYASU et al. 1986). Today, it most frequently means that the only pathognomonic sign of hemangiomas on CT, namely the globular enhancement in the hepatic-arterial phase, is missing. However, this is most probably not because the hemangioma is atypical, but because of technical limitations, either because the hemangioma is too small and globular enhancement (or the bright dot) is not detected, or because the hemangioma is not imaged with optimal delay after the contrast medium injec-

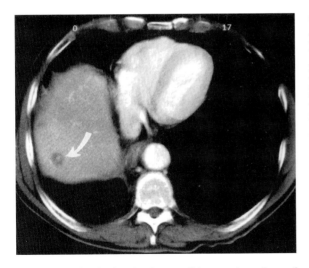

Fig. 7.12. The bright dot sign in a small hemangioma (*curved arrow*) imaged in the hepatic-arterial phase

tion. Thus, the appearance of hemangioma may depend on whether it is located cranially or caudally in the liver and in which direction scanning is performed (Fig. 7.14). If timing is not adequate, the hyperattenuation of globular enhancement may have already faded, for example, without complete filling-in yet having been achieved. Thus, the hemangioma appears as a hypointense lesion with an irregular border, which is very similar to a metastasis. Such a situation, which is particularly troublesome in an oncologic patient, occurs frequently when combined chest and abdominal scanning is performed (Fig. 7.15). Beginning the study at the liver with double-phase CT, before proceeding to the chest, is a way to avoid confusion.

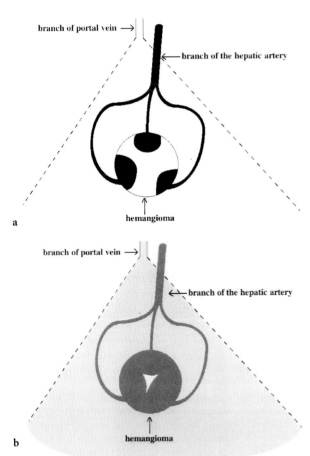

Fig. 13a, b. Contrast enhancement of a hemangioma. a Hepatic-arterial phase showing globular enhancement of the hemangioma, due to contrast medium flowing into vascular spaces. b Portal-venous phase, with progressive filling-in of the hemangioma

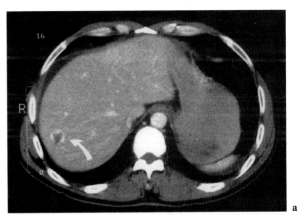

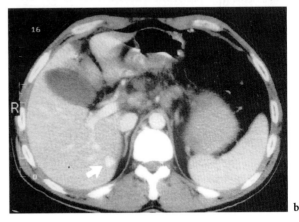

Fig. 14a, b. Different enhancement patterns of hemangiomas depending on their cranio-caudal location in the liver. Scanning is performed cranio-caudally. a A small hemangioma (*curved arrow*) in segment VII (cranial) imaged in the early hepatic-arterial phase shows characteristic globular enhancement. b A second hemangioma (*arrow*) in segment VI, of about the same size as the one in segment VII, was imaged later during the same sequence and appears homogeneously enhanced

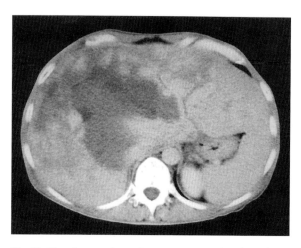

Fig. 15. Giant hemangioma. Postcontrast scan in a late phase. The appearance is worrying and could easily be confused with a malignant necrotic tumor

7.5
Other Imaging Modalities

The features of hemangiomas on other imaging modalities have been well described. Angiography has a typical appearance, but is seldom performed as a diagnostic procedure.

At ultrasonography the appearance may be very variable, a hyperechoic lesion being the most frequent finding, but this appearance is not specific.

Radiolabelled red-blood cell scintigraphy is a very specific modality (BIRNBAUM et al. 1990; DWIGHT and OATES 1994). However, its sensitivity is low, and owing to poor spatial resolution, only quite large hemangiomas can be confidently detected (>1.5–2 cm). This technique should not be used for the characterization of small hepatic lesions.

Magnetic resonance (MR) imaging is currently the best technique for the characterization of liver tumors, including hemangiomas. The appearance of the latter on native MR images, especially on T2-weighted images (high, water-like signal intensity) is typical but not pathognomonic. Therefore, the use of contrast medium is considered mandatory for MR imaging of the liver, both for detection and for characterization of the lesions. The pharmacodynamics of nonspecific gadolinium chelates is the same as that of iodinated contrast media. However, because of the inherent greater contrast sensitivity and the more compact shape of the contrast medium bolus, thanks to the relatively small amount injected, enhancement is more conspicuous and occurs faster in dynamic MR imaging than in spiral CT. Therefore

globular enhancement is better demonstrated with the former.

Beside nonspecific contrast media, several hepato-specific contrast media (gadolinium–Bopta, gadolinium–EOB–DTPA, manganese–DPDP, superparamagnetic iron oxide particles) have been developed. At present there is no consensus as to which contrast medium is the most appropriate for liver imaging.

However, with superparamagnetic iron oxide particles (SPIO), hemangiomas show a characteristic positive enhancement on T1-weighted images (T1 effect), which is very useful for differentiating them from other tumors, such as metastases or hepatocellular carcinomas (GRANGIER et al. 1994).

7.6
Conclusion

Double-spiral acquisition has increased the sensitivity of CT for detecting focal liver lesions. However, characterization of small lesions is often difficult and is one of the major daily problems encountered in liver imaging. On the other hand, the characterization of hemangiomas larger than 1.5–2 cm is very well performed with double-spiral CT, so that no other modality is needed. We consider this technique, in view of its availability, a good choice for reaching a definite diagnosis following discovery of an atypical lesion on ultrasonography. For smaller lesions, MR imaging is more appropriate. The choice of MR contrast medium is still a matter of debate. We favor SPIO particles.

Acknowledgements. The authors thank Mr. Orlando Domingos for the photographic work, Chantal Derenel for typing the manuscript, and Catherine Tairraz for the drawings.

References

Birnbaum BA, Weinreb JC, Megibow AJ, Sanger JJ, Lubat E, Kanamuller H, Noz ME, Bosniak MA (1990) Definitive diagnosis of hepatic hemangiomas: MR imaging versus Tc-99m-labeled red blood cell SPECT. Radiology 176:95–101

Bonaldi VM, Bret PM, Reinhold C, Atri M (1995) Helical CT of the liver: value of an early hepatic arterial phase. Radiology 197:357–363

Choi BI, Han MC, Park JH, Kim SH, Han MH, Kim CW (1989) Giant cavernous hemangioma of the liver: CT and MR imaging in 10 cases. AJR Am J Roentgenol 152:1221–1226

Dwight MA, Oates E (1994) Hepatic hemangioma in cirrhotics with portal hypertension: evaluation with Tc-99 m red blood cell SPECT. Radiology 191:115–117

Ellis JV, Salazar JE, Gavant ML (1985) Pedunculated hepatic hemangioma. An unusual cause for anteriorly displaced retroperitoneal fat. J Ultrasound Med 4:623–624

Ferrucci JT (1990) Liver tumor imaging: current concepts. AJR Am J Roentgenol 155:473–484

Fouchard I, Rosenau L, Calès P, Allory P (1994) Survenue d'hémangiomes hépatiques au cours de la grossesse. Gastroenterol Clin Biol 18:512–515

Frederick MG, McElaney BL, Singer A, Park KS, Paulson EK, McGee SG, Nelson RC (1996) Timing of parenchymal enhancement on dual-phase dynamic helical CT of the liver: how long does the hepatic arterial phase predominates? AJR Am J Roentgenol 166:1305–1310

Gaa J, Saini S, Ferrucci JT (1991) Perfusion characteristics of hepatic cavernous hemangioma using intravenous CT angiography (IVCTA). Eur J Radiol 12:228–233

Graham E, Cohen AW, Soulen M, Faye R (1993) Symptomatic liver hemangioma with intra-tumor hemorrhage treated by angiography and embolization during pregnancy. Obstet Gynecol 81:813–816

Grangier C, Tourniaire J, Mentha G, Schiau R, Howarth N, Chachuat A, Grossholz M, Terrier F (1994) Enhancement of liver hemangiomas on T1-weighted MR SE images by superparamagnetic iron oxide particles. J Comput Assist Tomogr 18:888–896

Hanafusa K, Ohashi I, Himeno Y, Suzuki S, Shibuya H (1995) Hepatic hemangiomas: findings with two-phase CT. Radiology 196:465–469

Hanafusa K, Ohashi I, Gomi N, Himeno Y, Wakita T, Shibuya H (1997) Differential diagnosis of early homogeneously enhancing hepatocellular carcinoma and hemangioma by two-phase CT. J Comput Assist Tomogr 21:361–368

Hihara T, Araki T, Katou K, Odashima H, Ounishi H, Kachi K, Uchiyama G (1990) Cystic cavernous hemangioma of the liver. Gastrointest Radiol 15:112–114

Hollett MD, Jeffrey RB Jr, Nino-Murcia M, Jorgensen MJ, Harris DP (1995) Dual-phase helical CT of the liver: value of arterial phase scans in the detection of small (≤1.5 cm) malignant hepatic neoplasms. AJR Am J Roentgenol 164:879–884

Iqbal N, Saleem A (1997) Hepatic hemangioma: a review. Tex Med 93:48–50

Ito K, Honjo K, Matsumoto T, Tanaka R, Nakada T, Nakanishi T (1992) Distinction of hemangiomas from hepatic tumors with delayed enhancement by incremental dynamic CT. J Comput Assist Tomogr 16:572–577

Jang HJ, Choi BI, Kim TK, Yun EJ, Yun EJ, Kim KW, Han JK, Han MC (1998) Atypical small hemangiomas of the liver: «bright dot» sign at two-phase spiral CT. Radiology 208:543–548

Jones EC, Chezmar JL, Nelson RC, Bernardino ME (1992) The frequency and significance of small (≤15 mm) hepatic lesions detected by CT. AJR Am J Roentgenol 158:535–539

Karhunen PJ (1986) Benign hepatic tumours and tumour like conditions in men. J Clin Pathol 39:183–188

Leslie DJ, Johnson CD, Johnson CM, Ilstrup DM, Harmsen WS (1995) Distinction between cavernous haemangioma of the liver and hepatic metastases on CT: value of contrast enhancement patterns. AJR Am J Roentgenol 164:625–629

Mitsudo K, Watanabe Y, Saga T, Dohke M, Sato N, Minami K, Shigeyasu M (1995) Nonenhanced hepatic cavernous hemangioma with multiple calcifications: CT and pathologic correlation. Abdom Imaging 20:459–461

Morley JE, Myers JB, Sack FS, Kalk F, Epstein EE, Lannon J (1974) Enlargement of cavernous haemangioma associated with exogenous administration of oestrogens. S Afr Med J 48:695–697

Nghiem HV, Bogost GA, Ryan JA, Lund R, Freeny PC, Rice KM (1997) Cavernous hemangiomas of the liver: enlargement over time. AJR Am J Roentgenol 169:137–140

Oliver JH III, Baron RL (1996) Helical biphasic contrast-enhanced CT of the liver: technique, indications, interpretation, and pitfalls. Radiology 201:1–14

Outwater EK, Ito K, Siegelman E, Martin CE, Bhatia M, Mitchell DG (1997) Rapidly enhancing hepatic hemangiomas at MRI: distinction from malignancies with T2-weighted images. J Magn Reson Imaging 7:1033–1039

Quinn SF, Benjamin GG (1992) Hepatic cavernous hemangiomas: simple diagnostic sign with dynamic bolus CT. Radiology 182:545–548

Schwartz LH, Gandras EJ, Colangelo SM, Ercolani MC, Panicek DM (1999) Prevalence and importance of small hepatic lesions found at CT in patients with cancer. Radiology 210:71–74

Scribano E, Loria G, Ascenti G, Vallone A, Gaeta M (1996) Spontaneous hemoperitoneum from a giant multicystic hemangioma of the liver: a case report. Abdom Imaging 21:418–419

Semelka RC, Brown ED, Ascher SM, Patt RH, Bagley AS, Li W, Edelman RE, Shoenut JP, Brown JJ (1994) Hepatic hemangiomas: a multi-institutional study of appearance on T2-weighted and serial gadolinium-enhanced gradient-echo MR images. Radiology 192:401–406

Shimada M, Matsumata T, Ikeda Y, Urata K, Hayashi H, Shimizu M, Sugimachi K (1994) Multiple hepatic hemangiomas with significant arterioportal venous shunting. Cancer 53:304–307

Soyer P, Levesque M (1995) Haemoperitoneum due to spontaneous rupture of hepatic haemangiomatosis: treatment by superselective arterial embolization and partial hepatectomy. Aust Radiol 39:90–92

Takayasu K, Moriyama N, Shima Y, Muramatsu Y, Yamada T, Makuuchi M, Yamasaki S, Hirohashi S (1986) Atypical radiographic findings in hepatic cavernous hemangioma: correlation with histologic features. AJR Am J Roentgenol 146:1149–1153

Takayasu K, Makuuchi M, Takayama T (1990) Computed tomography of a rapidly growing hepatic hemangioma – case report. J Comput Assist Tomogr 14:143–145

Van Hoe L, Baert AL, Gryspeerdt S, Vandenbosh G, Nevens F, Van Steenbergen W, Marechal G (1997) Dual-phase helical CT of the liver: value of an early-phase acquisition in the differential diagnosis of noncystic focal lesions. AJR Am J Roentgenol 168:1185–1192

Weimann A, Ringe B, Klempnauer J, Lamesch P, Gratz KF, Prokop M, Maschek H, Tusch G, Pichlmayr R (1997) Benign liver tumors: differential diagnosis and indications for surgery. World J Surg 21:983–990

Winograd J, Palubinskas AJ (1977) Arterial-portal venous shunting in cavernous hemangioma of the liver. Radiology 122:331–332

8 Adenoma and Focal Nodular Hyperplasia

V. Vilgrain

CONTENTS

8.1   Introduction 99
8.2   Technical Considerations for the Imaging Protocol
        for Helical CT of Hepatocellular Tumors 99
8.2.1   Vascularity of the Lesions 99
8.2.2   Hepatocellular Origin 100
8.2.3   Contour 100
8.2.4   Multiple Lesions 100
8.3   Focal Nodular Hyperplasia 100
8.3.1   Clinical Background 100
8.3.2   Pathology 100
8.3.3   Helical CT 100
8.3.4   FNH Associated with Other Lesions 103
8.3.5   Follow-up 104
8.4   Hepatocellular Adenoma 104
8.4.1   Clinical Background 104
8.4.2   Pathology 105
8.4.3   Helical CT 105
8.4.4   Adenomas Associated with Other Lesions 107
8.5   Advantages and Pitfalls of Helical CT Compared
        with Other Imaging Modalities 108
8.5.1   Advantages of Helical CT 108
8.5.2   Disadvantages of Helical CT 108
8.6   Impact of CT on the Management of Patients 108
8.7   Conclusion 109
        References 109

8.1
Introduction

Focal nodular hyperplasia (FNH) and hepatocellular adenoma (HA) are among the most common benign hepatic neoplasms encountered in clinical practice. These lesions have some features in common: they arise from the normal hepatocytes; they are often recognized as incidental hepatic masses during imaging for nonspecific symptoms; and they are observed mainly in women in the third to fifth decades of life. However, their pathogenesis and natural history are different (Cherqui et al. 1995). FNH is not

V. Vilgrain, MD; Department of Radiology, Hôpital Beaujon, F-92118 Clichy Cedex, France

directly related to oral contraceptive intake and complications are very rare, whereas HA is often induced by oral contraceptive intake and can have severe complications, such as hemorrhage and malignant transformation. Recognition of these two tumors is crucial, because asymptomatic FNH with typical findings on imaging will not be resected, whereas resection is the treatment of choice for HA. Therefore, the role of noninvasive imaging is essential to differentiate typical FNH from other hepatocellular tumors.

8.2
Technical Considerations for the Imaging Protocol for Helical CT of Hepatocellular Tumors

A chapter in this book is dedicated to the different imaging protocols for helical CT of liver. Therefore, we will merely highlight some specific keys to optimization of the detection and the characterization of benign hepatocellular lesions: vascularity of the lesions, hepatocellular origin, contours, and multiple lesions.

8.2.1
Vascularity of the Lesions

Both FNH and HA are hypervascular lesions and are mainly supplied by the hepatic arteries. Vascularization of the normal liver arises from both the hepatic arteries and the portal vein, but the latter provides the prominent part of the supply (2/3 of the total liver blood flow). Therefore it is essential to study the liver in the arterial phase of contrast enhancement to obtain a high contrast of density between the hypervascular lesions and the normal liver and in the portal phase of contrast enhancement, where the contrast differences between lesions and normal liver are slight.

8.2.2
Hepatocellular Origin

Because both FNH and HA contain mainly normal hepatocytes, contrast between lesions and normal liver is minimal, especially on precontrast CT scans. Visualization of the lesions may require narrow density windows.

8.2.3
Contour

Some HAs may have true peripheral capsules, which are barely seen on precontrast images and at the early phase of contrast enhancement. Delayed contrast enhancement is therefore mandatory to optimize helical CT examination.

8.2.4
Multiple Lesions

Benign hepatocellular tumors are often multiple or associated with other liver lesions. It is essential to make a careful reading of the entire liver at the different acquisitions.

8.3
Focal Nodular Hyperplasia

8.3.1
Clinical Background

FNH accounts for approximately 8% of all primary hepatic tumors and is the second most common benign liver tumor (CRAIG et al. 1989). FNH occurs in both sexes and at all ages and is found most commonly in women (80–95% of cases) in their third and fourth decades of life. Oral contraceptive use is associated with FNH, but the role of oral contraceptives in the occurrence of the lesion has not been demonstrated. They may promote growth and complications (CRAIG et al. 1989). FNH is thought to be a hyperplastic response to increased blood flow in an arterial malformation rather than a true neoplasm (WANLESS et al. 1985). Various vascular abnormalities, such as telangiectases, hereditary hemorrhagic telangiectasia, arteriovenous malformation, and anomalous venous drainage may be associated with it, especially in patients with multiple FNH (HABER et al. 1995). It seems that the FNH-to-HA ratio has changed in the past years. There were nearly equal

numbers of FNHs and HAs before 1985 (CRAIG et al. 1989; CHERQUI et al. 1995). Since 1989, a dramatic increase in the number of patients with FNH has been observed, whereas the number of patients with HA has not changed (CHERQUI et al. 1995). This increase could be caused by a higher detection rate of FNH because of the wider availability and improved quality of US examinations (CHERQUI et al. 1995).

FNH is usually an incidental finding at autopsy, and only one-third of cases are discovered because of clinical symptoms such as mild epigastric pain or discomfort and/or a palpable abdominal mass (CHERQUI et al. 1995).

8.3.2
Pathology

A FNH is a well-circumscribed mass, characterized by a central fibrous scar with surrounding nodules of hyperplastic hepatocytes and small bile ductules. The lesion is usually solitary (80%) and measures less than 5 cm in diameter (CRAIG et al. 1989). Occasionally, a FNH is pedunculated. Macroscopically, the majority of lesions have a central stellate scar, with radiating fibrous septa dividing the lesion into nodules. More rarely, the scar may be absent or located eccentrically (VILGRAIN et al. 1992). The margin is sharp, often lobulated, and no capsule is present (CRAIG et al. 1989). Hemorrhage and necrosis are rare.

Microscopy shows that the central fibrotic zone is dense connective tissue, which contains blood vessels with thick walls. Thick-walled arteries are also seen along the septa extending from the center to the periphery. Marked proliferation of biliary structures surrounded by inflammatory cells is observed within and at the periphery of the fibrous septa. Kupffer cells are also seen within the lesion. Occasionally, fatty change and bile formation may be detected.

In summary, FNH contains all of the components of normal liver but lacks normal hepatic architecture.

8.3.3
Helical CT

8.3.3.1
Typical Findings

On precontrast CT scans, FNH is demonstrated as a focal hypodense or isodense mass. A central hypodense scar is depicted in only one-third of the cases (Fig. 8.1A) (SHAMSI et al. 1993). Calcifications within the central scar are very rare and observed in only about 1% of the cases (CASEIRO-ALVES et al. 1996).

In all the published series, the lesions have most often been hypodense (PROCACCI et al. 1992; SHIRKHODA et al. 1994; MATHIEU et al. 1986). The hypoattenuation of the lesion may be explained by the aberrant architecture of the proliferating hepatocytes. Diffuse lesion hyperdensity developing in a nonfatty liver has never been reported.

Because of the prominent arterial supply to FNH, the lesion enhances rapidly in the arterial phase of contrast-enhanced CT and the lesion-to-liver contrast is high (Fig. 8.1B). The lesion contour is well demarcated and may be lobulated. At that time, the central scar is hypodense and appears more evident than on unenhanced CT scans. Central arteries are easily detected, and visualization of the vessels oc-curs more often than with dynamic incremental CT [22% in the series reported by MATHIEU et al. (1986) versus 80% in the series reported by CHOI and FREENY (1998)] (Fig. 8.1B). Central arteries may be associated with septal arteries and small arteries surrounding the periphery of the lesion. In the portal phase of contrast-enhanced CT, lesion enhancement decreases and the lesion may be either iso- or slightly hyperdense relative to normal liver (Fig. 8.1C). Small FNHs may be barely visible, whereas large FNHs are visualized because of a misshapen liver contour, displacement of adjacent vessels, or depiction of a relatively hypoattenuating central scar (BUETOW et al. 1996). Fibrous septa are more rarely observed than the central scar, and their densitometric features are identical to those of the central scar (Fig. 8.2) (PROCACCI et al. 1992).

On delayed images of the liver obtained at 10–15 min, FNHs are isodense relative to normal liver and, in most cases, central scars appear hyperattenuating

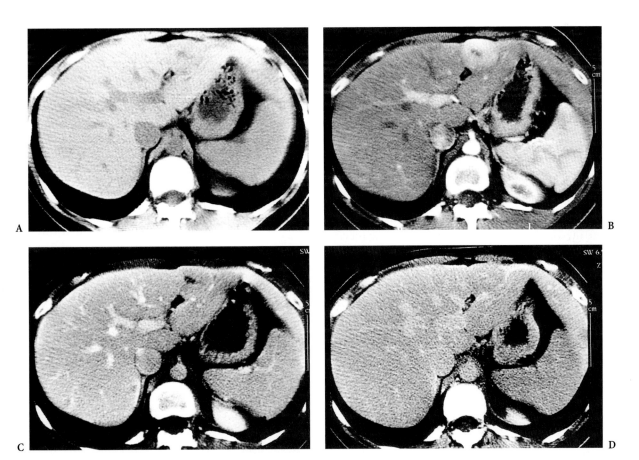

Fig 8.1A–D. Typical focal nodular hyperplasia (FNH). **A** On pre-contrast CT scan the lesion is isodense to the liver. Note the central low attenuation corresponding to the central scar. **B–D** The lesion is hypervascular at the arterial phase (**B**) and a central artery is seen. At the portal phase and on delayed scan, the lesion is isodense to the liver (**C, D**). Note the enhancement of the scar on the delayed scan

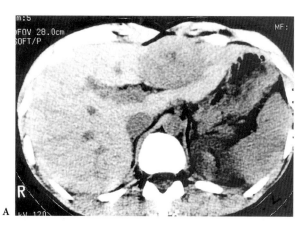

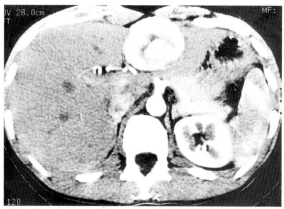

Fig. 8.2A, B. Typical FNH with fibrous septa. **A** On precontrast CT scan the lesion is hypodense relative to the liver and contains a more hypodense scar. The fibrous septa are not visible. **B** In the arterial phase of the contrast medium injection, central scar and fibrous septa are easily detected

owing to delayed washout of contrast material from the myxomatous stroma of the central scar relative to the surrounding hepatocytes (Fig. 1D) (BUETOW et al. 1996).

8.3.3.2
Atypical Findings

8.3.3.2.1
LACK OF CENTRAL SCAR

In earlier reports, central scars were depicted on CT in about 30–40% of FNH cases (MATHIEU et al. 1986; PROCACCI et al. 1992; SHAMSI et al. 1993), whereas in a series studied with triphasic helical CT, scars were seen in more than 80% of cases (CHOI and FREENY 1998). Reasons for a better depiction of the central scar are optimization of the contrast medium protocol and the thin collimation used with helical CT. However, radio-pathologic studies have demon-

strated that even pathological examination reveals no scar in some cases of FNH (Fig. 8.3) (VILGRAIN et al. 1992).

8.3.3.2.2
ATYPICAL SCARS

Occasionally, scars remain hypodense or isodense on delayed scans. This finding is observed in about 20% of cases (CHOI and FREENY 1998).

8.3.3.2.3
LESION ENHANCEMENT

All FNHs are hypervascular at the arterial phase of the enhancement, but lesion enhancement may vary at the portal phase or on delayed images. Hypodensity of the mass may be seen on delayed phase images or on both portal vein and delayed phase images, but hyperdensity of the mass on the portal vein phase or on both portal vein and delayed phase images may also be seen (CHOI and FREENY 1998). There is no known explanation for FNH cases with rapid washout or delayed contrast enhancement.

8.3.3.2.4
CAPSULE-LIKE RIM

Although FNH is a nonencapsulated lesion, capsule-like enhancement may be observed on portal vein and on delayed phase scans in about 25–36% of cases (Fig. 8.4) (PROCACCI et al. 1992; CHOI and FREENY 1998). This finding may also be observed on MR imaging. The distinction between a true capsule and a capsule-like rim can be difficult; however, a capsule-like rim is more irregular and less continuous than a true capsule.

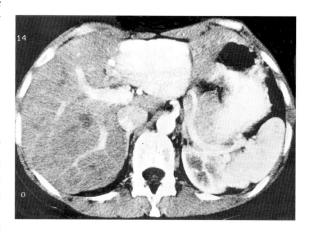

Fig. 8.3. FNH with no scar detected. CT scan in the arterial phase of the contrast medium injection, demonstrating a hypervascular and homogeneous lesion with no central element

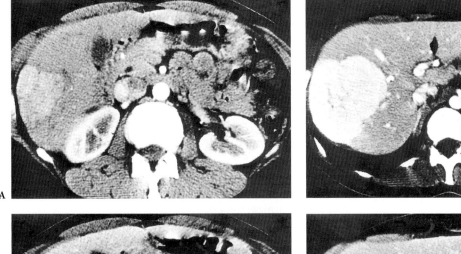

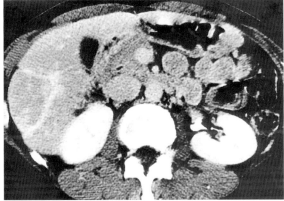

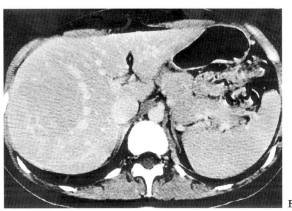

Fig. 8.4A, B. FNH with capsule-like rim. **A** In the arterial phase of the contrast medium injection, the lesion is well delineated. **B** On delayed scan the lesion is surrounded by a hyperdense capsule-like rim

Fig. 8.5A, B. FNH with draining veins. In the arterial phase of the contrast medium injection (**A**) the lesion is homogeneous and lobulated and central arteries are seen. On delayed scans (**B**), the lesion is isodense relative to the liver and draining peripheral veins are observed

8.3.3.2.5
EARLY DRAINING VEINS
Draining veins are commonly observed in malignant neoplasms, particularly hepatocellular carcinoma, but may be also seen in some FNH. They were seen in 3 of the 12 cases in the series of CHOI and FREENY (1998) (Fig. 8.5).

8.3.3.2.6
FNH WITH ADJACENT PARENCHYMAL CHANGES
The hypervascularity of FNH may cause localized prominent arterial supply in the vicinity of the lesion. This finding is observed at the arterial phase of the enhancement and appears as hyperattenuation of normal liver surrounding the lesion. In most such cases, dilatation of a lobar or segmental artery is seen.

Very occasionally, large FNH are responsible for vascular compression (portal vein or hepatic veins)

and transient alterations in the enhancement of normal liver may be detected. These abnormalities are not observed on unenhanced scans or on delayed scans.

FNH with prominent fatty infiltration surrounding the lesion has been reported in one paper (EISENBERG et al. 1995).

8.3.4
FNH Associated with Other Lesions

FNH is mainly a solitary lesion, however multiple lesions are observed in 20–30% of the cases (Fig. 8.6). The ability of helical CT in demonstrating small foci of hypervascularization will perhaps help to recognize multiple FNH more often.

FNH is associated with hepatic hemangiomas and in the study reported by MATHIEU et al. 1989, both

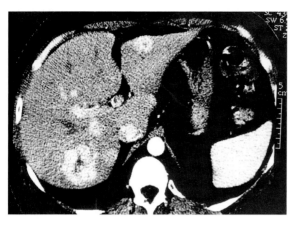

Fig. 8.6. Multiple FNH. Multiple and disseminated hypervascular lesions are seen within the liver. All these lesions correspond to FNH

lesions were seen in 23% the cases. For some authors, multiple FNH are more often associated with hemangiomas than are solitary FNH (WANLESS et al. 1989).

Also, FNH may be associated with other extrahepatic vascular abnormalities (WANLESS et al. 1989). Such association supports the concept that multiple FNHs may occur in a syndromic form and are induced by an irregular arterial supply in the liver with localized hyperperfusion.

By contrast, FNH are very rarely reported in association with hepatic adenoma. Association of FNH with fibrolamellar hepatocellular carcinoma is more controversial. For some authors, fibrolamellar carcinoma represents the malignant counterpart of FNH (VECCHIO et al. 1984); however, no malignant transformation has been observed. In a few cases, regenerative hyperplasia surrounding fibrolamellar carcinoma has been described (SAUL et al. 1987; SAXENA et al. 1994).

8.3.5
Follow-up

Follow-up of FNH cases is poorly reported in the literature, because resection was performed in most cases in the past. Because FNH is a benign tumor with no malignant potential, surgical resection should be performed only in doubtful cases or in symptomatic patients. Discontinuation of oral contraception is generally recommended, because increased lesion diameter after using oral contraceptives has been reported (NAKAMUTA et al. 1994). In most cases, FNH remains stable, but regression, disappearance and recurrence after resection have all been described (PAIN et al. 1991; ROSS et al. 1976).

8.4
Hepatocellular Adenoma

8.4.1
Clinical Background

HA is a rare primary benign tumor of hepatocellular origin. Since the introduction of oral contraceptives in 1960 the incidence of HA has increased, and oral contraceptives and androgen steroid therapy are known to be causative agents (MERGO and ROS 1998). The risk of developing HA while using oral contraception has changed in past years, probably because of the various concentrations in estrogens. In the studies including women who took contraceptive pills with a high estrogen content the risk in such women was elevated, being 34-fold that in nonusers, whereas in a case-control study including women who took low estrogen contraceptive pills their risk was increased by a factor of 3 (ROOKS et al. 1979; FLÉJOU et al. 1994). HA can also develop spontaneously or be associated with underlying metabolic disease, such as type I glycogen storage disease, galactosemia, tyrosinemia, and diabetes mellitus. HA is mostly seen in women in their third and fourth decades of life. Compared with FNH, symptoms are often associated with HA and include abdominal pain or, more rarely, spontaneous hemorrhage. Blood liver tests are often abnormal, and a significant increase in serum alkaline phosphatase activity or serum aminotransferase activity is noted in one-third of cases (CHERQUI et al. 1995).

In contrast to FNH, the diagnosis of HA is of clinical important, because it can be associated with life-threatening hemorrhage and because it can undergo malignant transformation to hepatocellular carcinoma. Hepatocellular carcinoma arising in HA has been reported in patients with and in patients without underlying metabolic disease. Therefore, when the diagnosis of HA is made, it should be treated by liver resection.

8.4.2
Pathology

HA is typically a solitary, well-circumscribed, often encapsulated lesion that is composed of hepatocytes arranged in cords and occasionally forms bile (CRAIG et al. 1989).

Necrosis, hemorrhage, and rupture are frequent in large tumors. This tumor may be pedunculated. On microscopy cytoplasmic changes may be noted, such as cholestasis, peliosis hepatis, or fatty hepatocytes that are sometimes prominent.

Blood vessels are mostly seen at the margins, and arteries within the hepatocellular adenoma are closely accompanied by veins (CRAIG et al. 1989). In most tumors a fibrous capsule is seen at the periphery; it is composed of collagenous connective tissue.

Malignant change is recognized by nodule-within-nodule growth and by the presence of large trabeculae (CRAIG et al. 1989). Anabolic steroid-associated hepatocellular adenoma may be difficult to differentiate from hepatocellular carcinoma, because cytologic atypia are present in both (CRAIG et al. 1989). Multiple hepatocellular adenomatosis is characterized by the presence of numerous HA. The macroscopical findings consist in multiple bulging nodules up to 5 cm in diameter and prominent surface vascularity (CRAIG et al. 1989).

8.4.3
Helical CT

To our knowledge, no large series of patients with HA studied by helical CT has been published. Therefore, most of the following findings were described following detection with a conventional CT unit. On precontrast CT scans, HA are mostly hypodense relative to the liver (67–86%) (Fig. 8.7A) (MATHIEU et al. 1986; WELCH et al. 1985). In 14–22%, the lesions appear spontaneously and diffusely hyperdense to the liver (MATHIEU et al. 1986; WELCH et al. 1985). However, hyperdense foci within lesions related to acute hemorrhage are identified in 15–43% of cases (KERLIN et al. 1983; WELCH et al. 1985). Hemorrhagic lesions may be associated with subcapsular hematoma. In rare cases, an area of fat density may be identified in the center of lesions, as well as hyperdensity resulting from calcifications (MATHIEU et al. 1986). HAs are very rarely isodense to the liver on unenhanced CT scans (MATHIEU et al. 1986).

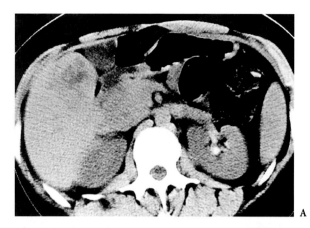

A

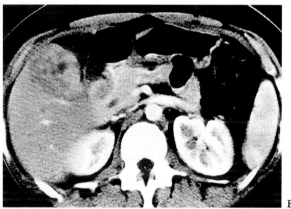

B

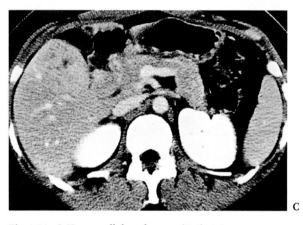

C

Fig. 8.7A–C. Hepatocellular adenoma (HA). **A** On precontrast CT scan the lesion is hypodense to the liver. **B** In the arterial phase of the contrast enhancement heterogeneous hypervascularization is detected. This lesion may mimic FNH but no enhancement of the central area is noted on portal phase images (**C**)

HAs are less often homogeneous than FNHs at CT (Fig. 8.7). Lesion homogeneity is observed in less that one half of lesions and is mainly seen in lesions smaller than 4 cm in diameter (MATHIEU et al. 1986).

On postcontrast CT scans, most lesions show significant enhancement during the arterial phase, decreasing during the portal phase until they become iso- or hypodense relative to the liver (Figs. 8.7, 8.8). However, in some lesions containing predominant fatty metamorphosis, necrosis, or hemorrhage the lesions may enhance only slightly or not at all (Figs. 8.9, 8.10). In a series of noncystic focal lesions examined by dual-phase helical CT, four patients with HA were enrolled and all HAs were predominantly hyperdense in the arterial phase: three were homogeneous and one had peripheral enhancement (VAN HOE et al. 1997). On portal vein phase images, two adenomas were hypodense with peripheral enhancement, one was hypodense and heterogeneous, and one was hyperdense and homogeneous. In this series, three adenomas out of four showed a pattern similar to that seen in FNH on arterial phase images and a different pattern from that seen in FNH on portal vein phase images (VAN HOE et al. 1997). This finding is quite interesting, but the low number of

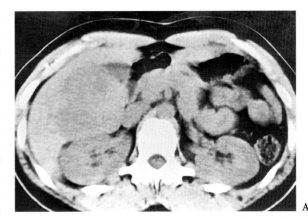

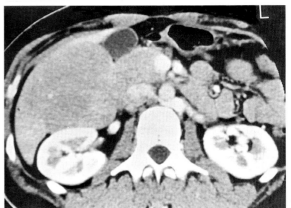

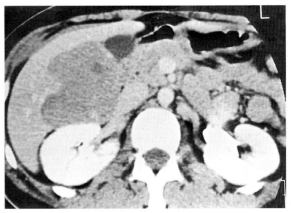

Fig. 8.9A–C. Hypovascular HA. A On precontrast CT scan the lesion is hypodense to the liver. At the arterial phase and at the portal phase of the contrast medium injection (B, C) the lesion remains hypodense

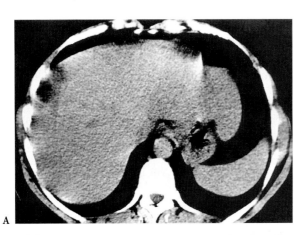

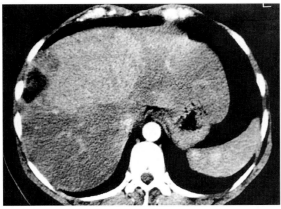

Fig. 8.8A, B. HA. A On pre-contrast CT scan the lesion is isodense to the liver. B At the arterial phase the lesion shows significant enhancement but contains a peripheral low density area corresponding to fat

patients does not allow any conclusion. Furthermore, no intratumoral hemorrhage, necrosis or fatty changes were detected in the patients in that study.

In contrast to FNH, when zones hypodense relative to HA are detected on CT they do not enhance on delayed images, because these zones correspond to bands of necrosis (MATHIEU et al. 1986). Delayed

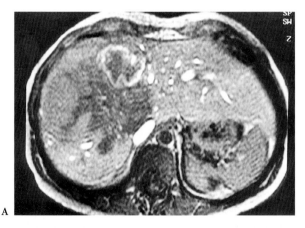

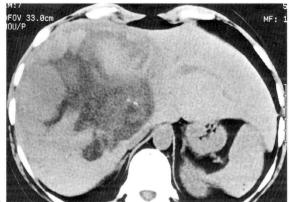

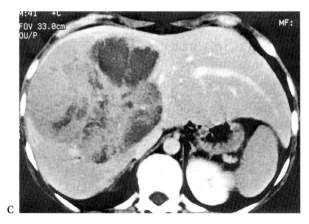

Fig. 8.10A–C. HA with hemorrhagic changes. **A** T1-weighted MR image demonstrating heterogeneous lesion with hemorrhage. **B** Pre-, **C** postcontrast CT scans revealing a heterogeneous lesion with hemorrhagic foci

images allow the depiction of peripheral capsule in some cases of HA by showing a continuous hyperdense rim. In summary, HAs are mostly hypervascular lesions that enhance predominantly on arterial phase images; they are easy to differentiate from typical FNH, because the spoke-wheel pattern, central scar, and central feeding vessels are usu-

ally not observed (VAN HOE et al. 1997): and they may resemble HCC, because both lesions are often heterogeneous, and clinical data and laboratory values are helpful in telling them apart.

8.4.4
Adenomas Associated with Other Lesions

8.4.4.1
Adenomatosis

Adenomatosis has been defined by the presence of at least 10 HAs in an otherwise normal liver and has been regarded as a distinct entity on the basis of the following: it affects men as well as women; adenomatosis does not seem to be related to oral contraceptive use; and increases in serum alkaline phosphatase and γ-glutamyl transpeptidase are common (FLÉJOU et al. 1985).

On imaging, two distinct patterns are observed: one with multiple small lesions that are often homogeneous and hypodense owing to the high content of fat and one with both small and large lesions together. The large lesions may be heterogeneous, with hemorrhagic or necrotic changes. This entity has to be differentiated from multiple hepatocellular carcinomas. To our knowledge, there have been no reports of malignant transformation in patients with adenomatosis.

8.4.4.2
Hepatic Adenoma and FNH

There are several reports in the literature concerning an association of HA and FNH (CHEN and BOCIAN 1983; GRANGÉ et al. 1987). Although no clear explanation has been proposed for the mechanism of this association, some authors have suggested a possible role of congenital heart disease or abnormal secretion of sex steroids. In these observations, HA and FNH were admixed or were located separately within the liver. We have observed a case of multiple HAs surrounded by areas of focal nodular hyperplasia in a patient who had a congenital portohepatic shunt (KAWAKATSU et al. 1994). A possible mechanism could have been increased hepatocellular proliferation induced by a larger number of hepatic arteries than normal. Similarly to our case, some authors have reported the coexistence of HA and nodular regenerative hyperplasia, which suggests a common pathogenesis (Nguyen et al. 1986).

8.4.4.3
Follow-up

The recommended treatment for HAs is surgical resection, because of the possibility of hemorrhage or the remoter possibility of transformation into hepatocellular carcinoma. However, a few follow-up studies in the literature have documented regression of HAs after cessation of oral contraceptive use (Kawakatsu et al. 1997; Bühler et al. 1982). Complete regression of HA has been observed, and the mean duration varies from 4 to 9 years (Kawakatsu et al. 1997). In all the reported cases, the oral contraceptives concerned were high-dose estrogen preparations.

8.5
Advantages and Pitfalls of Helical CT Compared with Other Imaging Modalities

8.5.1
Advantages of Helical CT

Helical CT offers an excellent opportunity for detection and characterization of focal liver lesions during the arterial, portal vein, and delayed phases. Previous studies have shown that this technique allows improved detection of hypervascular hepatic neoplasms because most hepatic tumors receive most of their blood from the hepatic artery and not from the portal vein system. Van Hoe et al. (1997) have demonstrated that the addition of arterial phase images significantly improves the characterization of focal hepatic lesions and that arterial phase images were most valuable in the subjective diagnosis of FNH and HA. Furthermore, the helical CT technique allows complete coverage of the liver at the arterial phase of the enhancement. It makes it possible to detect multiple lesions, such as multiple FNH or multiple HAs. Therefore we think that helical CT has numerous advantages over conventional CT.

Helical CT also has some advantages over MR imaging, because helical CT permits thin collimation slices and thin increments and has a high spatial resolution. Small structures, such as small lesions, or depiction of the central feeding artery or a spoked-wheel pattern are probably better seen on helical CT images than on MR images.

8.5.2
Disadvantages of Helical CT

General disadvantages of helical CT are the greater radiation exposure because multiple acquisitions are performed and the need for iodinated contrast medium. Another disadvantage of helical CT compared with MR imaging is the lower sensitivity in depiction macroscopic and microscopic changes within the tumor, such as fatty infiltration, necrotic or hemorrhagic changes, and intratumoral peliosis. However, to our knowledge no studies comparing the diagnostic efficacy of helical CT and MR imaging in benign hepatic neoplasms are available.

8.6
Impact of CT on the Management of Patients

Although US is a useful tool for the detection of liver tumors, findings on Doppler sonography are not sufficiently characteristic to allow a specific diagnosis. Compared with US studies, helical CT and MR imaging may show more specific findings. The diagnosis of typical FNH can be made on helical CT or MR imaging with a specificity of almost 100%. In those lesions, helical CT or MR imaging are very useful imaging modalities and histological confirmation is not necessary. In other cases, the findings are those encountered in primary hepatic tumors but are not characteristic of FNH. Histological diagnosis is the needed, and tissue may be obtained percutaneously. To increase confidence in the diagnosis, the specimen should be large enough and should be compared with normal liver. The standard procedure is a percutaneous biopsy under US guidance, with an 18-G cutting needle. Some authors claim that the risk of bleeding after biopsy is higher in the case of hypervascular tumors and prefer a laparoscopic approach. Finally, in some other cases, features of the lesion on helical CT are strongly atypical of FNH and may be suggestive of HA, because the lesions are heterogeneous, encapsulated or contain fat, necrosis or hemorrhage. However, we have to bear in mind that the imaging features of HA are very similar to those of hepatocellular carcinoma.

8.7
Conclusion

In conclusion, helical CT is a very useful tool for the detection and characterization of liver lesions. To optimize this technique in hepatic lesions, arterial phase imaging is required as well as thin collimation. The goal of this technique is to differentiate FNHs, which are benign and uncomplicated lesions, from HAs and hepatocellular carcinomas which are potentially malignant or malignant and require surgical resection.

References

Buetow PC, Pantongrag-Brown L, Buck JL, Ros PR, Goodman ZD (1996) From the archives of the AFIP. Focal nodular hyperplasia of the liver: radiologic-pathologic correlation. Radiographics 16:369–388

Bühler H, Pirovino M, Akovbiantz A, Altorfer J, Weitzel M, Maranta E, Schmid M (1982) Regression of liver cell adenoma. A follow-up study of three consecutive patients after discontinuation of oral contraceptive use. Gastroenterology 82:775–782

Caseiro-Alves F, Zins M, Mahfouz AE, Rahmouni A, Vilgrain V, Menu Y, Mathieu D (1996) Calcification in focal nodular hyperplasia: a new problem for differentiation from fibrolamellar hepatocellular carcinoma. Radiology 198:889–892

Chen KTK, Bocian JJ (1983) Multiple hepatic adenomas. Arch Pathol Lab Med 107:274–275

Cherqui D, Rahmouni A, Charlotte F et al (1995) Management of focal nodular hyperplasia and hepatocellular adenoma in young women: a series of 41 patients with clinical, radiological, and pathological correlations. Hepatology 22:1674–1681

Choi CS, Freeny PC (1998) Triphasic helical CT of hepatic focal nodular hyperplasia: incidence of atypical findings. AJR 170:391–395

Craig JR, Peters RL, Edmondson HA (1989) Tumors of the liver and intrahepatic bile ducts. In: Armed Forces Institute of Pathology (ed) Atlas of tumor pathology, 2nd ser, fasc 26. Armed Forces Institute of Pathology, Washington

Eisenberg LB, Warshauer DM, Woosley JT, Cance WG, Bunzendahl H, Semelka RC (1995) CT and MRI of hepatic focal nodular hyperplasia with peripheral steatosis. J Comput Assist Tomogr 19:498–500

Fléjou JF, Barge J, Menu Y, Degott C, Bismuth H, Potet F, Benhamou JP (1985) Liver adenomatosis. An entity distinct from liver adenoma? Gastroenterology 89:1132–1138

Fléjou JF, Pignon JP, Lê MG, Belghiti J, Barge J, Bismuth H, Benhamou JP (1994) Liver cell adenoma, focal nodular hyperplasia and oral contraceptive use: a French case-control study in young women (abstract). Hepatology 20:280A

Grangé, JD, Guéchot J, Legendre C, Giboudeau J, Darnis F, Poupon R (1987) Liver adenoma and focal nodular hyperplasia in a man with high endogenous sex steroids. Gastroenterology 93:1049–1413

Haber M, Reuben A, Burrell M, Oliverio P, Salem RR, West AB (1995) Multiple focal nodular hyperplasia of the liver associated with hemihypertrophy and vascular malformations. Gastroenterology 108:1256–1262

Kawakatsu M, Vilgrain V, Belghiti J, Fléjou JF, Nahum H (1994) Association of multiple liver cell adenomas with spontaneous intrahepatic portohepatic shunt. Abdom Imaging 19:438–440

Kawakatsu M, Vilgrain V, Erlinger S, Nahum H (1997) Disappearance of liver cell adenoma: CT and MR imaging. Abdom Imaging 22:274–276

Kerlin P, Davis GL, McGill DB, Weiland LH, Adson MA, Sheedy PF II (1983) Hepatic adenoma and focal nodular hyperplasia: clinical, pathologic, and radiologic features. Gastroenterology 84:994–1002

Mathieu D, Bruneton JN, Drouillard J, Caron Pointreau C, Vasile N (1986) Hepatic adenomas and focal nodular hyperplasia: dynamic CT study. Radiology 160:53–58

Mathieu D, Zafrani ES, Anglade MC, Dhumeaux D (1989) Association of focal nodular hyperplasia and hepatic hemangioma. Gastroenterology 97:154–157

Mergo PJ, Ros PR (1998) Benign lesions of the liver. Radiol Clin North Am 36:319–331

Nakamuta M, Ohashi M, Fukutomi T, Tanabe Y, Hiroshige K, Nakashima O, Nawata H (1994) Oral contraceptive-dependent growth of focal nodular hyperplasia. J Gastroenterol Hepatol 9:521–523

Nguyen TD, Oakes D, Fogel MR, Williams L, Sherck JP, Kozar M (1986) Hepatocellular adenoma and nodular regenerative hyperplasia of the liver in a young man. J Clin Gastroenterol 8:478–482

Pain JA, Gimson AES, Williams R, Howard ER (1991) Focal nodular hyperplasia of the liver: results of treatment and options in management. Gut 32:524–527

Procacci C, Fugazzola C, Cinquino M et al (1992) Contribution of CT to characterization of focal nodular hyperplasia of the liver. Gastrointest Radiol 17:63–73

Rooks JB, Ory HW, Ishak KG, Strauss LT, Greenspan JR, Paganini AH, Tyler CW (1979) The cooperative liver tumor study group. Epidemiology of hepatocellular adenoma. JAMA 242:644–648

Ross D, Pina J, Mirza M, Golvan A, Ponce L (1976) Regression of focal nodular hyperplasia after discontinuation of oral contraceptives. Ann Intern Med 85:203–204

Saul SH, Titelbaum DS, Gansler TS, Varello M, Burke DR, Atkinson BF, Rosato EF (1987) The fibrolamellar variant of hepatocellular carcinoma. Its association with focal nodular hyperplasia. Cancer 60:3049–3055

Saxena R, Humphreys S, Williams R, Portmann B (1994) Nodular hyperplasia surrounding fibrolamellar carcinoma: a zone of arterialized liver parenchyma. Histopathology 25:275–278

Shamsi K, de Schepper A, Degryse H, Deckers F (1993) Focal nodular hyperplasia of the liver: radiologic findings. Abdom Imaging 18:32–38

Shirkhoda A, Farah MC, Bernacki E, Madrazo B, Roberts J (1994) Hepatic focal nodular hyperplasia: CT and sonographic spectrum. Abdom Imaging 19:34–38

Van Hoe L, Baert AL, Gryspeerdt S, Vandenbosh G, Nevens F, Van Steenbergen W, Marchal G (1997) Dual-phase helical CT of the liver: value of an early-phase acquisition in the differential diagnosis of noncystic focal lesions. AJR 168:1185–1192

Vecchio FM, Fabiano A, Ghirlanda G, Manna R, Massi G (1984) Fibrolamellar carcinoma of the liver: the malignant counterpart of focal nodular hyperplasia with oncocytic change. Am J Clin Pathol 81:521–526

Vilgrain V, Fléjou JF, Arrivé L et al (1992) Focal nodular hyperplasia of the liver: MR imaging and pathologic correlation in 37 patients. Radiology 184:1–6

Wanless IR, Mawdsley C, Adams R (1985) On the pathogenesis of focal nodular hyperplasia of the liver. Hepatology 5:1194–1200

Wanless IR, Albrecht S, Bilbao J, Frei JV, Heathcote EJ, Roberts EA, Chiasson D (1989) Multiple focal nodular hyperplasia of the liver associated with vascular malformation of various organs and neoplasia of the brain: a new syndrome. Mod Pathol 2:456–462

Welch TJ, Sheedy PF II, Johnson CM et al (1985) Focal nodular hyperplasia and hepatic adenoma: comparison of angiography, CT, US, and scintigraphy. Radiology 156:593–595

9 Hepatocellular Carcinoma

R. Lencioni, D. Cioni, C. Bartolozzi

CONTENTS

9.1   Introduction   *111*
9.2   Spiral CT Features of Hepatocellular
        Carcinoma   *111*
9.2.1   Small Hepatocellular Carcinoma   *111*
9.2.2   Advanced Hepatocellular Carcinoma   *113*
9.2.3   Unusual CT Features of Hepatocellular
        Carcinoma   *115*
9.3   Angiographically Assisted Spiral
        CT Techniques   *117*
9.3.1   Spiral CT Arteriography   *118*
9.3.2   Spiral CT during Arterial Portography   *120*
9.3.3   Lipiodol Spiral CT   *120*
9.4   Screening   *120*
9.5   Differential Diagnosis   *122*
9.5.1   In Cirrhotic Liver   *122*
9.5.2   In Noncirrhotic Liver   *123*
9.6   Staging   *124*
9.7   Assessment of Tumor Response   *127*
        References   *130*

9.1
Introduction

Hepatocellular carcinoma (HCC) is one of the most common malignancies in the world, with an estimated incidence of about 1,000,000 cases per year throughout the world (Lencioni and Bartolozzi 1997). This tumor is the seventh most common cancer in men and the ninth most common cancer in women. HCC varies considerably among the various geographic areas in incidence, etiology, and clinicopathologic features. While this neoplasm is very common in the South-East of Asia and in sub-Sa-

R. Lencioni, MD; Division of Diagnostic and Interventional Radiology, Department of Oncology, University of Pisa, Via Roma 67, I-56125 Pisa, Italy
D. Cioni, MD; Division of Diagnostic and Interventional Radiology, Department of Oncology, University of Pisa, Via Roma 67, I-56125 Pisa, Italy
C. Bartolozzi, MD;Professor and Chairman; Division of Diagnostic and Interventional Radiology, Department of Oncology, University of Pisa, Via Roma 67, I-56125 Pisa, Italy

haran Africa, it is relatively rare in the United States and in the North of Europe. The South of Europe is characterized by a medium to high incidence of HCC. In Western countries and in Japan, HCC emerges in cirrhotic livers in more than 90% of cases. In fact, patients with liver cirrhosis have long been identified as a high-risk group for the development of HCC. The yearly incidence of HCC in cirrhotic patients may reach 3–5%, and HCC is recognized as the principal cause of death in these patients (Colombo et al. 1991; Lencioni et al. 1995a).

Since the mid-1970s, recognition of the close association of HCC with cirrhosis has stimulated the development of clinical programs for the early detection of HCC in cirrhotic patients (Oka et al. 1990; Peteron et al. 1994). Owing to widespread screening programs, increasing numbers of asymptomatic tumors have been detected at a treatable stage. Hence, interest in accurate diagnosis and staging of this kind of malignancy has substantially increased. Spiral CT currently plays a major part in the diagnostic and therapeutic management of patients with HCC (Rummeny and Marchal 1997). This article will focus on spiral CT features of HCC and on the usefulness of dual-phase spiral CT for screening, differential diagnosis, staging, and evaluation of response to treatment of HCC.

9.2
Spiral CT Features of HCC

9.2.1
Small HCC

Following recent progress in early diagnosis, various new items of information on the pathomorphologic characteristics and developmental process of early-stage HCC have been obtained through histological examination of resected lesions, explanted livers, and autopsy specimens (Choi et al. 1993; Takayasu et al. 1990, 1995a, b). Currently, HCC is thought to develop through two main pathways: de novo carcinogenesis and multistep progression. Multistep development is considered to be the most frequent model of hepatocarcinogenesis in cirrhotic livers. This model includes the transition from frankly benign nodules (large regenerative nodules or macroregenerative nodules) through equivocal lesions (dysplastic nodules or borderline lesions) and early HCC (very well-differentiated Edmondson grade 1 tumor) to, finally, overt HCC (advanced tumor classed as Edmondson grade 2 or greater) (KANAI et al. 1987; NAKAKUMA et al. 1993).

HCC usually develops as a focus of well-differentiated cancer within a dysplastic lesion. When the tumor grows to 1–1.5 cm in diameter de-differentiation of well-differentiated cancer cells occurs: cancer tissue at lower histological grades proliferates within the well-differentiated cancerous nodule (early advanced HCC), replaces the well-differentiated tissue that has weak proliferative activity, and then starts to grow expansively, developing into advanced HCC (KIM et al. 1998a).

Along with progression from regeneration to cancer, hepatocellular nodular lesions show a change in the blood supply. In fact, the intranodular portal blood supply tends to decrease, while the intranodular arterial supply, in contrast, tends to increase during the development from a benign to a malignant lesion. Macroregenerative and dysplastic nodules, like early HCC, have a predominantly portal blood supply, while overt HCC lesions are supplied almost exclusively by hepatic arterial branches. The neoangiogenesis of nontriadal arteries, that is the pathologic substratum of tumor hypervascularity, relates to the presence of HCC tissue of grade 2 (Edmondson) or greater (LENCIONI et al. 1996a, b; TAKAYAMA et al. 1990).

The different blood supply to the lesion is the single most important CT feature that may help differentiate among small hepatocellular lesions that have emerged in a cirrhotic liver (HOLLETT et al. 1995). In fact, small, overt HCC tumors show a typical hypervascular pattern, with clear-cut enhancement in the predominantly arterial phase and rapid wash-out in the portal venous phase (Fig. 9.1) (BONALDI et al. 1995; CHOI et al. 1996). In contrast, early-stage HCC and regenerative or dysplastic lesions fail to exhibit this feature and appear isoattenuating or hypoattenuating relative to surrounding liver parenchyma on dual-phase spiral CT images (Fig. 9.2) (LENCIONI et al. 1996).

Morphologically, small HCC tumors less than 3 cm in their greatest dimension usually show a nodu-

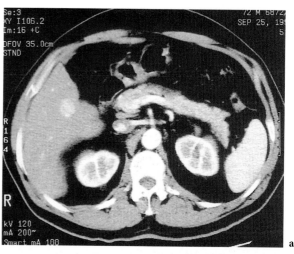

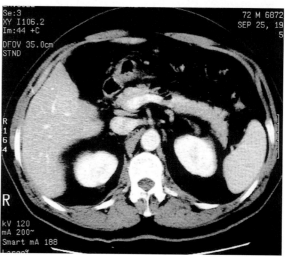

Fig. 9.1a,b. Small, overt, hepatocellular carcinoma (HCC). The tumor shows clear-cut hypervascular pattern and stands out in the arterial phase spiral CT image (**a**) against the faintly enhanced liver parenchyma. Rapid wash-out of contrast medium is observed in the portal venous phase image (**b**), in which the lesion is not detectable

lar configuration and can be divided into four types: single nodular type, single nodular type with extranodular growth, contiguous multinodular type, and poorly demarcated nodular type.

Small, classic, nodular-type HCC is a sharply demarcated lesion that may or may not be encapsulated. Pathologically, a tumor capsule is seen in about 50–60% of small HCC lesions. The CT detection rate of the capsule is low in small tumors because the capsule is thin and poorly developed. The capsule is seen as a peripheral rim that is hypoattenuating on unenhanced and arterial phase contrast-enhanced images, and hyperattenuating on delayed contrast-enhanced images (Fig. 9.3) (Ros et al. 1990). The

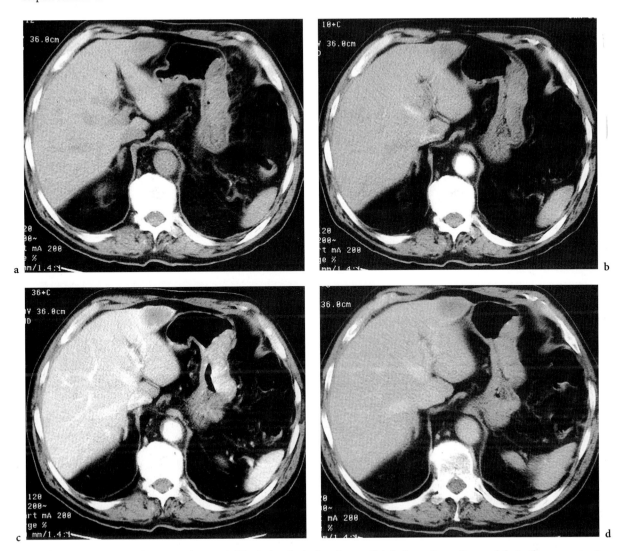

Fig. 9.2a–d. Early-stage, hypovascular HCC. The lesion is depicted as a slightly low-attenuating nodule in the precontrast spiral CT image (**a**). The lesion fails to enhance in the arterial phase image (**b**), and appears definitely hypoattenuating with respect to surrounding liver parenchyma in the portal venous phase (**c**) and in the delayed phase (**d**)

single nodular type with extranodular growth, the contiguous multinodular type, and the poorly demarcated nodular type show a nodular configuration with an irregular or unclear margin on CT images (Fig. 9.4) (FERNANDEZ and REDVANLY 1998; UEDA et al. 1995; MATSUI et al. 1991).

9.2.2
Advanced HCC

Advanced HCC lesions are classified into three major types: expansive nodular type, infiltrative type, and diffuse type.

The typical expansive type of HCC is a sharply demarcated lesion, which can be unifocal or multifocal. Typical features of expansive-type HCC include tumor capsule and internal mosaic architecture. Most expansive HCC lesions have a well-developed fibrous capsule. The capsule may be depicted by CT in up to 70–80% of large, encapsulated lesions on macroscopic pathological examination. The fibrous capsule is demonstrated by CT as a hypoattenuating rim that enhances in the delayed phase (Fig. 9.5) (Ros et al. 1990). Internal mosaic architecture is characterized by components separated by thin fibrous septa (Fig. 9.6). The different components may show various attenuation index on CT images, par-

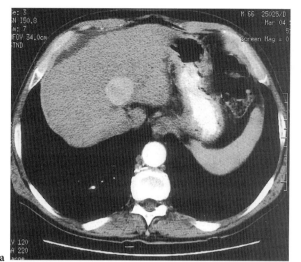

tion of neoplastic thrombosis of the portal vein is a crucial factor for staging and prognosis (CHOI 1995). Infiltrative HCC may create a massive involvement of the liver, replacing large parts of the parenchyma. The diffuse type is by far the most unusual presentation of HCC. This type is characterized by numerous small nodules scattered throughout the liver. The nodules do not fuse with each other and are visualized as diffusely distributed hypodense lesions.

In addition to these morphological features, HCC has the typical tendency to give rise to small or minute satellite nodules ("daughter" lesions), which are frequently located in the vicinity of the main tumor (Fig. 9.9). These nodules represent intrahepatic

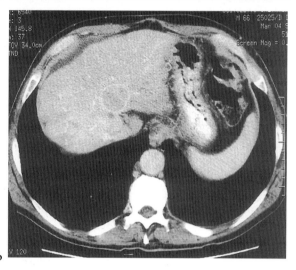

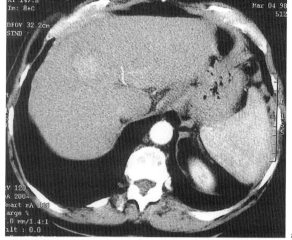

Fig. 9.3a, b. Small, encapsulated HCC. The lesion is well depicted in the arterial phase spiral CT image (a). In the portal venous phase, a peripheral rim of enhancement corresponding to the capsule is observed (b)

ticularly if areas of well-differentiated tumor with different degrees of fatty metamorphosis are present. Internal septa show delayed enhancement similar to that of the fibrous capsule (YOSHIKAWA et al. 1992).

The infiltrative type of HCC is characterized by an irregular and indistinct tumor–nontumor boundary. This type is demonstrated as a mainly segmental uneven hypodense area with unclear margins (Fig. 9.7). Strands of the tumor extend into surrounding tissue and frequently invade vascular structures, particularly portal vein branches. HCC, in fact, has a great propensity for invading and growing into the portal vein, eliciting tumor thrombi (Fig. 9.8). Identifica-

Fig. 9.4a, b. Small, poorly demarcated HCC. The tumor appears hyperdense in the arterial phase (a) and slightly hypodense in the portal venous phase (b) of the spiral CT study. The lesion shows nodular configuration with an irregular and unclear margin

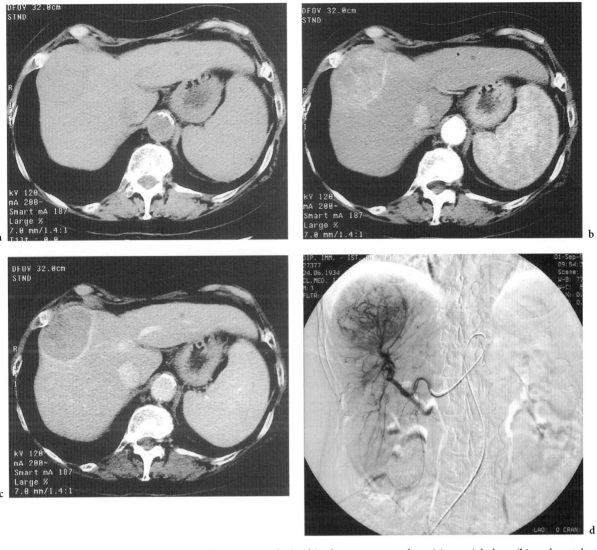

Fig. 9.5a–d. Large, encapsulated HCC. Spiral CT images obtained in the precontrast phase (a), arterial phase (b), and portal venous phase (c). The capsule is depicted as a low-attenuating rim in the precontrast image, with definite enhancement in the portal phase. Digital subtraction angiography (d) confirms large, uninodular, expansive type HCC with typical basketwork pattern

metastases, which have usually developed via the portal vein branches. Identification of these satellite lesions is of the utmost importance for therapeutic planning, and is one of the most challenging issues in HCC patients (CHOI et al. 1997). Satellite lesions should be distinguished from multiple small HCC tumors caused by multicentric development. Such a distinction is important, since the presence of intrahepatic metastases indicates a more advanced stage and is associated with a worse prognosis. In the case of multicentric development, multiple small tumors may exhibit different enhancement patterns on spiral CT, reflecting different degrees of tumor differentiation (FERNANDEZ and REDVANLY 1998; UEDA et al. 1995).

9.2.3
Unusual CT Features of HCC

Unusual histopathologic characteristics of HCC may modify the typical CT appearance of this tumor. These unusual histopathologic characteristics include marked fatty change, massive necrosis, abundant fibrous stroma (sclerosing-type HCC), sarcomatous change, copper accumulation, and calcifications (FREENY et al. 1992).

When fatty metamorphosis is severe, CT usually shows areas of negative attenuation values within the tumor, allowing diagnosis of the fat component. When the degree of fatty deposition differs among

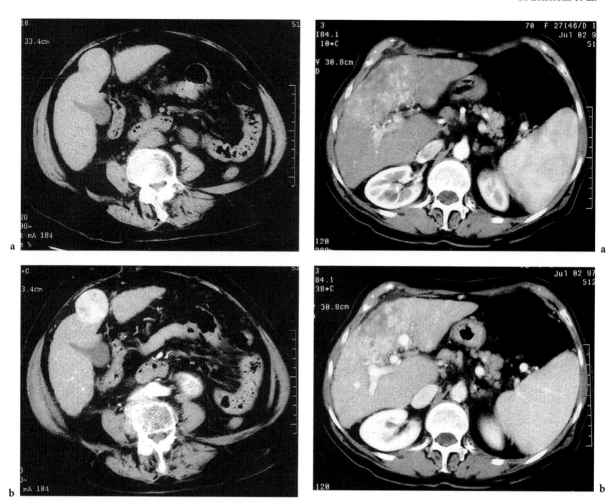

Fig. 9.7a, b. Infiltrative type HCC. The tumor is depicted by arterial phase (**a**) and portal venous phase (**b**) spiral CT images as an area with irregular borders and heterogeneous enhancement which extends in strands into surrounding tissue

Fig. 9.6a–c. HCC with internal mosaic architecture and intratumoral septa. Spiral CT images obtained in the precontrast phase (**a**), arterial phase (**b**), and portal venous phase (**c**). Different components of the tumor show various degrees of attenuation. Internal fibrous septa are depicted as they enhance in the portal venous phase

internal portions of the tumor the mosaic architecture can be visualized and the diagnosis of HCC made (Fig. 9.10) (YOSHIKAWA et al. 1988). However, in the case of diffuse fatty metamorphosis of the lesion, differential diagnosis from lipomatous tumors may not be achieved by CT.

Spontaneous massive necrosis within HCC shows up as a nonenhanced area, in a similar way to other necrotic tumors (Fig. 9.11). HCC with abundant fibrous stroma (sclerosing type HCC) demonstrates hypovascularity on arterial phase CT images and shows delayed enhancement (YAMASHITA et al. 1993). The same enhancement pattern may be seen in HCC with sarcomatous change, which is a very rare histotype. These CT features are commonly seen in lesions with a rich fibrous component, such as

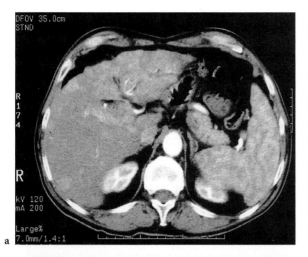

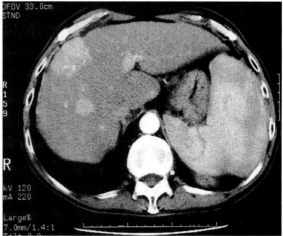

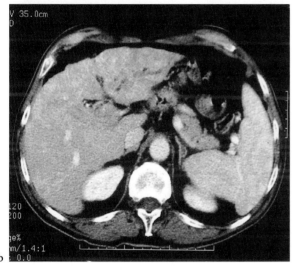

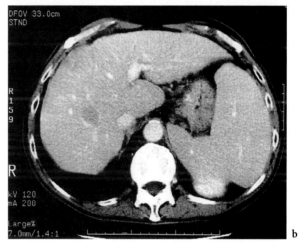

Fig. 9.8a, b. Infiltrative type HCC. Spiral CT images obtained in arterial (**a**) and in the portal venous phase (**b**). The tumor replaces a large part of the liver parenchyma, invading the portal vein branches and eliciting neoplastic thrombosis. Satellite lesions are also observed

Fig. 9.9a, b. HCC. The main tumor and the daughter nodule are well depicted in the arterial phase spiral CT image (**a**). In the portal venous phase (**b**), the main tumor appears slightly hypoattenuating, while the satellite lesion is definitely hypodense with respect to surrounding liver parenchyma

confluent hepatic fibrosis in cirrhotic liver and cholangiocellular carcinoma.

Deposition of copper and copper-binding protein has been recognized in some HCC lesions, resulting in increased attenuation on precontrast CT images (KITAGAUA et al. 1991). The presence of calcifications is uncommon in HCC, being detected in about 0.2–1% of tumors. Calcifications, however, are not rare in fibrolamellar carcinoma and in mixed cholangiocellular–hepatocellular carcinoma.

9.3
Angiographically Assisted Spiral CT Techniques

The combination of spiral CT and angiography allows the performance of accurate CT studies for detection and characterization of HCC (KANEMATSU et al. 1999; RUBIN et al. 1993). There are three combinations of spiral CT and angiography: spiral CT during the injection of contrast material into the hepatic artery (spiral CT arteriography), spiral CT during arterial portography, and spiral CT performed

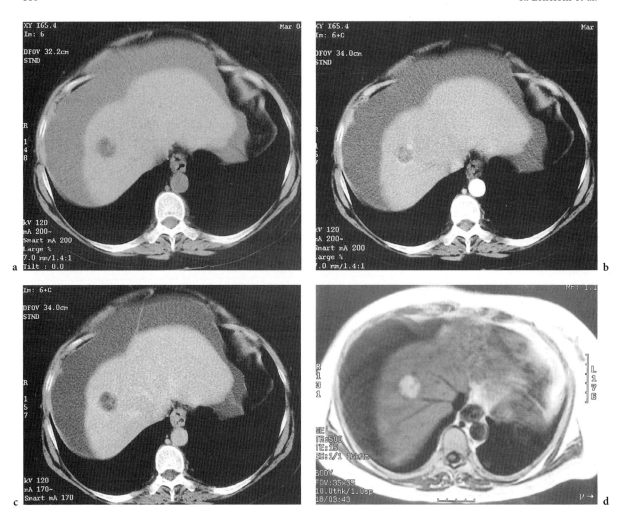

Fig. 9.10a–d. HCC with fatty metamorphosis. Spiral CT images obtained in the precontrast phase (**a**), arterial phase (**b**), and portal venous phase (**c**). The lesion appears definitely hypoattenuating in the precontrast image due to intratumoral fatty change. Spin echo T1-weighed magnetic resonance image (**d**) shows the lesion as a high intensity nodule, resulting from intratumoral fatty accumulation

after the intraarterial injection of iodized oil (Lipiodol spiral CT). These invasive procedures are currently used in selected cases, especially when a surgical therapeutic approach is being considered (NELSON et al. 1990; SMALL et al. 1993; SOYER et al. 1994).

9.3.1
Spiral CT Arteriography

In spiral CT arteriography (spiral CTA), contrast material is injected directly into the proper or common hepatic artery or, if this is not possible, into the celiac artery. This technique is based on the fact that all but a very few HCC tumors are fed from the hepatic artery. On spiral CTA images, HCC lesions show high-attenuation blushes compared with the surrounding normal liver and stand out against the faintly enhanced normal parenchyma (TAKAYASU et al. 1995a, b; UEDA et al. 1998).

With spiral CTA, even small but overt HCC tumors are well depicted. However, early-stage, well-differentiated HCC tumors with immature neovascularity fail to enhance and are not distinguished from liver parenchyma. Moreover, variations in vascular anatomy, flow-related artifacts, and altered hemodynamics resulting from the associated chronic liver disease can significantly change the patterns of enhancement and produce both false-negative and false-positive results (NOVICK and FISHMAN 1998).

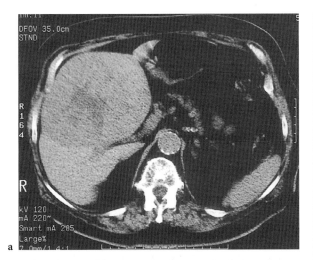

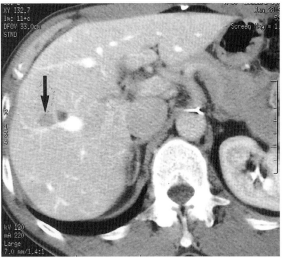

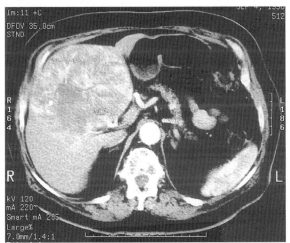

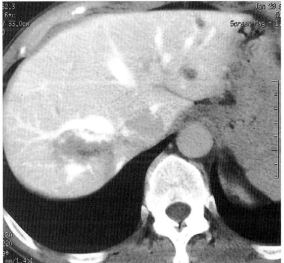

Fig. 9.12a, b. Spiral CT during arterial portography. The only one tumor deposit is indicated by the arrow (**a**). All the other tiny defects are caused by small cysts, while the large lesion at the right hepatic dome corresponds to hepatic hemangioma (**b**)

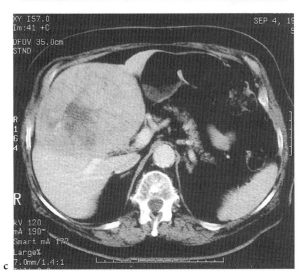

Fig. 9.11a–c. Large HCC with internal necrosis. The necrotic portion is depicted as a low-attenuating area in the precontrast spiral CT image (**a**), which fails to enhance in the arterial (**b**) and the portal (**c**) phases

9.3.2
Spiral CT during Arterial Portography

CT during arterial portography (spiral CTAP) is based on the reverse pathologic substratum with respect to CTA, that is, on the fact that almost no HCC tumors are fed by the portal vein. This procedure produces dense enhancement of portal venous blood, so that the arterially supplied overt HCC lesions are highlighted as negative defects. The liver is markedly increased in attenuation, and even small tumor deposits may be depicted as definitely hypodense areas.

Many reports have shown that this technique has a very high detection rate for small, overt HCC tumors (HORI et al. 1998). Well-differentiated, early-stage HCC lesions, however, maintain a portal blood supply (although usually decreased relative to that of normal liver or regenerative nodules) and may exhibit a faint hypodensity with respect to liver parenchyma, being hardly detectable (MERINE et al. 1990). Moreover, CTAP lacks specificity, as almost every focal lesion in the liver, including benign lesions such as hemangiomas and small cysts, assumes the same hypoattenuating appearance and therefore may simulate tumor (Fig. 9.12) (MATSUI et al. 1994). Moreover, this technique has the drawback that nontumorous portal vein perfusion defects unrelated to tumor deposits can occur as a result of altered hemodynamics, particularly in the presence of liver cirrhosis (KANEMATSU et al. 1998). In fact, false-positive rates as high as 20–30% have been reported, making CTAP unreliable for the correct prediction of positive tumor involvement (BLUEMKE et al. 1995; KANEMATSU et al. 1997).

9.3.3
Lipiodol Spiral CT

Lipiodol is the iodinated ethyl ester of the fatty acid of poppyseed oil and contains 37–38% of iodine by weight. When Lipiodol is injected into the hepatic artery most of the iodized oil droplets flow into HCC lesions by virtue of the increased blood supply to the tumor. Once deposited in the tumor, the Lipiodol droplets disappear at a far slower rate than those deposited in the normal liver tissue. In fact, while iodized oil undergoes rapid wash-out from the non-cancerous liver parenchyma, usually being no longer detectable 3–4 weeks after the intraarterial injection, it remains within HCC nodules for months or years.

The reason for the selective and prolonged retention of Lipiodol in HCC lesions has yet to be fully clarified. Some authors suggested that trapping of the oil in the irregular, tortuous, and poorly contractile vessels of the tumor and the abnormally increased permeability of these vessels may be involved. Moreover, it has been postulated that the slow disappearance of lipiodol from HCC lesions may be explained by the absence of lymphatic vessels and Kupffer cells in the tumor tissue.

On spiral CT scans acquired 3–4 weeks after intraarterial injection of Lipiodol, HCC lesions appear as highly hyperattenuating areas compared with nontumorous liver tissue (TOUREL et al. 1995). Many published reports have shown that Lipiodol CT has a high detection rate for tiny HCC nodules (MERINE et al. 1990). Findings on Lipiodol spiral CT are quite specific for the diagnosis of HCC, provided that correct diagnostic criteria are used. Small, rounded, circumscribed areas of dense Lipiodol retention on spiral CT scans obtained 3–4 weeks after intraarterial injection of the iodized oil have 90% positive predictive value for being true satellite neoplastic foci in the clinical setting of a cirrhotic patients with HCC (Fig. 9.13) (BISOLLON et al. 1998; CHOI et al. 1997; LENCIONI et al. 1997a, b).

9.4
Screening

Extensive screening for HCC was made possible by the application of widely available diagnostic methods, such as assays for serum alpha-fetoprotein (AFP) and real-time ultrasonography (US) (OKA et al. 1990; PETERON et al. 1994).

The use of US as the imaging modality of choice for screening has become widely accepted, although US examination of the entire liver is sometimes impossible because of patient's habitus, intervening bones, or colonic interposition, especially in small cirrhotic livers (DODD et al. 1992). Conventional CT performed with nonspiral scanners has not proved to have any substantial advantage over US for early detection of HCC. In fact, the sensitivity of conventional CT in the detection of small HCC lesions was inferior to that of US in most published series.

The increasing availability of spiral scanners opens up new prospects for HCC screening (OLIVER and BARON 1996). Spiral CT does have a high detection rate for small, overt, hypervascular HCC lesions (ROFFLETT et al. 1995; TUBLIN et al. 1999). Spiral CT

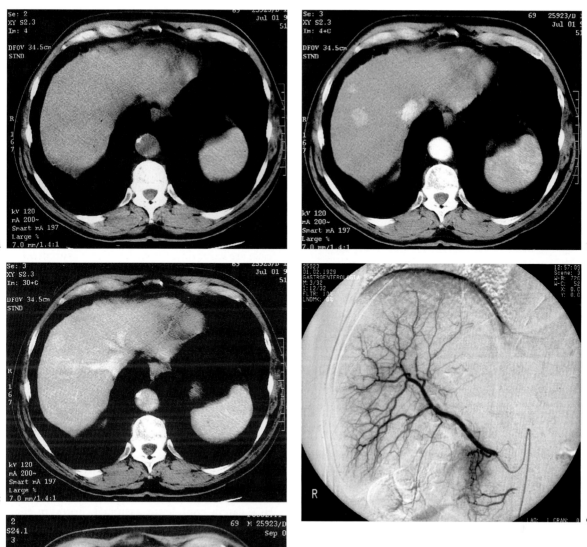

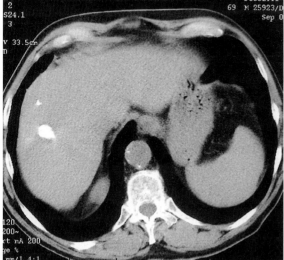

Fig. 9.13a–e. Small HCC with satellite lesion. Spiral CT images obtained in the precontrast phase (**a**), arterial phase (**b**), and portal venous phase (**c**). The two lesions are well depicted in the arterial phase image. Following digital subtraction angiography (**d**), anticancer-iodized oil emulsion is injected at the level of the proper hepatic artery. Unenhanced spiral CT scan obtained 4 weeks later demonstrates Lipiodol retention within the two neoplastic nodules (**e**)

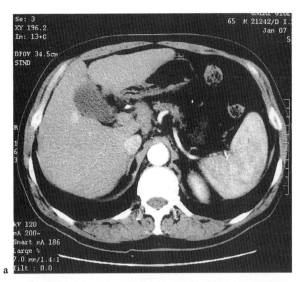

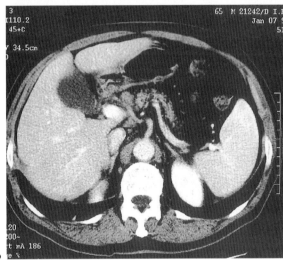

Fig. 9.14a, b. Small HCC. Spiral CT images acquired in the arterial (**a**) and the portal venous phase (**b**). Despite the small size, the lesion shows clear-cut hypervascular pattern. The tiny tumor nodule was undetectable by ultrasound

scan therefore guarantee an objective and comprehensive survey of the liver parenchyma, detecting small tumors for which timely therapeutic intervention is necessary, as hypervascularity testifies that these lesions have already started their progression toward advanced HCC (Fig. 9.14). The use of spiral CT could be recommended in high-risk patients, such as those with abnormally high (above 200 ng/ml) or increasing AFP levels and negative US findings (BARTOLOZZI et al. 1996; TAKAYASU et al. 1990).

9.5
Differential Diagnosis

The differential diagnosis of a suspected HCC raises different issues in the setting of a nodular lesion detected in a patient with liver cirrhosis or in the case of a tumor that has developed in an otherwise normal liver.

9.5.1
In Cirrhotic Liver

Currently, efforts are directed at diagnosing HCC that has developed in cirrhotic livers at an early, preclinical stage. To this end, patients with chronic liver disease are carefully followed, with measurement of AFP level and US examination performed at regular intervals. Hence, particular attention is directed at characterizing even very small nodules detected by US screening. Every solid focal liver lesion that emerges in a cirrhotic liver should be regarded as an HCC unless a different diagnosis has been confirmed (OHTOMO et al. 1993).

If the lesion show a typical hypervascular pattern, with clear-cut enhancement in the predominantly arterial phase and rapid wash-out in the portal venous phase, the diagnosis of HCC is very likely (Figs. 9.1, 9.14) (UEDA et al. 1995). If the additional features of a peripheral rim of delayed enhancement (corresponding to the capsule) (Fig. 9.3) or internal mosaic architecture are seen (Fig. 9.6), the diagnosis of HCC can be confidently assumed (BONALDI et al. 1995; CHOI et al. 1996). Biopsy confirmation may not be required in such instances. Mosaic architecture should not be confused with uneven CT densities in tumors caused by degeneration, necrosis, or bleeding (LEE et al. 1997; MITSUKAKI et al. 1996).

If these typical morphological features of HCC are not depicted, HCC must be differentiated from other hypervascular lesions that are occasionally found in cirrhotic livers. These include small hemangiomas and hypervascular metastases (KIM et al. 1998b; LEE et al. 1997; OLIVER et al. 1997).

Hemangiomas usually appear as low-attenuating lesions on precontrast CT images and show peripheral nodular or globular enhancement in arterial-phase images with progressive centripetal fill-in. Prolonged enhancement is typically seen in the delayed phase (HANAFUSA et al. 1997). On the other hand, classic HCC nodules are usually opacified throughout the entire tumor on arterial phase images, and become hypodense in the delayed phase. Tiny hemangiomas, however, sometimes exhibit the same homogeneously hypervascular pattern as small HCC. In these cases, differential diagnosis may not be possible by CT and further investigation with MRI is recommended (GRANGIER et al. 1994).

Hepatic metastases are uncommon in the clinical setting of a cirrhotic patient, and hypervascular metastases resembling HCC are uncommon among hepatic metastases (OLIVER et al. 1997). Nevertheless, this diagnostic dilemma may occur if the patient has a clinical history of extrahepatic malignancy or there is any clinical or laboratory suspicion of an extrahepatic tumor. In these cases, imaging findings alone may not allow a differential diagnosis and biopsy may be recommended.

The detection of a small hypovascular lesion in a cirrhotic liver may be due to either a dysplastic/well-differentiated hepatocellular nodule (Fig. 9.2) or, less frequently, to a non-cirrhosis-related lesion, such as an hepatic metastasis or an atypical hemangioma with persistent low attenuation at two-phase spiral CT (JANG et al. 1998).

Differentiation among the histologically varied grades of dysplastic and well-differentiated neoplastic hepatocellular lesions is not possible by CT. It has to be considered, however, that reliable clear-cut differentiation between dysplastic lesions and early-stage well-differentiated cancer is not possible by means of either imaging modalities or biopsy, as dysplastic nodules may contain microscopic foci of HCC. In keeping with new information on hepatocarcinogenesis, dysplastic nodules are now regarded as lesions with high malignant potential (KRINSKY et al. 1998). Therefore, these borderline lesions are currently considered eligible for interventional procedures such as percutaneous ethanol injection or radiofrequency thermal ablation, as small HCC nodules are.

Hypovascular metastases may exhibit peculiar features, such as necrotic center and vascular rim. Enhanced rims of neovascularity, or peripheral high-density rims resulting from congested, dilated sinusoids outside a hypovascular tumor may be best depicted in arterial-phase images. Prolonged enhancement is sometimes seen in the center of metastases in delayed scans. The combination of delayed and prolonged central enhancement producing a mass with high central density and relatively low peripheral density strongly suggests metastatic carcinoma (MATSUI et al. 1991).

9.5.2
In Noncirrhotic Liver

HCC that has developed in a noncirrhotic liver is usually not diagnosed until it is in an advanced stage, as no US investigation has been performed. Differential diagnosis is then usually more difficult, as a number of different entities must be taken into account.

If the tumor has an expansive growth, typical features suggesting HCC, such as tumor capsule and internal mosaic architecture (including areas of fatty degeneration), may be observed. In infiltrating lesions, invasion of portal vein branches may suggest HCC. Differential diagnosis of HCC in noncirrhotic livers includes a variety of benign and malignant entities (OLIVER et al. 1996; VAN HOE et al. 1997; GROSSHOLZ et al. 1998).

Expansive HCC lesions without signs of vascular invasion should first be distinguished from benign tumors. These include hemangioma, focal nodular hyperplasia, and hepatocellular adenoma.

Hemangiomas are well-demarcated masses that are hypodense with respect to normal liver and typically show peripheral nodular or globular enhancement in arterial-phase images with progressive centripetal fill-in. Prolonged enhancement is typically seen in the delayed phase. Large hemangiomas rarely fill in completely, however, as central regions of fibrosis or thrombosis remain hypodense (HANAFUSA et al. 1997).

Focal nodular hyperplasia and hepatocellular adenoma typically occur in young patients, and predominantly in females. Focal nodular hyperplasia usually has a typical biphasic enhancement on spiral CT: in the arterial phase the peripheral portion of the lesion shows clear-cut enhancement, becoming definitely hyperdense relative to adjacent hepatic parenchyma, while the central portion, which corresponds to the stellate scar, does not enhance. In the delayed-phase images, the peripheral portion of the lesion appears isodense relative to the surrounding normal liver, while the central scar demonstrates late enhancement. Hepatocellular adenoma is depicted as a nonspecific well-defined mass; areas of increased density may be observed on unenhanced scans, corresponding to recent intratumoral hemorrhage.

HCC that has emerged in noncirrhotic liver should also be distinguished from other kinds of malignancy. In addition to metastases and rare primary tumors, these include intrahepatic cholangiocellular carcinoma and fibrolamellar carcinoma.

Intrahepatic cholangiocellular carcinoma, originating in small intrahepatic ducts, represents 10% of all cholangiocarcinomas. It is the second most common primary malignancy and is usually seen in the seventh decade. There is no association between cholangiocarcinoma and liver cirrhosis. Characteristically, an abundant fibroblastic stroma is present in this tumor, which histologically is a sclerosing adenocarcinoma. Two CT configurations predominate in cholangiocarcinoma (TILLICH et al. 1998). The first is a well-defined hypodense mass with a slightly denser internal component on unenhanced scans. Injection of contrast medium produces prominent enhancement of the large internal component. The second appearance is that of a hypodense mass of variable homogeneity (sometimes with low-attenuating internal regions) and variable shape and sharpness of contour showing peripheral enhancement. Septated or streaked internal enhancement may be seen. Delayed scans may show accumulation of contrast medium within the tumor after wash-out from the normal liver, which seems to correlate with the fibrous component. Proximal biliary dilatation is often present in either of the two configurations of the disease, while is relatively uncommon in HCC (Ros et al. 1988).

Fibrolamellar carcinoma represents only 2% of hepatocellular malignancies. Typically, this neoplasm occurs in young people and is not associated with underlying cirrhosis. Most often, fibrolamellar carcinoma appears as a solitary, large, firm, circumscribed mass with lobulated borders. More than two thirds of reported cases have involved the left lobe. A prominent central fibrous scar with radiating fibrous septa may be present. The scar usually does not enhance after contrast administration, although accumulation of contrast in delayed scans, resembling the behavior of the central stellate scar commonly seen in focal nodular hyperplasia, has been reported. The major CT clue to the diagnosis of fibrolamellar carcinoma is the presence of central stellate or trabecular calcifications, which is seen in 30–70% of cases. In HCC, calcifications may occur in the sclerosing type, which is characterized by intense fibrosis: this kind of malignancy, however, typically arises in older patients.

9.6 Staging

Accurate staging is necessary to determine the best treatment method for HCC. Spiral CT is an ideal technique for staging, as it provides reliable detection of both intrahepatic and extrahepatic spread of the tumor. Staging of HCC includes the assessment of (a) number, size, location, and characteristics of the tumor nodules; (b) vascular invasion by the tumor; and (c) extrahepatic metastases. All these factors should be accurately evaluated, as they affect therapeutic options as well as patient's prognosis.

Dual-phase spiral CT provides accurate assessment of the number and size of HCC lesions, enabling identification of even small intrahepatic metastatic nodules. These tiny tumor deposits are usually hypervascular, in fact, like the main tumor, and are therefore well depicted in the arterial phase images (OI et al. 1996). The availability of spiral scanners has substantially restricted the indications for more complex and invasive angiographically assisted CT techniques, such as CTAP or Lipiodol CT, for detection of satellite lesions. However, if a surgical therapeutic approach is being considered, more precise preoperative staging by Lipiodol CT is still recommended (Fig. 9.15) (BISOLLON et al. 1998; CHOI et al. 1997; LENCIONI et al. 1997).

The CT location of the segment in which the tumor exists is determined in relation to hepatic and intrahepatic portal veins. The segmental location is usually determined on portal venous phase spiral CT images, in which intrahepatic veins are well opacified (FASEL et al. 1996). However, particularly when a small lesion is located at the boundary of the segments, it is not easy to determine segmental anatomy. When compared with authentic anatomical territories seen at anatomical examination, CT determination of portal venous territories within the liver was often found to be inaccurate (FASEL et al. 1998). CTAP, providing accurate delineation of the peripheral intrahepatic portal vein branches, results in more correct depiction of the complex and variable anatomical reality, and may be the ideal CT technique to determine the segmental or subsegmental location of a focal lesion.

The characteristics of the lesion, particularly with regard to the type of tumor growth (expanding or infiltrating), are usually well defined by spiral CT. CT identification of the tumor capsule is accurate in large tumors, but is less reliable in small lesions, which usually have a thin and poorly developed fibrous capsule (OLIVER et al. 1996).

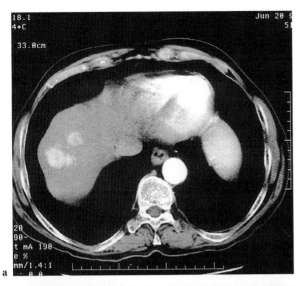

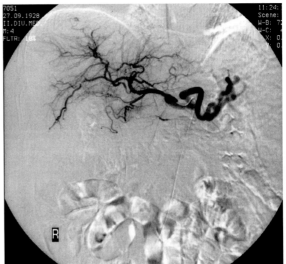

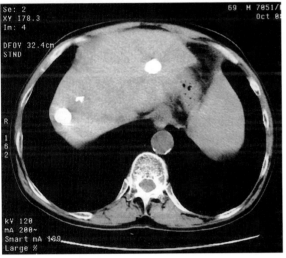

Fig. 9.15a–c. Multinodular HCC. Spiral CT acquired in the arterial phase (a) demonstrates two nodular lesions consistent with HCC. Following the angiographic study (b), anticancer iodized oil emulsion is injected into the proper hepatic artery. Subsequent unenhanced spiral CT study (c) obtained 4 weeks later confirms the two tumor nodules and shows an additional lesion undetected by previous examinations

Vascular invasion by the tumor is a crucial staging factor. A tendency to grow into the portal veins, eliciting tumor thrombi, is a feature peculiar to HCC. Spiral CT allows accurate identification of tumor thrombi in the main portal veins (NOVICK and FISHMAN 1998). Tumor thrombi are shown as solid masses in the blood vessels, with marked hypervascularity often seen on arterial phase spiral CT images. Arteriovenous shunting may be present within thrombi. The hepatic segment in which the feeding portal vein is obstructed demonstrates hyperperfusion abnormality on arterial phase CT images, as a result of arterial compensation and lack of dilution of the enhanced arterial blood with the unenhanced portal blood (Fig. 9.16). Reliable identification of tumor invasion in peripheral (segmental or subsegmental) portal vein branches is not possible with spiral CT and requires the use of CTAP. CTAP visualizes portal vein perfusion defects caused by thrombi as wedge-shaped hypodense areas including the tumor (CHOI 1995).

Lymphatic metastases in HCC are not common. They can be seen in about 10–15% of autopsy cases, especially in the hepatic hilar lymph nodes. Extrahepatic hematogenous metastases are usually associated with advanced-stage tumors. The lung is the most common site of metastases, followed by the bone and the adrenal gland. CT is valuable for the diagnosis of adenopathies and distant metastatic disease, except for bone metastases.

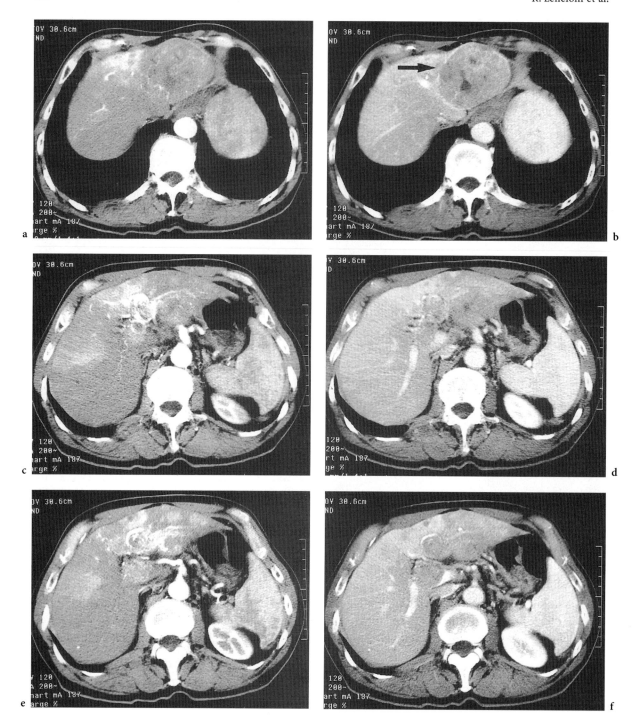

Fig. 9.16a–f. HCC with invasion of the portal vein and arterioportal shunting. Spiral CT images obtained in the arterial (**a**) and in the portal phase (**b**) show large HCC with extracapsular invasion (*arrow*). Spiral CT images obtained at two different caudal levels in the arterial (**c, e**) and in the portal phases (**d, f**) demonstrate tumor invasion into the portal vein and arterioportal shunting

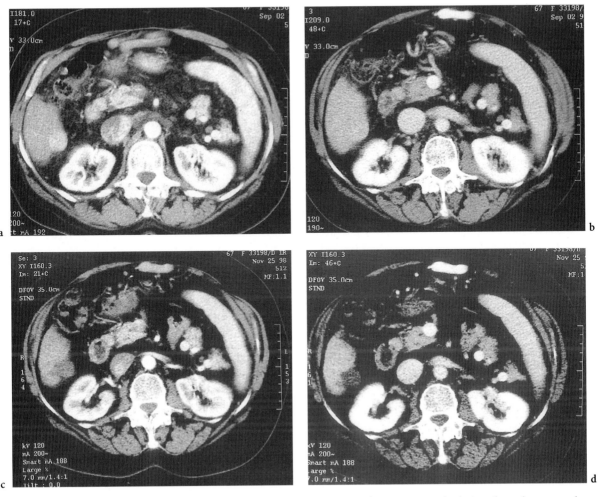

Fig. 9.17a–d. Small HCC treated with radiofrequency thermal ablation. Before treatment, the lesion shows hypervascular pattern and stands out in the arterial phase spiral CT image (**a**), while is undetectable in the portal venous phase, being isodense to liver (**b**). After percutaneous ablation, the tumor no longer enhances in both the arterial (**c**) and the portal phase (**d**) as a result of complete coagulation necrosis

9.7
Assessment of Tumor Response

Interventional procedures involving percutaneous tumor ablation have gained an increasingly important role in the treatment of HCC (LENCIONI et al. 1995a–c, 1997). After interventional therapies, diagnostic imaging has the key role in determining whether the treated lesion is completely ablated or contains areas of residual viable neoplastic tissue (LENCIONI et al. 1995b; BARTOLOZZI et al. 1998). This is particularly important, since in the case of incomplete necrosis of the lesion the treatment can be repeated and tumor ablation can be further pursued (BARTOLOZZI and LENCIONI 1996; BARTOLOZZI et al. 1995).

Spiral CT is recognized as the standard imaging modality for evaluating the response of HCC to interventional treatments. With spiral CT, lesions successfully treated by either percutaneous ethanol injection (PEI) or radiofrequency thermal ablation appear as hypoattenuating, nonenhancing areas in both the arterial and the portal venous phases (Fig. 9.17). In contrast, in the case of partial necrosis the areas of residual viable neoplastic tissue can be easily recognized as they stand out in the arterial phase against the faintly enhanced normal liver parenchyma and the unenhanced areas of coagulation necrosis (Fig. 9.18) (BARTOLOZZI et al. 1994a, b; LENCIONI et al. 1994).

If the imaging assessment of the outcome of therapy is performed shortly after the procedure,

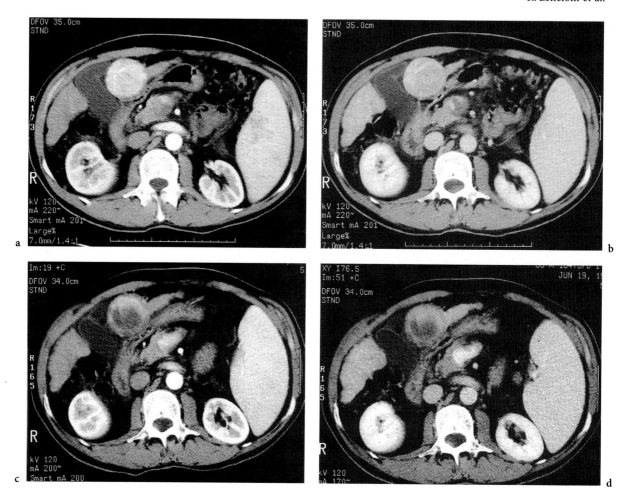

Fig. 9.18a–d. HCC with partial response after percutaneous ethanol injection. Before treatment, the tumor is definitely hyperattenuating in the arterial phase spiral CT image (**a**) and isoattenuating relative to liver parenchyma in the portal phase image (**b**). After therapy, a large area of necrosis which fails to enhance in both the arterial (**c**) and the portal phases (**d**) is depicted in the central portion of the tumor, while small residual viable tumor shows persistent arterial enhancement

however, spiral CT may show the presence of a peripheral halo surrounding the treated lesion. This halo, which may be irregular in shape and thickness, enhances predominantly in the arterial phase. This feature is due to the inflammatory reaction along the periphery of the area of coagulation necrosis, and is more pronounced after thermal ablation. The enhancing halo is depicted for several days after treatment, and has usually disappeared at later follow-up studies. It is of course of the utmost importance to be aware of this feature, to prevent misinterpretation of a peripheral inflammatory reaction associated with successful ablation as tumor progression. To make a reliable assessment, it is crucial to compare pretreatment and posttreatment studies performed according to the same technical examination protocol.

The enhancement pattern of the tumor-bearing area must be carefully examined to assess the out-

come of therapy. In particular, the finding of a wedge-shaped area of increased enhancement during the arterial phase in the vicinity of the treated lesion must be differentiated in terms of whether residual or recurrent infiltrative type of HCC is involved or whether a hyperperfusion abnormality is present. Hyperperfusion abnormalities following PEI may be caused by PEI-induced chemical thrombosis in the peripheral portal vein branches surrounding the lesion or by microscopic arteriovenous shunts produced by needle injury (LENCIONI et al. 1995a,c). Distinction between tumor progression and hyperperfusion abnormalities may be difficult, and requires accurate comparison of pretreatment and posttreatment studies (BECKER et al. 1997).

After transcatheter arterial oily chemoembolization, the degree of Lipiodol retention within the lesion shown by spiral CT helps predict the outcome

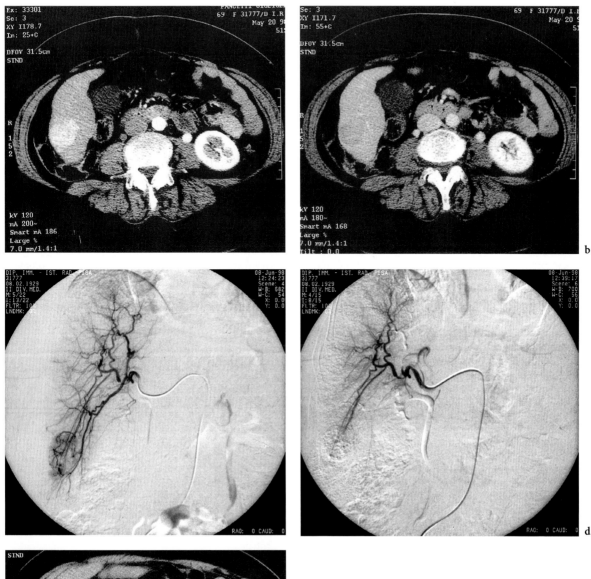

Fig. 9.19a–d. HCC treated with transcatheter arterial chemoembolization. Before treatment, the lesion is hyperdense in the arterial phase (**a**) and hypodense in the portal phase (**b**). Digital subtraction angiography confirms uninodular hypervascular tumor (**c**). After chemoembolization, devascularization of the tumor is seen angiographically (**d**). Unenhanced spiral CT performed 4 weeks later shows dense and homogeneous retention of iodized oil (**e**). Complete necrosis was shown at pathological examination of the resected specimen

of therapy: in fact, complete and homogeneous concentration of Lipiodol is usually associated with a favorable response to therapy, whereas partial and heterogeneous retention of iodized oil indicates a mi- nor response or no response (Fig. 9.19). However, limited persistence of tumor after treatment may sometimes be difficult to assess by CT, because the high attenuation of the iodized oil trapped within the lesion may not allow a confident interpretation of contrast-enhanced spiral CT studies (BARTOLOZZI et al. 1994b; LENCIONI et al. 1998).

A standard follow-up protocol for HCC patients who have undergone interventional procedures includes AFP level measurement and dual-phase spiral CT performed at 3- to 4-month intervals. Patients must be studied to diagnose either recurrences of the treated tumors or recurrences caused by the emergence of new nodular lesions. Complete response is considered to be obtained when no enhancing areas are seen at the level of the treated lesion at spiral CT, reduction in size persists during the follow-up, and serologic markers remain stable.

References

Bartolozzi C, Lencioni R (1996) Ethanol injection for the treatment of hepatic tumours. Eur Radiol 6:682–696

Bartolozzi C, Lencioni R, Caramella D, et al (1994a) Treatment of hepatocellular carcinoma with percutaneous ethanol injection: evaluation with contrast-enhanced MR imaging. AJR Am J Roentgenol 162:827–831

Bartolozzi C, Lencioni R, Caramella D, et al (1994b) Hepatocellular carcinoma: CT and MR features after transcatheter arterial embolization and percutaneous ethanol injection. Radiology 191:123–128

Bartolozzi C, Lencioni R, Caramella D, et al (1995) Treatment of large hepatocellular carcinoma: transcatheter arterial chemoembolization combined with percutaneous ethanol injection versus repeated transcatheter arterial chemoembolization. Radiology 197:812–818

Bartolozzi C, Lencioni R, Caramella D, Palla A, Bassi AM, Di Candio G (1996) Small hepatocellular carcinoma. Detection with US, CT, MR imaging, DSA, and Lipiodol-CT. Acta Radiol 37:69–74

Bartolozzi C, Lencioni R, Ricci P, Paolicchi A, Rossi P, Passariello R (1998) Hepatocellular carcinoma treatment with percutaneous ethanol injection: evaluation with contrast-enhanced color Doppler US. Radiology 209:387–393

Becker CD, Grossholz M, Mentha G, et al (1997) Ablation of hepatocellular carcinoma by percutaneous ethanol injection: imaging findings. Cardiovasc Intervent Radiol 20:204–210

Bisollon T, Rode A, Baricel B, et al (1998) Diagnostic value and tolerance of Lipiodol computed tomography for the detection of small hepatocellular carcinoma: correlation with pathologic examination of explanted livers. J Hepatol 28:491–496

Bluemke DA, Soyer P, Chan B, et al (1995) Spiral CT during arterial portography: techniques and application. RadioGraphics 15:633–637

Bonaldi VM, Bret PM, Reinhold C, Atri M (1995) Helical CT of the liver: value of an early hepatic arterial phase. Radiology 197:357–363

Choi BI (1995) Vascular invasion by hepatocellular carcinoma. Abdom Imaging 20:277–278

Choi BI, Takayasu K, Han MC, et al (1993) Small hepatocellular carcinomas and associated nodular lesions of the liver: pathology, pathogenesis and imaging findings. AJR Am J Roentgenol 160:1177–1187

Choi BI, Cho GM, Han JK, ct al (1996) Spiral CT for the detection of hepatocellular carcinoma: relative value of arterial and late phase scanning. Abdom Imaging 21:440–444

Choi BI, Lee HJ, Han JK, Choi DS, Seo JB, Han MC (1997) Detection of hypervascular nodular hepatocellular carcinomas: value of triphasic helical CT compared with iodized-oil CT. AJR Am J Roentgenol 168:219–224

Colombo M, De Franchis R, Del Ninno, et al (1991) Hepatocellular carcinoma in Italian patients with cirrhosis. N Engl J Med 325:675–680

Dodd GD, Miller WJ, Baron RL et al (1992) Detection of malignant tumors in end-stage cirrhotic livers: efficacy of sonography as a screening technique. AJR Am J Roentgenol 159:727–733

Fasel JH, Gailloud P, Terrier F, Mentha G, Sprumont P (1996) Segmental anatomy of the liver: a review and a proposal for an international working nomenclature. Eur Radiol 6:834–837

Fasel JH, Selle D, Evertsz CJ, Terrier F, Peitgen HO, Gailloud P (1998) Segmental anatomy of the liver: poor correlation with CT. Radiology 206:151–156

Fernandez MP, Redvanly RD (1998) Primary hepatic malignant neoplasms. Radiol Clin North Am 36:333–348

Freeny PC, Baron RL, Teefey SA (1992) Hepatocellular carcinoma: reduced frequency of typical findings with dynamic contrast enhanced CT in a non Asian population. Radiology 185:143–148

Grangier C, Tourniaire J, Mentha G, et al (1994) Enhancement of liver hemangiomas on T1-weighted MR SE images by superparamagnetic iron oxide particles. J Comput Assist Tomogr 18:888–896

Grossholz M, Terrier F, Rubbia L, et al (1998) Focal sparing in the fatty liver as a sign of an adjacent space-occupying lesion. AJR Am J Roentgenol 171:1391–1395

Hanafusa K, Ohashi I, Gomi N, Himeno Y, Wakita T, Shibuya H (1997) Differential diagnosis of early homogeneously enhancing hepatocellular carcinoma and hemangioma by two-phase CT. J Comput Assist Tomogr 21:361–368

Hollett MD, Jeffry RB Jr, Nino-Murcia M, et al (1995) Dual-phase helical CT of the liver: value of arterial phase scans in the detection of small (<1.5 cm) malignant hepatic neoplasms. AJR Am J Roentgenol 164:879–884

Hori M, Murakami T, Kim T, et al (1998) Sensitivity of double-phase helical CT during arterial portography for detection of hypervascular hepatocellular carcinoma. J Comput Assist Tomogr 22:861–867

Jang HJ, Choi BI, Kim TK, et al (1998) Atypical small hemangiomas of the liver: "bright dot" sign at two-phase spiral CT. Radiology 208:543–548

Kanai T, Hirohashi S, Upton M, et al (1987) Pathology of small hepatocellular carcinoma: a proposal for a new gross classification. Cancer 60:810–819

Kanematsu M, Oliver JH III, Carr B, Baron RL (1997) Hepatocellular carcinoma: the role of helical biphasic contrast-enhanced CT versus CT during arterial portography. Radiology 205:75–80

Kanematsu M, Kondo H, Enya M, Yokoyama R, Hoshi H (1998) Nondiseased portal perfusion defects adjacent to the right ribs shown on helical CT during arterial portography. AJR Am J Roentgenol 171:445–448

Kanematsu M, Hoshi H, Yamawaki Y, et al (1999) Angiographically assisted helical CT of the liver. AJR Am J Roentgenol 172:97–105

Kim SR, Hayashi Y, Matsuoka T, et al (1998a) A case of well-differentiated minute hepatocellular carcinoma with extrahepatic metastasis. J Gastroenterol Hepatol 13:892–896

Kim TK, Choi BI, Han JK, Chung JW, Park JH, Han MC (1998b) Nontumorous arterioportal shunt mimicking hypervascular tumor in cirrhotic liver: two-phase spiral CT findings. Radiology 208:597–603

Kitagaua K, Matsui O, Kadoya M, et al (1991) Hepatocellular carcinomas with excessive copper accumulation: CT and MR findings. Radiology 180:623–628

Krinsky GA, Theise ND, Rofsky NM, Mizrachi H, Tepperman LW, Weinreb JC (1998) Dysplastic nodules in cirrhotic liver: arterial phase enhancement at CT and MR imaging – a case report. Radiology 209:461–464

Lee HM, Lu DS, Krasny RM, Busuttil R, Kadell B, Lucas J (1997) Hepatic lesion characterization in cirrhosis: significance of arterial hypervascularity on dual-phase helical CT. AJR Am J Roentgenol 169:125–130

Lencioni R, Bartolozzi C (1997) Nonsurgical treatment of hepatocellular carcinoma. Cancer J 10:17–23

Lencioni R, Vignali C, Caramella D, et al (1994) Transcatheter arterial embolization followed by percutaneous ethanol injection in the treatment of hepatocellular carcinoma. Cardiovasc Intervent Radiol 17:70–75

Lencioni R, Bartolozzi C, Caramella D, et al (1995a) Treatment of small hepatocellular carcinoma with percutaneous ethanol injection: analysis of prognostic factors in 105 Western patients. Cancer 76:1737–1746

Lencioni R, Caramella D, Bartolozzi C (1995b) Hepatocellular carcinoma: use of color Doppler US to evaluate response to treatment with percutaneous ethanol injection. Radiology 194:113–118

Lencioni R, Caramella D, Sanguinetti F, Battolla L, Falaschi F, Bartolozzi C (1995c) Portal vein thrombosis after percutaneous ethanol injection for hepatocellular carcinoma: value of color Doppler sonography in distinguishing chemical and tumor thrombi. AJR Am J Roentgenol 164:1125–1130

Lencioni R, Mascalchi M, Caramella D, Bartolozzi C (1996a) Small hepatocellular carcinoma: differentiation from adenomatous hyperplasia with color Doppler US and dynamic Gd-DTPA-enhanced MR imaging. Abdom Imaging 21:41–48

Lencioni R, Pinto F, Armillotta N, Bartolozzi C (1996b) Assessment of tumor vascularity in hepatocellular carcinoma: comparison of power Doppler US and color Doppler US. Radiology 201:353–358

Lencioni R, Pinto F, Armillotta N, et al (1997a) Long-term results of percutaneous ethanol injection therapy for hepatocellular carcinoma in cirrhosis: a European experience. Eur Radiol 7:514–519

Lencioni R, Pinto F, Armillotta N, et al (1997b) Intrahepatic metastatic nodules of hepatocellular carcinoma detected at Lipiodol-CT: imaging-pathologic correlation. Abdom Imaging 22:253–258

Lencioni R, Paolicchi A, Moretti M, et al (1998) Combined transcatheter arterial chemoembolization and percutaneous ethanol injection for the treatment of large hepatocellular carcinoma: local therapeutic effect and long-term survival rate. Eur Radiol 8:439–444

Matsui O, Kadoya M, Kameyama T, et al (1991) Benign and malignant nodules in cirrhotic livers: distinction based on blood supply. Radiology 178:493–497

Matsui O, Takahashi S, Kadoya M, et al (1994) Pseudolesion in segment IV of the liver at CT during arterial portography: correlation with aberrant gastric venous drainage. Radiology 193:31–35

Merine D, Takayasu K, Wakao F (1990) Detection of hepatocellular carcinoma: comparison of CT during arterial portography with CT after intraarterial injection of iodized oil. Radiology 175:707–710

Mitsukaki K, Yamashita Y, Ogata I et al (1996) Multiple phase helical-CT of the liver for detecting small hepatomas in patients with liver cirrhosis: contrast-injection protocol and optimal timing. AJR Am J Roentgenol 167:753–757

Nakakuma Y, Terada T, Ueda K, et al (1993) Adenomatous hyperplasia of the liver as a precancerous lesion. Liver 13:1–9

Nelson RC, Chezmar JL, Sugarbaker TH, et al (1990) Preoperative localization of focal liver lesions to specific liver segments: utility of CT during arterial portography. Radiology 176:89–94

Novick SL, Fishman EK (1998) Portal vein thrombosis: spectrum of helical CT and CT angiographic findings. Abdom Imaging 23:505–510

Oi H, Murakami T, Kim T, et al (1996) Dynamic MR imaging and early-phase helical CT for detecting small intrahepatic metastases of hepatocellular carcinoma. AJR Am J Roentgenol 166:369–374

Oka H, Kurioka M, Kim K, et al (1990) Prospective study of early detection of hepatocellular carcinoma in patients with cirrhosis. Hepatology 12:680–687

Oliver JH III, Baron RL (1996) Helical biphasic contrast-enhanced CT of the liver: technique, indications, interpretation and pitfalls. Radiology 201:1–14

Oliver JH III, Baron RL, Federle MP, et al (1996) Detecting hepatocellular carcinoma: value of unenhanced or arterial phase CT imaging or both, used in conjunction with conventional portal venous phase contrast-enhanced CT imaging. AJR Am J Roentgenol 167:71–77

Oliver JH III, Baron RL, Federle MP, Jones BC, Sheng R (1997) Hypervascular liver metastases: do unenhanced and hepatic arterial phase CT images affect tumor detection? Radiology 205:709–715

Ohtomo K, Baron RJ, Dodd GD, et al (1993) Confluent hepatic fibrosis in advanced cirrhosis: appearance at CT. Radiology 188:31–35

Pateron D, Ganne N, Trinchet J, et al (1994) Prospectiv study of screening of hepatocellular carcinoma in Caucasian patients with cirrhosis. J Hepatol 20:65–71

Rofflett MD, Jeffrey RB, Nino Murcia M, et al (1995) Dual phase helical CT of the liver: value of arterial phase scans in the detection of small (< 1.5 cm) malignant hepatic neoplasms. AJR Am J Roentgenol 164:879–884

Ros PR, Buck JL, Goodman ID, et al (1988) Intrahepatic cholangiocarcinoma: radiologic-pathologic correlation. Radiology 167:689–693

Ros PR, Murphy BJ, Back JL, et al (1990) Encapsulated hepatocellular carcinoma: radiologic findings and pathological correlation. Gastrointest Radiol 15:233–237

Rubin GD, Dake MD, Napel SA, et al (1993) Three dimensional spiral CT angiography of the abdomen: initial clinical experience. Radiology 186:147–152

Rummeny EJ, Marchal G (1997) Liver imaging. Clinical applications and future perspectives. Acta Radiol 38:626–630

Small WC, Mehard WB, Langmo LS, et al (1993) Preoperative determination of the resectability of hepatic tumors; efficacy of CT during arterial portography. AJR Am J Roentgenol 161:319–322

Soyer P, Bluemke DA, Bliss DF, et al (1994) Surgical segmental anatomy of the liver: demonstration with spiral CT during arterial portography and multiplanar reconstruction. AJR Am J Roentgenol 163:99–103

Takayama T, Makuuchi M, Hirahashi S, et al (1990) Malignant transformation of adenomatous hyperplasia to hepatocellular carcinoma. Lancet 336:1150–1153

Takayasu K, Moriyama N, Muramatsu Y, et al (1990) The diagnosis of small hepatocellular carcinomas: efficacy of various imaging procedures in 100 patients. AJR Am J Roentgenol 155:49–54

Takayasu K, Muramatsu Y, Furukawa H, et al (1995a) Early hepatocellular carcinoma: appearance at CT during arterial portography and CT arteriography with pathologic correlation. Radiology 194:101–105

Takayasu K, Furukawa H, Wakao F, et al (1995b) CT diagnosis of early hepatocellular carcinoma: sensitivity, findings, and CT pathologic correlation. AJR Am J Roentgenol 164:885–890

Tillich M, Mischinger HJ, Preisegger KH, Rabl H, Szolar DH (1998) Multiphasic helical CT in diagnosis and staging of hilar cholangiocarcinoma. AJR Am J Roentgenol 171:651–658

Tourel PG, Pageaux GP, Coste V, et al (1995) Small hepatocellular carcinoma in patients undergoing liver transplantation: detection with CT after injection of iodized oil. Radiology 197:377–380

Tublin ME, Tessler FN, Cheng SL, Peters TL, McGovern PC (1999) Effect of injection rate of contrast medium on pancreatic and hepatic helical CT. Radiology 210:97–101

Ueda K, Kitigawa K, Kadoya M, et al (1995) Detection of hypervascular hepatocellular carcinoma by using spiral volumetric CT: comparison of US and MR imaging. Abdom Imaging 20:547–554

Ueda K, Matsui O, Kawamori Y, et al (1998) Differentiation of hypervascular hepatic pseudolesions from hepatocellular carcinoma: value of single-level dynamic CT during hepatic arteriography. J Comput Assist Tomogr 22:703–708

van Hoe L, Baert AL, Gryspeerdt S, et al (1997) Dual-phase helical-CT of the liver: value of an early phase acquisition in the differential diagnosis of non-cystic focal lesions. AJR Am J Roentgenol 169:1185–1192

Yamashita Y, Fan ZM, Yamamoto H, et al (1993) Sclerosing hepatocellular carcinoma: radiologic findings. Abdom Imaging 18:347–351

Yoshikawa J, Matsui O, Takashima T, et al (1988) Fatty metamorphosis in hepatocellular carcinoma: radiologic features in 10 cases. AJR Am J Roentgenol 151:717–720

Yoshikawa J, Matsui O, Kadoya M, et al (1992) Delayed enhancement of fibrotic areas in hepatic masses: CT-pathologic correlation. J Comput Assist Tomogr 16:206–211

10 Perfusion Disorders

G. Verswijvel, L. Van Hoe, G. Marchal

CONTENTS

10.1   Introduction   *133*
10.2   Imaging Technique   *134*
10.3   Portal Venous Inflow Obstruction   *135*
10.4   Hepatic Venous Outflow Obstruction   *136*
10.5   Mediastinal or Thoracic Inlet Venous
        Obstruction   *137*
10.6   Coexistence of Hepatic Arterial and
        Portal Venous Obstruction   *138*
10.7   Focal Liver Lesions   *138*
10.7.1 Portal Venous Obstruction or Compression   *138*
10.7.2 Arterioportal Shunting Secondary to Focal
        Liver Lesions   *138*
10.7.3 Steal Phenomena by Hypervascular
        Tumours or 'Siphoning'   *140*
10.8   Perfusion Disorders Caused By
        Inflammatory Changes   *141*
10.9   Variants in the Hepatic Vascular Anatomy   *143*
10.10   Perfusion Disorders Related to Transjugular
        Intrahepatic Portosystemic Shunts   *143*
10.11   Unexplained Hepatic Perfusion Disorders   *146*
        References   *146*

10.1
Introduction

The liver, as the largest parenchymal organ in the abdomen (constituting 2.5% of the total body weight), is 'blessed' with a meritorious dual blood supply via the hepatic artery and the portal vein. It receives about 25–30% of the total cardiac output. The majority of the hepatic blood flow volume, i.e. 75–80%, is supplied by the portal vein and is nutrient-rich blood, and the remaining 20–25% comes from the hepatic artery, which supplies mainly oxygen-rich blood. However, each of these vessels is

G. Verswijvel, MD; Department of Radiology, University Hospital Gasthuisberg, Herestraat 49, B-3000 Leuven, Belgium
L. Van Hoe, MD; Department of Radiology, University Hospital Gasthuisberg, Herestraat 49, B-3000 Leuven, Belgium
G. Marchal, MD; Department of Radiology, University Hospitals K.U.L., Herestraat 49, B-3000 Leuven, Belgium

responsible for about 50% of the total hepatic oxygen supply (Takayasu and Okuda 1997a).

The hepatic artery and its branches divide and further subdivide in the liver, their smaller rami being associated with those of the portal vein, which also divide in the liver. The smallest microvascular unit of the liver is the hepatic acinus, representing a cluster of parenchymal cells grouped around terminal branches of the hepatic arteriole and portal venule, as described by Rappaport in 1973. Blood is delivered to the liver initially via the hepatic artery, and approximately 19 s later by the portal vein (Baron 1994). The former delivery phase is known as the 'hepatic arterial phase' (HAP), and the latter, as the 'portal venous phase' (PVP). The blood is then conveyed from the liver to the inferior vena cava via the hepatic veins. The HAP and PVP can be studied elegantly by mean of double-phase (or dual-phase) contrast-enhanced spiral-computed tomography (SCT) (Marchal and Baert 1992; Bonaldi et al. 1995) (Fig. 10.1). The early hepatic arterial phase corresponds to the first passage of contrast material from the aorta into the hepatic artery and its branches. Since the blood supplied via the hepatic artery is 30% at most of the total amount, the contrast will be diluted by the nonopacified portal venous blood, resulting in only moderate enhancement of the liver parenchyma. The liver density will increase further during the second portal venous phase (Marchal 1992; Marchal and Baert 1992).

Perfusion disorders, reflecting a haemodynamic change in the normal blood supply to the liver, are defined as 'any disturbance of homogeneous enhancement of the liver during either the hepatic arterial phase or the portal venous phase at double phase SCT' (Gryspeerdt et al. 1997). Numerous causes are known to be related to hepatic perfusion disorders: portal venous inflow obstruction, hepatic venous outflow obstruction, mediastinal or thoracic venous inlet obstruction, focal liver lesions, inflammation, placement of a transjugular intrahepatic portosystemic shunt (TIPS) and hepatic vascular anatomical variants. However, sometimes the background of

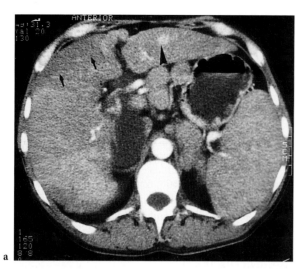

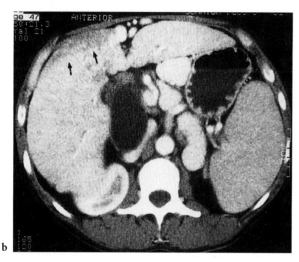

Fig. 10.1 a HAP shows a focal area of high attenuation (*arrowheads*) in the left lobe of the liver in a patient with liver cirrhosis. A subcapsular region of low attenuation is seen in the anterior part of the right lobe (*arrows*). **b** PVP image shows isodensity of the previously high attenuation area, with the surrounding parenchyma (final diagnosis was a hepatocellular carcinoma). The subcapsular wedge-shaped area of altered perfusion is still seen and has increased in density; it is due to confluent fibrosis. Note the large enhancing collateral vessels

certain perfusion disorders, as seen on dual-phase SCT, can (yet) not readily be explained.

In this chapter we describe and discuss the different groups of hepatic perfusion disorders detected by SCT. We attempt to demonstrate that careful analysis of the imaging features of perfusion disorders, which are not at random, is the key to the underlying cause. Recognition of certain types of attenuation differences caused by perfusion disorders will help to differentiate or to exclude underlying diseases, bearing in mind that perfusion disorders

sometimes are masters in mimicking tumour lesions (VAN BEERS et al. 1990). 'When the doors of perception are cleansed, man will see things as they truly are...' (William Blake).

10.2
Imaging Technique

Conventional incremental scanning requires approximately 1.5–2.5 min to image the entire liver. Therefore, with this type of scanners, biphasic injection protocols are necessary both (a) to obtain optimal contrast with high peak hepatic enhancement and (b) to delay the equilibrium phase (HEIKEN 1998). It becomes clear that it is not possible to scan the entire liver during both HAP and PVP phases of enhancement by mean of incremental scanning. In contrast, helical or spiral CT does have this ability. The entire liver can now be scanned during a single 19- to 29-s breath hold, allowing brilliant imaging of both vascular phases with elimination of motion artefacts and respiratory misregistration and resultant improved diagnostic performance, with single-phase injection protocols. Several studies have demonstrated improved detection of hepatic vascular disorders with the aid of dual-phase SCT (BONALDI et al. 1995; MURATA et al. 1995). This type of scanning requires optimization of the rate of injection of contrast material and of the delay between injection and the initiation of scanning (injection–scan delay time). A typical dual-phase SCT protocol for liver imaging consists of a uniphasic injection of 150 ml of iodinated contrast i.v. at 3–5 ml/s. This rapid injection rate maximizes hepatic arterial enhancement and separates optimal both HAP and PVP of parenchymal enhancement, which is necessary for adequate imaging studies (VAN HOE et al. 1997; HEIKEN 1998; HALAVAARA et al. 1996). The use of faster injection rates than 2 ml/s does not increase hepatic peak enhancement but may help to increase the magnitude of arterial enhancement (BAE et al. 1998). The optimal injection-scan delay time has to be the result of both extrinsic (volume of contrast injected and rate- and duration of injection) and intrinsic (patient weight, cardiac output, vascular conditions) factors. Therefore it is difficult to state this optimal injection–scan delay as an absolute number of seconds, but generally it is accepted that the first phase of scanning has to begin 20–25 s after the start of contrast injection (HEIKEN 1998). Images in the portal venous phase must be obtained during peak enhancement, i.e. after approximately 70–80 s, depending on the speed of contrast injection (if 'previous'-generation scanners are used than the portal venous phase should be initiated 'as soon as possible' after scanning the HAP, i.e. approximately 50–65 s after the start of contrast injection). As a consequence, images can be obtained during the arterial phase together with portal-venous phase images, during a single bolus injection. A pitch of 1–1.5 can be used to allow completion of each phase during the appropriate scanning time interval. The reconstruction interval (RI) depends on the slice thickness (ST) and table feed (TF). Semi-automated bolus-tracking software programs have been introduced by SILVERMAN and co-workers to individualize scanning protocols (SILVERMAN et al. 1996). Such bolus-tracking devices have proved their accuracy in timing the hepatic arterial phase and in advantaging the mean parenchymal enhancement in the portal venous phase (KOPKA et al. 1996).

10.3
Portal Venous Inflow Obstruction

Causes of obliteration of the portal vein can be extra- or intrahepatic. Extrahepatic portal venous obstruction can be the result of neoplastic involvement, thrombosis, extrinsic compression of the portal vein (e.g. by tumour or haematoma), congenital portal vein malformation, iatrogenic (e.g. splenectomy) or due to increased pressure on the hepatic parenchyma (e.g. by a subcapsular liver haematoma; TAKAYASU and OKUDA 1997). Intrahepatic (or prehepatic or presinusoidal) obliteration of the portal inflow can be due to narrowing of portal venules as a result of inflammation and fibrosis of the portal tract. Underlying causes can be cirrhosis, sarcoidosis, amyloidosis, Hodgkin's disease, chronic myelogenous leukaemia or schistosomiasis (TAKAYASU and OKUDA 1997).

In cases of obstruction of main portal venous inflow, extrinsic and intrinsic regulatory mechanisms will take effect, altering the hepatic blood supply to compensate the reduction in the portal supply (IMAEDA et al. 1991). In 1987 LAUTT and GREENWAY introduced the concept of the hepatic arterial buffer response as an important form of intrinsic blood flow regulation. If the portal blood flow is reduced, less adenosine, which is continuously secreted into the space of Mall (which surrounds the arterial resistance vessels and portal venules), is washed away, leading to dilatation of the hepatic artery and subsequently increasing the hepatic arterial inflow. In other words, when the blood flow through the portal vein is diminished or obstructed, the liver will try to compensate this shortening by reactively increasing its hepatic arterial blood supply. It can be described in a metaphor as a 'Robin Hood' phenomenon: stealing the blood from the rich (the arterial supply) and giving it to the poor (the portal supply).

This event can present itself via two different patterns. First, regional arterial inflow can be compensatorily increased in the area where portal inflow is reduced. This type of regulatory inflow compensation can be seen in the case of tumour thrombus, thrombo-embolus, and compression or stricture of the portal vein. It presents in the HAP image as a relatively homogeneous area of focal high attenuation with undefined borders, in a lobar, segmental or subsegmental distribution. The second pattern consists of a heterogeneous peripheral increase of arterial inflow, which is seen in the HAP image as multiple peripheral focal high attenuation areas, with unsharp borders, in a nonsegmental distribution (Fig. 10.2). This pattern has been reported in cases of cavernous transformation of the thrombosed main portal vein, where collateral vessels supply the central periportal regions better than the peripheral areas. The diminished blood supply to these peripheral regions will be compensated by the hepatic artery. Both phenomena are referred to as transient hepatic attenuation differences (THAD). This concept was described and defined by ITAI et al. in 1987 as 'attenuation differences of the liver appearing during bolus enhanced dynamic CT, not corresponding to mass lesions, and caused by locally altered haemodynamics.' Other causes of THAD are arterioportal shunting, steal phenomena by hypervascular tumours, hyperaemia, congestion and systemic-portal shunting (ITAI et al. 1982).

Neither pattern shows attenuation differences on PVP images, and usually no hepatic parenchymal density alterations will be seen on plain CT. There are other flow phenomena that can accompany portal venous thrombosis in certain circumstances. First, arterio-portal shunting can sometimes occur, for instance as a secondary phenomenon in hepatocellular carcinoma (HCC) complicated by portal thrombosis. This is seen on HAP images as enhancement of the affected portal branch during early arterial contrast enhancement (HEIKEN 1998). Second, owing to increased pressure in and dilatation of the vasa vasorum of the portal vein, a peripheral rim enhancement of the latter can be present on post-contrast images.

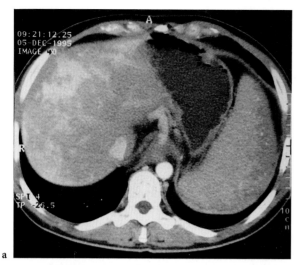

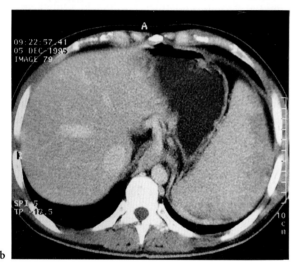

Fig. 10.2a, b. A patient with thrombosis of the main portal vein. **a** HAP image shows multiple areas of high attenuation, with unsharp borders, in the periphery of the right liver lobe. **b** These areas are isoattenuating with the surrounding parenchyma on PVP images

10.4
Hepatic Venous Outflow Obstruction

Hepatic venous outflow block can be due to Budd-Chiari syndrome (BAERT et al. 1989; MATHIEU et al. 1987), congestive right-sided cardiac failure (HOWARD et al. 1989), pericardial disease, mediastinal fibrosis and hepatic vein or IVC compression. Budd-Chiari syndrome, or hepatic veno-occlusive disease, was defined by LEEVY et al. in 1994 as an occlusion of the hepatic veins and their tributaries. However, as hepatic venous outflow block can also be caused by obstruction of the inferior vena cava above the entrance of the hepatic veins (TAKAYASU

and OKUDA 1997a), the definition of 'classic' Budd-Chiari syndrome has to be extended to describe related hepatic perfusion disorders.

Hepatic venous outflow obstruction will increase postsinusoidal intravascular pressure (hepatic venous hypertension), resulting in dilatation of the central veins and hepatic sinusoids. Hepatomegaly may be present. Stasis of blood in the sinusoids occurs, and eventually the flow in the portal vein may be reversed (MURATA et al. 1995; MATHIEU et al. 1987), turning the portal vein into the main hepatic draining branch. Hepatic lymphatic vessels will also increase in size and volume (ASPESTRAND et al. 1991). The latter, together with the inversion of the portal flow, may be the background of the diffuse, heterogeneous patchy enhancement on the HAP images, reflecting a 'mosaic' or reticular pattern (Fig. 10.3) (GRYSPEERDT et al. 1997; TAKAYSU and OKUDA 1997b). The abnormal enhancement can also be related to very slow blood flow secondary to hepatic venous obstruction or to hepatic venous hypertension (HOLLEY et al. 1989). MURATA and co-workers showed that since there is a relative increase in arterial supply and there is no dilution of the supplied contrast with portal blood, the occluded area can be hyperenhancing on the HAP images (MURATA et al. 1995). Initial PVP images, in contrast, can show prolonged existence of this patchy enhancement pattern, since the hepatofugal portal blood flow in the occluded area is delayed because of the small sinusoidal-portal vein pressure gradient. This prolonged enhancement will disappear approximately 5–10 min after contrast injection.

Although this abnormal enhancement pattern can be quite similar in patients with congestive heart failure, pericardial disease, mediastinal fibrosis or Budd-Chiari syndrome, there are important differences in the CT features of these different entities. Disproportionate enlargement of the caudate lobe is common in (partial and chronic) Budd-Chiari syndrome, occurring in up to 80% of cases (BAERT et al. 1983), whereas in passive hepatic congestion this phenomena only occurs in 8% (HOLLEY et al. 1989). In contrast to the marked heterogeneous enhancement of the remainder of the hepatic parenchyma, a more homogeneous, unaffected, enhancement of the caudate lobe can be seen in the case of Budd-Chiari syndrome, since the caudate lobe has its own draining veins, which are directly connected with the IVC and are usually spared from disease affecting the main hepatic veins (GRYSPEERDT et al. 1997; BAERT et al. 1983). Distension of the retrohepatic inferior vena cava (IVC) is always present in patients with

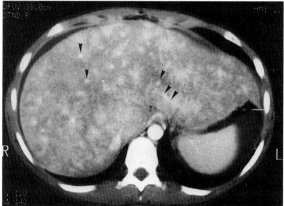

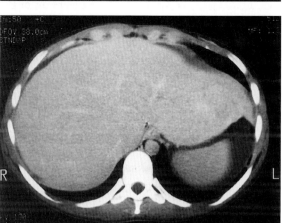

Fig. 10.3a, b. Hepatic venous outflow block in a patient with Budd-Chiari syndrome. **a** HAP image: a diffuse heterogeneous 'patchy' enhancement of the liver parenchyma is seen. Enhancement of small intrahepatic portal vein branches, which serve as draining veins, is also noted (*arrowheads*). Initial PVP images (not shown) revealed persistence of this patchy enhancement pattern. **b** On late (i.e. after 10 min) PVP images the prolonged enhancement has disappeared

congestive heart failure, while in the Budd-Chiari syndrome the retrohepatic IVC is usually narrow as a result of hypertrophy of the caudate lobe. The hepatic veins are not enhanced and do not contain thrombi in Budd-Chiari syndrome. On the other hand, in patients with congestive heart failure or pericardial disease, the hepatic vein orifices may be opacified by reflux of contrast from the IVC, or partial visualization of the hepatic veins (HOLLEY et al. 1989) can result from the same mechanism. Also, in patients with severe congestive heart failure prominent perivascular zones of diminished attenuation within the liver can occur secondary to perivascular lymphoedema (KOSLIN et al. 1988). Thrombotic hepatic veins in Budd-Chiari syndrome can present on CT as hypodense structures surrounded by rim en-

hancement owing to opacification of the vasa vasorum, a phenomena described by ZERHOUNI et al. in 1980. And last but not least, Budd-Chiari syndrome is classically associated with ascites.

Large right-sided adrenal tumours can sometimes cause compression of the right hepatic vein near its confluence with the IVC. As a consequence they can cause local perfusion disorders with attenuation differences similar to those seen in hepatic venous outflow obstruction from other causes (ITAI et al. 1995a).

10.5
Mediastinal or Thoracic Inlet Venous Obstruction

Obstruction of the thoracic inlet veins or superior vena cava can be caused by space-occupying lesions, granulomatous disorders, thrombosis or trauma (ENGEL et al. 1983). Four major interconnected collateral pathways between the superior and inferior vena cava exist: the azygos-hemiazygos route, the vertebral venous system (vertebral veins and vertebral venous plexus), the internal mammary veins and the lateral thoracic route (consisting of the lateral thoracic, thoraco-epigastric and superficial epigastric veins; ENGEL et al. 1983; GRYSPEERDT et al. 1997; ISHIKAWA et al. 1983). As a consequence, the hepatic blood supply will be increased in the case of obstruction of the thoracic inlet veins or superior vena cava. This phenomenon occurs because the azygos-hemiazygos veins and the vertebral venous system communicates with the IVC, and the lateral thoracic and internal mammary system interconnects with the superficial epigastric and paraumbilical veins, further communicating with the portal vein along the falciform ligament and ligamentum teres. The pattern of intrahepatic distribution will depend on quantitative and qualitative parameters of the interconnections between the umbilical and portal system. Strong enhancement on the HAP image can be seen in the hepatic region that receives extra blood supply via collateral pathways (best seen when contrast is injected in an antecubital vein in the arm). Most commonly this phenomena occur in the ventral part of the quadrate lobe (Fig. 10.4), but other distributions may also occur. Early enhancement of the IVC can be seen (due to collateral circulation with early enhancement of the azygos and hemiazygos veins). On PVP images the area involved will have equal attenuation to the surrounding liver

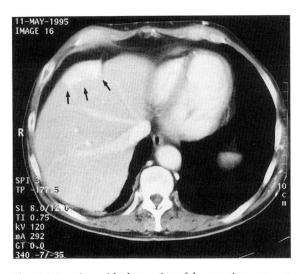

Fig. 10.4. A patient with obstruction of the superior vena cava secondary to a primary lung carcinoma. Late HAP image shows hyperattenuation of segment 4, or the quadrate lobe (*arrows*), and marked enhancement of the azygos and homozygous veins. As a consequence, early enhancement of the inferior vena cava can be seen

parenchyma. An interesting note is that this type of collateral supply can be responsible for a 'hot spot' in the liver on radionuclide scans (ENGEL et al. 1983).

10.6
Coexistence of Hepatic Arterial and Portal Venous Obstruction

Simultaneous obstruction of the arterial and the portal blood supply of any causation will result in an area of parenchymal infarction. Typical CT features of hepatic infarct are hypoattenuation of the involved area on plain and enhanced CT in an anatomical distribution (ITAI et al. 1995a,b).

10.7
Focal Liver Lesions

Focal liver lesions can alter the hepatic blood supply in three different ways: portal venous obstruction or compression, arterioportal shunting and steal phenomena. Each of these haemodynamic alterations can be present alone or can coexist with one or both other mechanisms. If a local or general perfusion disorder in the liver is seen, the possibility of a caus-

ative focal liver lesion should always be borne in mind (Itai et al. 1986a,b). It is becoming clear that these lesion-related flow-phenomena can only be studied adequately by mean of dual-phase SCT.

10.7.1
Portal Venous Obstruction or Compression

As discussed above, focal hepatic lesions can cause obstruction of portal venous inflow. This will alter the local hepatic blood supply, reactively increasing local hepatic arterial inflow, which will try to compensate for the reduction. As described earlier, this will be reflected on HAP images as a regional, subsegmental area of increased attenuation adjacent to the causative liver lesion (Fig. 10.5). On PVP images this region typically will not show any density difference from the surrounding hepatic parenchyma (ITAI et al. 1987). If these wedge-shaped perfusion disorders are noted on HAP images, one should always be aware that there may be an underlying focal lesion (Fig. 10.6, 10.7), which itself is not always clearly visualized, since even very small lesions can produce this type of flow alteration (GRYSPEERDT et al. 1997). The same perfusion disorders caused by focal hepatic lesions can of course be ascertained by means of magnetic resonance imaging (Fig. 10.8).

10.7.2
Arterioportal Shunting Secondary to Focal Liver Lesions

Focal liver lesions can directly induce arterioportal shunts or fistula via two major mechanisms. A shunting phenomenon can occur via a tumour thrombus in a portal vein (i.e. the 'transvasal type') or it can be generated in the tumour itself (i.e. the 'transtumoral type'; ITAI et al. 1995a,b; INOUE et al. 1998). These shunts will cause increased arterial inflow in the affected area. In addition, there may be a coexisting so-called transplexal route of blood supply via small peribiliary arterial branches (ITAI et al. 1995a,b). However, the exact role and impact of this transplexal support is not well understood. The phenomenon of arterioportal shunting can be detected on HAP images as areas of high attenuation. Its pattern differs from the portal venous obstruction type in that it is usually wedge-shaped and located peripheral to the underlying tumour (GRYSPEERDT et al. 1997). The portal vein will show early enhance-

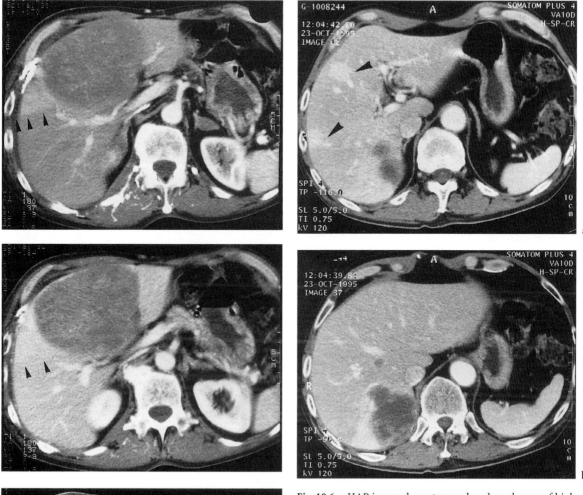

Fig. 10.6. a HAP image shows two wedge-shaped areas of high attenuation. These are due to small underlying metastases, which cannot be clearly seen (*arrowheads*). Note the large hypodense lesions, compatible with larger liver metastases. On PVP images the areas of altered perfusion are isoattenuating with the normal liver parenchyma (not shown). b A large metastasis in segment 6 is causing the same type of perfusion disorder adjacent to the inferior margin of the lesion

◁Fig. 10.5. a HAP image shows a triangular area of hyperattenuation adjacent to the border of a large hepatic tumour (*arrowheads*). b In the PVP and c on late images the area of altered perfusion shows the same density as the adjacent normal liver parenchyma

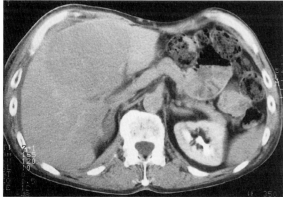

ment, a finding that is typical in cases of shunting (SUDHIR and TEAL 1989). This is an important feature in the differential diagnosis of other causes of transient high-attenuation phenomena. The affected area has normal attenuation characteristics on PVP images.

An interesting note is that huge tumours that cause obstruction of the ipsilateral main portal vein branch may cause early enhancement of the contralateral parenchyma and contralateral main portal vein branch, diagnostic of tumour-induced arterioportal shunting. On plain CT, the area involved in arterioportal shunting occasionally present as fanshaped or wedge-shaped areas of low density (ITAI et al. 1995a,b).

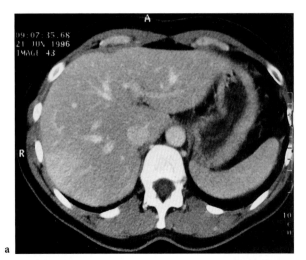

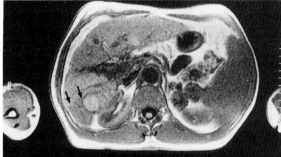

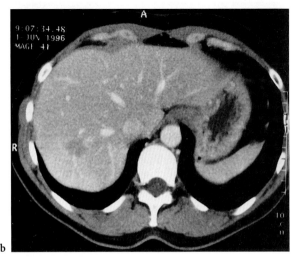

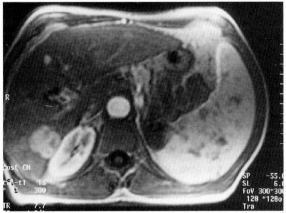

Fig. 10.8a,b. A patient with multifocal hepatocellular carcinoma. a T1-weighted TurboFLASH image: a large hyperintense lesion with hypointense rim is seen in segment 6; the posterior adjacent parenchyma (*arrows*) is slightly hypointense. b The latter shows increased attenuation after administration of gadolinium, owing to either portal venous obstruction by the tumour or arterioportal shunting

Fig. 10.7. a Early PVP image shows a triangular subcapsular high attenuation area in the right lobe. b PVP image, obtained at a different level, reveals an underlying focal liver lesion at the top of the area of altered perfusion

10.7.3
Steal Phenomena Caused by Hypervascular Tumours or 'Siphoning'

Siphoning or the siphonage phenomenon is caused by hypervascular tumours, which sometimes tend to attract or 'steal' blood from their surrounding (normal) parenchyma. The latter will appear as a hypoattenuating area surrounding the hyperattenuating tumour on the HAP images, as a consequence of the steal phenomenon (GRYSPEERDT et al. 1997; ITAI et al. 1995a,b). PVP images will not show any attenuation differences (Fig. 10.9). Siphoning can be seen on one or both sides of a hypervascular tumour (ITAI et al. 1995a,b).

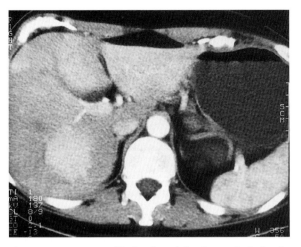

Fig. 10.9. A woman with focal nodular hyperplasia in the right liver lobe. a A hypervascular tumour is seen on the late HAP image. The parenchyma adjacent to the lesion is hypoattenuating (compare with the left lobe) possibly due to siphoning.

10.8
Perfusion Disorders Caused by Inflammatory Changes

Inflammatory conditions are associated with secondary arterial hyperaemia and concomitant increased local venous drainage. Abscess formation can be complicated with portal venous flow obstruction. Either phenomenon may be the underlying cause of perfusion disorders associated with inflammatory conditions. Acute cholecystitis (Fig. 10.10) or hepatic abscesses (Fig. 10.11) may be accompanied by transient increased attenuation of the liver parenchyma adjacent to the inflammatory focus on HAP images, as a result of the secondary changes mentioned above. On plain CT these areas are isodense in comparison with the surrounding

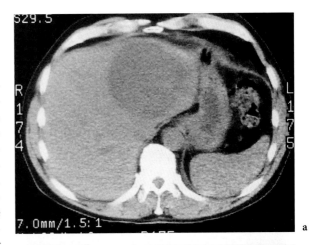

a

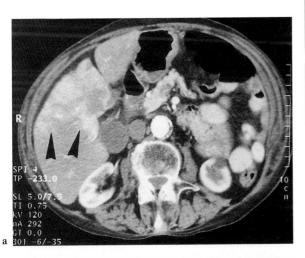

a

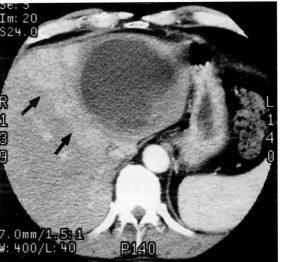

b

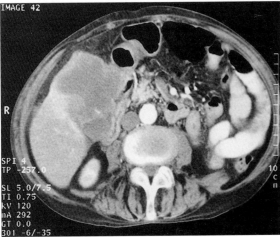

b

Fig. 10.10a, b. Acute cholecystitis accompanied with increased attenuation of the adjacent liver parenchyma on the HAP image (*arrowheads*)

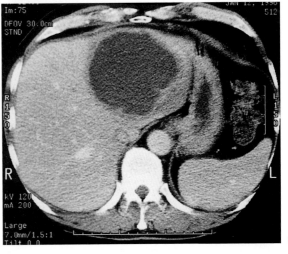

c

Fig. 10.11a–c. A 61-year old patient with an amoebic abscess in the left lobe of the liver. **a** Precontrast image: a large round hypodense lesion is seen. **b** HAP image shows an irregular area of high attenuation in the adjacent parenchyma (*arrows*). **c** This area of altered perfusion is isodense with the surrounding normal parenchyma on PVP images

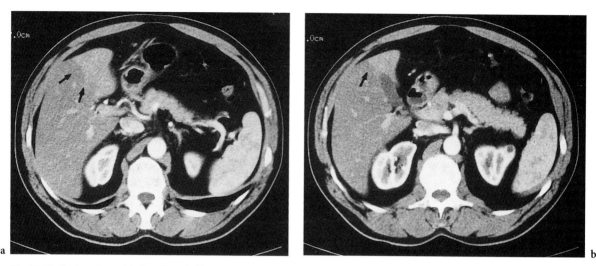

Fig. 10.12a, b. A patient with fatty liver infiltration with a 'skip area' in segment 4. This area is hyperattenuating on HAP images, owing to early inflow of blood via the systemic pathway (*arrows*) due to an altered vascular anatomy

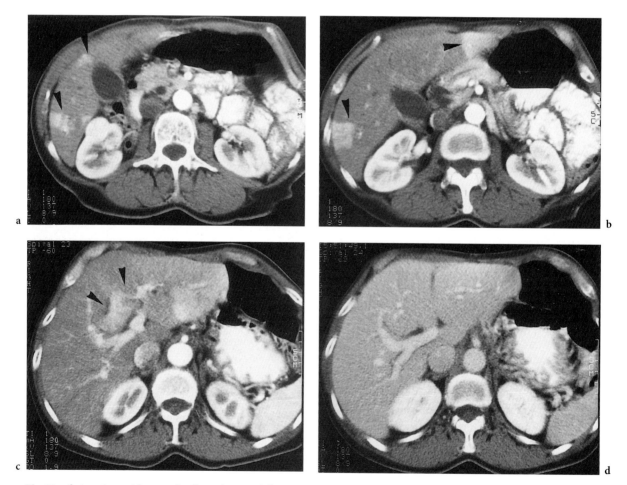

Fig. 13a–d. A patient with a renal cell carcinoma of the upper pole of the right kidney was referred for staging. **a–c** Several areas in the liver with high attenuation can be seen on the HAP images: **a** in the periphery of the liver, **b** near the gallbladder and **c** at the porta hepatis. **d** No density differences can be seen on PVP images. MRI did not reveal abnormalities

liver parenchyma; PVP images will show equal enhancement of the involved area (YAMASHITA et al. 1995).

10.9
Variants in the Hepatic Vascular Anatomy

A focal perfusion disorder can be seen in the liver parenchyma adjacent to the porta hepatis (segment IV). This is true if an aberrant right gastric venous system exists, draining systemic venous (i.e. nutrient-poor) blood from the gastric region into the hepatic sinusoids of segment IV. This type of aberrant inflow is also known as the 'third hepatic inflow tract' (MARCHAL et al. 1986; MATSUI et al. 1995). In other words, this parenchymal area receives three types of blood: arterial hepatic blood, splanchnic (nutrient-rich) portal venous blood and systemic (nutrient-poor) venous blood. These local differences in vascular anatomy explain why this area usually remains unaffected in the case of fatty liver infiltration, causing MARCHAL and co-workers to describe it in 1986 as a 'skip area'. Since the hepatic inflow of blood via the systemic pathway may be earlier than inflow of portal venous blood, the area may show marked hyperattenuation on late HAP images (MATSUI et al. 1995) and present as local 'perfusion defects' on helical CT with arterial portography (Figs. 10.12–10.14). Another focal perfusion disorder

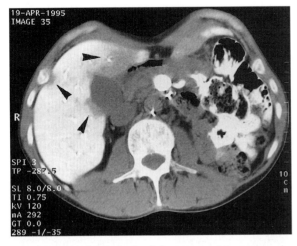

Fig. 10.14. Spiral CT obtained during arterial portography showing several low attenuation areas: near the gallbladder and in the subcapsular region (*arrowheads*). These 'pseudolesions' are compatible with areas that predominantly receive systemic venous blood, rather than portal blood

can occur in the presence of superior vena cava obstruction, where the area of aberrant perfusion is usually located in the ventral part of the liver (TRIGEAUX et al. 1996).

Other anatomical variants that can induce hepatic perfusion disorders are direct communications between portal systemic and capsular or accessory cystic veins. Nontumoral portal perfusion defects attributable to cholecystic venous drainage were described by YOSHIMITSU et al. in 1997 in their report of a study in which iodinated contrast was superselectively injected into the cholecystic artery during helical CT examination. Cholecystic venous blood usually entered peripheral portal branches of liver segment V and segment IV, but though to a lesser degree, other pathways to other segments were also seen (I, VI, VIII, II and VII in declining order of frequency). Subsequently the cholecystic venous blood drained into the hepatic veins (most frequently the middle, and less frequently the right hepatic vein).

10.10
Perfusion Disorders Related to Transjugular Intrahepatic Portosystemic Shunts

Placement of a transjugular intrahepatic portosystemic shunt(TIPSS) as a treatment for portal hypertension alters portal haemodynamics by flow redistribution. Portal venous flow to the liver will decrease and, via compensatory mechanisms, hepatic arterial velocity will increase (FOSHAGER et al. 1995; SURRATT et al. 1993). The size of the hepatic artery can even be increased after TIPSS placement. The flow alterations caused by a TIPPS are very heterogeneous. Segmental portal branches may show flow reversal, while others show stagnant flow and others maintain normal flow pattern (GRYSPEERDT et al. 1997). The main portal vein serves as a conduit for shunted blood to the stent. If flow reversal in a portal branch is apparent, it is due to blood diversion from the liver to the shunt (FOSHAGER et al. 1995).

These altered hepatic haemodynamics are translated on double-phase SCT into very heterogeneous perfusion patterns. Both HAP and PVP images will show a diffuse heterogeneous, pseudonodular, hepatic attenuation pattern (Fig. 10.15). This pattern is not specific and does not reflect patency of the TIPSS.

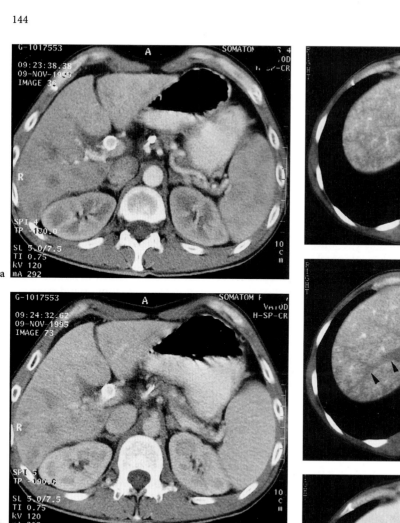

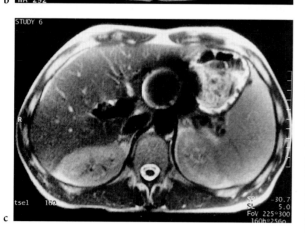

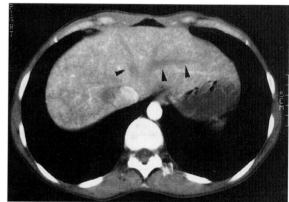

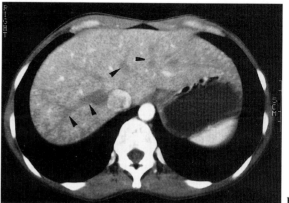

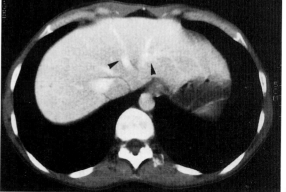

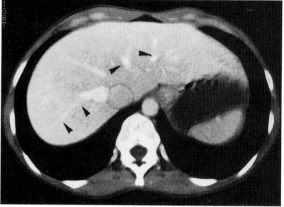

Fig. 10.15a–c. A patient with liver cirrhosis and encephalopathy, treated with a transjugular intrahepatic portosystemic shunt (TIPSS). HAP image (**a**) shows multiple areas of low attenuation in segment VI of the right liver lobe, which persist on PVP images (**b**). They are due to an altered hepatic enhancement, which accompanies TIPSS placement. MRI (**c** T2-weighted image) did not reveal any underlying focal liver lesion. Note the large metallic artefact caused by the TIPSS

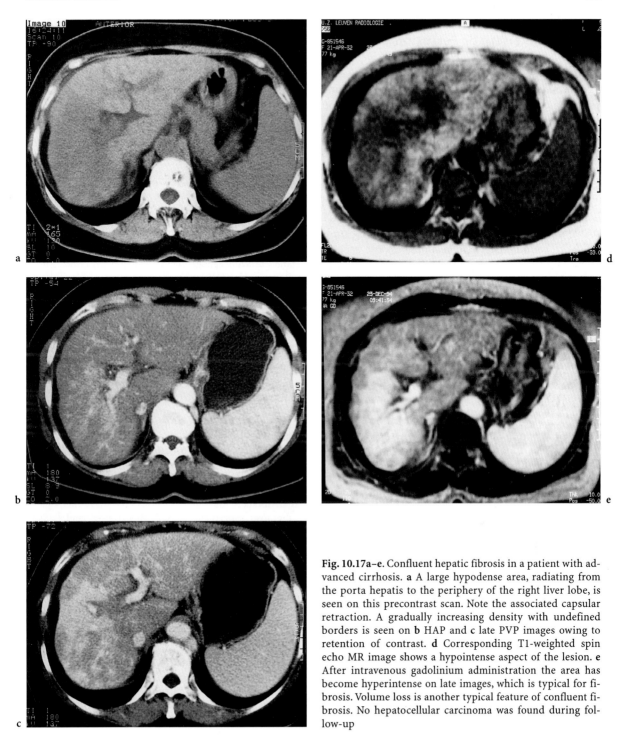

Fig. 10.17a–e. Confluent hepatic fibrosis in a patient with advanced cirrhosis. **a** A large hypodense area, radiating from the porta hepatis to the periphery of the right liver lobe, is seen on this precontrast scan. Note the associated capsular retraction. A gradually increasing density with undefined borders is seen on **b** HAP and **c** late PVP images owing to retention of contrast. **d** Corresponding T1-weighted spin echo MR image shows a hypointense aspect of the lesion. **e** After intravenous gadolinium administration the area has become hyperintense on late images, which is typical for fibrosis. Volume loss is another typical feature of confluent fibrosis. No hepatocellular carcinoma was found during follow-up

◁ **Fig. 10.16a–d.** Unexplained perfusion disorder in a patient presenting with severe epigastric pain. **a, b** HAP images show heterogeneous attenuation of the parenchyma in both lobes, traversed by the nonenhanced hepatic veins (*arrowheads*). **c, d** PVP images do not reveal any flow abnormality. No underlying causative factor could be found by other imaging modalities. A hypothetical reason is slower hepatic venous flow owing to Valsalva

10.11
Unexplained Hepatic Perfusion Disorders

If a perfusion disorder is seen on dual phase SCT one should always question what the underlying pathologic condition could be. Hepatic perfusion disorders can present both in anatomical and nonanatomical distributions, depending on their underlying cause. One should be aware that sometimes no clear-cut radio-pathological explanation can be found. Therefore, in cases where there is any doubt about the importance or impact of certain perfusion disorders, follow-up dual-phase SCT scans or further evaluation with other imaging studies (ultrasound, magnetic resonance) are recommended (Fig. 10.16). And of course, another priority is to differentiate perfusion disorders from lesion-confined flow phenomena (Fig. 10.17).

References

Aspestrand F, Schrumpf E, Jacobsen M, Hanssen L, Endresen K (1991) Increased lymphatic flow from the liver in different intra- and extrahepatic diseases by CT. J Comput Assist Tomogr 15:550–554

Bae KT, Heiken JP, Brink JA (1998) Aortic and Hepatic peak enhancement at CT: effect of contrast medium injection rate-pharmacokinetic analysis and experimental porcine model. Radiology 206(62):455–464

Baert AL, Fevery J, Marchal G et al. (1989) Early diagnosis of Budd-Chiari syndrome by computed tomography and ultrasonography: report of five cases. Gastroenterology 84:587–595

Baron RL (1994) Understanding and optimizing use of contrast material for CT of the liver. AJR Am J Roentgenol 163:323–331

Bonaldi VM, Bret PM, Reinhold C, Atri M (1995) Helical CT of the liver: value of an early hepatic arterial phase. Radiology 197:357–363

Engel IA, Auh YH, Rubenstein WA, Sniderman K, Whalen JP, Kazam E (1983) CT diagnosis of mediastinal and thoracic inlet venous obstruction. AJR Am J Roentgenol 141:521–526

Foshager MC, Ferral H, Nazarian GK, Castaneda-Zuniga WR, Letourneau JG (1995) Duplex sonography after portosystemic shunts (TIPS). AJR Am J Roentgenol 165:1–7

Gryspeerdt S, Van Hoe L, Marchal G, Baert A (1997) Evaluation of hepatic perfusion disorders with double-phase spiral CT. Radiographics 17:337–348

Halavaara JT, Hamberg LM, Leong FS, Hunter GJ, Gazelle GS, Wolf GL (1996) Functional CT with an experimental intravascular contrast agent in the assessment of liver vascular pathology. Acad Radiol 3:946–952

Heiken JP (1998) The liver. In: Lee J, Sagel S, Stanley R, Heiken JP (eds) Computed body tomography with MRI correlation, 3rd edn, vol/12. Lippincott-Raven, Philadelphia, pp 701–777

Holley HC, Koslin DB, Berland LL, Stanley RJ (1989) Inhomogeneous enhancement of liver parenchyma secondary to passive congestion: contrast-enhanced CT. Radiology 170:795–800

Howard CH, Bradley K, Lincoln LB et al (1989) Inhomogeneous enhancement of liver parenchyma secondary to passive congestion: contrast enhanced CT. Radiology 170:795–800

Imaeda T, Sone Y, Yamawaki Y, Seki M, Goto H (1991) Liver hypertrophy and portal hypertension in association with tumor thrombus in the portal vein: CT findings. J Comput Assist Tomogr 15:542–549

Inoue E, Fujita M, Hosomi N, Sawai Y, Hashimoto T et al (1998) Double phase CT arteriography of the whole liver in the evaluation of hepatic tumors. J Comput Assist Tomogr 22:64–68

Ishikawa T, Clark RA, Tokuda M, Ashida H (1983) Focal contrast enhancement on hepatic CT in superior vena caval and brachiocephalic vein obstruction. AJR Am J Roentgenol 140:337–338

Itai Y, Furui S, Ohtomo K, Kokubo T, Yamauchi T, Minami M, Yashiro N (1986a) Dynamic CT features of arterioportal shunts in hepatocellular carcinoma. AJR Am J Roentgenol 146:723–727

Itai Y, Ohtomo K, Kokubo T, Yamauchi T, Minami M, Yashiro N, Araki T (1986b) CT of hepatic masses: significance of prolonged and delayed enhancement. AJR Am J Roentgenol 146:729–733

Itai Y, Hachiya J, Makita K, Ohtomo K, Kokubo T, Yamauchi T (1987) Transient hepatic attenuation differences on dynamic computed tomography. J Comput Assist Tomogr 11:461–465

Itai Y, Eguchi N, Murata S, Kurosaki Y (1995a) Segmented areas of increased attenuation in the liver caused by right adrenal tumors: CT features. J Comput Assist Tomogr 19:959–962

Itai Y, Murata S, Kurosaki Y (1995b) Straight border sign of the liver: spectrum of CT appearances and causes. Radiographics 15:1089–1102

Kopka L, Rodenwaldt J, Fischer U, Mueller DW, Oestmann JW, Grabbe E (1996) Dual-phase CT of the liver: effects of bolus tracking and different volumes of contrast material. Radiology 201:321–326

Koslin BB, Stanley RJ, Berland LL et al (1988) Hepatic perivascular lymphedema: CT appearance. AJR Am J Roentgenol 150:111–113

Lautt WW, Greenway CV (1987) Conceptual review of the hepatic vascular bed. Hepatology 7:952–963

Leevy CM, Sherlock S, Tygstrup N, Zetterman R (1994) Diseases of the liver and biliary tract. Standarization of nomenclature, diagnostic criteria and prognosis. Raven, New York

Marchal G, Tshibwabwa-Tumba E, Verbeken E, Van Roost W, Van Steenbergen W, Baert A, Lauwerijns J (1986) "Skip-Areas" in hepatic steatosis: a sonographic-angiographic study. Gastrointest Radiol 11:151–157

Marchal G (1992) Contributions to tissue characterization in US, CT and MRI. Thesis submitted for the degree of 'doctor in medical sciences'. Catholic University of Louvain, faculty of Medicine, Belgium

Marchal G, Baert AL (1992) Dynamic CT of the liver. Radiologe 32:211–216

Mathieu D, Vasile N, Menu Y, Van Beers B, Lorphelin JM, Pringot J (1987) Budd-Chiari syndrome: dynamic CT. Radiology 165:409–413

Matsui O, Kadoya M, Yoshikawa J, Gabata T, Takahashi S et al. (1995) Aberrant gastric venous drainage in cirrhotic livers: imaging findings in focal areas of liver parenchyma. Radiology 197:345–349

Murata S, Itai Y, Asato M, Kobayashi H, Nakajima K, Eguchi N et al (1995) Effect of temporary occlusion of the hepatic vein on dual blood supply in the liver: evaluation with spiral CT. Radiology 197:351–356

Rappaport AM (1973) The microcirculatory hepatic unit. Microvasc Res 6:212–228

Silverman PM, Roberts SC, Ducic I et al (1996) Assessment of a technology that permits individualized scan delays on helical hepatic CT: a technique to improve efficiency in use of contrast material. AJR Am J Roentgenol 167:79–84

Sudhir K, Teal JS (1989) Discrepant sulfur colloid and radioparticle liver uptake in superior vena cava obstruction. Case report. J Nucl Med 30:113–116

Surratt RS, Middleton WD, Darcy MD, Melson GL, Brink JA (1993) Morphologic and hemodynamic findings at sonography before and after creation of a transjugular intrahepatic portosystemic shunt (TIPS). Cardiovasc Intervent Radiol 16:275–279

Takayasu K, Okuda K (1997a) Anatomy of the liver. In: Takayasu K, Okuda K (eds) Imaging in liver disease. Oxford University Press, Oxford, pp 1–49

Takayasu K, Okuda K (1997b) Portal hypertension. In: Takayasu K, Okuda K (eds) Imaging in liver disease. Oxford University Press, Oxford, pp 355–389

Trigeaux J, Lacrosse M, Daube A (1996) Venous return by the paraumbilical and hepatic veins in case of superior vena cava obstruction. Abdominal Imaging 21:504–506

Van Hoe L, Baert AL, Gryspeerdt S, Vandenbosch G, Nevens F, Van Steenbergen W, Marchal G (1997) Dual-phase helical CT of the liver: value of an early-phase acquisition in the differential diagnosis of noncystic focal lesions. AJR Am J Roentgenol 168:1185–1192

Van Beers B, Pringot J, Gigot JF, Dautrebande J, Mathurin P (1990) Nontumorous attenuation differences on computed tomographic portography. Gastrointest Radiol 15:107–111

Yamashita K, Jun Jin M, Hirose Y, Morikawa M, Sumioka H, Itoh K, Konish J (1995) CT finding of transient focal increased attenuation of the liver adjacent to the gallbladder in acute cholecystitis. AJR Am J Roentgenol 164:343–346

Yoshimitsu K, Honda H, Kaneko K, Kuroiwa T, Irie H, Chijiiwa K, Takenaka K, Masuda K (1997) Anatomy and clinical importance of cholecystic venous drainage: helical CT observations during injection of contrast medium into the cholecystic artery. AJR Am J Roentgenol 169:505–510

Zerhouni EA, Barth KH, Siegelmann SS (1980) Demonstration of venous thrombosis by computed tomography. AJR 134:753–758

Focal Liver Lesions:
Role of Spiral CT and Controversies

11 The Case for Ultrasonography

R. Lencioni, D. Cioni, L. Crocetti, C. Bartolozzi

CONTENTS

11.1   Introduction   151
11.2   Characterization of Incidental Liver Lesions   151
11.3   Detection and Characterization of Hepatocellular
        Carcinoma in Cirrhotic Patients   152
11.4   Detection and Characterization of Hepatic
        Metastases in Oncologic Patients   153
        References   154

11.1
Introduction

Ultrasonography (US) is the preferred routine hepatic imaging method throughout the world: it is easy to perform and largely accessible, and it has a low cost. Acceptance by the patient is good to excellent, which is mandatory for a technique dedicated to routine survey. Moreover, even though high-level equipment is required to perform such cutting-edge techniques as harmonic imaging, adequate diagnostic examinations can be performed with low- or medium-priced devices.

The liver is exceptionally well suited to evaluation by means of US, especially for the detection of focal lesions. Unfortunately, while US findings can help characterize some focal liver lesions, there is enough variability and overlap in the US appearance of benign and malignant liver tumors to make a definite distinction problematic in several instances. With

R. Lencioni, MD; Division of Diagnostic and Interventional Radiology, Department of Oncology, University of Pisa, Via Roma 67, I-56125 Pisa, Italy
D. Cioni, MD; Division of Diagnostic and Interventional Radiology, Department of Oncology, University of Pisa, Via Roma 67, I-56125 Pisa, Italy
L. Crocetti, MD; Division of Diagnostic and Interventional Radiology, Department of Oncology, University of Pisa, Via Roma 67, I-56125 Pisa, Italy
C. Bartolozzi, MD; Professor and Chairman, Division of Diagnostic and Interventional Radiology, Department of Oncology, University of Pisa, Via Roma 67, I-56125 Pisa, Italy

recent advances in the Doppler US technology and the introduction of echo-enhancing agents, the potential for US to add information in the analysis of focal liver lesions is substantially improved. However, whether new Doppler US studies will help distinguish among focal liver lesions – thus reducing the need for more expensive imaging examinations – is still a matter of debate.

In this chapter, we will discuss the diagnostic effectiveness of US relative to that of spiral CT in the following clinical scenarios: (a) characterization of incidental liver lesions; (b) detection and characterization of hepatocellular carcinoma in cirrhotic patients; and (c) detection and characterization of hepatic metastases in oncologic patients.

11.2
Characterization of Incidental Liver Lesions

Incidental liver lesions are lesions discovered by chance during a routine US examination of the abdomen performed in patients with neither known hepatic disease nor any history of malignancy. In the past few years, incidental liver lesions have been detected with increased frequency, as a result of the widespread use of US as first diagnostic step in patients with abdominal troubles.

The detection of an unexpected hepatic mass may be a real dilemma for both clinicians and radiologists. Many questions arise after its detection. Is it benign or malignant? Should biopsy be attempted in every case? Which is the best scheme for diagnosing such a lesion? The choice of an appropriate diagnostic work-up should take into account the potential clinical efficacy as well as the cost of the various imaging techniques. If we consider the cost of a liver US examination equal to 1, the cost of a contrast-enhanced Doppler US study can be estimated at 2, that of a contrast-enhanced spiral CT study at 4–5, and that of a contrast-enhanced MR imaging study at 6–

8. The first question is, therefore, when US by itself can provide a reliable diagnosis, thus avoiding the necessity for additional tests.

US usually allows a confident diagnosis in the case of cystic lesions with regular thin walls and homogeneous liquid content. Benign nonparasitic cysts of the liver are in fact a very common finding, occurring in 3–6% of healthy subjects over 60 years (GAINES and SAMPSON 1989). In contrast, cystic malignancies (both primary and secondary) are infrequent and usually associated with clinical symptoms. In some geographic areas where hydatid disease is an endemic disorder, however, the possibility of a uniloculated parasitic cyst, without the typical US features of hydatid cysts (wall thickening, parietal calcifications, presence of daughter cysts or collapsed membranes) cannot be excluded. Therefore, an accurate serologic evaluation of the patient may be required.

The detection of a solid mass opens up a wider range of differential diagnoses and requires a careful analysis of the US features of the lesion that can be useful in determining whether it is benign or malignant in nature. The most common benign lesions in the liver are hepatic hemangiomas, with a frequency at autopsy of up to 7% (GIBNEY et al. 1987; MOODY and WILSON 1993). They are usually solitary, but may be multiple in up to 10% of cases. Since hemangiomas are usually asymptomatic, they are often detected as incidental findings. About 70–80% of hemangiomas show a typical US pattern, characterized by an homogeneous hyperechoic appearance with well-defined margins and posterior acoustic enhancement (GIBNEY et al. 1987). A small hypoechoic area may be seen centrally, but not a peripheral hypoechoic halo. If a liver lesion has this classic US appearance, no further work-up is usually necessary, provided that the patient has (a) normal liver function tests; (b) no clinical symptoms referable to the liver; and (c) no known primary tumor.

However, the remaining 20–30% of hepatic hemangiomas do not show this typical pattern, and may appear as hypo-isoechoic lesions or show heterogeneous internal echogenicity (MIRK et al. 1982; MOODY and WILSON 1993). Reasons for variable US features include fibrosis, thrombosis, hemorrhagic necrosis, and myxomatous change. Moreover, a hemangioma can be seen as a hypoechoic mass when surrounded by diffusely fatty liver. Although some of these atypical hemangiomas may show a suggestive US morphology (solid tumor with an echogenic border and partially hypoechoic internal pattern), US is not an entirely reliable indicator of their nature. There are other lesions, particularly focal nodular hyperplasia or hepatocellular adenoma, that may exhibit similar features.

In these instances in which the US features of the lesion are nonspecific, further imaging evaluation is absolutely necessary. Color Doppler US, especially when the power mode is used in combination with echo-enhancers, may be useful to evaluate the vascular architecture and the hemodynamic characteristics of hepatic lesions. Doppler US studies may provide useful information in cases of incidentally detected benign hypervascular lesions, especially focal nodular hyperplasia (BARTOLOZZI et al. 1997). However, Doppler US is still considered not entirely reliable for diagnosing hepatic hemangiomas. Since it can be estimated that many of the lesions with a nonspecific US appearance are represented by hemangiomas with atypical US pattern, additional testing with spiral CT or MR imaging may be required in several instances. For the same reasons, the use of US-guided biopsy immediately after the detection of an incidental lesion should be strongly discouraged.

In other cases, the lesion may show US features highly suggestive of malignancy, such as peripheral hypoechoic halo, vascular invasion, and evidence of extrahepatic spread. In these instances, to maximize the cost effectiveness of the procedure, US-guided percutaneous biopsy could also be performed immediately after the detection of the lesion, if clinical and laboratory findings do not prove helpful in attempts to determine the nature of the neoplasm (BRET et al. 1986). Additional imaging studies will be performed, if indicated, after the biopsy to delineate the lesion further before a specific therapy is started or to search for a primary neoplasms if a diagnosis of metastatic disease has been established.

11.3
Detection and Characterization of Hepatocellular Carcinoma in Cirrhotic Patients

Hepatocellular carcinoma (HCC) is one of the most common malignancies in the world, with an estimated worldwide incidence of about 1,000,000 cases per year. This tumor is the seventh most common cancer in men and the ninth most common cancer in women. In Western countries, as well as in Japan, HCC emerge in cirrhotic livers in more than 90% of cases (COLOMBO et al. 1991). Patients with liver cirrhosis have long been identified as being a high-risk group for the development of HCC. The yearly incidence of HCC in cirrhotic patients may reach 3–5%, and HCC is recognized as the principal cause of death for these patients (COLOMBO et al. 1991). Since the mid-1970s, the recognition of the close association of HCC with cirrhosis has stimulated the development of clinical programs for the early detection of HCC in cirrhotic patients.

US, in combination with measurement of the serum level of alpha fetoprotein (AFP) has been the method of choice for screening high-risk patient populations in many countries. This resulted in great success in detecting early-stage, asymptomatic tumors, with approximately 20–30% of the HCC nodules currently detected being less than 2 cm in diameter and 50–60%, less than 5 cm in diameter. In patients with liver cirrhosis and a nodular lesion detected by US screening, color Doppler US may help differentiate HCC from nonneoplastic hepatocellular lesions, such as macroregenerative or dysplastic nodules (CHOI et al. 1993). Along with progression from regeneration to cancer, in fact, hepatocellular nodular lesions show a change in the blood supply: the intranodular portal blood supply tends to decrease and, in contrast, the intranodular arterial supply tends to increase during the transition from benign to malignancy (MATSUI et al. 1991). Hence, small, overt HCC tumors show a typical hypervascular pattern on color Doppler US, with intratumoral and peritumoral vessels showing pulsatile flow at spectral analysis (CHOI et al. 1996; LENCIONI et al. 1996b). After administration of US contrast agents, HCC shows clear-cut early enhancement in the arterial phase (BARTOLOZZI et al. 1998). In contrast, regenerative or dysplastic lesions fail to exhibit these hypervascular features and usually do not show internal blood flow on Doppler studies.

Although the use of US as the imaging modality of choice for screening is widely accepted, adequate thorough US examination of the entire liver is sometimes impossible because of patient's habitus, intervening bones, or colonic interposition, especially in small cirrhotic livers (DODD et al. 1992). The increasing availability of spiral CT scanners may open new prospects for HCC screening. Spiral CT has, in fact, demonstrated very high detection rates for small, overt, hypervascular HCC lesions (CHOI et al. 1997; HORI et al. 1998). Spiral CT can therefore guarantee an objective and comprehensive survey of the liver parenchyma, detecting small tumors that need timely therapeutic intervention. The use of spiral CT could be especially recommended in high-risk patients, such as those with abnormal (above 200 ng/ml) or increasing AFP levels, and negative US findings.

Once the diagnosis of HCC has been established, accurate staging is necessary to determine the best treatment method for this tumor. In particular, precise assessment of the number, size, and location of tumor deposits in the liver is of the utmost importance, because of the tendency of HCC to cause small or minute intrahepatic metastatic nodules. Unfortunately, the US detection rate of such tiny satellite lesions is low. In contrast, spiral CT and dynamic MR imaging are ideal techniques for this purpose, as small intrahepatic metastatic nodules are usually hypervascular, like the main tumor, and are therefore well depicted in the arterial phase images of contrast-enhanced studies (HORI et al. 1998; VAN HOE et al. 1997; LENCIONI et al. 1996a). As a matter of fact, the availability of spiral CT scanners and ultrafast MR imaging sequences has substantially restricted the indications for more complex and invasive angiographically assisted techniques, such as CT during arterial portography (CTAP) and CT following the intraarterial injection of iodized oil (Lipiodol CT) for staging of HCC (LENCIONI et al. 1997).

11.4
Detection and Characterization of Hepatic Metastases in Oncologic Patients

Metastatic disease of the liver is one of the most common and troublesome issues in oncology. In a summary of several autopsy series, 24–36% of patients who died of malignancy had liver involvement. Liver metastases were present in 65% of patients with colon carcinoma, 47% of patients with rectal carcinoma, 61% of patients with breast carcinoma, 40% of patients with lung carcinoma, and 45% of patients with gastric carcinoma (WILKES 1973). Indeed, metastatic lesions are by far the most common malignant lesion in the liver.

Twenty years ago, the discovery of metastatic deposits in the liver was nearly equivalent to a death sentence, and there was accordingly little enthusiasm for developing screening programs designed to detect them. However, results of a number of studies by aggressive surgical oncologists have demonstrated that, at least for colorectal cancer, there has been a clear-cut improvement in 5-year survival (20–40% increase) when successful removal of the metastatic burden can be accomplished (HUGHES et al. 1988). These percentages also seem to apply to patients with metastases from endocrine tumors, sarcomas, and even gastric cancer. More recently, interventional therapies also proved able to destroy small tumor deposits in the liver, thereby enhancing the number of cases suitable for curative treatment (LENCIONI et al. 1998b).

The tasks of diagnostic radiology in patients with known extrahepatic primary malignancy include: (a) global patient detection: does the liver contain tumor deposits?; (b) individual lesion detection: how many lesions are there?; (c) individual lesion characterization: what is the nature of the masses seen?; and (d) staging to settle the question of local treatment: if it is cancerous, can the disease be treated by partial hepatectomy or interventional therapy?

In clinical practice these functions are rarely confused, although they may not necessarily be performed in every case. In certain instances, a decision as to global status of the patient (cancerous liver or not) suffices; in others, detailed lesion-by-lesion detection, differential diagnosis of individual nodules, and mapping of the anatomic extensions of malignant disease is required. Many methods are now available to answer the questions, including a variety of CT and MR imaging techniques as well as transabdominal, intraoperative, and laparoscopic US. The usefulness of these techniques may vary across institutions because of local bias or expertise or both.

Our approach is to start with screening US. US may be sufficient in the instances in which numerous, obviously malignant hepatic lesions are demonstrated. If further diagnostic assessment is required to clarify equivocal US findings, show additional lesions, or evaluate extrahepatic disease, we usually prefer spiral CT to MR imaging, because of the lower cost and superior detection of extrahepatic disease. However, there are situations in which we prefer MR imaging to CT as the second diagnostic step. These include: (a) patients with a contraindication to the use of a reasonable volume bolus of iodinated contrast material, regardless of the reason; (b) patients with diffuse fatty infiltration of the liver or in whom there is a question of focal fat versus tumor; (c) patients with equivocal lesion(s) on preliminary CT; and (d) differential diagnosis of small lesions (typically hemangioma versus metastasis). MR imaging with use of hepato-specific agents or CTAP are reserved for patients who are potential candidates for partial hepatectomy after noninvasive imaging studies to assess their eligibility for surgery (LENCIONI et al. 1998a). In these cases, laparoscopic or intraoperative US will complete the diagnostic work-up before resection.

References

Bartolozzi C, Lencioni R, Paolicchi A, Moretti M, Armillotta N, Pinto F (1997) Differentiation of hepatocellular adenoma and focal nodular hyperplasia of the liver: comparison of power Doppler imaging and conventional color Doppler sonography. Eur Radiol 7:1410–1415

Bartolozzi C, Lencioni R, Ricci P, Paolicchi A, Rossi P, Passariello R (1998) Hepatocellular carcinoma treatment with percutaneous ethanol injection: evaluation with contrast-enhanced color doppler US. Radiology 209:387–393

Bret PM, Fond A, Casola G, et al (1986) Abdominal lesions: a prospective study of clinical efficacy of percutaneous fine-needle biopsy. Radiology 159:345–346

Choi BI, Takayasu K, Han MC, et al (1993) Small hepatocellular carcinomas and associated nodular lesions of the liver: pathology, pathogenesis and imaging findings. AJR Am J Roentgenol 160:1177–1187

Choi BI, Kim TK, Han JK, Chung JW, Park JH, Han MN (1996) Power versus conventional color Doppler sonography: comparison in the depiction of vasculature in liver tumors. Radiology 200:55–58

Choi BI, Lee HJ, Han JK, Choi DS, Seo JB, Han MC (1997) Detection of hypervascular nodular hepatocellular carcinomas: value of triphasic helical CT compared with iodized-oil CT. AJR Am J Roentgenol 168:219–224

Colombo M, De Franchis R, Del Ninno, et al (1991) Hepatocellular carcinoma in Italian patients with cirrhosis. N Engl J Med 325:675–680

Dodd GD, Miller WJ, Baron RL, et al (1992) Detection of malignant tumors in end-stage cirrhotic livers: efficacy of sonography as a screening technique. AJR Am J Roentgenol 159:727–733

Gaines PA, Sampson MA (1989) The prevalence and characterization of simple hepatic cysts by ultrasound examination. Br J Radiol 62:335–337

Gibney RG, Hendin AP, Cooperberg PL (1987) Sonographically detected hepatic hemangiomas: absence of change over time. AJR Am J Roentgenol 149:953–957

Hori M, Murakami T, Kim T, et al (1998) Sensitivity of double-phase helical CT during arterial portography for detection of hypervascular hepatocellular carcinoma. J Comput Assist Tomogr 22:861–867

Hughes KS, Rosenstein RB, Songhorbodi S, et al (1988) Resection of the liver for colorectal carcinoma metastases: a multi-institutional study of long-term survivors. Dis Colon Rectum 31:1–4

Lencioni R, Mascalchi M, Caramella D, Bartolozzi C (1996a) Small hepatocellular carcinoma: differentiation from adenomatous hyperplasia with color Doppler US and dynamic Gd-DTPA-enhanced MR imaging. Abdom Imaging 21:41–48

Lencioni R, Pinto F, Armillotta N, Bartolozzi C (1996b) Hepatocellular carcinoma: comparison of power Doppler US and color Doppler US for the assessment of tumor vascularity. Radiology 201:353–358

Lencioni R, Pinto F, Armillotta N, et al (1997) Intrahepatic metastatic nodules of hepatocellular carcinoma detected at Lipiodol-CT: imaging-pathologic correlation. Abdom Imaging 22:253–258

Lencioni R, Donati F, Cioni D, Paolicchi A, Cicorelli A, Bartolozzi C (1998a) Detection of colorectal liver metastases: prospective comparison of unenhanced and ferumoxides-enhanced MRI at 1.5 T, dual-phase spiral CT, and spiral CTAP. MAGMA 6:98–102

Lencioni R, Goletti O, Armillotta N, et al (1998b) Radio-frequency thermal ablation of liver metastases with a cooled-tip electrode needle: results of a pilot clinical trial. Eur Radiol 8:1205–1211

Matsui O, Kadoya M, Kameyama T, et al (1991) Benign and malignant nodules in cirrhotic livers: distinction based on blood supply. Radiology 178:493–497

Mirk P, Rubaltelli L, Bazzocchi M, et al (1982) Ultra-sonographic patterns in hepatic hemangiomas. J Clin Ultrasound 10:373–378

Moody AR, Wilson SR (1993) Atypical hepatic hemangioma: a suggestive sonographic morphology. Radiology 188:413–417

van Hoe L, Baert AL, Gryspeerdt S, et al (1997) Dual-phase helical-CT of the liver: value of an early phase acquisition in the differential diagnosis of non-cystic focal lesions. AJR Am J Roentgenol 169:1185–1192

Wilkes RA (1973) Secondary tumours of the liver, 3rd edn. Butterworths, London, pp 175–183

12 The Case for Spiral CT

B. Marincek

CONTENTS

12.1   Introduction   157
12.2   Single-Phase Contrast-Enhanced CT   157
12.3   Dual-Phase Contrast-enhanced CT   157
12.4   Conclusions   158
        References   158

12.1 Introduction

Spiral CT represents a major advancement in liver imaging. Because this technology significantly reduces the total scanning time and enables the acquisition of a contiguous set of images in a single breathhold, respiratory misregistration is avoided, which improves the detection of small focal liver lesions. An even greater advantage of the increased image acquisition speed is the ability to optimize timing for contrast-enhanced imaging (Baron 1994). The more precise delivery of intravenous contrast agents allows complete studies at optimum vessel opacification. Because conventional incremental CT requires 2 min or more to scan the liver, arterial phase imaging is never achieved, which requires the ability to image the entire liver in approximately 20 s. Such timing can be critical for detection and characterization of hypervascular liver tumors.

In patients with suspected focal liver lesions, accurate clinical information is essential for selection of the appropriate imaging protocol. Two basic protocols are used: single-phase (portal venous phase) contrast-enhanced CT for the assessment of lesions that are hypovascular relative to liver, and dual-phase (hepatic arterial and portal venous phase) contrast-enhanced CT if hypervascular lesions are suspected.

B. Marincek, MD; Institute of Diagnostic Radiology, University Hospital Zurich, Rämistrasse 100, CH-8091 Zurich, Switzerland

12.2 Single-Phase Contrast-Enhanced CT

Because the liver parenchyma receives approximately 80% of its blood supply from the portal venous system and lesion conspicuity is generally greatest during peak parenchymal enhancement, imaging during the portal venous phase of enhancement is desirable (Bluemke et al. 1995). Hypovascular hepatic metastases, such as those arising from colonic carcinoma, represent the majority of hypovascular lesions. They are best imaged during the portal venous phase when there is peak enhancement of the hepatic parenchyma. Contrast-enhanced spiral CT in the portal phase has a sensitivity of 91% for detection of hepatic metastases greater than 1 cm in size and compares favorably with CT scan arterial portography, once thought the gold standard in the detection of liver neoplasms (Kuszyk et al. 1996).

12.3 Dual-Phase Contrast-Enhanced CT

Common hypervascular liver lesions include benign (focal nodular hyperplasia, hepatocellular adenoma) and malignant tumors (hepatocellular carcinoma, hypervascular metastases from breast carcinoma, renal cell carcinoma, neuroendocrine tumors [islet cell, carcinoid], sarcomas, thyroid carcinoma, and melanoma); metastases from breast carcinoma or renal cell carcinoma can also be hypovascular in nature. These tumors, unlike liver parenchyma, receive their blood supply predominantly from the hepatic arteries. They enhance early during the arterial phase and may become isodense with liver parenchyma during the portal phase, particularly those less than 1.5 cm in size (Hollett et al. 1995). Because of this, hypervascular lesions may remain undetected or may be incorrectly diagnosed if only portal venous phase images are evaluated. In one study, hepatic arterial phase imaging depicted additional nodules of hepatocellular carcinoma in 33% of patients, and in 11% the tumors were only seen on arterial phase images (BARON et al. 1996). Furthermore, arterial phase imaging was helpful in demonstrating arterial supply to portal venous thrombus, thereby confirming tumor invasion into vascular structures.

In a recent study, however, arterial phase images introduced new diagnostic dilemmas because not all lesions seen on the arterial phase alone were caused by hepatocellular carcinoma or metastases, even in patients with malignancies; several lesions represented benign abnormalities including focal nodular hyperplasia (MILLER et al. 1998). Another potential disadvantage of dual-phase contrast-enhanced CT is the occurrence of nontumorous arterioportal shunts, which can be a cause of pseudolesions in cirrhotic liver mimicking hypervascular tumors (KIM et al. 1998). Finally, biphasic spiral CT is still less sensitive than CT arterial portography (CTAP; KANEMATSU et al. 1997). With spiral CTAP, an overall sensitivity greater than 90% is reported for tumor detection, as opposed to 80% for dynamic spiral CT scanning, although these figures fall to nearer 50% for detecting tumors less than 1 cm in size (KUSZYK et al. 1996).

There is some controversy about the necessity of routine unenhanced scanning. Because some hypervascular lesions may become isodense during conventional bolus dynamic scanning, routine unenhanced scanning has been advocated in patients with known or suspected hypervascular malignancies (BRESSLER et al. 1987). Unenhanced scans may be an important adjunct to portal venous phase imaging and obviate the need for arterial phase scanning in patients with hypervascular metastases (OLIVER et al. 1997). On the other hand, in a recent study encompassing 102 patients the unenhanced phase was not routinely necessary for detection of liver metastases; no patient had a lesion that was detectable on unenhanced phase images that was not identifiable on either hepatic arterial or portal venous phase images (MILLER et al. 1998).

Dual-phase contrast-enhanced imaging can be helpful in characterizing liver lesions, particularly with hemangioma. The attenuation of enhancing portions of hemangiomas should always be the same as that of vessels such as the aorta (in the arterial phase) or portal vein (in the portal venous phase and later; OLIVER and BARON 1996). On delayed imaging, the contrast diffuses into the large blood-filled chan-nels, yielding a centripetal pattern of enhancement with time. Delayed scans are also useful in showing the increased attenuation relative to liver associated with cholangiocarcinoma (LACOMIS et al. 1997).

Recent developments in MR imaging, such as the use of liver-specific contrast agents and dynamic scanning, have underlined the role of the modality in the detection and characterization of liver lesions. Dynamic Gd-enhanced MRI can diagnose hepatic hemangiomas with 100% specificity and 95% accuracy if the typical enhancement pattern of peripheral hyperintense nodules followed by progressive centripetal enhancement is seen (WHITNEY et al. 1993). MR images, when enhanced with the paramagnetic hepatobiliary contrast agent MnDPDP, may reveal early foci of well-differentiated hepatocellular carcinoma not depictable by spiral CT (DONATI et al. 1998).

12.4
Conclusions

Thus, the optimal imaging modality for focal liver lesions is still controversial, despite the advent of spiral CT. In practical terms, patients with potential liver metastases are first examined by ultrasound, unless there is a lesion for which CT staging is being performed anyhow. It remains open to debate whether CT or MRI should be used when ultrasound is equivocal (e.g. hemangioma) or when detailed information is required (as in cirrhosis, rising alphafetoprotein, or possible hepatocellular carcinoma).

MRI is probably more suitable for the characterization of focal liver lesions than CT, but the latter remains the modality of choice at many institutions because of cost and time considerations. The role of MRI may again expand with the use of liver-specific contrast agents.

References

Baron RL (1994) Understanding and optimizing use of contrast material for CT of the liver. AJR Am J Roentgenol 163:323–331

Baron RL, Oliver JH, Dodd GD et al (1996) Hepatocellular carcinoma: evaluation with biphasic, contrast-enhanced, helical CT. Radiology 199:505–511

Bluemke DA, Soyer P, Fishman EK (1995) Helical (spiral) CT of the liver. Radiol Clin North Am 33:863–886

Bressler EL, Alpern MB, Glazer GM et al (1987) Hypervascular hepatic metastasis: CT evaluation. Radiology 162:49–51

Donati F, Lencioni R, Cioni D et al (1998) Detection of hepatocellular carcinoma in liver cirrhosis: MnDPDP-enhanced MRI vs dual-phase spiral CT. MAGMA 6 [Suppl 1]:23

Hollett MD, Jeffrey RB, Nino-Murcia M et al (1995) Dualphase helical CT of the liver: value of arterial phase scans in the detection of small (<1.5 cm) malignant hepatic neoplasms. AJR Am J Roentgenol 164:879–884

Kanematsu M, Hoshi H, Imaeda T et al (1997) Detection and characterization of hepatic tumors: value of combined helical CT hepatic arteriography and CT during arterial portography. AJR Am J Roentgenol 168:1193–1198

Kim TK, Choi BI, Han JK et al (1998) Nontumorous arterioportal shunt mimicking hypervascular tumor in cirrhotic liver: two-phase spiral CT findings. Radiology 208:597–603

Kuszyk BS, Bluemke DA, Urban BA et al (1996) Portal-phase contrast-enhanced helical CT for the detection of malignant hepatic tumors: sensitivity based on comparison with intraoperative and pathologic findings. AJR Am J Roentgenol 166:91–95

Lacomis JM, Baron RL, Oliver JH et al (1997) Cholangiocarcinoma: delayed CT contrast enhancement patterns. Radiology 203:98–104

Miller FH, Butler RS, Hoff FL et al (1998) Using triphasic helical CT to detect focal hepatic lesions in patients with neoplasms. AJR Am J Roentgenol 171:643–649

Oliver JH, Baron RL (1996) Helical biphasic contrast-enhanced CT of the liver: technique, indications, interpretation, and pitfalls. Radiology 201:1–14

Oliver JH, Baron RL, Federle MP et al (1997) Hypervascular liver metastases: do unenhanced and hepatic arterial phase CT images affect tumor detection? Radiology 205:709–715

Whitney WS, Herfkens RJ, Jeffrey RB et al (1993) Dynamic breath-hold multiplanar spoiled gradient-recalled MR imaging with gadolinium enhancement for differentiating hepatic hemangiomas from malignancies at 1.5 T. Radiology 189:863–870

13 Liver: Role of Helical CT and Controversies: the Case for MRI

M. Taupitz, B. Hamm

CONTENTS

13.1   Introduction   *161*
13.2   Technical Considerations   *161*
13.3   Contrast Agents   *162*
13.4   Results and Discussion   *162*
        References   *164*

13.1
Introduction

The advent of the helical technique has undoubtedly led to an enormous expansion of the diagnostic potential of computed tomography (CT). As a consequence, there is a need to redefine the role of CT in the diagnostic assessment of the liver with reference to both detection and characterization of focal liver lesions. However, a great leap forward has also been made in magnetic resonance (MR) imaging. State-of-the-art MR imaging units, just like CT, allow imaging of the entire liver during a single breath-hold. The use of new coil techniques provides high-quality images with excellent contrast and depiction of small details despite extremely fast image acquisition. These advances are of particular interest when combined with bolus injection of contrast agents, both in CT and in MR imaging. With both modalities, it has thus become possible to examine the entire liver during the arterial phase as well as during the portal-venous phase at a high resolution. This article presents the technical features of state-of-the-art MR imaging and the examination protocol for liver imaging and focuses on recent clinical results.

M Taupitz, MD; Department of Radiology, Universitäts-klinikum Charité, Medizinische Fakultät der Humboldt-Universität zu Berlin, Schumannstrasse 20/21, D-10117 Berlin, Germany
B. Hamm, MD; Department of Radiology, Universitäts-klinikum Charité, Medizinische Fakultät der Humboldt-Universität zu Berlin, Schumannstrasse 20/21, D-10117 Berlin, Germany

13.2
Technical Considerations

The following factors have markedly expanded the diagnostic spectrum of MR imaging in recent years, especially with regard to abdominal examinations (Fujita et al. 1994). All major manufacturers of high-field MR imaging units have developed so-called high-performance gradient systems. The most important features of these gradient systems are a maximal gradient amplitude between 20 and 25 mT/m together with a minimal rise time of approximately 600 µs to reach the maximal gradient amplitude; in units with special equipment this time may be reduced further to as low as 300 µs. Even higher gradient amplitudes are theoretically feasible with further technical sophistication, but they are of no use in a clinical setting, since they may lead to nerve stimulation of the patient being examined. The practical clinical benefit resulting from these advances in abdominal imaging is a dramatic shortening of examination times. With the new imagers, a multi-section set of liver images can be acquired in about 20 s instead of the 6–10 min required with conventional technique. Such an examination can be performed during breath-hold, which eliminates otherwise very troublesome respiratory artifacts. Furthermore, examinations can be performed in sequential single-section technique with an acquisition time of 1 s or less for each section. All kinds of motion artifacts, regardless of their physiological origin (respiration, peristalsis, vascular pulsations), are thus effectively suppressed. In terms of physics, a shortening of the acquisition time is always associated with a reduction of the signal-to-noise ratio, which in turn leads to a lower image quality with a poorer visualization of anatomical details. It is here that the second important technical advance in MR imaging plays a role, namely the introduction of so-called torso or body phased-array coils. Such coils consist of a combination of four to six semiflexible surface coils which receive the signal directly at the body surface. The body phased-array coils have an improved signal-to-noise ratio compared with conventional whole-body coils, which ensures an excellent image quality obtained with the fast imaging techniques despite their short acquisition times.

13.3
Contrast Agents

MR imaging of the liver is highly advantageous from the aspect of the use of contrast agents, since not only conventional, unspecific contrast agents are available for clinical practice, but also various organ-specific agents with totally different mechanisms of action. Other substances are presently in the preclinical and clinical trial phases. As in CT, the conventional, unspecific agents used for MR imaging are low-molecular water-soluble compounds with distribution in the interstitial space after intravenous injection and rapid renal elimination. Since MR imaging is more sensitive to contrast agents, the contrast agent doses required are rather low relative to those needed for CT (about 10–20 ml of a gadolinium-containing contrast agent in MR imaging versus 100–150 ml of an iodine-containing contrast agent in CT). Liver MR imaging can thus also be performed in patients with an intolerance to iodine-containing contrast agents. The liver is examined using a heavily T1-weighted multi-section gradient-echo sequence during breath-hold. Unenhanced imaging is followed by acquisition at about 10 and 60 s and also at 2, 5, and 10 min after bolus injection of the contrast agent. With this protocol, both the arterial and portal-venous phases and several late phases are covered. Besides the classic, so-called ionic agents (e.g., Magnevist, Dotarem), so-called nonionic or low-osmolality contrast agents (e.g., Omniscan, Prohance) have been developed to improve acute tolerance and to thus allow the administration of higher doses. Compared with the use of ionic and nonionic agents in CT, however, these developments are of little practical relevance owing to the intrinsically better tolerance of MR contrast agents.

The tissue-specific contrast agents for the liver are subdivided into two groups: (1) superparamagnetic iron oxide particles with uptake by the Kupffer's cells of the liver, which predominantly shorten T2 relaxation times and thus reduce the signal intensity of normal liver tissue; (2) low-molecular agents with accumulation in the hepatocytes and biliary excretion, which reduce T1 relaxation times and thus increase the signal intensity of normal liver tissue. Preparations from both groups have been approved for clinical use. Others with even better tolerance, easier application, and better efficiency in their signal-changing effects are in the clinical trial phase. The examination protocol for superparamagnetic iron oxide particles comprises unenhanced T1- and T2-weighted sequences as well as proton-density-weighted or moderately T2-weighted delayed sequences in spin-echo technique or turbo-spin-echo technique for substances that are administered by slow infusion (e.g. Endorem, Feridex). The very sensitive T2*-weighted gradient-echo sequences can also be used for postcontrast imaging. Besides unenhanced T1- and T2-weighted imaging, the protocol for hepatobiliary contrast agents includes a delayed postcontrast T1-weighted study for substances that are administered by slow infusion (e.g. Teslascan). When substances that can be administered as bolus injections are used, a dynamic study can be performed in addition to depict perfusion characteristics of the liver pathology. Such contrast agents include Resovist as a superparamagnetic contrast medium and Multihance or Eovist as hepatobiliary contrast media.

13.4
Results and Discussion

Numerous studies have shown that conventional unenhanced MR imaging is superior to conventional incremental CT in the detection and characterization of focal liver lesions (HEIKEN et al. 1989; RUMMENY et al. 1992; SEMELKA et al. 1992; SITZMANN et al. 1990). The advent of the helical technique in CT and the introduction of the new gradient technology in combination with fast sequences in MR imaging requires a reconsideration of the respective capacities of these two modalities. Of particular importance is the differentiation of hypovascularized malignant liver tumors (typically metastases from colorectal cancer and pancreatic cancer) from hypervascularized ones (metastases from renal cell cancer, breast cancer, islet cell cancer, melanoma, and sarcoma or hepatocellular carcinoma as a primary liver tumor). Truly hypovascularized benign liver tumors do not exist. Special cases are avascular cystic liver lesions, abscesses or hemorrhages, on the one hand, and liver hemangioma with the typical hyperintense fill-in on the other. Hypervascularized benign liver tumors comprise focal-nodular hyperplasia and adenoma. How, then, does bi-phasic helical CT compare to multi-phase MR imaging? There are as yet no clear-cut results as to which of these two techniques is superior in the detection of hypovascular liver lesions. In MRI the possibility of examining the entire liver during the arterial and portal-venous perfusion phases is of minor significance for the identification of hypovascular liver tumors. The data available suggest that contrast-enhanced MR imaging has no advantage over plain MRI in the detection of hypovascularized lesions (HAMM et al. 1997). The situation is rather different for the detection of hypervascularized lesions by bi- or multi-phasic volume-covering examinations with either CT or MR imaging. Studies by FUJITA et al. (1994) demonstrated that helical CT during the arterial phase is superior to conventional CT in detecting hypervascularized lesions, especially small ones. Similar results were reported by HOLLETT et al. (1995), who compared bi-phasic helical CT, that is helical CT with inclusion of an arterial phase, with helical CT during the portal-venous phase alone. For the case of MR imaging, a significant advantage, especially in the detection of small hypervascular lesions, has been demonstrated for the volume-covering examination during the arterial perfusion phase relative to examination during the portal-venous phase and to unenhanced MR imaging (OI et al. 1996; YAMASHITA et al. 1996). Regarding the comparison of MR imaging with helical CT, YAMASHITA et al. (1996), OI et al. (1996) and MURAKAMI et al. (1995) found MR imaging to be superior to helical CT in the detection of small hypervascularized lesions. All these studies were performed in patients with multiple foci of HCC. The question that arises here is the reason for the suggested advantage of MR imaging versus helical CT, both performed during the arterial perfusion phase. One factor is certainly the high sensitivity of MR imaging to the contrast agents; a further factor might be the well-defined, compact bolus administered in MR imaging. A further difference between MR imaging and CT is the simultaneous data acquisition of the entire volume in the majority of 2D techniques used with MR imaging, which means that the contrast agent dynamics are identical in the most cranial and the most caudal section. In contrast, sequential measurement of the volume, as in CT, is always associated with the problem that the first sections are acquired too early and/or the last sections too late for an arterial perfusion phase. There is potential for further development of both modalities. In MR imaging, the sequences can be further improved, for example by the introduction of 3D techniques for a better spatial resolution. In CT, multi-detector systems will enable the acquisition of individual perfusion phases with a better temporal resolution in the future. With this technique, it will become possible, for instance, to scan the entire liver during the purely arterial phase. However, at present there is nothing in CT comparable to the tissue- or liver-specific contrast agents for MR imaging presently in clinical use or in an advanced clinical trial phase, although some liver-specific contrast agents for CT are presently undergoing preclinical or early clinical trials. With the administration of tissue-specific contrast agents, the sensitivity in the detection of focal liver lesions can be increased to the level of CT-AP, but with a markedly higher specificity than that of CT-AP (JOERGENSEN et al. 1997; MUELLER et al. 1997; VAN DEN HEUVEL et al. 1997).

Regarding the characterization of liver lesions, the high soft-tissue contrast is a decisive advantage of MR imaging over CT even in the unenhanced examination (LÜNING et al. 1991). The characterization of focal liver lesions is further significantly improved by dynamic MR imaging after bolus administration of a gadolinium-containing contrast agent (HAMM et al. 1994). The volume-covering sequences available today provide an optimal technique for examination of the entire liver both for detection and for characterization of lesions. Additional delayed sequences will further improve diagnostic accuracy, for example by depicting the characteristic peripheral wash-out of metastases (MAHFOUZ et al. 1994), the delayed enhancement of cholangiocellular carcinomas, or the centripetal fill-in phenomenon of hemangiomas (HAMM et al. 1990). The absence of radiation exposure is a decisive advantage of MR imaging, especially in patients in whom there is no strong suspicion of malignancy.

Despite its many advantages, MR imaging also has a decisive drawback, namely that it is an organ-related examination procedure which, for instance, covers only the liver as part of an examination of the upper abdomen. With the tube performance now available, on the other hand, a bi-phasic or tri-phasic CT examination can be supplemented by an examination of the lower abdomen and of the chest, to yield a complete thoracoabdominal staging.

Summary. With the introduction of powerful gradient technology and faster pulse sequences, MR imaging has made a great leap forward in the diagnostic assessment of the liver, just as CT has with the possibility of bi- and tri-phasic examinations through the advent of the helical technique. The new techniques in MR imaging, when used in combination with the bolus injection of contrast material, improve the detection of hypervascularized liver lesions. In this respect, results suggest a superiority of MR imaging during the arterial perfusion phase over the corresponding helical CT examination. Regarding the detection of hypovascularized lesions, at present there appears to be no advantage of MR imaging versus CT resulting from the examination during the arterial or portal venous phase.

For lesion characterization, unenhanced MR imaging already offers advantages over CT, because of the high contrast spectrum. And this advantage becomes even more pronounced with the possibility of performing volume-covering, multi-phasic examinations, including delayed studies. With CT, the price to be paid for bi- and tri-phasic examinations is a marked increase in radiation exposure.

References

Fujita M, Kuroda C, Kumatani T, Yoshioka H, Kuriyama K, Inoue E, Kasugai H, Sasaki Y (1994) Comparison between conventional and spiral CT in patients with hypervascular hepatocellular carcinoma. Eur J Radiol 18:134– 136

Hamm B, Mahfouz AE, Taupitz M, Mitchell DG, Nelson R, Halpern E, Speidel A, Wolf KJ, Saini S (1997) Liver metastases: improved detection with dynamic gadolinium-enhanced MR imaging? Radiology 202:677– 682

Hamm B, Fischer E, Taupitz M (1990) Differentiation of hepatic hemangiomas from metastases by dynamic contrast-enhanced MR imaging. J Comput Assist Tomogr 14:205– 216

Hamm B, Thoeni RF, Gould RG, Bernardino ME, Luning M, Saini S, Mahfouz AE, Taupitz M, Wolf KJ (1994) Focal liver lesions: characterization with nonenhanced and dynamic contrast material-enhanced MR imaging. Radiology 190:417– 423

Heiken, JP, Weyman PJ, Lee JK, Balfe DM, Picus D, Brunt EM, Flye MW (1989) Detection of focal hepatic masses: prospective evaluation with CT, delayed CT, CT during arterial portography, and MR imaging. Radiology 171:47– 51

Hollett, MD, Jeffrey RB Jr, Nino Murcia M, Jorgensen MJ, Harris DP (1995) Dual-phase helical CT of the liver: value of arterial phase scans in the detection of small (<or = 1.5 cm) malignant hepatic neoplasms. AJR Am J Roentgenol 164:879– 884

Joergensen M, Wilken J, Rosenthal H, Oldhafer KJ, Maschek H, Galanski MW (1997) Preoperative assessment of focal liver lesions: comparison of MR imaging with superparamagnetic iron oxide and double spiral CTAP. 83rd scientific assembly and annual meeting of the RSNA. Radiology 205 (P):371

Lüning M, Koch M, Abet L, Wolff H, Wenig B, Buchali K, Schopke W, Schneider T, Muhler A, Rudolph B (1991) The accuracy of the imaging procedures (sonography, MRT, CT, angio-CT,nuclear medicine) in characterizing liver tumors. Fortschr Rontgenstr 154:398– 406

Mahfouz AE, Hamm B, Wolf KJ (1994) Peripheral washout: a sign of malignancy on dynamic gadolinium-enhanced MR images of focal liver lesions. Radiology 190:49– 52

Mueller D, Kopka L, Fischer U, Grabbe EH (1997) Imaging of focal liver lesions with fast SPIO-MR imaging in comparison with triple phase helical-CT. 83rd scientific assembly and annual meeting of the RSNA. Radiology 205 (P):371

Murakami T, Kim T, Oi H, Nakamura H, Igarashi H, Matsushita M, Okamura J, Kozuka T (1995) Detectability of hypervascular hepatocellular carcinoma by arterial phase images of MR and spiral CT. Acta Radiol 36:372– 376

Oi H, Murakami T, Kim T, Matsushita M, Kishimoto H, Nakamura H (1996) Dynamic MR imaging and early-phase helical CT for detecting small intrahepatic metastases of hepatocellular carcinoma. AJR Am J Roentgenol 166:369– 374

Rummeny EJ, Wernecke K, Saini S, Vassallo P, Wiesmann W, Oestmann JW, Kivelitz D, Reers B, Reiser MF, Peters PE (1992) Comparison between high-field-strength MR imaging and CT for screening of hepatic metastases: a receiver operating characteristic analysis. Radiology 182:879– 886

Semelka RC, Shoenut JP, Kroeker MA, Greenberg HM, Simm FC, Minuk GY, Kroeker RM, Micflikier AB (1992) Focal liver disease: comparison of dynamic contrast-enhanced CT and T2-weighted fat-suppressed, FLASH, and dynamic gadolinium-enhanced MR imaging at 1.5 T. Radiology 184:687– 694

Sitzmann, JV, Coleman J, Pitt HA, Zerhouni E, Fishman E, Kaufman SL, Order S, Grochow LB, Cameron JL (1990) Preoperative assessment of malignant hepatic tumors. Am J Surg 159:137– 142discussion 142– 143

Van Den Heuvel AG, Van Der Sijp JR, Kruijt R, Oudkerk M (1997) Liver metastases: preoperative evaluation with CTAP and ferumoxide-enhanced T1-weighted and T2-weighted imaging. 83rd scientific assembly and annual meeting of the RSNA. Radiology 205 (P):371

Yamashita Y, Mitsuzaki K, Yi T, Ogata I, Nishiharu T, Urata J, Takahashi M (1996) Small hepatocellular carcinoma in patients with chronic liver damage: prospective comparison of detection with dynamic MR imaging and helical CT of the whole liver. Radiology 200:79– 84

14 Synthesis

F. Terrier

The relative advantages of US, CT, and MRI for liver imaging have been the subject of numerous contradictory scientific papers, and this debate is not yet over. Indeed, although large liver tumors are now very accurately detected with all three imaging methods, nodules less than 1–2 cm across remain difficult to detect and even more troublesome to characterize, and present a major challenge.

CT arterial portography has long been considered the most sensitive technique for detecting focal liver lesions. However, it is an invasive and cumbersome procedure. In addition, it is fraught with a large number of false-positive results. Thus, clinically irrelevant perfusion defects caused by local heterogeneity of portal flow may be difficult to differentiate from genuine tumors. Furthermore, on CT arterial portography, all tumors appear as hypoattenuating lesions, regardless of their nature. Because of the high prevalence of benign liver lesions, especially small cysts and hemangiomas, a highly sensitive imaging technique should also be accurate in lesion characterization. This is obviously not the case for CT arterial portography. For all these reasons, and despite the fact that CT arterial portography has been strongly advocated in the literature as the reference technique for the detection of liver metastases, its use has been rather limited and is now further decreasing, as a consequence of the steady improvement of the noninvasive imaging techniques.

Intraoperative US is another technique that, in experienced hands, is very sensitive. However, because of the particular setting in which it is used, it will not be discussed here.

One of the major problems in defining the role of MRI arises from the enormous disparity in equipment and imaging protocols. As a consequence of the rapid technical developments in this field, there are innumerable combinations of field strengths and pulse sequences, not to mention the different types of contrast media now available for liver imaging. Thus the performance of MRI and its accessibility differ greatly from center to center, depending on local resources, the type of equipment, experience and strategic options.

In contrast, the standard of CT equipment is quite uniform and the imaging protocols are well established, so that there is not much difference in the quality of CT examinations among the various centers.

Many authors now consider that MRI has become equivalent (or even superior) to CT for detecting focal liver lesions. However, this statement is valid only for state-of-the-art high-field equipment in combination with an intravenous contrast medium. The choice of contrast medium, however, is another hot topic. In our opinion, T1-weighted hepato-specific contrast media (for example manganese-DPDP) are the most helpful for improving sensitivity, but this remains controversial.

For the characterization of focal liver lesions, most authors agree that MRI is superior to CT for two reasons (1) the much higher soft-tissue contrast of MRI, allowing demonstration of subtle changes in signal intensity induced by contrast media (native images are unreliable for accurate lesion characterization); and (2) the availability of hepato-specific MRI contrast media, which has opened up new perspectives both for detection and for characterization (however, further work is still needed to evaluate their potential fully).

The advent of spiral technology has greatly improved the performance of CT. A further breakthrough is also expected in the very near future from multi-array detectors. Thus, using optimized imaging protocols such as double-phase CT, high sensitivity and accurate characterization can be achieved in the vast majority of cases. One definite advantage of CT over MRI is that the entire chest and abdomen, including the pelvis, can be studied in the same examination. This is of particular importance in oncologic patients.

F. Terrier, MD; Department of Radiology, Division de Radiodiagnostie et Radiologie Interventionnelle, Hôpital Cantonal, Rue Micheli-du-Crest 24, CH-1211 Genève 14, Switzerland

Color and power Doppler followed by 2nd harmonic imaging combined with the use of echogenic contrast media have made US into a highly sophisticated technique. However, its weaknesses of operator dependence and relatively low reproducibility persists. Nevertheless, it is the most appropriate technique for screening and follow-up purposes, for example in a check for liver metastases and hepatocellular carcinoma as part of the standard work-up in oncologic patients and in patients with liver cirrhosis, respectively. It is also useful for rapid confirmation of a strong clinical suspicion of advanced neoplastic disease of the liver. US is, of course, much used for abdominal surveys in numerous clinical situations. Because focal liver lesions, especially cysts and hemangiomas, are frequently found incidentally during such examinations, it is particularly important to reach a definite and correct diagnosis in the same session to avoid needless expensive or even invasive modalities, such as percutaneous liver biopsy. In this setting, the new developments in US, in particular echogenic contrast media, may be of value if they can make further investigations unnecessary. Otherwise, they will only add another burden to the growing health care costs.

In conclusion, CT is still the prime modality for liver imaging, allowing detection of primary and secondary tumors with high sensitivity and specificity. In some circumstances, absolute certainty is mandatory. This is the case, for example, when a diagnosis of hemangioma or FNH is made. Indeed, these tumors need no treatment and no follow-up. Nevertheless, there is the risk of mistaking a malignant tumor for a benign one at a stage when it could still be cured. Sometimes such a definite diagnosis is not possible with CT. Contrast-enhanced MRI then becomes the method of choice, because of its greater potential for lesion characterization. However, there is still no agreement on the imaging protocol and type of contrast medium. MRI is also indicated in the preoperative work-up of those patients with primary or secondary liver tumors, in whom the results of imaging will have a major impact on the decision as to whether or not to operate. In this situation, the technique with the highest sensitivity and specificity should be used.

Although US is considered inferior to CT and MRI in performance, it is the most adequate technique as a screening method and for follow-up, mostly because of its low cost, wide availability and absence of irradiation.

Pancreas and Biliary Ducts

15 Tailoring the Imaging Protocol

V.M. Bonaldi

CONTENTS

15.1   Introduction   *169*
15.2   Contrast Dynamics and Dosage   *169*
15.2.1 Vascular Supply of Pancreas and Bile Ducts   *170*
15.2.2 Parameters Influencing the Time–
        Attenuation Curve of the Pancreas   *170*
15.2.3 Practical Considerations for an Optimal
        CT Imaging Protocol   *170*
15.3   Single- or Multiple-Phase CT After Intravenous
        Bolus of Iodinated Contrast Medium   *172*
15.3.1 Single-Phase CT Imaging Protocols   *172*
15.3.2 Double-Phase CT Imaging Protocols   *172*
15.4   Selection of Collimation, Reconstruction Interval
        and Pitch with Regard to Indications   *173*
15.4.1 Basic Questions Applicable to All Patients   *173*
15.4.2 Applications to Pancreatic Adenocarcinomas   *174*
15.4.3 Application to Islet Cell Tumours   *174*
15.4.4 Application to Cystic Tumours   *174*
15.4.5 Application to Inflammatory Conditions
        of the Pancreas   *174*
15.4.6 Application to Diseases of the Bile Tract   *175*
15.5   Conclusion   *175*
        References   *176*

15.1
Introduction

As mentioned in previous chapters of this book, the helical (spiral) CT technique is now the imaging method of choice for abdominal examinations, particularly in pancreatic diseases (WYATT and FISHMAN 1994). Spiral CT allows a continuous volume of data to be obtained during a single breathhold. Reliable examinations with gapless coverage of the abdominal organs that are normally mobile during breathing can be performed by this technique. Because spiral CT acquisition is very fast, it can be completed within the phase of maximum parenchymal enhancement after intravenous injection of iodinated contrast medium, as long as care is taken to

V.M. BONALDI, MD; Département d'Imagerie Médicale, Hôpital Universitaire de L'Archet II, Route de St Antoine de Ginestière, Boite Postale 79, F-06202 Nice Cedex 03, France

select an appropriate delay between the injection and the initiation of CT scanning.

Thin collimation is needed for an effective search for pancreatic cancer, since depiction of small neoplasms remains the major indication for examinations in this anatomical area. Thanks to continuous improvements in CT X-ray tubes, slices as thin as 3 mm are feasible, as are spiral sequences with as long as 100 s duration, with enough high energy per slice to image anatomical areas as thick as the abdomen. The increased power dissipation needed in the X-ray tube for such demanding imaging protocols has been the incentive for major developments in heat dissipation and detector resistance. All these advances in spiral CT technology have allowed the use of the multi-phase technique, resulting in a large number of publications documenting its value in daily clinical practice. As a consequence of this evolution, the number of images that have to be dealt with daily has also increased tremendously and is becoming a serious concern.

Numerous interacting factors have to be considered at the time the CT imaging protocol of the pancreas has to be defined. They derive from the CT instrumental parameters, from requirements and limitations of the parameters of the contrast medium injection protocol, and also from the intrinsic haemodynamics and the general condition of the patient. An in-depth knowledge of all these factors and how they interact, allowing an appropriate selection of the imaging parameters, is a prerequisite for a successful examination of pancreas and bile ducts.

15.2
Contrast Dynamics and Dosage

The goal of the intravenous injection of iodinated contrast medium in CT is to increase the image contrast between normal and pathologic tissues. Indeed, in most cases, enhancement of tumour tissue is delayed with respect to the normal parenchyma of the pancreas. This being the case, the hypothesis has been proposed that detection of pancreas lesions becomes better with intensifying enhancement of the normal parenchyma. This does not relate to islet cell tumours, which are characteristically hypervascular and which require a specific imaging protocol.

15.2.1
Vascular Supply of Pancreas and Bile Ducts

The rich vascularization of the pancreas accounts for the intense increase in attenuation of the normal parenchyma after intravenous injection of contrast medium. Maximum parenchymal contrast attenuation is reached earlier for the pancreas than for the liver after injection, since the hepatic blood supply originates mainly from the portal vein. In contrast to the liver, the pancreas has an exclusive arterial blood supply, which originates from the coeliac and superior mesenteric arteries and which is grossly distributed in three zones. For the head of the pancreas, the blood supply comes from the pancreatic arcades; these are formed by superior and inferior anterior and posterior pancreatico-duodenal branches of the gastroduodenal and superior mesenteric artery, respectively. The body of the pancreas is supplied by the dorsal pancreatic artery, whereas the transverse pancreatic artery and branches of the splenic artery supply the tail of the gland. Each of the intrapancreatic arteries anastomoses freely with adjacent vessels, all combining to form a fine arterial network.

The pancreas is drained by multiple veins, which roughly correspond to the arteries: the anterior and posterior superior pancreatico-duodenal veins drain the head, whereas the transverse pancreatic vein drains the body and tail of the pancreas.

The cystic artery usually arises from the right hepatic artery in the angle between the common hepatic duct and the cystic duct. It divides into a superficial and a deep branch that arborize on the respective surfaces of the gallbladder. The bile ducts are supplied by several fine sinuous arteries from nearby larger arteries (ROUVIÈRE and DELMAS 1997).

Peripancreatic vessels are key anatomical landmarks in the staging of pancreatic carcinomas, since vascular invasion represents a contraindication for any attempt at surgical resection (WYATT and FISHMAN 1994; ZEMAN et al. 1995). As a result of the continuous advances in the performance of spiral CT, small veins surrounding the pancreas can now be visualized, which is helpful in the staging of pancreatic cancer (IBUKURO et al. 1996; VEDANTHAM et al. 1998).

15.2.2
Parameters Influencing the Time–Attenuation Curve of the Pancreas

From the site of injection in a peripheral vein of the arm or the forearm, the bolus of contrast medium reaches the arterial circulation of the body via the pulmonary circulation. Several factors affect contrast enhancement after injection of the contrast medium into the limb. Some of them are patient related, whereas others result from the modalities of contrast medium administration. Schematically, these factors can be divided into two groups:

- The first group is related to haemodynamics, such as the patient's cardiac and splanchnic outputs, and to the state of the arm vein into which the injection is given. The rate at which the contrast medium is injected plays here a major role. Factors in this group influence the time to peak of the pancreas time–attenuation curve after injection of the dye: The faster the rate of injection and the greater the cardiac output, the earlier the peak of contrast enhancement.
- The second group includes factors affecting the transfer of the contrast medium from the vascular to the interstitial compartment. These factors are the iodine content of the contrast medium, the total injected volume of contrast medium and the volume of the distribution compartment in the patient, the last factor being closely related to the patient's body weight. Factors of this second group preferentially determine the values of the maximum enhancement obtained after injection. The degree of parenchymal enhancement and the peak of the time–attenuation curve are directly related to the amount of iodine administered (DEAN et al. 1980; CLAUSSEN et al. 1984; BONALDI et al. 1996).

15.2.3
Practical Considerations for an Optimal CT Imaging Protocol

15.2.3.1
Native CT Scan and Oral Contrast Medium

In order to delineate the pancreas from adjacent anatomical structures, a sufficient volume of oral contrast medium (generally 750–1000 ml) is given to the patient between 30 and 60 min prior to the CT examination. This oral contrast medium may be a water-soluble iodinated agent (positive contrast medium) or a negative contrast medium, such as plain water (in our institution, we favour the first approach). In addition, an antispasmodic agent can be injected immediately before the CT examination, to reduce motion artefacts from bowel peristalsis (VALETTE 1995).

A 19- to 22-gauge catheter is placed into an antebrachial vein before the patient is positioned on the CT table, in order to ensure safe injection at rates varying from 2 to 5 ml/s, depending on the indications.

The patient is given a careful explanation of how to hold his or her breath in such a way that the inspiration volume is the same during every step of the scanning protocol (e.g. scout view, unenhanced and single- or multi-phase scans after the injection of contrast medium). Since an optimal technique is mandatory for the detection of small lesions, we use successive fast clusters of slices in preference to a helical technique when patients are obviously unable to hold their breath or to understand the basic requirements of the imaging protocol.

After the scout view has been carried out, a precontrast helical acquisition is first achieved in order to localize the pancreas and to depict calcium originating from stones in the ducts or from plaques in the walls of arterial vessels. We usually perform this precontrast study from the dome of the liver to the iliac crests, by using 10-mm thick slices. The level of the more distal slices of the pancreas is noted, as this will serve as the landmark for the enhanced sequence(s). With due consideration for the observation that the maximum liver contrast enhancement occurs later than the enhancement peak of the pancreas, we favour the "bottom-up" direction for the postcontrast sequence(s). Patients are asked to hyperventilate deeply before and during the beginning of the injection to enable them to maintain apnoea throughout the entire pancreatic acquisition(s). If needed, the liver portion not included in the pancreatic sequences can be scanned by means of an additional sequence immediately after a short pause for breath recovery.

15.2.3.2
Amount of Intravenously Injected Contrast Medium

Once intravenously injected, the iodinated contrast medium is delivered throughout the entire volume of biodistribution in the patient's body. The ratio between this distribution volume and the amount of contrast administered determines the maximum enhancement of the normal parenchyma. This consideration emphasizes that doses of contrast medium should be calculated as fractions of the patients' weight (KORMANO et al. 1983; HEIKEN et al. 1995). Indeed, the use of the same fixed dose to obese and normal-weight patients without reference to their body weight, leads to significant differences in the contrast enhancement of organs, and subsequently in lesion depiction.

We usually inject a dose of 2 ml/kg body weight of contrast medium (generally with a content of 300 mg I /ml), unless known renal failure imposes the necessity to reduce either the dose or the concentration of the iodinated contrast medium.

15.2.3.3
Rate of Injection and Delay Before Scan Initiation

As has been extensively demonstrated for the liver, there is a theoretical time after injection at which both pathologic and normal tissues reach similar contrast enhancement values (equilibrium phase). The same phenomenon applies in the pancreas, although is has not been so much studied as in the liver. Care must therefore be taken to scan the entire pancreas before this critical phase occurs. Adequate combination of contrast medium injection and initiation of the spiral CT sequence is therefore essential for successful examination of the pancreas. The purpose is to acquire the data during the optimal temporal window (COX et al. 1991), when the lesions are optimally detectable. As already mentioned, the higher the injection rate, the earlier the maximum enhancement of the pancreas parenchyma. However, as demonstrated in two studies conducted by BRET and colleagues (BONALDI et al. 1996; GARCIA et al. 1996) on the liver and the pancreas, respectively, a faster contrast injection rate does not result in an increase of the peak, but rather in shortening of the plateau of the time–enhancement curve, with a subsequent theoretical risk of scanning the pancreas outside the optimal temporal window.

15.3
Single- or Multiple-Phase CT After Intravenous Bolus of Iodinated Contrast Medium

The choice among the large range of scanning protocols using the helical technique that are now available has to be made with due consideration for the clinical situation encountered and for the particular type of scanner used. Indeed, the slice collimation and the injection protocol have to be selected according to the type of lesions that the investigators expect to find. Conversely, the parameters required by the scanning protocol have to be adapted to the capacities of the CT scanner:

- On the one hand, the major challenge for CT examination of the pancreas is still cancer: pancreatic tumours have to be depicted in the earliest possible stage and, once diagnosed, must be staged as resectable or nonresectable tumours. In this clinical condition, the key parameters, as underlined by MEGIBOW (1992), are an appropriate slice thickness and an optimal injection protocol. With the most recent refinements of the helical scanners reducing constraints attributable to X-ray tube heating, double-phase protocols have become feasible, with adequate slice thickness and without the need for a long delay for tube cooling between the two acquisition phases (LU et al. 1997; GRAF et al. 1997; KEOGAN et al. 1997; DIEHL et al. 1998).
- On the other hand, larger lesions, such as the majority of pancreatic inflammatory diseases and some cystic neoplasms, do not require the use of such thin slices or of multiphase imaging protocols.

15.3.1
Single-Phase CT Imaging Protocols

As mentioned above, there are many conditions in which a single-phase CT imaging protocol is sufficient in terms of diagnostic or staging relevance for pancreatic disease. Thus, in the majority of inflammatory diseases, the questions the CT examination has to answer are related to the extent of necrosis or haemorrhage in the pancreatic loge (assessed by comparing pre- and postcontrast images) and to the size of the peripancreatic fluid collections (BALTHAZAR et al. 1990; JOHNSON et al. 1991). Following a native CT scan, we generally perform the enhanced CT sequence by using 5- to 7-mm-thick

slices in the caudo-cranial direction. When follow-up examinations have to be repeated in case of pancreatitis, we favour protocols including 10-mm-thick slices with an mAs value as low as possible. A pitch up to 1.5:1 has also been suggested for this specific kind of follow-up (HOPPER et al. 1998).

15.3.2
Double-Phase CT Imaging Protocols

Double-phase imaging has become increasingly accessible as a result of the continuous improvements in helical CT technology. Initially feasible only with thick slices for liver examination (BONALDI et al. 1995; HOLLETT et al. 1995), this technique has been progressively combined with thinner slices. Hence, the contrast enhancement behaviour of the pancreas can now be studied twice after injection of the contrast medium, first during the early arterial phase, and then during the later venous phase. However, during the programming of the CT imaging protocol, the overall features of the time–enhancement curve must be kept in mind, in order to maintain the time of both sequences within the optimal temporal window.

Three-dimensional CT angiography (3D-CTA) has been an important application of helical CT since the earliest times of its use. It has been presented as an alternative to standard angiography, with the advantage of being non-invasive and coupled with the cross-sectional information on organs routinely derived from CT (BLUEMKE and CHAMBERS 1995). This volume rendering imaging method is much appreciated by surgeons, because it obviates the need for paging through the various sections of axial or other uniplanar images. In a recent study comparing conventional axial helical CT and 3D-CT angiographic images, RAPTOPOULOS et al. (1997) demonstrated the additional value of 3D-CTA in predicting the resectability of pancreatic tumours.

3D-CTA requires both thin slices and high mAs values to get subtle details. Therefore, it was not routinely included in two-phase protocols until recently, because of the prohibitive delay needed for tube cooling between the two spiral acquisitions. Owing to the variations in the time–enhancement curve, which are dependent on the injection rate (i.e. the faster the rate, the earlier the peak and the narrower the optimal temporal window), the performance of a double-phase spiral CT protocol challenges the operator's skill:

– On the one hand, optimal 3D-CTA preferably requires injection rates faster than 4.5 ml/s (Winter et al. 1996). For such fast injection rates, automated bolus delivery by means of a power electric injector is essential. The reason why such a fast rate is needed is two-fold. First, it helps to ensure the first pass of a minimally diluted bolus through the target vasculature. Second, it facilitates differentiation between arteries and veins, and also between arteries and parenchyma, providing that CT-angio data are obtained early enough after the contrast medium injection. It should not be forgotten that many pitfalls can be encountered during the generation of 3D maximum intensity projection (3D-MIP) images. Among these, insufficient separation in attenuation between vessels and surrounding anatomy (e.g. vessels and parenchyma) remains the principal drawback of this postprocessing imaging technique, because MIP images are based on selecting attenuation values lying above a predetermined threshold. This is one of the reasons why water should be used in preference to barium or iodine-based oral contrast medium.

– On the other hand, the parenchyma of the pancreas is intensively enhanced during the early phase after contrast medium injection, with a rapid wash-out because of its rich arterial blood supply (Bonaldi et al. 1996). Increasing the speed of the injection subsequently decreases the optimal temporal window for the examination of the parenchyma. Hence, for keeping optimal conditions during the two sequences, the shortest intersequence delay possible is mandatory.

As was addressed in Sect. 15.2.2 the patient's haemodynamics can considerably modify the time-to-peak pancreatic enhancement. In a study conducted with the aim of defining how to improve prediction of the optimal scanning delay in spiral CT angiography, Van Hoe and colleagues (1995) have shown the usefulness of injecting a test bolus.

At the time of writing, questions remain about the accurate injection protocol for optimal assessment of both the pancreatic parenchyma and the arterial and venous anatomical landmarks. However, it can already easily be predicted that with the tremendous progress going on in helical scanning technology, the use of multi-phase protocols will continue to expand.

15.4
Selection of Collimation, Reconstruction Interval and Pitch with Regard to Indications

Emphasis is put on the skilful evaluation of the different interacting factors to allow selection of the optimal parameters of the spiral CT imaging protocol according to the type of the lesions the radiologist is asked to demonstrate. Specific pancreatic diseases are described in other chapters of this book.

15.4.1
Basic Questions Applicable to All Patients

First of all, the radiologist should evaluate the patient's general condition in order to detect any limitations inherent to the patient:

1. Is the patient able to keep his or her breath held satisfactorily for the time required to cover the target area? If the answer is no, we usually abandon the attempt to use helical acquisition because of the risk of poor image quality and decreased pertinence of the diagnosis. A fast dynamic cluster technique is preferred in such cases. An alternative is to use two successive spiral sequences, with the intersequence delay permitting a short period of breathing before the next breath-hold. However, this technique involves a risk of missing information since the depth of the breath-hold during the successive sequences or clusters is often not the same.

2. Is the quality of the vein that has been punctured for contrast medium injection adequate for the injection speed that has to be used for the optimal single-, double-, or angio-phase required by the clinical indication? If the answer is no, the speed of injection and the corresponding imaging protocol must be modified.

3. Do the technical capabilities of the available CT scanner allow the protocol that the radiologist wants to perform? If a double-phase examination can only be achieved at the price of a considerable decrease in image quality or with a prohibitive delay for tube cooling between the two sequences, a single-phase protocol may be more adequate. Otherwise, the second spiral CT sequence will not yield any pertinent information, but only lead to unnecessary irradiation.

4. Will the available storage memory of the CT scanner be sufficient for the entire protocol that has to be achieved? Nothing is more frustrating than

having to wait between two consecutive sequences for the purpose of rendering memory space available.

15.4.2
Applications to Pancreatic Adenocarcinomas

Once the basic questions detailed above have been answered, the critical concern in the search for a pancreas tumour, particularly if 3D-CTA post-processing is required, is to image the pancreas with a collimation as thin as possible, a pitch as low as possible (preferentially 1:1 or lower) and mAs values as high as possible, since details as subtle as very small tumours, vascular invasion or lymphadenopathy have to be looked for. High spatial resolution requires narrow collimation and relatively slow patient translation. However, slow table motion limits the amount of anatomical coverage that can be obtained in a given time interval. In order to compensate for the limitations imposed by the heating of the X-ray tube, pitches greater than 1:1 have been advocated. However, whereas narrower collimation favours higher spatial resolution, increase in pitch favours artefacts. Several manufacturers impose use of a higher pitch as soon as a double-phase sequence is planned. Fortunately, the CT scanner in current use in our institution does not require this kind of concession (AVE1, Philips Medical Systems, The Netherlands). We actually perform such examinations by using 140 kV, 225 mAs, 3- to 5-mm thin slices and a pitch of 1:1. A 1-s scan time is used, in order to optimize acquisition during the peak enhancement after bolus injection of contrast medium.

A major advantage of applying spiral CT in the work-up of tumours is the arbitrary reconstruction interval that this technique allows, when the images are calculated after the data have been acquired. URBAN and colleagues have demonstrated the usefulness of overlapping cross-sectional reconstructions for such a purpose (URBAN et al. 1993). This overlapping also allows optimal 3D or 2D multiplanar reformatted images when needed. We generally use a 50% overlap when such postprocessing is performed.

15.4.3
Application to Islet Cell Tumours

The islet cells of the pancreas may give rise to a wide variety of functional tumours, the symptoms of which result from the hormone activity. These tumours include vipomas, insulinomas, gastrinomas, glucagonomas and somatostatinomas, which all are usually of small size at the time they are searched for. Islet cell tumours also can be non functional, and as such can be of larger size by the time they are detected. Because these tumours are classically hypervascular, there is a considerable gain to use a double-phase sequence, with the first sequence carried out during a real arterial phase (CHUNG et al. 1997). For the depiction of small tumours, small field-of-view targeted reconstructions are of interest (NISHIHARU et al. 1998).

15.4.4
Application to Cystic Tumours

Microcystic and mucinous neoplasms both demonstrate neovascularity in solid components, alternating with areas of avascular cystic spaces. The differentiation between the solid and cystic components and the precise demonstration of the respective arrangement of both tissues in the tumour are exquisitely well obtained by double-phase spiral CT . Although it is not always possible to distinguish between malignant and benign tumours in this group of cystic lesions by CT, the sunburst-type septations of the microcystic tumours is well demonstrated during an early arterial phase. The cystic tumours tend to be larger than adenocarcinomas or islet-cell tumours at the time of presentation. Therefore, they can usually be examined with 5-mm-thick slices.

15.4.5
Application to Inflammatory Conditions of the Pancreas

In contrast to what has been underlined above for the search of small neoplasms, pathologic changes that have to be sought by CT in acute inflammatory conditions are large: initial work-up of acute pancreatitis, in fact, must appreciate the extent of peripancreatic exudation (often large) and the proportion of the gland that is necrotic. Whereas studies focused on the use of double-phase protocols are still lacking, it can reasonably be predicted that areas of low enhancement within the pancreatic gland would be optimally analysed by the use of an early-phase CT sequence. Initial diagnosis and assessment of the severity of acute pancreatitis could then theoretically be optimized. At the time the complications of acute pancreatitis occur, helical CT will help to delineate aneurysms as well as the hypervascular rim of phlegmons and collected abscesses.

15.4.6
Application to Diseases of the Bile Tract

The gapless volume of data derived from spiral CT is exquisitely useful for detecting small stones of the common bile duct. In this condition, reconstructions using overlapping sections are of major interest.

For similar reasons, small cholangiocarcinomas can be more accurately diagnosed when such overlapping images are generated.

15.5 Conclusion

As the result of continuous improvements in CT technology, imaging protocols suggested today will probably be outdated within the next few years. However, the reader of this chapter and the user of

spiral CT should remember that thinner and thinner slices are becoming available and should be used for the purpose of depicting small cancers. Overlap of 50% in reconstructions has been shown to increase both the confidence in and the rate of detection of parenchymal lesions.

Iodinated contrast medium should be given in doses calculated as a fraction of the patient's body weight in order to ensure sufficient difference in attenuation between lesions and normal parenchyma. With slow or medium rates of injection (e.g. 2–3 ml/s), intravenous administration of contrast medium allows the spiral CT sequence to be performed during a relatively prolonged optimal temporal window. Similarly, when examination of both arterial and venous phases of the examination are required, common injection rates of 2–3 m/s can still be used, with both sequences included within the optimal temporal window of imaging. When the examination is specifically performed for the purpose of demonstrating arterial anatomy, higher rates over 4.5 ml/s should be used. As a consequence, the delay between contrast medium injection and initiation of CT scan should be shortened (Table 1).

Table 1. Summary guide of CT and injection protocols parameters depending on specific requirements for pancreas examinations. All information given relates to CT examinations of 30 s duration. Conditions of the cardiac output and the quality of the veins used for injection of contrast medium can significantly alter the time-to-peak occurrence (*CM* contrast medium, *BW* body weight, *ICT* islet cell tumours)

Examination type	Thickness of CT sections	Reconstruction overlap[a]	Volume of CM	Rate of injection	Delay between CM injection and initiation of CT scanning	Additional considerations
Single-phase protocols						
Routine work-up	5–7 mm	50%	2 ml/kg BW	2 ml/s	55 s	
Follow-up pancreatitis	10 mm	50%	2 ml/kg BW	2 ml/s	55 s	Pitch can be superior to 1
Pancreatic cancer search	3–5 mm	50%	2 ml/kg BW	2 ml/s	55 s	Oral water contrast
Dual-phase protocols						
For early and late phases of parenchyma attenuation	5 mm	50%	2 ml/kg BW	3 ml/s	35/80 s	
Three-dimension imaging protocols						
Study of arterial vasculature or ICT	3–5 mm	50%	2 ml/kg BW	+4.5 ml/s	30 s	Oral water contrast
Study of venous and arterial vasculature	3–5 mm	50%	2 ml/kg BW	3 ml/s	50 s	Oral water contrast

[a]Reconstruction overlap superior to 50% is advised for optimal 2D multiplanar reconstructions

Acknowledgements. I should like to express my gratitude to Patrice M. Bret for his unstinting support during my fellowship and my thanks to Robin Walsh for revisions of the current manuscript.

References

Balthazar EJ, Robinson DL, Megibow AJ, Ranson JH (1990) Acute pancreatitis: Value of CT in establishing prognosis. Radiology 174:331–336

Bluemke DA, Chambers TP(1995) Spiral CT angiography: an alternative to conventional angiography. Radiology 195:317–319

Bonaldi VM, Bret PM, Atri M, Garcia P, Reinhold C (1996) A comparison of two injection protocols using helical and dynamic acquisitions in CT examinations of the pancreas. Am J Roentgenol (AJR) 167:49–55

Bonaldi VM, Bret PM, Reinhold C, Atri M (1995) Spiral CT of the liver: Value of an early hepatic arterial phase. Radiology 197:357–363

Chung MJ, Choi BI, Han JK, Chung JW, Han MC, Bae SH (1997) Functioning islet cell tumor of the pancreas: Localization with dynamic spiral CT. Acta Radiol 38:135–138

Claussen CD, Bander D, Pfretzscher C, Kalender WA, Schorner W (1984) Bolus geometry and dynamics after intravenous contrast medium injection. Radiology 153:365:368

Cox IH, Foley WD, Hoffmann RG (1991) Right window for dynamic hepatic CT. Radiology 170:18–21

Dean PB, Violante MR, Mahoney JA (1980) Hepatic CT contrast enhancement: effect of dose, duration of infusion and time elapsed following infusion. Invest Radiol 15:158–161

Diehl SJ, Lehmann KJ, Sadick M, Lachmann R, Georgi M (1998) Pancreatic cancer: value of dual-phase helical CT in assessing resectability. Radiology 206:373–378

Garcia P, Bonaldi VM, Bret PM, Liang LL, Atri M, Reinhold C (1996) Effects of rate of contrast medium injection on hepatic enhancement at CT. Radiology 199:185–189

Graf O, Boland GW, Warshaw AL, Fernandez-del-Castillo C, Hahn PF, Mueller PR (1997) Arterial versus portal venous helical CT for revealing pancreatic adenocarcinoma: conspicuity of tumor and critical vascular anatomy. Am J Roentgenol (AJR) 169:119–123

Heiken JP, Brink JA, McClennan BL, Sagel SS, Crowe TM, Gaines MV (1995) Dynamic incremental CT: effect of volume and concentration of contrast material and patient weight on hepatic enhancement. Radiology 195:353–357

Hollett MD, Jeffrey RBJr, Nino-Murcia M, Jorgensen MJ, Harris DP (1995) Dual-phase helical CT of the liver: value of arterial phase scans in the detection of small (_1.5 cm) malignant hepatic neoplasms. Am J Roentgenol 164:879–884

Hopper KD, Keeton NC, Kasales CJ et al (1998) Utility of low mA 1.5 pitch helical versus conventional high mA abdominal CT. Clin Imag 22:54–59

Ibukuro K, Tsukiyama T, Mori K, Inoue Y (1996) Peripancreatic veins on thin-sections (3 mm) helical CT. AJR Am J Roentgenol 167:1003–8

Johnson CD, Stephens DH, Sarr MG (1991) CT of acute pancreatitis: Correlation between lack of contrast enhancement and pancreatic necrosis. AJR Am J Roentgenol 156:93–95

Keogan MT, McGermott VG, Paulson EK, Sheafor DH, Frederick MG, DeLong DM, Nelson RC (1997) Pancreatic malignancy: effect of dual-phase helical CT in tumor detection and vascular opacification. Radiology 205:513–518

Kormano M, Kaarina P, Soimakallio S, Kivimäki T (1983) Dynamic contrast enhancement of the upper abdomen: effect of contrast medium and body weight. Invest Radiol 18:364–367

Lu DS, Reber HA, Krasny RM, Kadel BM, Sayre J (1997) Local staging of pancreatic cancer: criteria for unresectability of major vessels as revealed by pancreatic-phase, thin-section helical CT. AJR Am J Roentgenol 168:1439–1443

Megibow AJ (1992) Pancreatic adenocarcinoma: designing the examination to evaluate the clinical questions. Radiology 183:297–303

Nishiharu T, Yamashita Y, Ogata I, Sumi S, Mitszaki K, Takahashi M (1998) Spiral CT of the pancreas: the value of small field-of-view targeted reconstruction. Acta Radiol 39:60–63

Raptopoulos V, Stter ML, Sheiman RG, Vrachliotis TG, Gougoutas CA, Movson JS (1997) The use of helical CT and CT angiography to predict vascular involvement from pancreatic cancer: correlation with findings at surgery. AJR Am J Roentgenol 168: 971–977

Rouvière H, Delmas A (1997) Pancreas, vaisseaux et nerfs. In: Anatomie humaine descriptive, topographique et fonctionnelle, vol II. Masson, Paris, pp 467–468

Urban BA, Fishman EK, Kuhlman JE, Kawashima A, Hennessey JG, Siegelman SS (1993) Detection of focal hepatic lesions with spiral CT: comparison of 4 and 8 mm interscan spacing. AJR Am J Roentgenol 160:783–785

Valette PJ (1995) Collection d'imagerie radiologique, anatomie du pancréas normal. In: Imagerie du pancréas. Masson, Paris, pp 27–33

Van Hoe L, Marchal G, Baert AL, Gryspeerdt S, Mertens L (1995) Determination of scan delay time in spiral CT-angiography: utility of a test bolus injection. J Comput Assist Tomogr (JCAT) 19:216–220

Vedantham S, Lu DS, Reber HA, Kadell B (1998) Small peripancreatic veins: improved assessment in pancreatic cancer patients using thin-section pancreatic phase helical CT. AJR Am J Roentgenol 170:377–383

Winter TC, Nghiem HV, Schmiedl UP et al (1996) CT angiography of the visceral vessels. Semin Ultrasound CT MRI 17:339–351

Wyatt SH, Fishman EK (1994) Spiral CT of the pancreas. Semin Ultrasound, CT MRI 15:122–132

Zeman RK, Silverman PM, Ascher SM, Patt RH, Cooper C, Al-Kawas F (1995) Helical (spiral) CT of the pancreas and biliary tract. Radiol Clin North Am 33:887–902

16 Benign and Malignant Biliary Stenoses

M. Bezzi, L. Broglia

CONTENTS

16.1   Introduction   177
16.2   Normal Bile Ducts   177
16.3   Bile Duct Neoplasms   178
16.3.1   Benign Neoplasms   178
16.3.2   Cholangiocarcinoma   178
16.4   Inflammatory Disease   182
16.4.1   Recurrent Cholangitis   182
16.4.2   Primary Sclerosing Cholangitis   183
16.5   Benign Postoperative Strictures   183
          References   186

16.1 Introduction

Spiral scanning has much improved spatial and contrast resolution in computed tomography (CT) by making it possible to acquire a continuous volume within a single breath-hold and to avoid respiratory misregistration artifacts. These advantages have increased the efficacy of CT in the study of the biliary tree, especially as regards lesion detection and the distinction between malignant and benign causes of biliary obstruction (Reiman et al. 1987). Arterial and venous phase contrast studies allow evaluation of vascular involvement and increase our confidence in assessing tumor resectability. In addition, from images reconstructed with at least 50% overlap, the radiologist may obtain reformatted images of the biliary tree in any plane for ideal depiction of anatomical and pathological findings.

Our spiral CT protocol is tailored according to the nature of the lesion suspected. However, we generally acquire 5-mm-thick sections, with a pitch of 1.0–1.6 and a 4-mm reconstruction interval. A total volume of 120–150 ml of intravenous contrast medium is injected at a rate of 3.5 ml/s. A more detailed discussion of tailored imaging protocols can be found in other chapters of this book.

Selective opacification of the biliary tree may be obtained with intravenous administration of contrast media secreted into the bile. This technique requires image postprocessing with Multiplanar Reformation (MPR) and Multiple Intensity Projection (MIP) in order to obtain cholangiographic images not so different from those obtained using MR cholangiography, ERCP or PTC. However, this technique suffers from the same limitation as intravenous cholangiography, with suboptimal opacification of the biliary system in patients with high bilirubin levels.

16.2 Normal Bile Ducts

Nondilated intrahepatic bile ducts are generally not identified because they are smaller than 1 mm in size. The main right and left hepatic ducts appear as thin tubular structures approximately 1 mm in diameter, running anterior to the right and left portal vein branches and converging toward the hepatic duct, anterior to the common portal trunk.

Patients with suspected intrahepatic lithiasis and cholangitis who have previously undergone sphincterotomy or biliary-enteric anastomosis may present with gas bubbles in the bile ducts, which can easily be differentiated from the presence of air in the portal system: gas in the venous system is peripheral, close to the hepatic capsule, while pneumobilia is more centrally located.

When air is seen in nondilated biliary ducts, a check of the patient's history for previous sphincterotomy or surgery is mandatory. If the history is unremarkable, pneumobilia may be suggestive of a spontaneous biliary-enteric fistula: this may be the consequence of cholelithiasis with chronic cholecystitis, where inflammation produces migration of the

M. Bezzi, MD; Istituto di Radiologia – III Cattedra, Università degli Studi di Roma "La Sapienza", Policlinico Umberto I, Viale Regina Elena 324, I-00161 Rome, Italy
L. Broglia, MD; Istituto di Radiologia – III Cattedra, Università degli Studi di Roma "La Sapienza", Policlinico Umberto I, Viale Regina Elena 324, I-00161 Rome, Italy

stone in the bowel lumen through gallbladder wall erosion (SAUERBREI et al. 1992).

16.3
Bile Duct Neoplasms

16.3.1
Benign Neoplasms

Benign bile duct neoplasms, such as adenoma, papilloma and cystadenoma, are rare pathologic conditions (KANE 1988), occurring in approximately 0.1% of surgical series (BURHANS and MYERS 1971).

Papilloma and adenomas appear as intraluminal masses with a broad base, generally growing within the larger ducts or in the periampullary region and causing obstructive jaundice (McINTYRE and CHENG 1968). Papilloma may be multiple, and it usually appears as a small filling defect in the ducts. Adenoma is generally single, and since it consists of glandular structures may often be hypodense (RICHTER and GRENACHER 1997).

The adenoma of the papilla of Vater is included in this group since it originates from the cholangiocellular epithelium (Fig. 16.1). Such a tumor of the distal CBD must be differentiated from neoplasms of the pancreatic head, from ampullary carcinoma and even from duodenal carcinoma. Adequate technique is extremely important in order to identify and characterize the lesion correctly. Some authors suggest to acquire thin-slice spiral scanning with water distention of the duodenum combined with pharmacological hypotonia by intravenous administration of N-butylscopolamine bromide (RICHTER and GRENACHER 1997). This technique, with water used as a negative intraluminal contrast agent, allows visualization of the ampullary mass within the duodenal lumen and differentiation of the mass from the distended duodenal wall. We believe that positive intraluminal contrast agents are also effective in demonstrating the lesion (Fig. 16.1).

Cystadenomas originating from the biliary tree are rare and occur mainly in middle-aged women. These tumors are often incidentally discovered during routine liver examination. At pathology the lesions present as well-circumscribed, intrahepatic, bulky, multilocular cystic masses consisting of multiple cysts containing mucinous fluid and lined by well-vascularized septa. Cyst walls may be irregular and show nodules or calcifications (DEVANEY et al. 1994).

At CT the tumor appears as a well-circumscribed, intrahepatic lobulated or multilocular hypodense lesion, characterized by density values higher that those of simple liver cysts, probably because of mucin content. After intravenous contrast injection the solid septa, the peripheral capsule, and the nodules on the wall show enhancement, with a behavior similar to that of cystadenocarcinoma (Fig. 16.2). It is almost impossible to differentiate between these two forms by CT criteria, and needle biopsy is often useless, because benign areas can exist in cystadenocarcinoma. At histology these two forms may be distinguished on the basis of the cuboidal epithelial inner lining, which is unicellular in benign lesions and pluricellular in cystadenocarcinoma (DEVANEY et al. 1994).

Differential diagnosis of these tumors includes intrahepatic cyst, hydatid cysts, abscesses, hematomas and, although extremely rare, hamartomas and cystic teratomas of the liver.

16.3.2
Cholangiocarcinoma

Although rare, this is one of the most common neoplastic causes of biliary obstruction. Jaundice generally occurs when the tumor is relatively small, and differential diagnosis against lithiasis or other causes of benign biliary stenosis is required.

It may be associated with congenital abnormalities of the biliary system, such as Caroli's disease, or with inflammatory conditions, such as sclerosing cholangitis (RITCHIE et al. 1974).

Cholangiocarcinoma originates from epithelial cells of the biliary duct and may develop at any level within the biliary system, either intra- or extra-hepatically.

According to the level of origin, cholangiocarcinoma can be subdivided into several subgroups:
a) Intrahepatic cholangiocarcinoma
b) Klatskin's tumor (hilar cholangiocarcinoma)
c) Cholangiocarcinoma of the common hepatic or common bile ducts
d) Ampullary carcinoma

Intrahepatic cholangiocarcinoma may be very small and should be suspected when dilated bile ducts are seen, at a segmental or subsegmental level, in patients with normal extrahepatic bile ducts and when other causes of biliary obstruction have been ruled out. In these patients with small tumors no other CT findings may be observed.

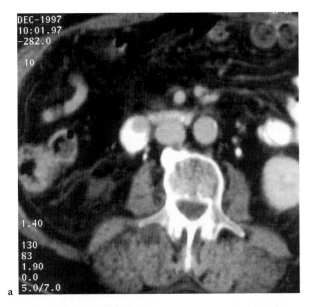

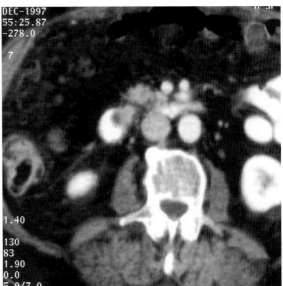

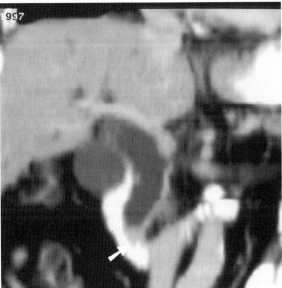

Fig. 16.1a–c. Ampullary adenoma. **a, b** CT scans obtained after iodinated oral contrast media and duodenal hypotonia show a small soft tissue density mass protruding into the duodenum at the level of the papilla. A small portion of the lesion (**b**) is hypodense because of dilated mucinous glands; this finding is typical of ampullary tumors. **c** Coronal MPR demonstrates dilation of the CBD and the papillary location of the obstructing mass (*arrow*) better

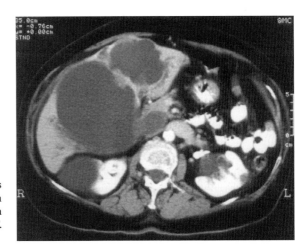

Fig. 16.2. Biliary cystadenoma. Multiloculated cystic mass with multiple septa and solid tumor nodules arising from both the wall and the septa. Differential diagnosis between cystadenoma and cystadenocarcinoma is not possible by CT. (Courtesy of Prof. P. Rossi, University of Rome, Italy)

In some cases the tumor grows before producing obstruction; in such instances a hepatic mass is identified on CT images. The findings on dynamic contrast-enhanced images are not so typical as to allow correct characterization of the lesions. During arterial and portal venous phases the lesion generally appears with a thin, mild, incomplete rim-like contrast enhancement combined with a low intra-tumoral attenuation with amorphous areas of slightly high attenuation (KIM et al. 1997) (Fig. 16.3). Delayed post-equilibrium phase, acquired between 6 and 30 min after the intravenous injection of contrast medium, seems to be more accurate in the diagnosis of this tumor. In fact, in a recent study performed on 47 patients affected by peripheral cholangiocarcinoma, 74% of patients with one or multiple lesions showed hyperdensity on delayed enhanced phase, with attenuating values similar to those of vessels (LACOMIS et al. 1997).

About one third of cholangiocarcinomas can be highly hypervascular in early phases, because they maintain an adenomatous structure with high cellularity. As with any other intrahepatic masses of possibly malignant origin, the definitive diagnosis should be obtained with image-guided biopsy.

"Klatskin" tumor (KLATSKIN 1965) can be radiologically divided into three types: infiltrative, exophytic and polypoid (CHOI et al. 1989).

Infiltrating tumors are the most common type (78% of Choi's series); they tend to grow along the bile duct wall, are usually ill-defined on cross-sectional imaging and become manifest as a focal biliary stricture on cholangiography. Exophytic tumors are well-defined masses with outward extension beyond the duct wall and spread into the surrounding structures.

Polypoid tumors are the least common type (8% of Choi's series) and present as an intraluminal mass.

On conventional CT the accuracy of tumor detection is extremely low, because of the small size of the lesion, which is not directly visible at the hepatic hilum; the diagnosis is often based on indirect signs, such as nonunion of dilated intrahepatic ducts at the hepatic hilum with a normal extrahepatic biliary duct (MEYER and WEINSTEIN 1983) or diffuse enhancement around the hepatic hilum. Results with spiral CT seem to be promising: infiltrative tumors appear as small masses or as focal wall thickening that obliterates the lumen. The wall is often hyperdense in both arterial and venous phase images; more rarely it can be hypoattenuating. Exophytic tumors show early peripheral enhancement, while they tend to become hypodense in the venous phase (HAN et al. 1997).

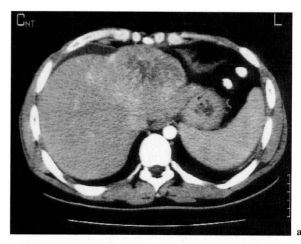

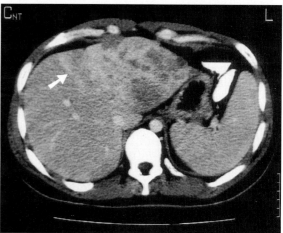

Fig. 16.3a, b. Cholangiocellular carcinoma of the left lobe. CT scans obtained during i.v. injection of contrast medium (**a** arterial, **b** venous phases at two different levels). Typical CT appearance: poorly defined margins, central hypodense areas, focal areas of hypervascularity at the periphery. Intrahepatic metastases (*arrow*) are seen (**b**)

Although the resectability criteria used by surgeons differ, a cholangiocarcinoma can be considered unresectable when the main portal vein or both the portal vein branches are infiltrated. Infiltration of both intrahepatic branches of the hepatic artery is rare and more difficult to demonstrate, and again it is associated with unresectability. Unilateral portal vein or hepatic artery involvement may be considered compatible with resection by some surgical groups.

The most difficult evaluation to be made at CT is the assessment of the extension of tumor within the intrahepatic biliary radicles. Direct cholangiography is superior to CT in this respect, as reported by HAN et al. (1997), who have compared the results of spiral CT with those of cholangiography. In this study the authors were able to evaluate the level and the extent of the tumor correctly by spiral CT in 63% of cases. Underestimation was reported to be due to the superficial spread of the tumor, whereas overestimation was due to failure to identify the ductal confluence or to biliary anatomical variances (HAN et al. 1997).

Cholangiocarcinoma of the common hepatic and common bile duct is also called ductal carcinoma (BRAASCH 1973; DALLA PALMA et al. 1980).

When the tumor has a polypoid growth pattern, CT shows a soft tissue mass within the dilated duct, which is easily differentiated from nonradiopaque biliary stones or mud, since it has higher attenuation values (Fig. 16.4).

Infiltrating forms of ductal cholangiocarcinoma at early stages, like hilar cholangiocarcinoma, are usually not seen on CT. As the tumor grows with its typical parietal spread along the longer axis of the duct, it usually reaches a size that is symptomatic and often detectable at the same time, usually at the T2 tumor stage. When an accurate technique is used a small mass can be demonstrated, often showing early enhancement (Fig. 16.5). This does not entail a definite diagnosis of cholangiocarcinoma, since other nonneoplastic conditions, such as benign postoperative strictures, may present a similar pattern.

The differential diagnosis must also include other malignant conditions, such as lymphadenopathy

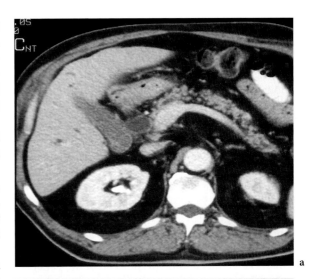

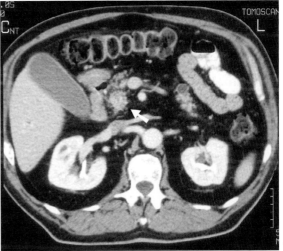

Fig. 16.5a, b. Carcinoma of the distal common bile duct. a CT scan above the pancreatic head shows dilatation of common bile duct. b Scan at the level of the pancreatic head shows a 20-mm tumor mass (*arrow*), hyperdense compared with the surrounding pancreatic head parenchyma, which presents fatty degeneration. The lesion is confined within the pancreas

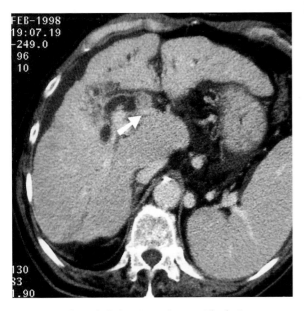

Fig. 16.4. Polypoid cholangiocarcinoma. The lesion appears as a soft tissue mass (*arrow*) heterogeneous in density after contrast enhancement, localized within the common bile duct

and peritoneal spread to the porta hepatis from other abdominal primary neoplasms.

Ampullary carcinoma is difficult to demonstrate, since, due to its primary site at the papilla of Vater, it may be confused with duodenal carcinoma or juxtapapillary pancreatic carcinoma. The presence of a small tumor should be suspected whenever dilatation of the common bile duct and Wirsung duct is seen. Since these findings may also be found with inflammation of the ampulla, with small benign tumors and with inflammation of the head of the pancreas, the diagnosis is achieved only by ERCP and biopsy.

Larger lesions appear on CT as intraduodenal masses associated with dilated bile ducts, dilated Wirsung duct and an overdistended gallbladder. A hypodense pattern may be seen, as in ampullary adenoma, secondary to intratumoral mucin production. However, more commonly the density is that of a soft tissue mass, because of tumor cellularity, with an increase in attenuation values after injection of contrast medium (Fig. 16.6).

As explained above, definitive tissue diagnosis is provided by endoscopy and endoscopic biopsy. The role of CT in the imaging work-up is mainly aimed at local staging of the lesion and disclosure of any distant spread of disease. CT is particularly useful in establishing the infiltration of the duodenal wall (T2 tumors) and the invasion of the head of the pancreas (T3 tumors).

16.4
Inflammatory Disease

16.4.1
Recurrent Cholangitis

Recurrent cholangitis is an inflammatory condition of the biliary system that is due to recurrent biliary obstructions and secondary ascending bacterial infection. Symptoms are biliary colic, fever, chills and jaundice. It is usually related to previous surgery on the biliary system, or it may represent a complication of choledocholithiasis, congenital abnormalities and even neoplasms.

Repeated episodes of inflammation cause progressive damage of the ductal wall, with loss of parietal elasticity. This can be the reason for persistent abnormal dilatation even after removal of the obstructive cause (e.g. after stone removal) and can also explain why ductal ectasia can be seen independently of the presence of a mechanical obstruction; it can involve the biliary system either above or below a stone. CT can demonstrate the distribution of biliary dilatation, the presence of stones, biloma and abscesses as well as atrophy of the segments involved. Analysis of the segmental distribution of the dilatation may be particularly useful when percutaneous biliary drainage is planned.

Intrahepatic calculi are rarely radiopaque; they may be slightly denser than the bile or hepatic parenchyma on unenhanced CT, with a range of attenuation values between 20 and 160 HU (LIM 1991; CHAN et al. 1989). Since stones may become isodense

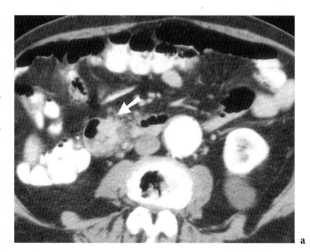

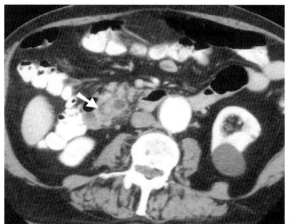

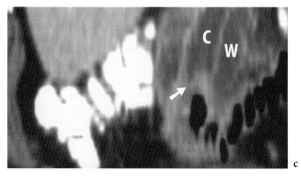

Fig. 16.6a–c. Ampullary carcinoma. **a** CT at the level of the papilla shows a relatively hyperdense soft-tissue mass (*arrow*) invading the duodenal wall and the head of the pancreas for less than 3 cm (stage T3). **b** At a higher level the mass clearly present a vegetation growing into the common bile duct (*arrow*). **c** Coronal reformatted image shows the mass (*arrow*) and dilatation of both common bile duct (*C*) and Wirsung's duct (*W*)

to surrounding structures on an enhanced scan, baseline pre-contrast images throughout the whole liver are usually recommended. The use of hyperdense oral contrast medium is not advised, since once refluxed into the biliary tree, it may obscure the presence of stones. CT may also be useful in distinguishing pneumobilia from intrahepatic stones when this differential diagnosis is questionable on US scans.

16.4.2
Primary Sclerosing Cholangitis

Primary sclerosing cholangitis (PSC) is a rare inflammatory disease of unknown etiology that causes multiple intra- and extrahepatic biliary strictures. It consists in chronic fibrosis and may lead to biliary cirrhosis. Between 50% and 80% of cases of PSC are associated with inflammatory bowel disease, mainly ulcerative colitis (CHAPMA and ARBORGH 1985). The disease may occur at any age, with a prevalence in young males.

CT is generally not helpful in diagnosing and staging the disease at the time of onset, because the typical cholangiographic findings, such as mural irregularities, annular strictures, pruning or beaded appearance of the intrahepatic bile ducts, are difficult to demonstrate. In later stages of the disease, when jaundice occurs, beaded cholangectasias, multisegmental intra- and extrahepatic biliary dilatation with different degrees of biliary dilatation among the liver segments, with sparing of some segments, are typical features (Fig. 16.7). Intrahepatic stones may be observed, although more rarely than in bacterial cholangitis. In these advanced cases the CT study is aimed at ruling out complications and other causes of obstructive jaundice.

Among the complications, CT may reveal the presence of cholangiocarcinoma, which is known to occur with increased frequency in patients with PSC (ROSEN and NAGORNEY 1991; RITCHIE et al. 1974). Spiral CT may be particularly helpful in this respect (CAMPBELL et al. 1998). CAMPBELL et al. suggest that thin-section spiral CT with bolus injection of contrast medium, completed with delayed acquisition, can improve the detection of soft tissue masses associated with the typical strictures of PSC with an accuracy of 74–83%. This can be particularly true for intrahepatic tumors, where cholangiography has poor sensitivity, since it can only demonstrate the narrowing of the duct.

At CT carcinoms, complicating PSC, appears as ill-defined mass surrounding or adjacent to the dilated ducts. Most masses are hypodense or of mixed attenuation compared with the liver parenchyma during the portal venous phase. CAMPBELL and co-workers report that 50% of cholangiocarcinoma appeared hyperdense when studied with delayed phase at 10–15 min, and they suggest that delayed scans should be included in the CT protocol of patients with PSC.

Biliary changes similar to those seen in PSC are reported in patients affected by AIDS. In fact some opportunistic organisms, such as *Cryptosporidium*, cytomegalovirus and *Candida albicans* (DOLMATCH et al. 1987; SCHNEIDERMAN 1988) produce cholangitis with elevated cholestasis parameters and bile duct dilatation even in the absence of mechanical obstruction. However, in AIDS patients, bile duct dilatation may also be caused by enlarged lymph nodes at the hepatic hilum, secondary to lymphoma or Kaposi's sarcoma.

16.5
Benign Postoperative Strictures

The majority of postoperative benign bile strictures are due to iatrogenic injuries caused during cholecystectomy. Other causes are damage from common bile duct instrumentation or ischemic lesions of the hepatic artery during other types of surgery.

While bile duct injuries usually present early in the postoperative period, obstructive jaundice and bile leak being the most common clinical signs, postoperative strictures may present months to years after surgery. Morbidity is high, and the clinical manifestation at onset generally consists in episodes of cholangitis; if they are untreated, secondary biliary cirrhosis or even hepatic failure may follow.

The diagnosis of benign postoperative stricture presenting weeks to months after cholecystectomy or other biliary surgery is often made on clinical presentation. In a large percentage of patients, however, symptoms may be so remote from previous surgery as to raise the suspicion of malignant biliary obstruction.

Abdominal ultrasound, MR cholangiography and spiral CT play an important role in determining the level of the stricture and in ruling out malignant causes of obstruction. In post-cholecystectomy strictures, the CT findings are those of intrahepatic ductal dilation. The ducts can be followed up to the site of the stricture, where they are suddenly interrupted, often at the level of surgical clips placed during laparoscopic surgery. In rare instances the scar tissue can be seen as a small soft tissue density that replaces the ductal structures (Fig. 16.8).

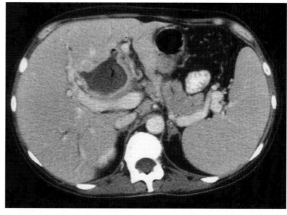

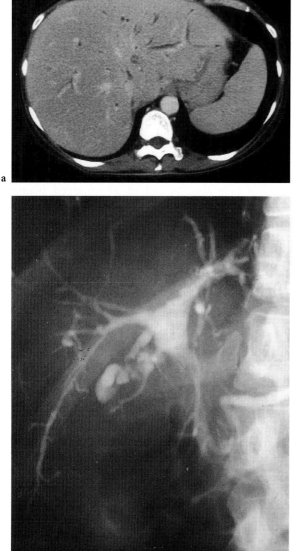

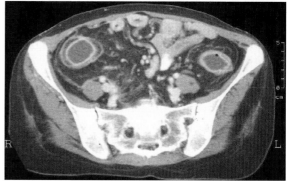

Fig. 16.7a–d. Primary sclerosing cholangitis (PSC) in patient with inflammatory bowel disease. a CT scan at the level of the intrahepatic ducts shows typical focal distribution of slightly dilated ducts, with some liver segments that are spared by the ductal abnormalities. b CT scan at the level of the common hepatic duct shows abnormal dilatation. There is some pneumobilia. c Endoscopic retrograde cholangiogram confirms abnormal dilatation of the common hepatic duct and changes in the intrahepatic ducts consistent with PSC, mainly in the left ductal system. d CT scan at the level of the pelvis shows thickening of the wall of the ascending and descending colon. The mucosa and the serosa are hyperdense and are separated by a relatively hypodense layer. Although these findings are more often found in cases of ulcerative colitis, this patient had biopsy-proven Crohn's disease of the colon

Once the diagnosis of obstructive jaundice is made, treatment is planned. However, since the options for treatment are decided mainly on the basis of the anatomical location and appearance of the stricture, cholangiography remains the definitive diagnostic test for patients with benign bile duct stenoses, and it is superior to CT in this respect. Currently, in our Institution we use magnetic resonance cholangiography (MRC) to obtain a noninvasive cholangiogram in such patients before they undergo surgical or nonoperative management. Although endoscopic retrograde cholangiopancreatography (ERCP) has been widely used, we believe that MRC may provide information superior to that yielded by

the endoscopic technique, because it allows visualization of the biliary ducts below and above the stricture. When all the information provided by US, CT and MRC are combined, the patient is then scheduled for a therapeutic percutaneous biliary drainage or ERCP.

Benign strictures can also occur at the level of a biliary-enteric anastomosis. CT, like US, allows evaluation of the patency of the anastomosis: the presence of gas in the bile ducts implies patency (but does not rule out of a partial stenosis), whereas bile duct dilatation without evidence of air will suggest a tight stenosis of the anastomosis (SAUERBREI et al. 1992) (Fig. 16.9). In certain instances CT may be su-

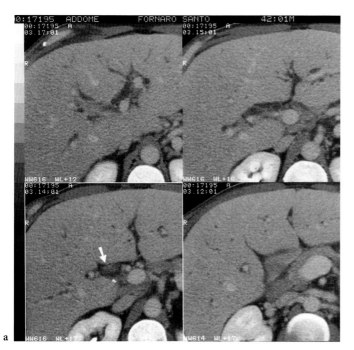
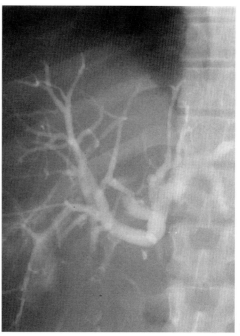

a

b

Fig. 16.8a, b. Benign stricture after laparoscopic cholecystectomy. **a** CT scans show dilated intrahepatic ducts (*top left*) and dilated left and right ducts at the level of the hilum (*top right*). Immediately below the confluence of the hepatic ducts the postoperative scar tissue appears as a small soft tissue mass, slightly hyperdense compared with the surrounding hilar fat, adjacent to a surgical clip (*arrow, bottom left*). The intrapancreatic CBD is of normal size (*bottom right*). **b** Percutaneous transhepatic cholangiogram confirms the presence of a tight stricture at the level of the confluence of the hepatic ducts (grade III lesion according to Bismuth's classification)

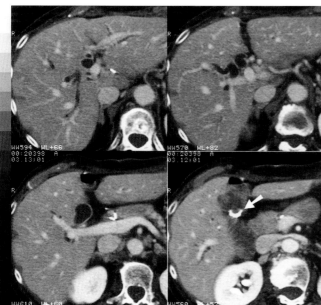
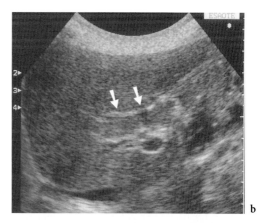
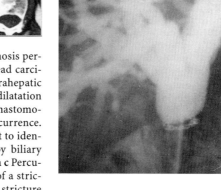

a

b

c

Fig. 16.9a, b. Stricture at the level of a biliary-enteric anastomosis performed after pancreatectomy in a patient with pancreatic head carcinoma. **a** Four CT scans at 1.5-cm intervals show dilated intrahepatic ducts and dilated common hepatic duct (*bottom left*); the dilatation stops at the level of the metallic suture used to construct the anastomosis (*arrow, bottom right*). There are no signs of local tumor recurrence. **b** The dilated common hepatic duct (*small arrows*) is difficult to identify by ultrasound, since the lumen is entirely occupied by biliary sludge that has the same echogenicity as the liver parenchyma **c** Percutaneous transhepatic cholangiogram confirms the presence of a stricture at the level of the biliary enteric anastomosis (grade II stricture according to Bismuth's classification)

perior to US in demonstrating the ductal dilatation, particularly when the ultrasound image is unclear because of the presence of stones, surgical clips, intraductal air or biliary sludge (Fig. 16.9).

Biliary anastomoses are often the result of surgery performed for pancreatic or biliary neoplasms. When jaundice or cholangitis present weeks or months after the operation, there is always the suspicion of a recurrent malignancy. In order to undertake the more appropriate treatment it is not so important to define the anatomical appearance of the stenosis, as it is in the case of postcholecystectomy strictures, as to confirm that there are no signs of recurrent neoplasm. In such cases CT is extremely useful, since it may reveal local soft tissue masses, metastatic nodes and peritoneal spread of disease. Therefore, the role of CT is to give the information necessary to decide whether the patient is affected by a benign complication of previous surgery and needs only a percutaneous dilatation or surgical revision of the anastomosis, or is facing a relapsing malignancy and needs oncological treatment.

References

Braasch JW (1973) Carcinoma of the bile duct. Surg Clin North Am 53:1217
Burhans R, Meyer RT (1971) Benign neoplasms of the extrahepatic biliary ducts. Am Surg 37:161–166
Campbell WL, Ferris JV, Holbert BL, Theate FL, Baron RL (1998) Biliary tract carcinoma complicating primary sclerosing cholangitis: evaluation with CT, cholangiography, US and MR imaging. Radiology 207:41–50
Chan FL, Man SV, Leong LLY, Fan ST (1989) Evaluation of recurrent pyogenic cholangitis with CT: analysis of 50 patients. Radiology 170:165–169
Chapma RWG, Arborgh BAM (1985) Primary sclerosing cholangitis: a review of its clinical features, cholangiography and hepatic histology. Gut 21:870–877
Choi B, Lee JH, Han MC, Kim SH, Yi JG, Kim CW (1989) Hilar cholangiocarcinoma: comparative study with sonography and CT. Radiology 172:689–692
Dalla Palma L, Rizzatto G, Pozzi-Mucelli RS, Bazzocchi M (1980) Gray-scale ultrasonography in the evaluation of carcinoma of the gallbladder. Br J Radiol 53:662
Devaney K, Goodman ZD, Ishak KG (1994) Hepatobiliary cystadenoma and cystadenocarcinoma: a light microscopic and immunohistological study of 70 patients. Am J Surg Pathol 18:1078–1091
Dolmatch BL, Liang FC, Federle MP, Jeffrey RB, Cello J (1987) AIDS-related cholangitis: radiographic findings in nine patients. Radiology 163:313–316
Han JK, Choi BI, Kim TK, Kim SW, Han MC, Yeon KM (1997) Hilar cholangiocarcinoma: thin-section spiral CT findings with cholangiographic correlation. Radiographics 17:1475–1485
Kane RA (1988) The biliary system. In: Kurtz AB, Goldberg BB (eds) Gastrointestinal ultrasonography. (Clinics in diagnostic ultrasound) Churchill Livingstone, Edinburgh, pp 75–137
Kim TK, Choi BI, Han JK, Jang HJ, Cho SG, Han MC (1997) Peripheral cholangiocarcinoma of the liver: two-phase spiral CT findings. Radiology 204:539–543
Klatskin G (1965) Adenocarcinoma of the hepatic duct at its bifurcation within the porta hepatis. Am J Med 38:241–256
Lacomis JM, Baron RL, Oliver JH, Nalesnik MA, Federle MP (1997) Cholangiocarcinoma: delayed CT contrast enhanced patterns. Radiology 203:98–104
Lim JH (1991) Oriental cholangiohepatitis pathologic, clinical, and radiologic features. AJR Am J Roentgenol 157:1–8
McIntyre JA, Cheng PZ (1979) Adenoma of the common bile duct causing obstructive jaundice. Can J Surg 11:215–218
Meyer DG, Weinstein BJ (1983) Klatskin tumors of the bile ducts: sonographic appearance. Radiology 148:803–804
Reiman TH, Balfe DM, Weyman PJ (1987) Suprapancreatic biliary obstruction. Radiology 163:49–56
Richter GM, Grenacher L (1997) CT of the biliary tree. In: Rossi P (ed) Biliary tract radiology. Springer, Berlin Heidelberg New York, pp 87–100
Ritchie JK, Allan RN, MaCartney J, Thompson H, Hawley PR, Cooke WT (1974) Biliary tract carcinoma associated with ulcerative colitis. QJM 43:263
Rosen CB, Nagorney DM (1991) Cholangiocarcinoma complicating primary sclerosing cholangitis. Semin Liver Dis 11:26–30
Sauerbrei EE, Nguyen KT, Nolan RL (1992) The bile ducts. In: Abdominal sonography. Raven Press, New York, pp 51–72
Schneiderman DJ (1988) Hepatobiliary abnormalities of AIDS. Gastroenterol Clin North Am 17:615–630

17 Choledocholithiasis and CT Cholangiography

B.E. Van Beers, J.H. Pringot

CONTENTS

17.1 Introduction: Clinical Context 187
17.2 Unenhanced Spiral CT 188
17.3 Spiral CT Cholangiography 189
17.3.1 Technique 189
17.3.2 Results 189
17.3.3 Imaging Before Laparoscopic
Cholecystectomy 191
17.4 Conclusion 193
References 193

17.1
Introduction: Clinical Context

Bile duct calculi can be classified into primary or secondary stones, depending on their site of origin. The majority of bile duct stones are secondary stones formed in the gallbladder, which then migrate into the extrahepatic biliary tree. These stones reflect the composition of gallbladder stones, i.e. predominantly cholesterol in 80% and black pigment in 20% (HAWES and SHERMAN 1995). The frequency of common bile duct stones increases with increasing age of the patient. Cystic duct diameter appears to be an important factor in the migration of gallbladder stones into the common bile duct. Primary stones form de novo in the bile ducts. These pigmented stones are brown or black and are often friable. Their pathogenesis depends on two main factors, which are biliary stasis and bacterial or parasitic infection. Predisposing conditions include congenital dilatation of the bile ducts (choledochal cyst and Caroli disease), sclerosing cholangitis, benign bile duct stenosis, and recurrent cholangitis including oriental cholangiohepatitis (CHAN et al.

B. E. VAN BEERS, MD, PhD; Department of Radiology, St-Luc University Hospital, Avenue Hippocrate 10, B-1200 Brussels, Belgium
J. H. PRINGOT, MD; Department of Radiology, St-Luc University Hospital, Avenue Hippocrate 10, B-1200 Brussels, Belgium

1989; DODD et al. 1997; KIM et al. 1995; LIM 1991; MILLER et al. 1995; SCHULMAN 1987).

It appears that the frequency of common bile duct stones seen at cholecystectomy has dropped in recent years (BARKUN et al. 1994). It was considered earlier that 10–15% of patients undergoing open cholecystectomy for cholelithiasis had concomitant bile duct stones. The corresponding range for the laparoscopic era is 5–10%. This decline possibly reflects a different patient population that presents earlier in the course of symptomatic gallstone disease.

The natural history of choledocholithiasis is variable. As with gallstones, some patients with bile duct stones remain asymptomatic for months or even years, but the majority of patients ultimately become symptomatic (HAWES and SHERMAN 1995). These patients present with biliary colic or a complication, such as cholangitis, obstructive jaundice, pancreatitis, or rarely, biliary cirrhosis. Small stones may pass spontaneously into the duodenum, but they are not always asymptomatic. Indeed, microlithiasis (defined as stones less than 3 mm in diameter) and sludge (defined as a suspension of cholesterol monohydrate crystals or calcium bilirubinate granules in a mucous matrix) may cause biliary colic or be the source of pancreatitis (HOUSSIN et al. 1983; LEE et al. 1992; ROS et al. 1991).

Several parameters may be used in combination in an attempt to predict the presence of common bile stones. These predictors include a previous history of jaundice or cholangitis, elevated serum bilirubin or alkaline phosphatase, and a dilated common bile duct found on ultrasound examination (BARKUN et al. 1994). However, all clinical, laboratory, and ultrasonographic findings may be normal in some patients with common bile duct stones (8% in the series of BARKUN et al.).

The introduction of laparoscopic cholecystectomy has renewed interest in preoperative detection of common bile duct stones. Indeed, the removal of calculi in the common bile duct during laparoscopy can be difficult (GIGOT et al. 1997a). If the surgeon has not acquired this skill, he needs either to convert to open laparotomy or to rely on endoscopic retrograde cholangiography with sphincterotomy and stone extraction (Jones and Soper 1994; Strasberg and Soper 1995). Endoscopic retrograde cholangiography and stone extraction can be performed before, during or after laparoscopic cholecystectomy, and the optimal timing remains the subject of debate. Intraoperative endoscopic stone extraction is not popular because of team co-ordination problems between endoscopists and surgeons and because of difficulties in cannulating the bile duct in the supine position, which leads to an increased risk of acute pancreatitis. Postoperative endoscopic stone extraction is not always successful, and another operation may be necessary if the endoscopic extraction fails. For this reason, preoperative endoscopic retrograde cholangiography and stone extraction may be the preferred technique. However, preoperative endoscopic cholangiography cannot be recommended as a routine diagnostic procedure for detection of bile duct stones, because it is invasive (Neuhaus et al. 1992). Use of a noninvasive imaging technique to detect biliary calculi is thus mandatory. Before cholecystectomy, this imaging technique should also detect any anatomic variations of the bile ducts that may increase the risk of bile duct injury during surgery. Anatomic variations include cystic duct variants, such as a spiral cystic duct, a low junction of the cystic duct, a short cystic duct, and a cystic duct entering a right hepatic duct, and aberrant right hepatic ducts draining directly into the common hepatic duct, the common bile duct, the cystic duct, or the gallbladder. For laparoscopic cholecystectomy, the most relevant variants are aberrant right hepatic ducts and short cystic ducts, especially when scleroatrophic cholecystitis is present (Gigot et al. 1997). The detection of anatomic variations might be especially important before laparoscopic cholecystectomy, as absence of three-dimensional perspective and loss of tactile sensation during laparoscopy have been considered factors that may contribute to the apparently higher prevalence of bile duct injuries after laparoscopic than after open surgery (Davids et al. 1993; Deziel et al. 1993; Gigot et al. 1997b; Goldberg and Mulvihill 1994).

17.2
Unenhanced Spiral CT

It is generally accepted that conventional CT depicts choledocholithiasis in approximately 75% of patients with this disorder (Amouyal et al. 1994; Baron 1987; Baron 1997). More recently, the use of unenhanced spiral CT has been advocated to detect common bile stones (Fig. 17.1), and a higher sensitivity of 88% has been reported (Neitlich et al. 1997). The increased sensitivity was related to the following factors. With spiral CT, all data can be acquired during a single breath hold, which prevents misregistrations between sections, and images can be reconstructed retrospectively in an overlapping fashion to reduce volume-averaging effects. In the study of Neitlich et al., a 5-mm slice thickness was used with a pitch of 1 and a reconstruction increment of 2 mm. No oral or intravenous contrast material was used. This was considered to be important, as several stones were diagnosed by a high attenuation ring in the bile duct, which could be confused with enhancement of the bile duct wall if contrast material were used. The authors also used narrow windows to maximize bile–soft tissue contrast.

Multiplanar volume reconstructions with minimum intensity projections may help in the detection of low-density stones (Raptopoulos et al. 1998).

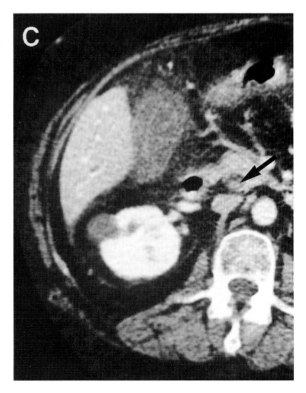

Fig. 17.1. Spiral CT scan obtained at the level of the distal common bile duct shows a stone with soft-tissue density (*arrow*) surrounded by a rim of hypodense bile

The approach of using unenhanced spiral CT to detect bile duct stones is similar to the approach of using unenhanced spiral CT to detect urinary tract calculi (SMITH et al. 1995). However, in contrast to urinary tract stones, which all have substantially higher attenuation values than surrounding soft tissue, gallstones appear isoattenuating with bile in about 15–25% of cases, as shown by in vitro studies (BARON et al. 1995; BRAKEL et al. 1990). It is thus expected that in large series of patients with common bile duct stones, the calculi will not be detected in 15–25% of patients (BARON 1997). Low-density intrahepatic stones may also remain undetected on CT (DODD et al. 1997; LIM 1995). Further in vivo studies are necessary to assess the role of unenhanced spiral CT in the detection of cholelithiasis.

17.3
Spiral CT Cholangiography

17.3.1
Technique

Spiral CT cholangiography consists of spiral CT scanning of the bile ducts after indirect opacification of the biliary tree with cholangiographic contrast agent (FLEISCHMANN et al. 1996; KLEIN et al. 1993; STOCKBERGER et al. 1994; VAN BEERS et al. 1994).

CT cholangiography was previously performed with conventional CT scanners (GREENBERG et al. 1983; ITAI et al. 1994; MUSANTE et al. 1982; PAIVANSALO et al. 1988; TOOMBS et al. 1981). However, the introduction of spiral CT has renewed interest in CT cholangiography, because it makes it possible to obtain thin slices without misregistration and allows high-resolution three-dimensional images of the biliary tree.

The opacification of the biliary tract is usually obtained by slow (30–60 min) intravenous infusion of an iodinated contrast agent with hepatobiliary excretion, such as iodipamide meglumine. The usual contraindications to the use of iodinated contrast agents should be observed. In addition, spiral CT cholangiography should not be performed in patients with hyperbilirubinemia. Indeed, the biliary excretion of the contrast agent is impaired in patients with serum bilirubin levels above 34–51 µmol/L (2–3 mg/dL) (STOCKBERGER et al. 1994; VAN BEERS et al. 1994). A high rate of adverse events has been reported after the administration of iodinated cholangiographic agents (GOODMAN et al. 1980). More recently these contrast agents have been reported to be safe when a slow infusion rate in used (DALY et al. 1987; DORENBUSCH et al. 1995; JOYCE et al. 1991). In two large series no major reactions occurred and minor reactions (mainly skin rash or itch) were observed in 0.5–0.7% of the cases (KWON et al. 1998; LINDSEY et al. 1997). However, as with other contrast agents, severe reactions to biliary contrast agents, such as dyspnea, sudden drop in blood pressure, cardiac arrest or loss of consciousness, can occur. Therefore, the use of drugs that are not entirely innocuous must be weighed against the potential positive information to be gained (GOLDBERG 1994).

After infusion of the contrast agent, spiral CT scanning of the bile ducts is performed, preferably in the inferosuperior direction, starting below the ampulla of Vater. Collimation of 2.5–5 mm and a pitch of 1–2 have been used (FLEISCHMANN et al. 1996; STOCKBERGER et al. 1996; VAN BEERS et al. 1995). The detection of small lesions (stones) is improved, and the quality of multiplanar images and three-dimensional displays is enhanced when the images are reconstructed at increments of less than half the distance traveled during one rotation of the tube through 360°(KALENDER et al. 1994).

Three-dimensional displays are useful for demonstration of the biliary anatomy, but only the transverse slices and multiplanar reconstructions are useful for the detection of bile duct stones (Fig. 17.2) (KLEIN et al. 1993; KWON et al. 1995; VAN BEERS et al 1994).

Three-dimensional displays are thus only one aspect of a spiral CT cholangiographic examination that would increase acceptance of this technique by endoscopists and surgeons. The major diagnostic information, however, lies in the transverse source images (FLEISCHMANN et al. 1996). For these transverse images, adequate windows (window width 500–800 HU, window level 70–150 HU) should be used to improve the detection of small stones in the opacified bile.

17.3.2
Results

Spiral CT cholangiography can be used for the detection of choledocholiths (Fig. 17.3). The reported sensitivity and specificity of spiral CT cholangiography for the detection of ductal stones before laparoscopic cholecystectomy are 85–89% and 96–

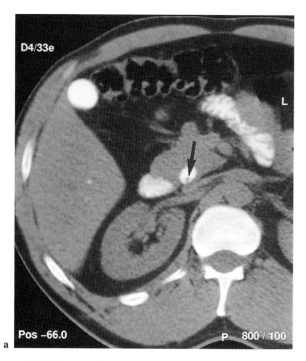

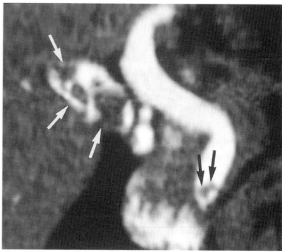

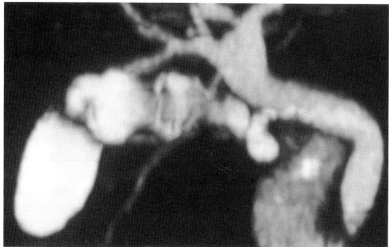

Fig. 17.2a–c. Spiral CT cholangiography performed before laparoscopic cholecystectomy for gallstones. **a** Transverse slice shows a hypodense stone (*arrow*) in the common bile duct. **b** Multiplanar reconstruction through the long axis of the common bile duct demonstrates two stones (*black arrows*). Gallstones (*white arrows*) are also seen. **c** Three-dimensional reconstruction (maximum intensity projection) shows the anatomy of the bile ducts, but the calculi are less clearly seen

100% respectively (GALEON et al. 1996a; KWON et al. 1998). A case of nonobstructing stone of the distal common duct that was not detected because it had the same attenuation as the enhanced bile has been reported (STOCKBERGER et al. 1994). The demonstration of common duct sludge has been reported in one case (FLEISCHMANN et al. 1996), but the precise sensitivity of spiral CT cholangiography in the detection of common duct microlithiasis and sludge is not known. Intrahepatic stones (Fig. 17.4) and retained or recurrent stones after cholecystectomy (Fig. 17.5) can also be detected with spiral CT cho-

langiography (VAN BEERS et al. 1995). In addition to the detection of stones, spiral CT cholangiography can be used for the detection of anatomic variations of the bile ducts before laparoscopic cholecystectomy (Fig. 17.6) (MURAKAMI et al. 1997; VAN BEERS et al. 1994). Moreover, absence of cystic duct and gallbladder opacification on CT cholangiography has been used to predict severe inflammation and adhesion around the gallbladder, precluding laparoscopic cholecystectomy (KWON et al. 1998).

The use of spiral CT cholangiography has also been reported for the assessment of choledochal

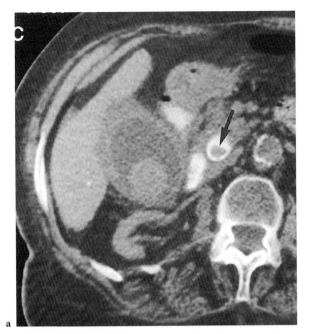

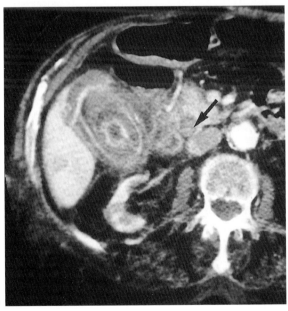

Fig. 17.3. a Spiral CT cholangiogram shows a hypodense stone (*arrow*) in the choledochus. The gallbladder contains a stone and is not opacified in this patient with acute cholecystitis. b The common bile duct stone (*arrow*) is less conspicuous on the spiral CT scan obtained without biliary enhancement in the same patient

cysts (Fig. 17.7) (GALEON et al. 1996b), the detection of traumatic and iatrogenic bile duct injuries (STOCKBERGER and JOHNSON 1997), the follow-up of bilio-digestive anastomoses (HAMADA et al. 1995), and the evaluation of patients with anicteric cholestasis (FLEISCHMANN et al. 1996; LACROSSE et al. 1996).

17.3.3
Imaging Before Laparoscopic Cholecystectomy

One of the main potential applications for spiral CT cholangiography is screening prior to laparoscopic cholecystectomy (GOLDBERG and MULVIHILL 1994). The need for routine imaging before cholecystectomy remains the subject of debate. Indeed, the frequency of asymptomatic common duct stones is low, especially in patients with normal results of hepatic tests, a history that is negative for jaundice, and normal-caliber bile duct at ultrasonography. In addition, bile duct lesions during open or laparoscopic cholecystectomy may be related to other causes than anatomic variations; in particular, the learning curve of the surgeon plays a role (ANDREN-SANDBERG et al. 1985). However, the difficulty of dealing with choledocholithiasis or anatomic variations in the bile ducts is greater during laparoscopic than during conventional cholecystectomy. In addition, operative cholangiography is sometimes difficult to perform during laparoscopic cholecystectomy (DAWSON et al. 1993). This has renewed interest in imaging prior to surgery. The value of spiral CT cholangiography before laparoscopic cholecystectomy should be compared with that of percutaneous ultrasonography, spiral CT, intravenous cholangiography, MR cholangiography, endoscopic ultrasonography, and endoscopic retrograde cholangiography. The following points should be considered:

- The detection rate of common bile duct stones with percutaneous ultrasonography is low, around 20–25% (AMOUYAL et al. 1994; PASANEN et al. 1992). The specificity of ultrasonography, however, exceeds 90%, and this method remains an important screening examination in patients with biliary stones.
- Spiral CT is generally not used for screening patients before laparoscopic cholecystectomy. Indeed, as discussed above, many biliary stones are hypodense or isoattenuating with bile and are difficult to detect with spiral CT (BARON 1997). In addition, bile duct variations can not be detected with ultrasonography or CT.
- Endoscopic retrograde cholangiography is often considered to be the gold standard for the detection of choledocholiths, but it is invasive and cannot be recommended for routine imaging before cholecystectomy (LO and CHEN 1996; NEUHAUS et al. 1992).
- Endoscopic ultrasonography is highly accurate in the detection of common bile duct stones, but it is also relatively invasive and it requires particular

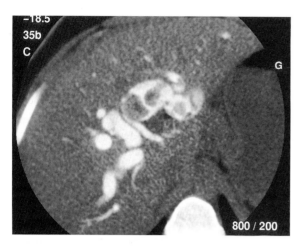

Fig. 17.4. Intrahepatic stones are demonstrated by spiral CT cholangiography in a patient with oriental cholangiohepatitis

skills that will prevent it from becoming widely available outside of referral centers (AMOUYAL et al. 1994; PASRICHA 1996; PRAT et al. 1996).

– Intravenous cholangiography is a classic method of assessing the biliary tree before cholecystectomy. However, intravenous cholangiography has been almost completely abandoned, especially in North America, because of concerns about its efficacy and safety (RHOLL et al. 1985; SCOTT et al. 1989). In contrast, several authors have reported recently that intravenous cholangiography is safe and has a sensitivity of more than 90% in preoperative screening for incidental common bile duct stones (DORENBUSCH et al. 1995; LINDSEY et al. 1997). However, the opacification of the bile ducts at intravenous cholangiography is often faint. Therefore, this method is not recommended for the detection of anatomic variations of the bile ducts (ALINDER et al. 1986; MAGLINTE and DORENBUSCH 1993; PATEL et al. 1993).

– Spiral CT cholangiography offers a far better contrast resolution than intravenous cholangiography and shows significantly more anatomic detail of the bile ducts (KLEIN et al. 1993; KWON et al. 1995). In addition, the problem of overlying bowel gas misinterpreted as choledocholithiasis does not occur with spiral CT cholangiography.

– Common bile duct stones and anatomic variations of the bile ducts can also be detected with MR cholangiography (FULCHER et al. 1998; HOLZKNECHT et al. 1998; TAOUREL et al. 1996). The great advantage of MR cholangiography over CT cholangiography is that administration of contrast medium is not required. However, the advantage of CT is its wider availability and lower cost. To the best of our knowledge, no study has been performed comparing the value and cost-effectiveness of spiral CT cholangiography and MR cholangiography before laparoscopic cholecystectomy.

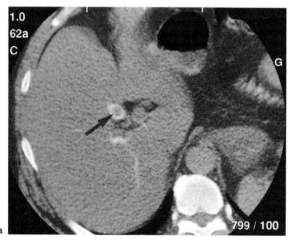

a

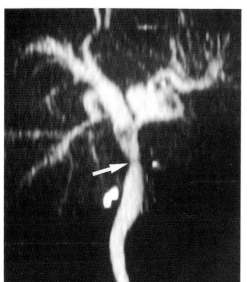

b

Fig. 17.5. a Spiral CT cholangiogram shows a stone (*arrow*) in the common hepatic duct of a patient with a history of cholecystectomy. **b** Three-dimensional reconstruction shows that the stone lies above an iatrogenic stricture of the common hepatic duct (*arrow*)

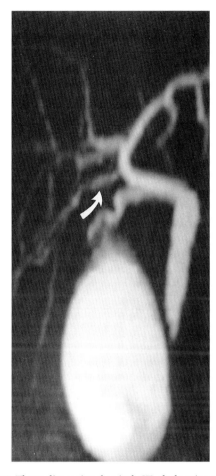

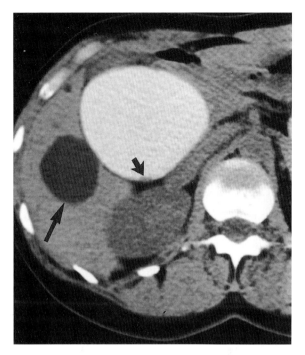

Fig. 17.7. CT cholangiogram in a patient with choledochal cyst. The huge choledochal cyst contains opacified bile and a small hypodense stone (*short arrow*). A hepatic cyst (*long arrow*) remains unenhanced

Fig. 17.6. Three-dimensional spiral CT cholangiogram obtained before laparoscopic cholecystectomy shows low insertion of a right hepatic duct (*curved arrow*) into the common hepatic duct. Patients with this anatomic variant have an increased risk of bile trauma during surgery

Acknowledgements. The authors are deeply grateful to Prof. J.F. Gigot for reviewing the manuscript and to Dr. R. Materne and Mrs. F. Martin for assistance in manuscript preparation.

17.4
Conclusion

There is no definite consensus on the best non-invasive technique for the diagnosis of bile duct stones. The detection with unenhanced spiral CT is limited by the frequency of low-density stones. Spiral CT cholangiography is a feasible method for the detection of biliary anatomic variations and bile duct stones before or after laparoscopic cholecystectomy. For these indications, spiral CT cholangiography might be an alternative to MR cholangiography, but this remains to be proven. The main limitation of spiral CT cholangiography is the need to use a cholangiographic contrast agent, since excretion of such agents is impaired in patients with hyperbilirubinemia and high-grade stenosis of the bile ducts.

References

Alinder G, Nilsson U, Lunderquist A, Herlin P, Holmin T (1986) Pre-operative infusion cholangiography compared to routine operative cholangiography at elective cholecystectomy. Br J Surg 73:383–387

Amouyal P, Amouyal G, Lévy P, et al (1994) Diagnosis of choledocholithiasis by endoscopic ultrasonography. Gastroenterology 106:1062–1067

Andrén-Sandberg A, Alinder G, Bengmark S (1985) Accidental lesions of the common bile duct at cholecystectomy. Pre- and perioperative factors of importance. Ann Surg 201:328–332

Barkun AN, Barkun JS, Fried GM, et al (1994) Useful predictors of bile duct stones in patients undergoing laparoscopic cholecystectomy. Ann Surg 220:32–39

Baron RL (1987) Common bile duct stones: reassessment of criteria for CT diagnosis. Radiology 162:419–424

Baron RL (1997) Diagnosing choledocholithiasis: how far can we push helical CT? Radiology 203:601–603

Baron RL, Rohrmann CA, Lee SP, Shuman WP, Teefey SA (1988) CT evaluation of gallstones in vitro: correlation with chemical analysis. AJR Am J Roentgenol 151:1123–1128

Brakel K, Laméris JS, Nijs HG, Terpstra OT, Steen G, Blijenberg BC (1990) Predicting gallstone composition with CT: in vivo and in vitro analysis. Radiology 174:337–341

Chan FL, Man SW, Leong LL, Fan ST (1989) Evaluation of recurrent pyogenic cholangitis with CT: analysis of 50 patients. Radiology 170:165–169

Daly J, Fitzgerald T, Simpson CJ (1987) Pre-operative intravenous cholangiography as an alternative to routine operative cholangiography in elective cholecystectomy. Clin Radiol 38:161–163

Davids PH, Ringers J, Rauws EA, de Wit LT, Huibregtse K, van der Heyde MN, Tytgat GN (1993) Bile duct injury after laparoscopic cholecystectomy: the value of endoscopic retrograde cholangiopancreatography. Gut 34:1250–1254

Dawson P, Adam A, Benjamin IS (1993) Intravenous cholangiography revisited. Clin Radiol 47:223–225

Deziel DJ, Millikan KW, Economou SG, Doolas A, Ko ST, Airan MC (1993) Complications of laparoscopic cholecystectomy: a national survey of 4,292 hospitals and an analysis of 77,604 cases. Am J Surg 165:9–14

Dodd GD, Niedzwiecki GA, Campbell WL, Baron RL (1997) Bile duct calculi in patients with primary sclerosing cholangitis. Radiology 203:443–447

Dorenbusch MJ, Maglinte DD, Micon LT, Graffis RA, Turner WW (1995) Intravenous cholangiography and the management of choledocholithiasis prior to laparoscopic cholecystectomy. Surg Laparosc Endosc 5:188–192

Fleischmann D, Ringl H, Schöfl R, et al (1996) Three-dimensional spiral CT cholangiography in patients with suspected obstructive biliary disease: comparison with endoscopic retrograde cholangiography. Radiology 198:861–868

Fulcher AS, Turner MA, Capps GW, Zfass AM, Baker KM (1998) Half-Fourier RARE MR cholangiopancreatography: experience in 300 subjects. Radiology 207:21–32

Galeon MH, De Pierre P, Gigot JF, Pringot JH (1996a) Spiral CT cholangiography in precholecystectomy work-up: correlation with surgical findings. Radiology 201(P):353

Galeon M, Deprez P, Van Beers BE, Pringot JH (1996b) Spiral CT cholangiography of choledochocele. J Comput Assist Tomogr 20:814–815

Gigot JF, Navez B, Etienne J, Cambier E, Jadoul P, Guiot P, Kestens PJ (1997a) A stratified intraoperative surgical strategy is mandatory during laparoscopic common bile duct exploration for common bile duct stones. Lessons and limits from an initial experience of 92 patients. Surg Endosc 11:722–728

Gigot JF, Etienne J, Aerts R et al (1997b) The dramatic reality of biliary tract injury during laparoscopic cholecystectomy. An anonymous multicenter Belgian survey of 65 patients. Surg Endosc 11:1171–1178

Goldberg HI (1994) Helical cholangiography: complementary or substitute study for endoscopic retrograde cholangiography. Radiology 192:615–616

Goldberg HI, Mulvihill SJ (1994) The radiologist's role in the new era of laparoscopic general surgery. AJR Am J Roentgenol 163:1302–1303

Goodman MW, Ansel HJ, Vennes JA, Lasser RB, Silvis SE (1980) Is intravenous cholangiography still useful? Gastroenterology 79:642–645

Greenberg M, Rubin JM, Greenberg BM (1983) Appearance of the gallbladder and biliary tree by CT cholangiography. J Comput Assist Tomogr 7:788–794

Hamada Y, Sato M, Sanada T, Tsuji M, Kogata M, Hioki K (1995) Spiral computed tomography for biliary dilatation. J Pediatr Surg 30:694–696

Hawes RH, Sherman S (1995) Choledocholithiasis. In: Haubrich WS, Schaffner F, Berk JE (eds) Bockus gastroenterology. Saunders, Philadelphia, pp 2745–2779

Holzknecht N, Gauger J, Sackmann M, et al (1998) Breathhold MR cholangiography with snapshot techniques: prospective comparison with endoscopic retrograde cholangiography. Radiology 206:657–664

Houssin D, Castaing D, Lemoine J, Bismuth H (1983) Microlithiasis of the gallbladder. Surg Gynecol Obstet 157:20–24

Itai Y, Ebihara R, Tohno E, Tsunoda HS, Kurosaki Y, Saida Y, Doy M (1994) Hepatic peribiliary cysts: multiple tiny cysts within the larger portal tract, hepatic hilum, or both. Radiology 191:107–110

Jones DB, Soper NJ (1994) Laparoscopic general surgery: current status and future potential. AJR Am J Roentgenol 163:1295–1301

Joyce WP, Keane R, Burke GJ, Daly M, Drumm J, Egan TJ, Delaney PV (1991) Identification of bile duct stones in patients undergoing laparoscopic cholecystectomy. Br J Surg 78:1174–1176

Kalender WA, Polacin A, Süss C (1994) A comparison of conventional and spiral CT: an experimental study on the detection of spherical lesions. J Comput Assist Tomogr 18:167–176

Kim OH, Chung HJ, Choi BG (1995) Imaging of the choledochal cyst. Radiographics 15:69–88

Klein HM, Wein B, Truong S, Pfingsten FP, Günther RW (1993) Computed tomographic cholangiography using spiral scanning and 3D image processing. Br J Radiol 66:762–767

Kwon AH, Uetsuji S, Yamada O, Inoue T, Kamiyama Y, Boku T (1995) Three-dimensional reconstruction of the biliary tract using spiral computed tomography. Br J Surg 82:260–263

Kwon AH, Inui H, Imamura A, Uetsuji S, Kamiyama Y (1998) Preoperative assessment for laparoscopic cholecystectomy. Feasibility of using spiral computed tomography. Ann Surg 227:351–356

Lacrosse M, De Ronde T, Nguyen P, et al (1996) Diagnostic value of spiral CT cholangiography (SCTC) in anicteric enzymatic cholestasis. Gastroenterology 110:A1245

Lee SP, Nicholls JF, Park HZ (1992) Biliary sludge as a cause of acute pancreatitis. N Engl J Med 326:589–593

Lim JH (1991) Oriental cholangiohepatitis: pathologic, clinical, and radiologic features. AJR Am J Roentgenol 157:1–8

Lindsey I, Nottle PD, Sacharias N (1997) Preoperative screening for common bile duct stones with infusion cholangiography. Review of 1000 patients. Ann Surg 226:174–178

Lo SK, Chen J (1996) The role of ERCP in choledocholithiasis. Abdom Imaging 21:120–132

Maglinte DD, Dorenbusch MJ (1993) Intravenous infusion cholangiography: an assessment of its role relevant to laparoscopic cholecystectomy. Radiol Diagn 34:91–96

Miller WJ, Sechtin AG, Campbell WL, Pieters PC (1995) Imaging findings in Caroli's disease. AJR Am J Roentgenol 165:333–337

Murakami T, Kim T, Tomoda K, Narumi Y, Sakon M, Monden M, Nakamura H (1997) Aberrant right posterior biliary duct: detection by intravenous cholangiography with helical CT. J Comput Assist Tomogr 21:733–734

Musante F, Derchi LE, Bonati P (1982) CT cholangiography in suspected Caroli's disease. J Comput Assist Tomogr 6:482–485

Neitlich JD, Topazian M, Smith RC, Gupta A, Burrell MI, Rosenfield AT (1997) Detection of choledocholithiasis: comparison of unenhanced helical CT and endoscopic retrograde cholangiopancreatography. Radiology 203:753–757

Neuhaus H, Feussner H, Ungeheuer A, Hoffmann W, Siewert JR, Classen M (1992) Prospective evaluation of the use of endoscopic retrograde cholangiography prior to laparoscopic cholecystectomy. Endoscopy 24:745–749

Päivänsalo M, Merikanto J, Lähde S, et al (1988) Radiographic diagnosis of bile duct cysts. Retrospective analysis of thirteen cases. Acta Radiol 29:657–660

Pasanen P, Partanen K, Pikkarainen P, Alhava E, Pirinen A, Janatuinen E (1992) Ultrasonography, CT, and ERCP in the diagnosis of choledochal stones. Acta Radiol 33:53–56

Pasricha PJ (1996) Endoscopic ultrasonography versus endoscopic retrograde cholangiography for common bile duct stones: erosion of the gold standard? Gastroenterology 111:829–830

Patel JC, McInnes GC, Bagley JS, Needham G, Krukowski ZH (1993) The role of intravenous cholangiography in preoperative assessment for laparoscopic cholecystectomy. Br J Radiol 66:1125–1127

Prat F, Amouyal G, Amouyal P, et al (1996) Prospective controlled study of endoscopic ultrasonography and endoscopic retrograde cholangiography in patients with suspected common-bileduct lithiasis. Lancet 347:75–79

Raptopoulos V, Prassopoulos P, Chuttani R, McNicholas MM, McKee JD, Kressel HY (1998) Multiplanar CT pancreatography and distal cholangiography with minimum intensity projections. Radiology 207:317–324

Rholl KS, Smathers RL, McClennan BL, Lee JK (1985) Intravenous cholangiography in the CT era. Gastrointest Radiol 10:69–75

Ros E, Navarro S, Bru C, Garcia-Pugés A, Valderrama R (1991) Occult microlithiasis in "idiopathic" acute pancreatitis: prevention of relapses by cholecystectomy or ursodeoxycholic acid therapy. Gastroenterology 101:1701–1709

Schulman A (1987) Non-Western patterns of biliary stones and the role of ascariasis. Radiology 162:425–430

Scott IR, Gibney RG, Becker CD, Fache S, Burhenne HJ (1989) The use of intravenous cholangiography in teaching hospitals: a survey. Gastrointest Radiol 14:148–150

Smith RC, Rosenfield AT, Choe KA, Essenmacher KR, Verga M, Glickman MG, Lange RC (1995) Acute flank pain: comparison of non-contrast-enhanced CT and intravenous urography. Radiology 194:789–794

Stockberger SM, Johnson MS (1997) Spiral CT cholangiography in complex bile duct injuries after laparoscopic cholecystectomy. J Vasc Interv Radiol 8:249–252

Stockberger SM, Wass JL, Sherman S, Lehman GA, Kopecky KK (1994) Intravenous cholangiography with helical CT: comparison with endoscopic retrograde cholangiography. Radiology 192:675–680

Stockberger SM, Sherman S, Kopecky KK (1996) Helical CT cholangiography. Abdom Imaging 21:98–104

Strasberg SM, Soper NJ (1995) Management of choledocholithiasis in the laparoscopic era. Gastroenterology 109:320–322

Taourel P, Bret PM, Reinhold C, Barkun AN, Atri M (1996) Anatomic variants of the biliary tree: diagnosis with MR cholangiopancreatography. Radiology 199:521–527

Toombs BD, Sandler CM, Conoley PM (1981) Computed tomography of the nonvisualizing gallbladder. J Comput Assist Tomogr 5:164–168

Van Beers BE, Lacrosse M, Trigaux JP, de Cannière L, De Ronde T, Pringot J (1994) Noninvasive imaging of the biliary tree before or after laparoscopic cholecystectomy: use of three-dimensional spiral CT cholangiography. AJR Am J Roentgenol 162:1331–1335

Van Beers BE, Lacrosse M, Trigaux JP, Pringot J (1995) Spiral CT of the bile ducts. J Belge Radiol 78:95–97

18 Spiral CT for the Diagnosis and Staging of Pancreatic Adenocarcinoma

O. Cay, V. Raptopoulos

CONTENTS

18.1   Introduction   197
18.2   Technical Considerations   197
18.2.1 Intravenous Contrast Material   197
18.2.2 Pitch and Collimation   198
18.2.3 CT Angiography   198
18.2.4 Image Processing   199
18.2.5 CT Cholangiopancreatoscopy   201
18.2.6 Virtual CTCP   202
18.3   Detection of Pancreatic Adenocarcinoma
        and Differential Diagnosis   203
18.3.1 Tumor Detection   204
18.3.2 CT Findings   204
18.3.3 Double Duct Sign   205
18.3.4 The Pancreatic Duct   206
18.3.5 Differential Diagnosis   207
18.4   Staging of Pancreatic Adenocarcinoma:
        Assessment of Resectability   207
18.4.1 Multiphase and High-resolution Scanning   208
18.4.2 Pancreatoduodenal Venous Arcade   209
18.4.3 Small Bowel Enhancement   209
18.4.4 Distal Metastasis   210
18.4.5 CT Angiography   210
18.4.6 Vascular Staging   210
18.5   Surgical Planning   211
        References   212

18.1 Introduction

Pancreatic cancer is the ninth most common malignancy in Europe and the United States and the fourth most frequent cause of death related to a malignancy. The prognosis is poor, and the diagnosis is made late. Surgery provides the only effective treatment, but in only 10–30% of patients is the condition amenable to resection at the time of diagnosis

O. Cay, MD; Department of Radiology, Beth Israel Deaconess Medical Center and Harvard Medical School, 330 Brookline Ave., Boston, MA 02215, USA
V. Raptopoulos, MD; Department of Radiology, Beth Israel Deaconess Medical Center and Harvard Medical School, 330 Brookline Ave., Boston, MA 02215, USA

(Freeny et al. 1988; Megibow et al. 1995; Warshaw et al. 1990; Warshaw and Fernandez-del-Castillo 1992). Computed tomography (CT) is the most useful modality for the evaluation of pancreatic neoplasms. It is used both for diagnosis and for preoperative selection of patients who may undergo radical pancreatoduodenectomy (Aspestrand and Kolmannskog 1992; Baker 1991; Freeny et al. 1988, 1993; Warshaw et al. 1990). The volumetric data acquisition and speed of spiral CT allows for image processing techniques including spiral CT angiography, CT cholangiopancreatography and virtual CT cholangiopancreatoscopy, which further enhance diagnosis and staging (Bluemke and Chambers 1995; Prassopoulos et al. 1998; Raptopoulos et al. 1998).

18.2 Technical Considerations

Both helical or axial incremental scanning can be used to study a pancreatic mass, although technical factors differ in each of these methods (Bluemke et al. 1995; Freeny et al. 1993). Various single or multiphase scanning protocols may be used. Because the pancreas is a well-vascularized organ with a rich arterial supply, vascular phase scanning may be optimal for evaluation of pancreatic tumors (Diehl et al. 1998; Tublin et al. 1999). We found milk used as oral contrast agent in evaluation of the pancreas superior to no oral contrast, water, or conventional high-density oral contrast agents (Thompson et al. 1999).

18.2.1 Intravenous Contrast Material

Typically, a 100- to 150-ml bolus of contrast material is administered at a rate of 3.5–6 ml/s for scanning during the arterial (20–30 s delay), portal venous

(55–70 s delay) and equilibrium (85–90 s delay) phases (Diehl et al. (1998). When the bolus is increased to 200 ml and scanning is carried out with a 60-s to 80-s delay, a hybrid phase usually provides optimal arterial and portal venous opacification during peak pancreatic (60 s delay) and hepatic (80 s delay) parenchymal enhancement (Raptopoulos et al. 1997). For patients in whom altered circulation time is suspected a test injection (7–10 cc) followed by production of a time–density curve can be used. Alternatively, automated scanning triggering programs are available, although we have not found these useful in clinical practice.

18.2.2
Pitch and Collimation

Helical scanning provides volumetric data, which can be presented not only as axial sections but also as multiplanar displays. In a dual-phase helical CT protocol, thin section (1-mm or 3-mm collimation) pancreatic phase images have been reported to provide better visualization of the small peripancreatic veins than thicker (5-mm or 7-mm collimation) hepatic phase images (Vadentham et al. 1998).

Pitch selection is crucial to accommodate scanning during a single breath-hold. The duration of each helix should be set at 20–25 s. We have found that breath-holding over 25 s frequently produces respiratory misregistration artifacts. To cover the desired cranial caudal length (Δ_z) we chose scanning parameters based on the simple formula:

$$\Delta_z = (\text{Rotations/s}) \times \text{Breath-hold} \times \text{Collimation} \times \text{Pitch}$$

For example, 15 cm can be covered using 1.25 rotations/s, a 20-s breath-hold, 3-mm collimation, and pitch of 2. To increase coverage, we prefer increasing the pitch rather than the collimation, because this achieves a better spatial resolution. If 3-mm collimation is used, with an increase in the pitch from 1 to 2, the effective slice thickness increases from 3 mm to 3.9 mm, which provides better resolution than 5-mm collimation. In the above example, increasing the collimation from 3 mm to 5 mm rather than increasing the pitch from 1 to 2 would mean the span of the helix would be 12.5 cm instead of 15 cm.

In arterial phase scanning we use thin collimation and high pitch. This is based on the need to scan over the pancreas only (short helix): the contrast is high (higher pitch is acceptable), and the arteries have a small caliber (need for high spatial resolution). In the portal venous phase we increase the collimation and decrease the pitch. This is based on the need to scan over the liver (longer helix): the contrast is lower (lower pitch is preferred), and the veins are larger (wider collimation is acceptable). Thus, for arterial phase scanning we use 3-mm collimation and a pitch of 1.5–2 for scanning the region of the pancreas only, 20 s after the initiation of contrast injection (3–5 ml/s). This is followed by portal venous scanning of the liver and pancreas 60 s after injection, using 5-mm collimation and a pitch of 1–1.5.

18.2.3
CT Angiography

Helical CT with CT angiography of the pancreas provides useful information about local vascular involvement in pancreatic carcinoma. Compared with conventional axial helical CT, the addition of CT angiography improves radiologists' ability to predict resectability of pancreatic tumors. Integrated helical CT with CT angiography is done as follows: a non-contrast-enhanced scan of the region of the pancreas with 7-mm collimation and pitch of 1 (for better low-contrast resolution) is done. If there is a gross mass invading the major vessels, with or without liver, peritoneal or lymph node metastasis, a conventional contrast enhanced scan of the abdomen is done with 150 ml intravenous contrast, 65 s delay, 5-mm collimation and a pitch of 1–1.5. If there is a mass without obvious vascular invasion or liver metastasis, a high intravenous bolus of 180–200 ml is given at 3–5 ml/s. Scanning of the pancreas starts at 60 s with 3-mm collimation and a pitch of 1.3–1.8. This is followed immediately with scanning of the abdomen too, with 5-mm collimation and a pitch of 1–1.5. If there is not an obvious mass or if a neuro-endocrine tumor is suspected, a bi-phasic scan is done to detect either a small non-contour-altering mass (best prognosis) or early hyperenhancing lesion with quick contrast washout (neuro-endocrine tumors). Thus, an arterial phase (20 s) pancreas scan with 3-mm collimation is followed by a portal venous phase (65 s) scan of the liver with 5-mm collimation. This will both assess hepatic parenchyma and provide adequate peripancreatic venous detail to assess vascular invasion.

The use of helical CT with CT angiography is not without problems, an important one being the increase in reconstruction and physician time. Although imaging of the vessels from multiple projections is a great advantage of CT angiography, routine views should be standardized. The availability of an infinite number of views may increase the amount of time spent per case while adding little or no information. The high rate and large amount of i.v. contrast required for CT angiography should also be considered. In addition to allergic reactions, many patients may have impaired renal function and/or cardiac reserve, while the use of nonionic contrast material increases the cost of the test further. This, however, may be compensated by the potential for decreasing additional tests. Because of the relatively high injection rate, the risk and extent of extravasation increases. Nonfilling of veins, especially the inferior vena cava and hepatic veins, may also produce some diagnostic difficulties. Because of the thin collimation, axial images may be photon depleted and the increased number of axial images may require additional time for hard-copy imaging and interpretation, and additional expense for film and storage.

18.2.4
Image Processing

Axial images are reconstructed at half to two thirds the collimation interval used for image processing. This can be done either prospectively or retrospectively. Hard copy of sequential axial images is made on film. The overlapping images are used for image processing. Spiral scanning with volumetric data acquisition can produce multiplanar models of both soft tissues and vessels about the pancreas (FISHMAN et al. 1992; R et al. 1997; ZEMAN et al. (1994). We have found Multiple Projection Volume Reconstructions (MPVR) most helpful and easy to produce. These are in essence thick slabs of tissue. Variable thickness can be selected and can be viewed with various renderings, such as Maximum Intensity Projections (MIP), Average or Minimum Intensity Projection (MinIP). The last is particularly helpful for better delineation of low-attenuation structures within the tissue block, such as the pancreatic duct. For best results, two interactive oblique models can provide optimal planes.

Shaded Surface Renderings (SSR) can be quickly produced (see Fig. 18.1A.) Since they depend on the attenuation threshold, a lot of information can be lost both by exclusion of lower attenuation structures and by oversegmentation of structures not touching each other (DILLON et al. 1993; RUBIN et al. 1993; STEHLING et al. 1994). They can, however, be used as road maps for multiplanar reformations (MPR) or MPVRs. Three-dimensional MIP render-

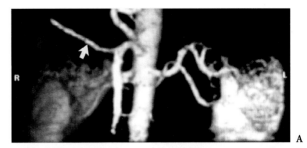

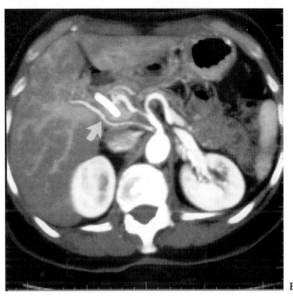

Fig. 18.1A, B. Replaced right hepatic artery from SMA. **A** CTA with shaded surface rendering shows origin of right hepatic artery from SMA (*arrow*), along with double renal arteries, bilaterally. Threshold was set at 160 HU, and the skeleton has been subtracted. **B** MIP MPVR shows replaced right hepatic artery's course (*arrow*) behind the portal vein

ings may be hampered by overlying high-attenuation structures such as the bones (NAPEL et al. 1992). Subtraction or manual segmentation techniques may be cumbersome. Since only the highest attenuation of a projection is seen, a lot of information is also lost. Furthermore, MIPs do not provide depth perception, and overlying structures need to be viewed from different angles (see Fig. 18.2). Newer workstations with increased computer power allow for Volume Renderings (VR). A range of densities is seen, and viewing through tissue is possible since transparencies are now possible (see Fig. 18.3C). Volume renderings produce more accurate and inclusive images than any other technique (JOHNSON et al. 1996).

Bone Subtraction. On the 3D images, we remove the skeleton by initially isolating it in another model

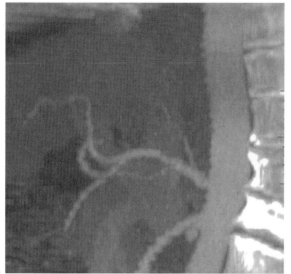

A

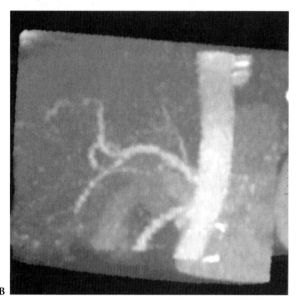

B

Fig. 18.2A, B. Three-dimensional MIP CTA shows right hepatic artery arising directly from the celiac axis. The skeleton in (**A**) was isolated by threshold and then subtracted to produce a less distracted image (**B**)

Fig. 18.3A–C. Large hypoenhancing pancreatic tumor not extending to the peripancreatic tissues. Common bile duct stent is present. Despite its size, adenocarcinoma was resected (see Tables 18.1, 18.2). **A** Axial image shows 4-cm heterogeneously enhancing mass (*arrow*) with hypoenhancing center in the head of the pancreas. There is a clear fat plane separating the mass from the SMV. **B** MinIP image shows mass producing obstruction to pancreatic duct (*arrow*) There is atrophy of the pancreatic body and tail. **C** CT angiogram (15 mm thick multiple projection volume reconstruction (MPVR)] shows flattening of one side of the superior mesenteric vein (SMV; *arrow*), but no concentric encasement (grade 2). As feared, tumor resection was technically difficult and the tumor recurred within 6 months

and using an attenuation threshold of approximately 160 H in the arterial and 140 H in the venous or combined arterial–venous phase. Subsequently, we subtract the skeleton from the intact 3D volume (see Figs. 18.1, 18.2). This allows unobstructed viewing of vessels from multiple angles without the accidental over segmentation that is common in manual techniques (RAPTOPOULOS et al. 1996).

For quick and satisfactory results, MPVRs are a most helpful and efficient image processing method. They are simple and accurate and require minimal training (see Figs. 18.1B, 18.3C, 18.4B.) Volume renderings are also produced rapidly and provide elegant and accurate true 3D images without loss of data, but are less widely available (see Figs. 18.4–18.8).Similarly, 3D MIP, surface renderings or curved

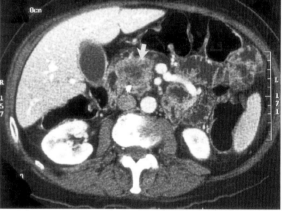

A

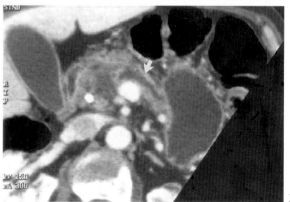

B

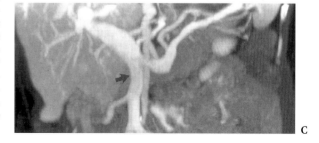

C

reformations are valuable methods; however, they are used less frequently since they require more time and have a longer learning curve.

18.2.5
CT Cholangiopancreatoscopy

This image post-processing technique improves CT visualization of the pancreatic and common bile ducts (RAPTOPOULOS et al. 1998). In selected patients, this technique may decrease the need for diagnostic endoscopic retrograde cholangiopancreatography (ERCP) after CT. Imaging of the pancreatic ducts is accomplished by applying minimum intensity to volume projections of selected thickness

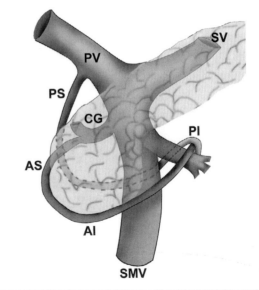

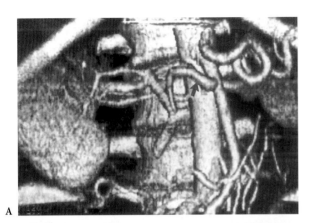

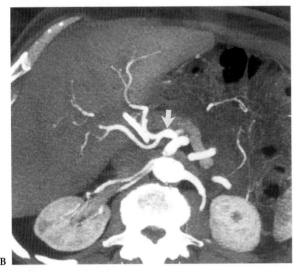

Fig. 18.4A, B. Replaced hepatic artery from SMA (*arrows*). **A** The origin of the vessel (*arrow*) is seen on volume rendering, while **B** the intrahepatic branching (*arrow*) is best seen on MIP MPVR. High resolution achieved with 1.25 mm collimation on a multidetector platform scanner

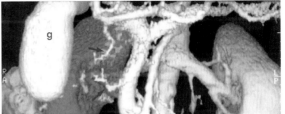

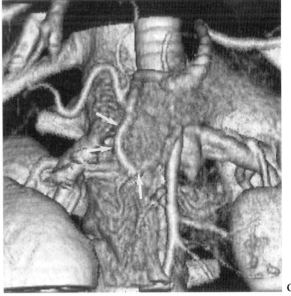

Fig. 18.5A–C. Pancreatoduodenal arcade. **A** Diagram of pancreatoduodenal venous (PDV) arcade connecting the SMV with the portal vein. SMV: superior mesenteric vein; PV: portal vein; SV: splenic vein; CG: gastrocolic trunk; AS: anterior superior PDV; PS: posterior superior PDV; AI: anterior inferior PDV; PI: posterior inferior PDV. **B** CTA (shaded surface rendering, SSR) of pancreatoduodenal venous arcade (*arrows*). Gallbladder (*g*) is seen due to contrast material from previous ERCP (endoscopic retrograde pancreatography). **C** CTA (volume rendering, VR) of arterial pancreatoduodenal arcade (*arrows*)

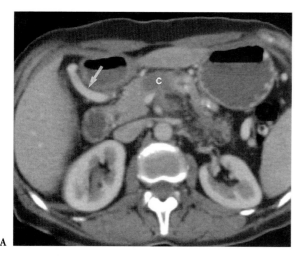

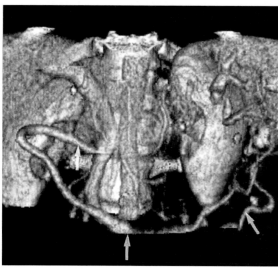

Fig. 18.6. A Pancreatic carcinoma (*c*) seen on axial image, producing occlusion of splenic vein and drainage via collaterals to gastrocolic trunk (*arrow*); **B** PDV (*arrows*) seen better on volume rendering CTA

(minIP MPVRs.) The best results are achieved when slab thickness does not exceed the thickness of the organ (see Fig. 18.9B.) A too thick volume may contain structures with attenuation lower than that of the bile and pancreatic fluid (e.g., peripancreatic fat). Conversely, too thin a slab may exclude some portion of the duct, resulting in oversegmentation and losing the projectional effect of a single image. We find it easier to use two interactive oblique "windows." A desirable slab is then selected by identifying the appropriate oblique plane and volume thickness. Once the duct is visualized on minIPs it can be used as a road map to produce average intensity oblique or curved (traced) reconstructions. In selected patients we found CT cholangio-

pancreatoscopy CTCP) helpful to demonstrate anatomic relationships among the ducts, delineate the type of obstruction and provide further information in equivocal or complicated images. Furthermore, minIP viewing of pancreatic parenchyma may make small, non-contour-altering tumors more conspicuous (see Fig. 18.10).

18.2.6
Virtual CTCP

Endoluminal virtual CTCP can help in assessment of the cause and relationships of pancreatic and distal common bile duct dilatation (Prassopoulos et al. 1998). After identification of the duct on a reference 2D image, endoluminal views are obtained by determining threshold differentials at the attenuation difference between duct fluid and soft tissue. We found

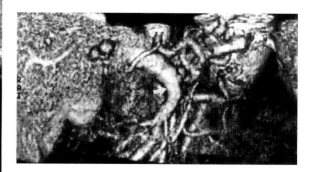

Fig. 18.7. CTA with volume rendering shows smooth displacement of SMV (*arrow*) by pancreatic mass without other vascular abnormality (grade 1). Tumor resection was uneventful

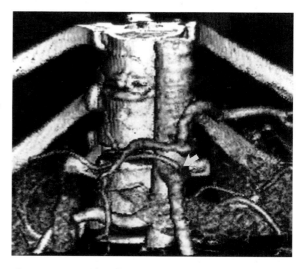

Fig. 18.8. CTA with volume rendering shows replaced right hepatic artery directly from the aorta (*arrow*)

that threshold values of 50–90 HU for the pancreatic duct and 30–60 HU for the intrapancreatic common bile duct worked best for most endoluminal views, and that a 30°–50°field of view was appropriate for simulation of endoscopic perspective. A smooth mode and light-and-shade technique are used to provide an in-relief effect that simulates endoluminal views. Endoluminal images constructed at 3- to 10-mm steps on a trajectory along the duct provide a fly-through sequence (see Fig. 18.11.)

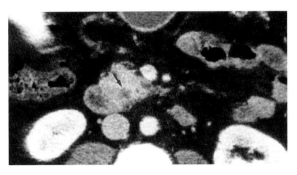

Fig. 18.10. Pancreatic adenocarcinoma measuring 1 cm (*arrow*), seen best on this 7-mm-thick minimum intensity projection (minIP). The fat plane to the great vessels is preserved (type A, grade 1; see Tables 18.1, and 18.2)

18.3
Detection of Pancreatic Adenocarcinoma and Differential Diagnosis

Radiologic diagnosis of pancreatic carcinoma in its earliest clinical stages is not always easy. With recent

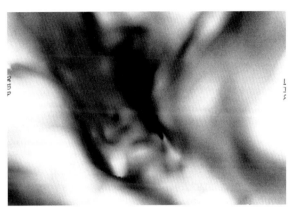

Fig. 18.11. Intraluminal view of pancreatic duct shows irregular narrowing and abrupt occlusion of the duct

developments in helical CT techniques, detection and staging of pancreatic tumors is improving. Despite the development of promising technologies such as magnetic resonance imaging (MRI) or endoscopic ultrasound (EUS), CT is still the most frequently utilized modality for detection and staging of pancreatic neoplasms (MÜLLER et al. 1994; ROSCH et al. 1992). CT is also endorsed by the Radiology Diagnostic Oncology Group (MEGIBOW et al. 1995).

Pancreatic adenocarcinoma is the most common neoplasm of the pancreas, comprising approximately 80% of all tumors arising from the epithelium of the pancreatic duct. The majority of pancreatic carcinomas have been found to be located in the head of the pancreas (60–65%), followed by the body and the tail, respectively. A small percentage (5–10%) of pancreatic tumors invade the pancreas diffusely (FREENY et al. 1993; WARSHAW and FERNANDEZ-DEL-CASTILLO 1992). The tumors arising in the head of the pancreas tend to produce symptoms earlier than those in the body, and the tail,

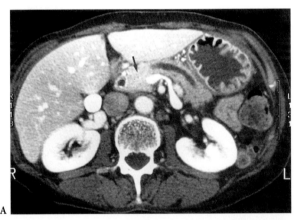

A

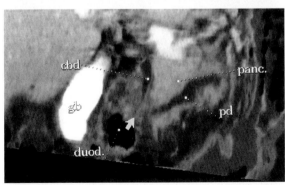

B

Fig. 18.9A, B. Double duct sign. A Axial image shows dilated pancreatic and common bile ducts, with a 2.3-cm thickness of normal pancreatic tissue separating them (*arrow*). B CTCP (oblique minIP MPVR) shows tapering of common bile duct (*cbd*) and abrupt obstruction of the pancreatic duct (*pd*) by infiltrating mass (*arrow*) in the head of pancreas (*duod.* duodenum, *gb* gallbladder)

because the head of the pancreas has an intimate anatomic relationship with the common bile duct and duodenum, so that a tumor in that region causes clinical symptoms even when it is not yet large. Conversely, even a large pancreatic tail tumor may present without clinical symptoms such as jaundice (FREENY et al. 1993; WARSHAW and FERNANDEZ-DEL-CASTILLO 1992; WARSHAW et al. 1990).

18.3.1
Tumor Detection

Early detection is imperative, especially since survival is directly related to tumor size. A 100% 6-year survival can be expected with tumors smaller than 1 cm. In comparison, the 6-year survival with masses larger than 4 cm is nil. Adenocarcinoma of the pancreas is best demonstrated on images obtained during the high blood perfusion phase with CT, while high concentrations of contrast material are present within the organ. It appears that peak vascular and parenchymal enhancement achieved with spiral CT may improve the sensitivity of CT scans in detecting pancreatic carcinoma, especially small tumors confined within the organ (BLUEMKE et al. 1995; FISHMAN et al. 1992; HOLLETT et al. 1995; KEOGAN et al. 1997; LU et al. 1996). These studies suggest that pancreatic tumor conspicuity is best achieved using a scanning delay of 30–70 s and injection rates of 2.5–4 ml/s. TUBIN et al. (1999) found a statistically significant and considerable difference in pancreatic enhancement when comparing 5 ml/s to 2.5 ml/s injection rates. With 2.5 ml/s the pancreas reached a peak attenuation of 65 HU at 69 s, as opposed to the 84 HU at 43 s achieved with 5 ml/s (Fig. 18.12). In the same study, the liver reached peak attenuation of 58 HU at 87 s with 2.5 ml/s and 75 HU at 63 s with 5 ml/s. Based on these observations it is hoped that high injection rates may facilitate tumor conspicuity with scanning at about 30 s delay after a 5 ml/s bolus of 150 ml of iodinated contrast material (Fig. 18.13). Repeat scanning of the liver at 60–70 s delay is then needed for best liver metastasis conspicuity.

It is suggested that increased conspicuity of tumor may be seen with minIPs (RAPTOPOULOS et al. 1998). Pancreatic adenocarcinoma is much less vascular than pancreatic tissue and usually appears as a hypoenhancing tumor relative to the surrounding parenchyma, although tumors may be relatively isodense with pancreatic parenchyma, showing little difference in attenuation without and with contrast enhancement. However, considering the range of at-

tenuation values, the minimal attenuation on enhanced scans may be substantially less in carcinoma than in the adjacent pancreas because of increased desmoplastic stroma (Fig. 18.10).

18.3.2
CT Findings

The CT appearance of pancreatic cancer varies, depending on intravenous contrast administration (BAKER 1991; FREENY et al. 1988; MEGIBOW et al. 1995). A small pancreatic tumor may be missed in a noncontrast study. If there is no extensive necrosis present, the tumor appears isodense to the normal parenchyma. If the tumor is large enough to cause distortion in the contour of the organ, a large

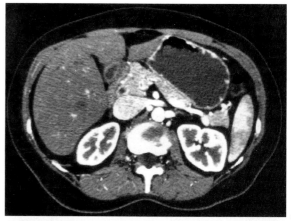

A

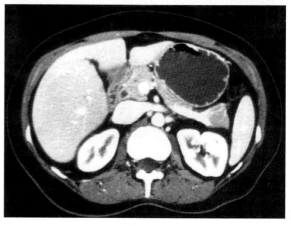

B

Fig. 18.12A, B. Axial images of normal pancreas obtained with 5 ml/s injection of i.v. contrast medium showing significant early enhancement and rapid washout. The liver enhancement lags behind the early pancreatic blush. **A** Arterial phase, images obtained 30 s after injection. **B** Portal venous image obtained 60 s after injection.

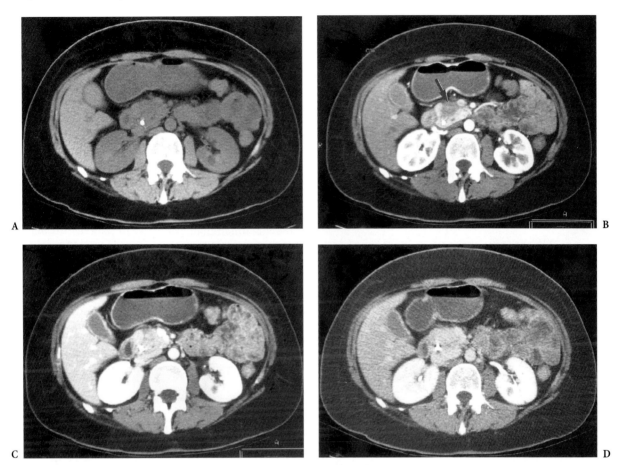

Fig. 18.13A–D. Small pancreatic adenocarcinoma, best appreciated in arterial phase. Stent is present in the common bile duct. Contrast 150 ml i.v. injected at 5 ml/s. High resolution is achieved with 1.25 mm collimation on a multidetector platform scanner. **A** Noncontrast scan shows prominent head of pancreas. **B** Arterial phase (30 s). Carcinoma (*arrow*) is seen as hypoenhancing mass compared to hyperenhancing pancreatic parenchyma. **C** Portal venous phase (60 s.) Carcinoma is less conspicuous, almost isodense with the pancreas. **D** Delayed phase (105 s.) Tumor is inconspicuous

isodense mass can be identified. If contrast material is administered, a hypoattenuating solid-appearing mass within the normal contour of the pancreas or, more frequently, a larger mass causing distortion of the contour of the organ will be seen (Fig. 18.13). The intrapancreatic margin of the tumor is usually well defined but is sometimes indistinct.

If there is ductal involvement, interruption of the main pancreatic duct, usually with upstream dilatation, is seen. This may be accompanied by parenchymal atrophy, cysts resulting from obstruction, or even changes compatible with acute pancreatitis. However, a few important signs are useful to differentiate acute pancreatitis from an infiltrating tumor, such as lack of peripancreatic inflammatory changes of the mesenteric fat or peripancreatic fluid collection, as well as other indicators suggesting local or distant invasion of the diffuse neoplastic process,

such as loss of fat plane posterior to the origin of the superior mesenteric artery or presence of peripancreatic lymphadenopathy.

Rounded prominence of the uncinate process anteriorly and posteriorly with no evidence of a mass should raise the question of presence of a small mass located in this region, especially if there is an upstream dilatation of the pancreatic duct (Fig. 18.14).

18.3.3
Double Duct Sign

Obstruction of the common bile duct will occur when there is a tumor located within the head of the pancreas or the ampulla causing a mass effect on the duct (Fig. 18.15). When dilatation and separation of both the common bile duct and the pancreatic duct

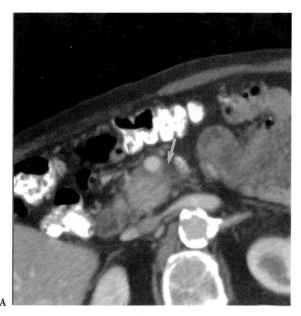

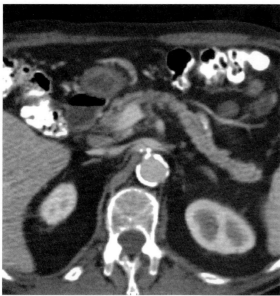

Fig. 18.14. A Large uncinate process of the head of the pancreas with relatively atrophic pancreatic body and tail. There is infiltration of the fat surrounding the SMV and extending to the superior mesenteric artery (SMA; *arrow*). Differential diagnosis includes focal pancreatitis and tumor. **B** Subsequent scan showed resolution of the peripancreatic exudate, but the enlargement of the head persisted for 1 year. Percutaneous biopsy did not reveal malignancy. Endoscopic ultrasound showed no distinct tumor

directly detected on CT) but often ampullary or duodenal carcinoma is present. Double duct sign may also result from intrapancreatic extension of cholangiocarcinoma, although less frequently.

18.3.4
The Pancreatic Duct

Dilatation of the pancreatic duct is a sensitive indicator of pancreatic disease, but not necessarily a pathognomonic sign for pancreatic carcinoma. Duodenal inflammatory disease or pancreatitis may also present with pancreatic ductal dilatation. Smooth dilatation of the duct has been attributed to a neoplastic process. However, in one third of patients with chronic pancreatitis, the main pancreatic duct demonstrated a similar configuration (KARASAWA et al. 1983). Similarly, a smoothly dilated pancreatic duct diameter greater than one half the width of the pancreatic gland was associated

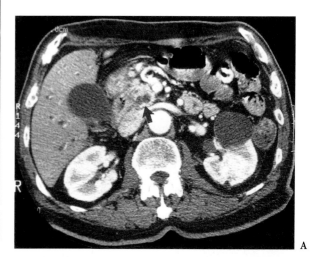

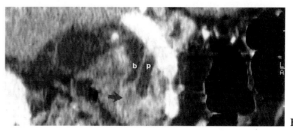

Fig. 18.15A, B. Dilated pancreatic and common bile ducts caused by small ampullary carcinoma. A stone could produce similar duct dilatation. **A** Axial image shows converging dilated ducts in head of pancreas (*arrow*). **B** cholangiopancreatography (CTCP; oblique minIP MPVR) shows dilated bile and pancreatic ducts (*b, p*) and a small ampullary mass

are found simultaneously, this is referred to as the double duct sign, and it is most commonly associated with pancreatic adenocarcinoma (Fig. 18.16). If both ducts are seen to be dilated up to the ampulla, the cause may be an obstructing calculus (only 60%

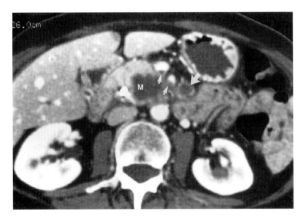

Fig. 18.16. Axial CT image shows pancreatic mass (*M*), adenocarcinoma, invading SMA and SMV (*small arrows*), and focal lymph node enlargement (*large arrow*) to the left side of the SMA. This is an unresectable tumor

with carcinoma in 90% of the patients. Abrupt cutoff of the pancreatic duct or the common bile duct is an important indicator suggesting that the termination of the ducts is most probably due to malignancy (STANLEY and SEMELKA 1998).

When no detectable mass is found on axial or helical incremental CT examination, endoscopic retrograde cholangiopancreatography (ERCP) or MR cholangiopancreatography (MRCP) is performed for further evaluation. One major advantage of both ERCP and MRCP is the availability of projectional imaging.

From spiral CT source images, three-dimensional images of a dilated biliary tree can be produced with shaded surface renderings using a narrow-range threshold at around water attenuation (ZEMAN et al. 1994). Recent results from our institution demonstrated that CTCP with minIP MPVRs is a feasible technique that markedly improves CT depiction of pancreatic and bile ducts and provides image quality approaching that of ERCP (RAPTOPOULOS et al. 1998). Comparison of conventional axial CT images with CTCP showed significant improvement in pancreatic duct visualization. Furthermore, for dilated ducts there was no significant difference between ERCP and CTCP in detection or characterization of the nature of any obstruction (RAPTOPOULOS et al. 1998). Duct obstruction caused by smooth narrowing due to an inflammatory stricture suggests pancreatitis, as against abrupt or irregular obstruction caused by a carcinoma (Figs. 18.3B, 18.9B). In addition, noncalcified intraluminal bile duct stones and a number of small tumors were more conspicuous on minIP images. Similarly, CTCP may help distinguish

cystic duct branches from cystic or necrotic tumors.

Virtual endoluminal CT cholangiopancreatoscopy can detect obstruction due to a mass causing abrupt and irregular occlusion (Fig. 18.11). In contrast, a stone is seen intraluminally and inflammation produces tapering with or without a beaded duct. Extrinsic compression can be also distinguished from intraluminal or mural abnormalities (PRASSOPOULOS et al. 1998).

18.3.5
Differential Diagnosis

Other entities that should be considered in the differential diagnosis of pancreatic adenocarcinoma are a mass arising on the basis of chronic pancreatitis, focal pancreatitis (Fig. 18.14), peripancreatic lymph nodes, pancreatic cysts, and other pancreatic tumors, such as acinar cell carcinoma, microcystic adenoma, mucinous cystic neoplasm, and lymphoma.

18.4
Staging of Pancreatic Adenocarcinoma: Assessment of Resectability

The only effective treatment of pancreatic carcinoma is surgical resection. For tumors in the tail, distal pancreatectomy and splenectomy are done. Although these are not particularly difficult operations, carcinoma in this location is diagnosed late, usually with extensive local invasion or distal metastasis rendering the mass unresectable. For carcinoma of the head, radical pancreatoduodenectomy (Whipple procedure) is done. This is a complicated operation and requires clear planes between the tumor and the great peripancreatic vessels, and also absence of lymph node or distal metastasis (WARSHAW and FERNANDEZ-DEL-CASTILLO 1992).

The diagnosis and staging of pancreatic adenocarcinoma are interrelated. The CT techniques best suited for diagnosis are usually appropriate for selection of surgical candidates. In addition, secondary features that establish the staging of the disease may call attention to the primary tumor or characterize it as a neoplasm. CT scanning has a 95% accuracy in predicting unresectability of pancreatic carcinoma, rarely requiring additional tests (FREENY et al. 1993; WARSHAW et al. 1990). However, CT is accurate in predicting resectability in only 66–78% of cases

(BLUEMKE et al. 1995; DIEHL et al. 1998; FREENY et al. 1993; WARSHAW et al. 1990). The major reasons for CT error are failure to detect small liver and peritoneal metastatic implants, metastatic lymphadenopathy, and encasement of the great vessels by tumor. Consequently, many surgeons routinely perform laparoscopy and laparoscopic biopsy before proceeding to radical pancreatectomy. However, detection of vascular encasement cannot be made laparoscopically; hence the need for angiography (ASPESTRAND and KOLMANNSKOG 1992; FREENY et al. 1988; WARSHAW et al. 1990). It is to this angle that CT with CT angiography adds significantly in the evaluation of pancreatic carcinoma, providing the potential for a "one-stop" test.

Although vascular encasement is not an absolute contraindication for resection, advanced knowledge of its existence is important, as it renders the prospect of resection more difficult. It requires careful planning and mobilization of available resources, including referral to more specialized centers. Furthermore, aborted pancreatoduodenectomy is associated with perioperative morbidity and prolonged recovery.

For pancreatic tumors, assessment of the superior mesenteric artery and vein (SMA and SMV) and of the portal vein (PV) is crucial for successful surgical excision (Fig. 18.16). Identification of tumor spread to the retroperitoneum, especially behind the SMA, is important, since direct intraoperative detection of this is usually not possible until the final stage of the operation (Fig. 18.17). Involvement of the liver and regional lymph nodes within the peripancreatic, periaortic, pericaval and periportal regions and peritoneal carcinomatosis are also determinant factors for unresectability, as is tumor spread to the contiguous organs.

Teardrop SMV is a recently described sign of unresectability (HOUGH et al. 1999). The vein appears tethered, and its shape changed from round to teardrop on axial images. Although low in sensitivity (43%) it has a 98% specificity in diagnosis and surgical staging of pancreatic head adenocarcinoma.

Identification of pathways of the tumor spread is crucial, especially when the tumor expands beyond the usual margins of pancreaticoduodenectomy (Fig. 18.18). Tumor invasion of the duodenum is usually not a contraindication for resection, because the tumor and the duodenum are removed together in the resected specimen. However, nodal staging is important and for this CT depends on size, which is a crude criterion. Early metastatic involvement can be encountered in normal-sized lymph nodes. Biopsy of a pancreatic mass or presumed spread in peri-

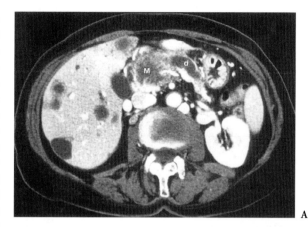

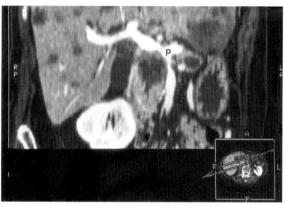

Fig. 18.17A, B. Unresectable pancreatic adenocarcinoma with vascular encasement and liver metastasis (*M*). **A** Axial image shows large hypodense mass in the head of pancreas. The pancreatic duct (*d*) is dilated and there are numerous metastatic nodules in the liver. **B** CT angiogram (maximum intensity projection – MIP – MPVR) shows irregular encasement at the origin of the portal vein (*p*). Vascular staging: type D, or grade 3 (see Tables 18.1, 18.2)

pancreatic tissues, lymph nodes, liver metastasis or other distant locations can yield the information necessary for assessment of resectability. Biopsy can be done percutaneously with CT or ultrasound guidance, with endoscopic ultrasound, or at laparoscopy.

18.4.1
Multiphase and High-resolution Scanning

The newer applications of helical CT include multiphase scanning after a single bolus injection of contrast material. This improves both tumor detection and characterization, while vascular imaging helps in assessing tumor resectability and surgical planning.

High-resolution scanning with 1.5-mm-thick noncontiguous images (5 mm slice intervals) has

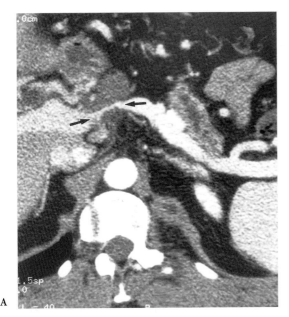

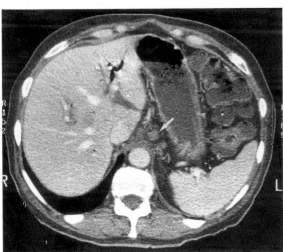

Fig. 18.18A, B. Spread of pancreatic adenocarcinoma rendering tumor unresectable. **A** CT angiography (CTA) (curved reconstruction) shows lymph nodes encasing the portal vein (*arrows*). **B** Axial image shows pre-aortic extension and left gastric lymph node enlargement (*arrow*)

been shown to predict resectability of pancreatic neoplasms accurately (FUHRMAN et al. 1994). New multidetector scanners can scan the liver and pancreas within one breath-hold with 1.25-mm collimation without the need for intervening gaps (Fig. 18.13).

In a recent study, DIEHL et al. (1998) reported that use of thin-section scanning of the pancreatic region with 3-mm collimation and a pitch of 1.6 (3-mm reconstruction increment) produced the best results for evaluation of pancreatic parenchyma and peripancreatic vessels. In this study, helical CT allowed

detection of pancreatic cancer in 97% of the patients where helical CT demonstrated a 91% accuracy in detection of unresectability with a negative predictive value of 79%. In a study by BLUEMKE et al. (1995), 7 (16%) of 43 patients with presumed resectable tumors on CT had undetected vascular encasement.

18.4.2
Pancreatoduodenal Venous Arcade

Recently, a number of papers have been published discussing abnormalities in the arcade (Fig. 18.5) of small arteries and veins surrounding the head of the pancreas and their value in staging cancer (MOODY and POON 1992; MORI et al. 1991, 1992; HOMMEYER et al. 1995; VADENTHAM et al. 1998). The pancreatoduodenal veins (PDV) produce an arcade of potential collateral connection of the portal vein and superior mesenteric vein (SMV).

Assessment is better made with high-resolution techniques. Asymmetric enlargement of one vein may be interpreted as a secondary sign of peripancreatic vein encasement of another major vein and may be the only sign of unresectability (Figs. 18.6, 18.19). However, the sensitivity of this sign is low and detection of abnormalities in these vessels is uncommon, even in patients with unresectable tumors (HOMMEYER et al. 1995).

18.4.3
Small Bowel Enhancement

A secondary sign of major vein encasement and unresectability is an increase in ratio of small bowel

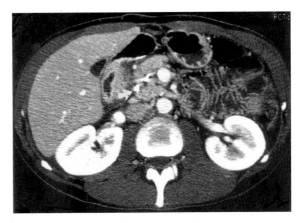

Fig. 18.19. Asymmetric enlargement of posterior inferior pancreatoduodenal vein (*arrow*) as the only overt finding in the presence of unresectable pancreatic adenocarcinoma. Stent is present in the common bile duct

wall over portal vein enhancement ratio to over 0.78 (0.78–1.21, mean 0.90.) In a recent study, there were significantly smaller ratios in patients with pancreatic head cancer without venous encasement (0.42–0.70, mean 0.52) or normal controls (0.26–0.62, mean 0.46) (SHEIMAN and RAPTOPOULOS 1996). Enhancement was determined as a smaller attenuation difference in the portal venous phase than in noncontrast scans. The increased ratio is attributed to decreased washout of contrast medium from the small bowel wall owing to the encasement of major venous drainage. There was also significantly higher small bowel enhancement (72±8 HU in patients with venous encasement as opposed to 60±10 HU for nonencased and 58±14 HU for normal controls.) Enhancement of the portal vein was significantly decreased in patients with encasement (82±18 HU against 122±22 HU in nonencased and 134±31 HU in normal controls.) Compared with axial images, increased ratios were shown to be another secondary sign of venous encasement and, on occasion, the only sign of nonresectability of a pancreatic head adenocarcinoma.

18.4.4
Distal Metastasis

With recent advancements in CT scanning, detection and staging of pancreatic tumor is improving (BLUEMKE et al. 1995; FUHRMAN et al. 1994; HOMMEYER et al. 1995; MOODY and POON (1992); MORI et al. 1991, 1992; ZEMAN et al. 1994). However, distal metastasis, especially when it takes the form of peritoneal implants, remains a problem. In a recent study, BLUEMKE et al. (1995), using state-of-the-art techniques, found unresectable disease due to undetected liver and peritoneal implants in nine (21%) of 43 patients considered to have locally resectable disease by CT. In our series, six (14%) patients undergoing planned laparoscopy before pancreatectomy had metastatic disease not detected on axial CT images (RAPTOPOULOS et al. 1997).

18.4.5
CT Angiography

The inability of CT to distinguish vascular encasement accurately may be due to insufficient vascular enhancement or the relatively decreased resolution of cross-sectional imaging along the longitudinal axis of the vessels. Thus, subtle changes in the caliber

of the major peripancreatic vessels, such as SMV, portal vein or superior mesenteric artery (SMA) may be missed. Some of these problems may be remedied with the use of helical CT and CT angiography, which increases vascular opacification, improves parenchymal enhancement and produces both conventional cross-sectional and angiographic images (RAPTOPOULOS et al. 1997). However, spiral CT angiography does not improve resolution and artifacts from image processing techniques, and involuntary motion may further degrade the z-axis resolution. This has improved markedly with the new multidetector CT platform, which provides 1.25-mm collimation but not at the expense of short z-axis coverage (Fig. 18.6).

For clinical evaluations, these degradations in resolution seem to be overcompensated by the angiographic display, which enhances the conspicuity of subtle alterations in vessel caliber. Helical CT angiography, by thus improving detection of vascular invasion, improves prediction of tumor resectability and thus the preoperative staging of carcinoma of the head of the pancreas.

Direct depiction of vascular encasement can be used to predict local resectability of pancreatic carcinoma of the head. We found vascular assessment on CT angiography helpful and accurate (RAPTOPOULOS et al. 1997). In 38 patients with surgical correlation there was exact, almost verbatim, correlation of the CT and operative notes describing the vessel–tumor relationship in 32 patients and minor differences in the reports of the remaining 6 patients.

18.4.6
Vascular Staging

In Table 18.1 a CTA grading system is presented, assessing the relationship of tumors to the great peripancreatic vessels (RAPTOPOULOS et al. 1997). Grades range from normal (grade 0) to completely occluded (grade 4). All tumors with grades 0 and 1 (loss of fat plane between tumor and vessel with or without smooth displacement of the vessel) were resectable (Figs. 18.4, 18.7). In contrast, all tumors with grade 3 (tumor around two sides of SMA or narrowing of SMV or PV) or grade 4 were nonresectable (Figs. 18.6, 18.17). Using this grading system, the predictive value for resectability (negative result) of axial CT was 70%, as against the 96% (P=0.02) achieved when CTA was added. Furthermore, spiral CTA helped predict technical difficulties encountered at surgery when dissecting along vascular planes in half the patients with grade 2 appearance, which shows flattening or slight irregularity of one side of any of the great vessels (Fig. 18.4). Others, however, with similarly good results did not find the addition of angiography all that helpful (DIEHL et al. 1998).

LOYER et al. (1996) devised a vascular grading system assessing the relationship between the tumor and the great vessels (Table 18.2). The abnormalities ranged from the presence of an intervening fat plane (type A) or pancreatic parenchyma (type B), indicating resectability, to tumor occluding a vessel (type F), indicating unresectability. Type C (tumor inseparable from vessel but with convex contour of the latter) does not reliably predict resectability. Similarly, tumor partially encircling a vessel (type D) indicates the need for vascular resection in almost half the patients.

18.5
Surgical Planning

Variants of hepatic and pancreatic vascular anatomy are common, and since their presence may alter surgical management, should be detected preoperatively. For example, an accessory or replaced right hepatic artery arises from either the celiac axis or the superior mesenteric artery, passes posterior to the portal vein and posterolateral to the bile duct in the hepatoduodenal ligament to reach the liver hilum. This variant occurs in 12–25% of patients. Replaced left hepatic arteries occur in approximately 10% of patients, and arise from the left gastric artery coursing in the gastrohepatic ligament through the fissure for ligamentum venosum into the umbilical fissure to supply the left liver. In-advance knowledge of the origin of the right hepatic artery is very important for radical pancreatoduodenectomy, since the surgeon is frequently working "blind" when dissecting pancreatic head tumor from the retroperitoneum. CT angiography can visualize the pancreatoduodenal arcade as well as vascular variants, providing preoperative guidance. Furthermore, thin section spiral CT scanning can depict areas that may require biopsy before resection, including lymph nodes, liver lesions or peritoneal nodules.

Table 18.1. CT angiography staging of pancreatic carcinoma. (Adapted from Raptopoulos et al. 1997)

Grade	Pancreatic vessels (SMA, SMV, PV)	Tumor resectability
0	Normal	Resectable
1	Loss of fat with or without smooth displacement of vessel	Resectable
2	Flattening or slight irregularity of one side of any vessel	Varying difficulty in resection; 8% unresectable
3	Tumor around two sides of vessel (artery). Narrowing of lumen (vein)	Unresectable or tumor in margins
4	Occluded vessel	Unresectable

Table 18.2. Vascular staging of pancreatic carcinoma. (Adapted from Loyer et al. 1996)

Type	Tumor–vessel relation	Tumor resectability
A	Intervening fat plane	Resectable
B	Intervening normal parenchyma	Resectable
C	Tumor inseparable but convex contours of vessel at contact	Not reliable prediction
D	Tumor partially encircling vessel	47% resectability with venous resection
E	Tumor completely encircling vessel	Unresectable
F	Tumor occluding vessel	Unresectable

References

Aspestrand F, Kolmannskog F (1992) CT compared to angiography for staging of tumors of the pancreatic head. Acta Radiol 33:556–560

Baker ME (1991) Pancreatic adenocarcinoma: are there pathognomonic changes in fat surrounding the superior mesenteric artery? Radiology 180:613–614

Bluemke DA, Chambers TP (1995) Spiral CT angiography: an alternative to conventional angiography. Radiology 195:317–319

Bluemke DA, Cameron JL, Hruban RH, et al (1995) Potentially resectable pancreatic adenocarcinoma: spiral CT assessment with surgical and pathologic correlation. Radiology 197:381–385

Diehl SJ, Lehmann KJ, Sadick M, Lachmann R, Georgi M (1998) Pancreatic cancer: value of dual-phase helical CT in assessing resectability. Radiology 206:373–378

Dillon EH, van Leeuwen MS, Fernandez MA, Mali WPT (1993) Spiral CT angiography. AJR Am J Roentgenol 160:1273–1278

Fishman EK, Wyatt SH, Ney DR, Kuhlman JE, Siegelman SS (1992) Spiral CT of the pancreas with multiplanar display. AJR Am J Roentgenol 159:1209–1215

Freeny PC, Marks WM, Ryan JA, Traverso LW (1988) Pancreatic ductal adenocarcinoma: diagnosis and staging with dynamic CT. Radiology 166:125–133

Freeny PC, Traverso LW, Ryan JA (1993) Diagnosis and staging of pancreatic adenocarcinoma with dynamic computed tomography. Am J Surg 165:600–606

Fuhrman GM, Charnsangavej C, Abbruzzese JL, et al (1994) Thin-section contrast-enhanced computed tomography accurately predicts the resectability of malignant pancreatic neoplasms. Am J Surg 167:104–113

Hollett MD, Jorgensen MJ, Jeffrey RB (1995) Quantitative evaluation of pancreatic enhancement during dual-phase helical CT. Radiology 195:359–361

Hommeyer SC, Freeny PC, Crabo LG (1995) Carcinoma of the head of the pancreas: evaluation of the pancreaticoduodenal veins with dynamic CT – potential for improved accuracy in staging. Radiology 196:233–238

Hough TJ, Raptopoulos V, Siewert B, Matthews JB (1999) Teardrop SMV: CT sign for unresectable carcinoma of the pancreas. AJR Am J Roentgenol (in press)

Johnson PT, Heath DG, Bliss DF, Cabral B, Fisman EK (1996) Three-dimensional CT: real-time interactive volume rendering. AJR Am J Roentgenol 167:581–583

Karasawa E, Goldberg HI, Moss AA, Federle MP, et al (1983) CT pancreatogram in carcinoma of the pancreas and chronic pancreatitis. Radiology 148:489–493

Keogan MT, McDermott VG, Paulson EK, et al (1997) Pancreatic malignancy: effect of dual-phase helical CT in tumor detection and vascular opacification. Radiology 205:513–518

Loyer EM, David CL, Dubrow RA, Evans DB, Charnsagavej C (1996) Vascular involvement in pancreatic adenocarcinoma: reassessment by thin-section CT. Abdom Imaging 21:202–206

Lu DSK, Vedantham S, Krasny RM, Kadell B, Berger WL, Reber HA (1996) Two-phase helical CT for pancreatic tumors: pancreatic versus hepatic phase enhancement of tumor, pancreas, and vascular structures. Radiology 199:697–701

Megibow AJ, Zhou XH, Rotterdam H, et al (1995) Pancreatic adenocarcinoma: CT versus MR imaging in the evaluation of resectability – report of the Radiology Diagnostic Oncology Group. Radiology 195:327–332

Moody AR, Poon PY (1992) Gastroepiploic veins: CT appearance in pancreatic disease. AJR Am J Roentgenol 158:779–783

Mori H, Miyake H, Aikawa H, et al (1991) Dilated posterior superior pancreatico-duodenal vein: recognition with CT and clinical significance in patients with pancreatico-biliary carcinomas. Radiology 181:793–800

Mori H, McGrath FP, Malone DE, Stevenson GW (1992) The gastrocolic trunk and its tributaries: CT evaluation. Radiology 182:871–877

Müller MF, Meyenberger C, Bertschinger P, Schaer R, Marincek B (1994) Pancreatic tumors: Evaluation with endoscopic US, CT, and MR imaging. Radiology 190:745–751

Napel S, Marks MP, Rubin GD, et al (1992) CT angiography with spiral CT and maximum intensity projection. Radiology 185:607–610

Prassopoulos P, Raptopoulos V, Chuttani R, McKee JD, McNicholas MMJ, Sheiman RG (1998) Development of virtual cholangiopancreatoscopy. Radiology 209:570–574

Raptopoulos V, Rosen MP, Kent KC, Kuestner LM, Sheiman RG, Pearlman JD (1996) Sequential helical CT angiography of aortoiliac disease. AJR Am J Roentgenol 166:1347–1354

Raptopoulos V, Steer ML, Sheiman RG, Vrachliotis TG, et al (1997) The use of helical CT and CT angiography to predict vascular involvement from pancreatic cancer: correlation with findings at surgery. AJR Am J Roentgenol 168:971–977

Raptopoulos V, Prassopoulos P, Chattani R, McNicholas MMJ, McKee JD, Kressel HY (1998) Multiplanar CT pancreatography and distal cholangiography with minimum intensity projections. Radiology 207:317–324

Rosch T, Braig C, Gain T, et al (1992) Staging of pancreatic and ampullary carcinoma by endoscopic ultrasonography: comparison with conventional sonography, computed tomography and angiography. Gastroenterology 102:188–199

Rubin DG, Dake MD, Napel SA, McDonnell CH, Jeffrey RB Jr (1993) Three-dimensional spiral CT angiography of the abdomen: initial clinical experience. Radiology 186:147–152

Sheiman RG, Raptopoulos V. (1996) Delayed intravenous contrast medium washout from the small bowel in patients with pancreatic carcinoma and splanchnic venous invasion. J Comput Assist Tomogr 20:924–929

Stanley JR, Semelka RC (1998) Pancreas. In: Lee JKT, Sagel SS, Stanley RJ, Heiken JP (eds) Computed body tomography with MRI correlation, 3rd edn. Lippincott-Raven, Philadelphia, 873–959

Stehling MK, Lawrence JA, Weintraub JL, Raptopoulos V (1994) CT angiography: expanded clinical applications. AJR Am J Roentgenol 163:947–955

Thompson SE, Raptopoulos V, Sheiman RG, McNicholas MMJ, Prassopoulos P (1999) Milk as a low attenuation oral contrast agent for abdominal helical CT. Radiology (in press)

Tublin ME, Tessler FN, Cheng SL, Peters TL, McGovern PC (1999) Effect of injection rate of contrast medium on pancreatic and hepatic helical CT. Radiology 210:97–101

Vadentham S, Lu DSK, Reber HA, Kadell B (1998) Small peripancreatic veins: improved assessment in pancreatic cancer patients using thin-section pancreatic phase helical CT. AJR Am J Roentgenol 170:377–383

Warshaw AL, Gu ZY, Wittenberg J, Waltham AC (1990) Preoperative staging and assessment of resectability of pancreatic cancer. Arch Surg 125:230–233

Warshaw AL, Fernandez-del-Castillo C (1992) Pancreatic carcinoma. N Engl J Med 326:455–465

Zeman RK, Davros WJ, Berman P, et al (1994) Three-dimensional models of the abdominal vasculature based on helical CT: usefulness in patients with pancreatic neoplasms. AJR Am J Roentgenol 162:1425–1429

Zeman RK, Berman PM, Silverman PM, et al (1995) Biliary tract: three-dimensional helical CT without cholangiographic contrast material. Radiology 196:865–867

19 CT of Endocrine and Cystic Tumors of the Pancreas

D. A. Bluemke, P. Soyer

CONTENTS

19.1   Introduction   215
19.2   CT Scanning Protocol   215
19.3   Pancreatic Mass: Differential Diagnosis   216
19.4   Islet Cell Tumors   216
19.4.1 Insulinoma   217
19.4.2 Gastrinoma   218
19.4.3 Other Functioning Tumors   219
19.5   Cystic Pancreatic Neoplasm   220
19.5.1 Serous Cystadenoma   220
19.5.2 Mucinous Cystic Neoplasm   222
19.5.3 Solid and Papillary Epithelial Neoplasm   224
19.5.4 Simple Pancreatic Cyst   224
19.5.5 Other Cystic Peripancreatic Masses   225
        References   225

19.1
Introduction

Computed tomography (CT) is the dominant imaging modality used for the diagnosis and staging of pancreatic disease. High-quality preoperative radiological evaluation is helpful in selecting patients who are candidates for surgery, and it has reduced the proportion of patients who undergo noncurative surgery for pancreatic tumors (Nordback et al. 1992). Helical CT provides excellent depiction of small vessels, high levels of parenchymal enhancement and lack of respiratory misregistration (Dupuy et al. 1992; Fishman et al. 1992), which is beneficial for the diagnosis of pancreatic tumors. In this discussion, CT features of endocrine and cystic pancreatic tumors and their differential diagnosis will be presented.

D. A. Bluemke, MD, PhD; Department of Radiology, The Johns Hopkins University School of Medicine, 600 North Wolfe Street, MRI 143, Baltimore, MD 21287-6953, USA
P. Soyer, MD, PhD; Department of Abdominal and Vascular Imaging, Hôpital Lariboisière Université, 2, rue Ambroise Paré, F-75475 Paris Cédex 10, France

19.2
CT Scanning Protocol

In the evaluation of pancreatic tumors, three factors should be considered. First, the tumor must be detected and characterized. Since these tumors may be small, this requires narrow collimation. Second, the effect of the tumor on the major vessels adjacent to the tumor must be assessed. This requires iodinated contrast material and bolus contrast administration (125–150 ml, 2–3 ml/s injection). Third, pancreatic tumors tend to metastasize early throughout the abdomen, but also frequently to the liver. Therefore, CT scanning must also provide adequate visualization of the abdomen, and particularly of the liver. Note that many endocrine tumors are hypervascular, and are best visualized during what may be considered the arterial dominant phase of hepatic enhancement.

These requirements are difficult to fulfill with dynamic CT, since a large scanning area, from the diaphragm to the pancreas, is required. Further, narrow collimation around the pancreas and high levels of contrast administration are needed. With helical CT, and particularly dual-phase scanning, an ideal CT scanning protocol can be achieved. Additionally, for islet cell tumors, noncontrast CT images of the pancreas are usually helpful to establish baseline CT attenuation values. Since many different types of scanners now exist, with varying capabilities, the principles of scanning for various types of capabilities are discussed below, in order of preference:

- If dual-phase helical scanning is available, arterial phase scanning at 25–30 s after contrast material administration is performed, using 3–4 mm collimation. Portal phase scanning of the liver is performed beginning at 60–70 s using 5–8 mm collimation. For suspected islet cell tumors, arterial phase scanning of the liver is also desirable.
- If single-phase helical scanning is available for a known or suspected small pancreatic or ampullary mass, 4 mm scanning of the pancreas is performed beginning approximately 30 s after con-

trast material injection. Usually however, complete staging of the liver and pancreas is required: CT scanning with 5–8 mm collimation, pitch of 1–1.5, is thus performed 60–70 s after contrast administration.

– If dynamic CT is available, again, the choice is whether to use small collimation for a small pancreatic mass, or whether to scan the liver and pancreas together. Collimation of 4–5 mm is adequate for a small pancreatic mass; 7–8 mm collimation is useful for the liver plus pancreas. In both cases, dynamic CT scanning must be started sooner after contrast material injection than with helical CT, because the duration of the scan is much longer relative to the injection duration. With dynamic CT, scanning should begin 30–40 s after the start of the contrast material injection.

19.3
Pancreatic Mass: Differential Diagnosis

Primary tumors of the pancreas take their origin from the various cell types of the pancreas. Tumors most commonly arise from epithelial cells of the pancreas; these include duct cells (duct cell adenocarcinoma), exocrine cells (pancreaticoblastoma, acinar cell carcinoma), and endocrine cells (islet cell tumors). Nonepithelial cell tumors include various sarcomas and tumors of the lymphatics and vessels. The solid and papillary epithelial cell tumor of the pancreas is of uncertain origin.

The differential diagnosis for pancreatic masses can be divided into solid and cystic masses and is presented in Table 19.1.

Table 1. Pancreatic mass: differential diagnosis (*MFH* malignant fibrous histiocytoma)

Solid pancreatic mass	Cystic pancreatic mass
Duct cell adeno-carcinoma	Mucinous cystic tumor
Endocrine tumors (islet cell tumors)	Serous cystadenoma
Nonepithelial MFH Sarcoma Lymphangioma	Solid and cystic papillary tumor
Secondary neoplasms Metastatic disease Lymphoma	Lymphangioma
Congenital: pancreas divisum	Pancreatic pseudocyst
Inflammatory: pancreatitis, fibrosis	Necrotic peripancreatic lymphadenopathy

19.4
Islet Cell Tumors

Islet cell tumors are tumors of the endocrine pancreas. These tumors are relatively rare, with an incidence of 0.4% per 100,000 population (ERIKSSON et al. 1990). Islet cell tumors arise from the neural crest cells, sharing biochemical similarities with other tumors of the APUD system (amine precursor uptake and decarboxylation). In general, these tumors have a much better prognosis for the patient than the more common pancreatic ductal carcinoma (ZOLLINGER 1985). Because many of these tumors secrete functioning hormones, they are symptomatic when small and are thus detected at an early stage.

Clinical presentation of patients depends on whether the islet cell tumor is functional or nonfunctional. Functional tumors elaborate excess hormones, resulting in particular clinical syndromes. An example of excess hormone production from an islet cell tumor is hypersecretion of gastrin in Zollinger-Ellison syndrome (ZOLLINGER and ELLISON 1955). Functional tumors may be benign or malignant; malignancy may be difficult to determine histologically, but is indicated by local invasion of adjacent structures as well as distant metastases. Patients with nonfunctional tumors have nonspecific clinical symptoms, such as dyspepsia or chronic abdominal pain (ERIKSSON et al. 1990). Nonfunctioning tumors tend to be large, bulky masses at the time of diagnosis, and metastases are more common. These tumors may also be discovered incidentally on CT examination of the abdomen. In general, both functioning and nonfunctioning islet cell tumors are slow growing, and the average overall survival from the time of diagnosis is 8.7 years. Average survival for patients with malignant tumors is 6.7 years; patients with benign tumors have a 10-year survival of 80% (ERIKSSON et al. 1990).

Islet cell tumors are commonly associated with multiple endocrine neoplasia (MEN). In these patients, multiple endocrine adenoma is an autosomal dominant condition. Patients have multiple tumors involving cells originating from the APUD system. MEN type I, or Wermer syndrome, is associated with parathyroid adenoma or hyperplasia in 90% of cases, and 80% have pancreatic islet cell tumors, usually gastrinomas. The pituitary gland is also involved, as are the adrenal cortex (40% of patients) and the thyroid (20%). Insulinoma or VIPoma is less commonly associated than gastrinoma. Islet cell tumors in MEN I have a less aggressive course than sporadically occurring tumors. Islet cell tumors in these patients also develop at an earlier age, and tend to be multiple and smaller. Associations between islet cell tumors and MEN type I are summarized in Table 19.2.

Table 2. Multiple endocrine neoplasia I

Organ	Abnormality
Parathyroid	Parathyroid adenoma or hyperplasia (90%)
Pancreas	Islet cell tumor (80%) Gastrinoma Insulinoma VIPoma
Pituitary gland	Adenoma (40%)
Thyroid gland	Thyroid tumor (20%)
Adrenal gland	Adrenal cortical tumors

Islet cell tumors may also be seen in association with Von Hippel-Lindau (VHL) disease. VHL is an inherited neurocutaneous dysplasia complex. Primary diagnostic criteria include more than one central nervous system (CNS) hemangioblastoma, one CNS hemangioblastoma plus one or more visceral components, or family history plus CNS hemangioblastoma. Retinal angioma is the earliest manifestation of the disease, and may be multiple in more than two-thirds of cases. Approximately 17% of patients with VHL have islet cell tumors (BINKOVITZ et al. 1990). Adrenal pheochromocytoma occurs in 10–17%; multiple simple cysts involve the pancreas, kidneys, liver, spleen or other organs. The second most common cause of death in this condition is related to renal cell carcinoma (30–50% of cases). VHL is also associated with serous cystadenoma of the pancreas.

Islet cell tumors are "hypervascular" tumors; with CT, the primary tumor is typically hyperattenuating relative to the rest of the pancreas (Fig. 19.1). Overall, dynamic CT demonstrates approximately 80% sensitivity for detection of islet cell tumors and appears to identify all malignant tumors (STARK et al. 1984). In the liver, the tumor is best detected during the arterial phase of hepatic enhancement. If dynamic CT only is available, noncontrast CT of the liver may be useful prior to contrast injection, since slow scanning results in equal tumor and liver enhancement, so tumors are isoattenuating to liver and not otherwise detected. PATTEN et al. (1993), however, found that the addition of noncontrast scans demonstrated only 1 additional neoplasm among 34 patients with hypervascular liver lesions.

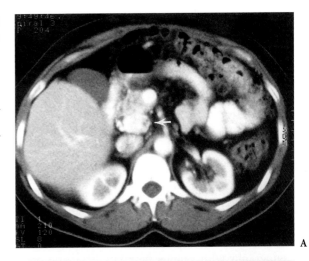

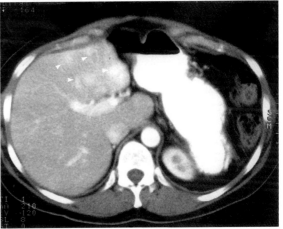

Fig. 19.1A, B. Islet cell neoplasm with hepatic metastasis. **A** Contrast-enhanced CT scan shows enhancing mass in the pancreatic head (*arrow*). **B** Images of the liver show multiple hypervascular metastases (*arrowheads*). The left lobe of the liver is absent owing to prior surgical resection

19.4.1
Insulinoma

Insulinoma is the most common islet cell tumor. These tumors occur in the 4th to 6th decade, with a male-to-female ratio of 2–3. Although the tumors may be multiple in 5–10% of cases, the tumor is most commonly (80–90%) a single benign adenoma. Approximately 5–10% of cases are malignant, with a similar number due to islet cell hyperplasia rather than tumor. The tumor is associated with multiple endocrine neoplasia (MEN) type I; patients with this condition usually have multiple lesions. Patients with insulinomas usually present when the tumors are small, usually less than 1.5 cm in size. Fasting glucose levels are less than <50 mg/dl, with hypoglycemia relieved by intravenous dextrose.

Insulinoma can occur in any part of the pancreas. Approximately 2–5% of tumors are ectopic and 10% are multiple. The majority of tumors (75%) cause symptoms of hypoglycemia while they are still less than 1.5 cm in size. The tumor is usually single, although 5–10% may be multiple or due to diffuse hyperplasia of islet cells. The tumors are evenly distributed throughout the body and tail of the pancreas.

CT detection of lesions involves identification of a hyperattenuating mass during bolus infusion of iodinated contrast medium (GUNTHER et al. 1983; STARK et al. 1984; Fig. 19.1). Small lesions are difficult to detect, and intraoperative ultrasound and/or angiography with venous sampling have also been used with a good rate of success for lesion localization (KRUDY et al. 1984). CT detection of lesions less than 1 cm is possible (STARK et al. 1984), although this demands rapid bolus infusion of contrast agent together with rapid CT scanning (SEMELKA et al. 1993).

Helical CT with 3–4 mm collimation and bolus injection of iodinated contrast medium appears to be more sensitive than nonhelical techniques for detection of small tumors (CHUNG et al. 1997; VAN HOE et al. 1995). Tumor conspicuity is improved by imaging during the arterial phase of contrast enhancement, although multi-phase helical technique may be helpful in some cases for tumor identification (VAN HOE et al. 1995). Delayed images (180 s after contrast administration) have not been shown to increase tumor detection (CHUNG et al. 1997; KOITO et al. 1997).

Dual-phase helical CT has recently been applied to insulinoma and islet cell tumor detection (KING et al. 1998; STAFFORD-JOHNSON et al. 1998). KING et al. demonstrated detection of six of seven small insulinomas of the pancreas, ranging in size from 6 to 18 mm, located in the incinate process (2), head (1), neck (2) and body (1) of the pancreas. All six tumors were identified in the arterial phase of enhancement, while only four were detected also in the arteriovenous phase. Results published by STAFFORD-JOHNSON et al. were similar, with demonstration tumor–normal pancreas attenuation difference of 32 HU in the arterial phase, but only 19 HU in the portal venous phase of enhancement (STAFFORD-JOHNSON et al. 1998).

19.4.2
Gastrinoma

Gastrinoma is the second most common islet cell tumor. These tumors are an exception to the generalization that most islet cell tumors are benign in nature, since 60% of gastrinomas are malignant and have metastasized by the time of diagnosis. The tumor causes Zollinger-Ellison syndrome (ZOLLINGER and ELLISON 1955), with pre- and postbulbar ulcers resulting from elevated gastrin levels and hypersecretion of gastric acid and malabsorption. Gastrinomas are often found in patients with MEN I syndrome; 20–40% of patients with Zollinger-Ellison syndrome have MEN I (ZOLLINGER 1985). In 50% of cases the site is in the pancreatic head or tail; the average size is 3–4 cm (Fig. 19.2). The tumor may be multiple and present with diffuse involvement of the pancreas.

Patients with gastrinoma present with peptic ulcer disease, but less than 1% of patients with peptic ulcer disease have gastrinoma. Associations of gastrinoma include atypical ulcers distal to the ampulla of Vater, hypersecretion and thickening of gastric folds in the fundus and gastric ulcers. Multiple ulcers are an additional feature that should suggest gastrinoma as a potential etiology for peptic ulcer disease.

CT imaging with helical or dynamic CT represents the primary diagnostic imaging method for these tumors. Tumors greater than 2 cm in size are readily localized with CT, although tumors less than 1 cm in diameter may not be detected. Large tumors may contain areas of calcification and central necro-

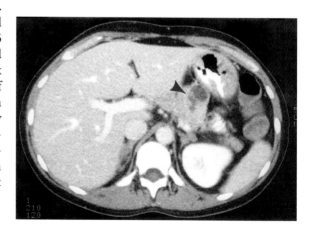

Fig. 19.2. Gastrinoma of the body and tail of the pancreas. Spiral CT scan shows a low attenuation mass with an internal septation (*arrowhead*). Moderate thickening of the stomach is also present

sis. Metastatic disease involves the liver, mesentery and lymph nodes.

Tumor metastases to the liver reflect the high degree of vascularity of the primary tumor and are best detected during the arterial phase of hepatic enhancement. If arterial phase scanning of the liver is not available, noncontrast images of the liver are recommended, since hypervascular tumors may become isoattenuating to the liver during the portal phase of hepatic enhancement (BONALDI et al. 1995; BRESSLER et al. 1987; PATTEN et al. 1993). Dual-phase helical CT likely obviates the need for noncontrast images of the liver.

19.4.3
Other Functioning Tumors

Glucagonoma is a rare islet cell tumor. It is malignant in 80% of cases, and is detected as a large mass 5–6 cm across (Fig. 19.3). Patients present with necrolytic migratory erythema affecting the buttocks, perineal area and thighs, as well as diabetes and weight loss. Diabetes mellitus, if present, is mild. Thromboembolism is reported in up to one third of cases.

VIPoma (vasoactive intestinal peptide) presents as WDHA syndrome (profuse watery diarrhea, hypokalemia and acidosis) (Fig. 19.4). The tumor size is 5–10 cm across when detected, and 50% of lesions are malignant. WDHA syndrome has been found associated with ganglioneuromas, ganglioblastomas and adrenal tumors, although it is most frequently associated with VIPoma of the pancreas. They are more frequently located in the body or tail of the pancreas.

Somatostatinoma is also a rare islet cell tumor. This tumor is a slow-growing mass, usually located in the pancreatic head, averaging 4 cm in size (ROBERTS et al. 1984). Somatostatin is a potent hormone inhibitor. This substance suppresses insulin, gastrin and pancreatic secretions. Patients present with diabetes, gallstones, weight loss, and low gastric acid output.

Nonfunctioning Islet Cell Tumors. These tumors are unusual because of their large size at presentation, usually 5–10 cm or more, with 30% of tumors reported to be larger than 10 cm (EELKEMA et al. 1984; Fig. 19.5). Nonfunctioning islet cell tumors do not result in clinical or laboratory manifestations of endocrinopathy. Nonfunctioning islet cell tumors are the third most common type of islet cell tumor fol-

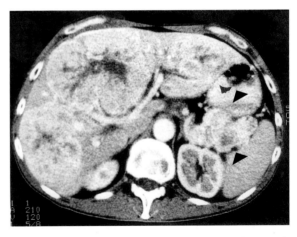

Fig. 19.3. Malignant glucagonoma. Spiral CT scan shows multiple enhancing masses throughout the liver. A large mass with similar enhancement characteristics is present in the pancreatic tail (*arrowheads*). Surgical biopsy revealed glucagonoma

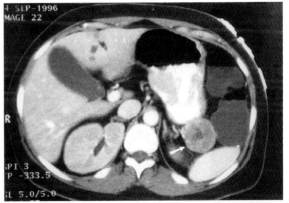

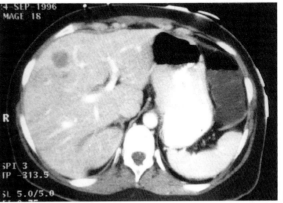

Fig. 19.4. A VIPoma of the pancreatic tail. An enhancing mass is present in the pancreatic tail. Although the appearance is nonspecific, this patient presented with a typical constellation of symptoms, including watery diarrhea, acidosis and hypokalemia. **B** A metastatic lesion was present in the liver. The mass is hypoattenuating on the portal phase image of the liver

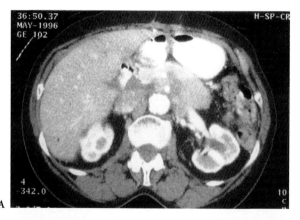

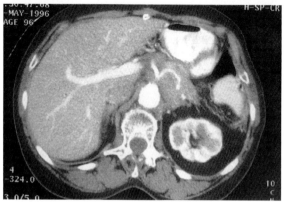

Fig. 19.5A, B. Nonfunctioning islet cell tumor. A retroperitoneal mass is seen extending upward from the pancreas (A) to encase the celiac axis (B)

lowing insulinoma and gastrinoma. One series at the Mayo Clinic indicated that nonfunctioning islet cell tumors were quite frequent, representing 50% of all islet cell tumors (THOMPSON et al. 1988). Patients may have a history of chronic abdominal pain or gastrointestinal bleeding. Symptoms result from a mass effect of the tumor on adjacent organs, and intestinal obstruction may result. The prognosis for patients with this tumor is the worst of the islet cell tumors, which is related to the large size at initial diagnosis.

CT features are those of a large, homogeneously enhancing mass centered in the retroperitoneum (EELKEMA et al. 1984; STAFFORD-JOHNSON et al. 1998). Approximately 20% of tumors will demonstrate areas of calcification, and low attenuation areas of necrosis may be seen. Approximately half of the patients will have metastatic disease to the liver at the time of diagnosis, with one third of patients demonstrating regional lymphadenopathy. Owing to the tumor size, both the pancreatic duct and the bile duct may be dilated. CT features of this mass are dis-

tinct, however, from those of duct adenocarcinoma of the pancreas (FUGAZZOLA et al. 1990; STAFFORD-JOHNSON et al. 1998).

Nonfunctioning islet cell tumors are much larger at initial presentation than duct adenocarcinomas. Additional features that suggest nonfunctioning islet cell tumor rather than adenocarcinoma are the lack of celiac and superior mesenteric arterial encasement and the presence of calcification.

19.5
Cystic Pancreatic Neoplasm

Cystic neoplasms of the pancreas account for 10–15% of pancreatic cysts (ZIRINSKY et al. 1984). They are of particular interest because they frequently occur in particular patient subgroups and differentiation among subtypes by CT directly affects patient management. Approximately 60–80% of subtypes of cystic neoplasms can be correctly categorized by CT (RHODES et al. 1993).

19.5.1
Serous Cystadenoma

This tumor has also been termed "microcystic adenoma." More than 80% are found in patients older than 60 years. Serous cystadenoma is more common in women than in men, with a female-to-male ratio reported as 3:2–9:2. Symptoms at presentation include chronic abdominal pain, gastrointestinal bleeding, weight loss and/or palpable abdominal mass of months' to years' duration (LOSER et al. 1990). CA 19-9, a serum marker associated with pancreatic malignancy, has been reported to be normal in patients with serous cystadenoma (LOSER et al. 1990). The prognosis is excellent, and the tumor can be aggressively and successfully treated by surgery. Accurate noninvasive imaging diagnosis is helpful and has a direct bearing on patient management, since high risk or elderly patients can be managed conservatively without surgery. Serous cystadenoma is a benign tumor with no malignant potential (BUCK and HAYES 1990; FRIEDMAN et al. 1983; ITAI et al. 1988).

At diagnosis, these tumors are typically 5–10 cm or more in size. They are composed of innumerable small cysts ranging in size from 1 mm to 2 cm, with an externally lobulated contour of the tumor mass (Fig. 19.6). High glycogen content in the small cysts

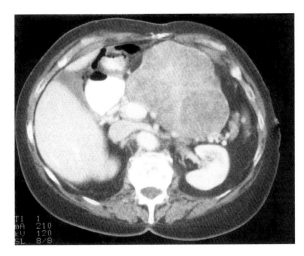

Fig. 19.6. Serous cystadenoma in an 82-year-old woman. Contrast-enhanced CT shows a large heterogeneously enhancing mass with a Swiss-cheese appearance centered on the pancreas. The peripheral margins of the mass are lobulated

is characteristic (COMPAGNO and OERTEL 1978a,b). The small cysts are separated by a thin connective tissue network that is evenly lined with cuboidal or flattened epithelial cells (FRIEDMAN et al. 1983; MINAMI et al. 1989). The cytoplasm of these lining cells frequently contains glycogen. A prominent central area of scarring has been described as usually present, and may calcify (Fig. 19.7; FRIEDMAN et al. 1983), although in one series of 16 patients only 2 serous cystadenomas showed central scarring (FRIEDMAN et al. 1983). Calcifications are typically central, and up to one third are visible on plain films of the abdomen. Central calcification is seen more frequently in serous cystadenoma than in any other pancreatic tumor (Fig. 19.8). Accordingly, the CT

appearance is that of a large hypodense mass; the appearance of the mass is reminiscent of a Swiss cheese or a honeycomb following contrast administration. SOYER et al. (1994) have evaluated the contrast-enhanced appearance of cystic pancreatic tumors. Intravenous contrast administration helped identify solid excrescences, and thick septations of cystic tumors that excluded the diagnosis of serous cystadenoma, being more characteristic of mucinous pancreatic tumors. Thirty-eight percent of serous cystadenomas have been described as having calcification on CT (JOHNSON et al. 1988). The external lobulation of the tumor is also well-depicted on CT.

In some cases, the many small cysts within this tumor, when it is 2–3 mm in size, may be difficult to visualize separately, and the tumor may appear as an heterogeneously enhancing solid mass. Nevertheless, upon histological examination, the innumerable small cysts readily identify the nature of this tumor. Conversely, five cases of a "macrocystic" variant of this serous tumor have been described in the pathological literature (LEWANDROWSKI et al. 1992; Fig. 19.9). The appearance of the lesion on CT is similar to that of pseudocyst or mucinous cystic neoplasm, although pathological examination revealed this tumor as a variant of serous cystadenoma, i.e., a tumor with large, rather than small cystic spaces (GOUHIRI et al., to be published; LEWANDROWSKI et al. 1992). Thickening of the wall suggested a solid excrescence in one case, but pathologically this represented hemorrhagic changes. Thus, although the majority of serous cystadenomas appear to have a typical CT appearance, the potential exists for misdiagnosis of some serous tumors due to overlap in CT appearance with mucinous cystic neoplasms.

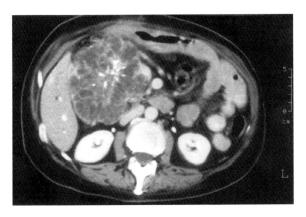

Fig. 19.7. Serous cystadenoma. Contrast-enhanced CT scan of a 61-year-old woman with chronic abdominal pain. A large lobulated cystic mass with many small cystic spaces is demonstrated in the pancreas. Central calcifications are present

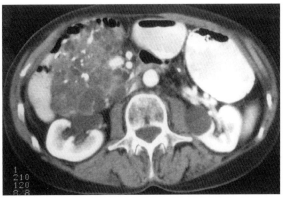

Fig. 19.8. Serous cystadenoma in a 61-year-old woman who presented with chronic abdominal pain. The mass shows innumerable small cysts and central calcifications

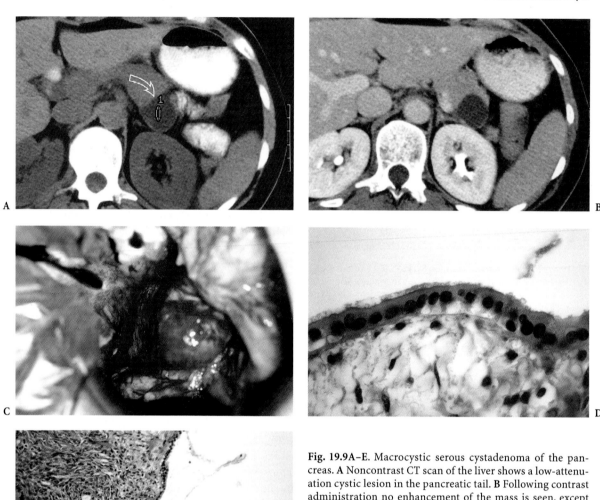

Fig. 19.9A–E. Macrocystic serous cystadenoma of the pancreas. **A** Noncontrast CT scan of the liver shows a low-attenuation cystic lesion in the pancreatic tail. **B** Following contrast administration no enhancement of the mass is seen, except for the thin cyst wall. **C** Operative view of the mass shows a well-defined, smooth-walled lesion in the pancreatic tail. **D** Microscopic view of the cyst-lining epithelium shows cuboidal epithelial cells with central nuclei. No mucin secreting cells were identified. +250 **E** Microscopic view shows a tiny cyst (*arrow*) measuring 2 mm in diameter located in the wall of the largest cyst. The small cyst is lined with epithelium similar to the large cyst. +52.5 (Reprinted from GOUHIRI et al., to be published)

19.5.2
Mucinous Cystic Neoplasm

Subtypes of mucinous cystic neoplasm are indistinguishable on CT, and include mucinous cystadenoma and cystadenocarcinoma (SOYER et al. 1994). These tumors are characterized by large cystic spaces filled with mucin of water attenuation on CT (Fig. 19.10). The clinical presentation is that of abdominal pain, with a palpable mass in the right upper quadrant (ERESUE et al. 1985). The majority of tumors are found in women (6:1 female-to-male ra-

tio), typically in the 40- to 60-year-old age range. CA 19–9 levels may be elevated (LOSER et al. 1990). Cystadenoma and cystadenocarcinoma are not readily distinguished by cytologic evaluation of fine-needle aspiration biopsy sampling, since undersampling of portions of the tumor containing carcinoma is likely (RHODES et al. 1993). Thus, all tumors are treated as potentially malignant. If distant metastases are not present, the possibility for cure exists if the tumor can be treated by complete local resection. In the case of incomplete resection, recurrence and/or malignant behavior appears inevitable. The 5-year survival for patients with mucinous cystic neoplasm is much better than that for pancreatic adenocarcinoma, and may be up to 50% (Friedman and Edmonds 1989; Friedman et al. 1983).

Mucinous adenocarcinomas tend to be large, many over 10 cm in size (Fig. 19.11). These typically occur in women (9 times as common as in men) aged 40–60 years. The tumors are treated surgically, but recurrence and malignant behavior are common, although survival is much better than for pancreatic ductal adenocarcinoma. Pathologically, the tumor has a smooth external surface and is composed of unilocular or multilocular large (>5 cm) cystic spaces. The cyst wall is relatively thin (1–2 mm) and shows evidence of calcification in 15–20% of cases. Within the large cystic spaces, smaller cysts measuring 1–4 cm may be present, as may solid papillary excrescences (Compagno and Oertel 1978a,b). The cells lining the cavity are mucin-producing columnar cells. These cells may be arranged in a single orderly layer, or may be stratified, forming papillae. Areas of carcinomatous change may be quite focal and small; thus, the tumor cannot be sufficiently sampled to confidently diagnose cystadenoma and exclude carcinoma.

The CT appearance, in contrast to serous cystadenoma, is that of large, thick-walled near water density cystic components 1–5 cm in size (Itai et al. 1982). The majority of tumors (85%) are located in the pancreatic tail, or in the body and tail (Figs. 19.11, 19.12). The external contour is ovoid and

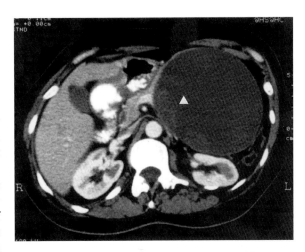

Fig. 19.11. Mucinous cystadenoma in a 49-year-old woman. Contrast-enhanced CT shows a large mass, centered on the pancreatic tail, with low attenuation but peripheral areas of increased density (*arrowhead*). The wall is well defined. Pathological examination showed no evidence of malignancy

smooth (Fig. 19.13). The cyst walls (1 mm to 2 cm) may contain areas of nodularity. Following intravenous contrast administration, both the cyst walls and any solid excrescences or papillary portions of the tumor will enhance (Soyer et al. 1994). The cysts contain mucin, and metastatic disease to the liver appears similar to simple liver cysts unless nodularity or septa are present. Central calcifications may also be present, but these are less common than with serous cystadenoma.

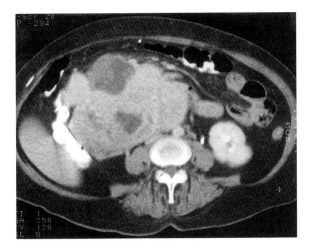

Fig. 19.10. Mucinous cystadenocarcinoma in a 71-year-old woman with a 17-cm mass in the mid-abdomen. Although large portions of the mass appear solid, several large cystic components are present

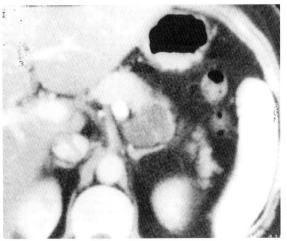

Fig. 19.12. Mucinous cystadenoma. Contrast-enhanced CT shows a well-circumscribed cystic mass in the distal pancreas. A small enhancing septation is present

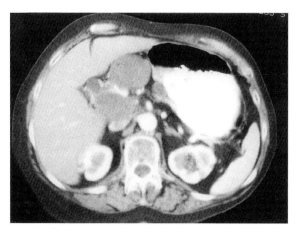

Fig. 19.13. Mucinous cystic neoplasm. Contrast-enhanced CT demonstrates a multilocular cystic mass extending from the pancreas toward the porta hepatis. The biliary duct is not dilated. Surgery revealed a low-grade malignant mucinous cystic neoplasm

19.5.3
Solid and Papillary Epithelial Neoplasm

This tumor is uncommon, but typically occurs in black females aged 10–50 years. The tumor is a low-grade malignancy that is curable by resection. Symptoms consists of chronic abdominal pain. The CT appearance is that of a large (10 cm) mass of intermediate attenuation that contains low-density areas and thick cyst walls that enhance with contrast (Fig. 19.14).

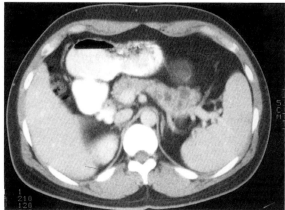

Fig. 19.15. Contrast-enhanced CT of the pancreas in a 29-year-old man with Von Hippel-Lindau disease shows multiple small cysts in the body and tail of the pancreas

19.5.4
Simple Pancreatic Cyst

Congenital simple cysts of the pancreas are rare, but may be solitary or multiple. Multiple pancreatic cysts are associated with Von Hippel-Lindau disease (Fig. 19.15). In these cases, pancreatic cysts are found in 72% of cases at autopsy, but much less frequently by CT. Pancreatic cystic disease is also associated with polycystic disease of the kidneys (Fig. 19.16; THOMSEN et al. 1997). This condition results

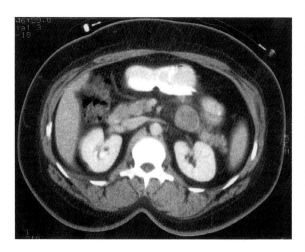

Fig. 19.14. Solid and papillary epithelial neoplasm in a 35-year-old woman. Contrast-enhanced CT scan shows nonspecific appearance of a mass located in the distal pancreas. At surgery, the tumor appeared well-demarcated and was gray white and red. More commonly, these tumors appear as large (10 cm) abdominal masses

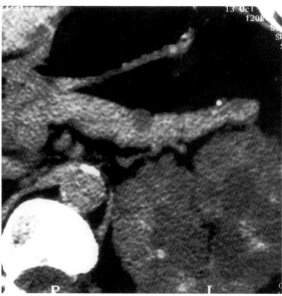

Fig. 19.16. Autosomal dominant polycystic renal disease in a 63-year-old man. Noncontrast CT scan shows a simple cyst in the pancreatic body. Hyperdense areas in the kidney are due to hemorrhagic cysts

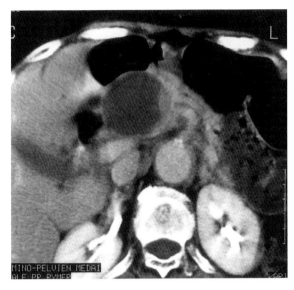

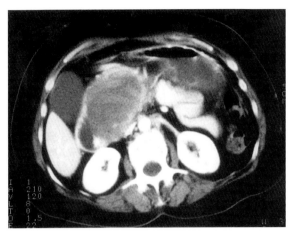

Fig. 19.17. Cystic metastasis in a 76-year-old white woman with a history of endometrial adenocarcinoma. Contrast-enhanced CT scan shows a cystic tumor of the pancreas suggestive of mucinous cystic neoplasm. Biopsy revealed metastatic disease

Fig. 19.18. Retroperitoneal leiomyosarcoma. Contrast-enhanced CT scan of the abdomen shows a heterogeneous mass with internal near-water attenuation central areas and peripheral solid, thick walls. The size and location of the mass caused biliary as well as pancreatic duct dilatation (not shown), which would be unusual for a primary pancreatic cystic neoplasm

in renal cyst formation in the kidneys in more than 80% of patients by the third decade of life. In 25–50% of patients associated cysts are detected in the liver by CT, although a much higher percentage of patients have pathologically identified hepatic cysts. Approximately 10% of patients have multiple pancreatic cysts. Multiple other organs, including the spleen, thyroid, ovaries, testis, and seminal vesicles may show cystic changes. Berry aneurysms of the cerebral arteries are present in approximately 10% of patients.

19.5.5
Other Cystic Peripancreatic Masses

Retroperitoneal masses near the pancreas may simulate a primary pancreatic neoplasm (Fig. 19.17). Large masses frequently show internal areas of degeneration with cystic change, potentially simulating a primary pancreatic neoplasm (Fig. 19.18). Low or water attenuation lymph nodes, in particular, associated with tuberculosis or mucinous neoplasms, may also simulate primary pancreatic neoplasms.

References

Binkovitz LA, Johnson CD, Stephens DH (1990) Islet cell tumors in Von Hippel-Lindau disease: increased prevalence and relationship to the multiple endocrine neoplasias. AJR Am J Roentgenol 155:501–505

Bonaldi VM, Bret PM, Reinhold C, Atri M (1995) Helical CT of the liver: value of an early hepatic arterial phase. Radiology 197:357–33

Bressler EL, Alpern MB, Glazer GM, Francis IR, Ensminger WD (1987) Hypervascular hepatic metastasis. Radiology 162:49–51

Buck JL, Hayes WS (1990) From the archives of the AFIP. Microcystic adenoma of the pancreas. Radiographics 10:313–322

Chung MJ, Choi BI, Han JK, Chung JW, Han MC, Bae SH (1997) Functioning islet cell tumor of the pancreas. Localization with dynamic spiral CT. Acta Radiol 38:135–138

Compagno J, Oertel JE (1978a) Microcystic adenomas of the pancreas (glycogen-rich cystadenomas): a clinicopathologic study of 34 cases. Am J Clin Pathol 69:289–298

Compagno J, Oertel JE (1978b) Mucinous cystic neoplasms of the pancreas with overt and latent malignancy (cystadenocarcinoma and cystadenoma). A clinicopathologic study of 41 cases. Am J Clin Pathol 69:573–580

Dupuy DE, Costello P, Ecker CP (1992) Spiral CT of the pancreas. Radiology 183:815–818

Eelkema EA, Stephens DH, Ward EM, Sheedy PF (1984) CT features of nonfunctioning islet cell carcinoma. AJR Am J Roentgenol 143:943–948

Eresue J, Drouillard J, Philippe JC, Guibert JL, Roux P, Tavernier J (1985) CT and US findings in pancreatic ductal tumours. A report of an unusual case and review of the literature. Eur J Radiol 5:40–42

Eriksson B, Arnberg H, Lindgren PG et al (1990) Neuroendocrine pancreatic tumours: clinical presentation, biochemical and histopathological findings in 84 patients. J Intern Med 228:103–113

Fishman EK, Wyatt SH, Ney DR, Kuhlman JE, Siegelman SS (1992) Spiral CT of the pancreas with multiplanar display. AJR Am J Roentgenol 159:1209–1215

Friedman AC, Edmonds PR (1989) Rare pancreatic malignancies. Radiol Clin North Am 27:177–190

Friedman AC, Lichtenstein JE, Dachman AH (1983) Cystic neoplasms of the pancreas. Radiological-pathological correlation. Radiology 149:45–50

Fugazzola C, Procacci C, Bergamo Andreis IA et al (1990) The contribution of ultrasonography and computed tomography in the diagnosis of nonfunctioning islet cell tumors of the pancreas. Gastrointest Radiol 15:139–144

Gouhiri M, Soyer P, Barbagelatta M, Rymer R (1998) Macrocystic serous cystadenoma of the pancreas: CT and endosonographic features. Abdom Imaging (to be published)

Gunther RW, Klose KJ, Ruckert K et al (1983) Islet-cell tumors: detection of small lesions with computed tomography and ultrasound. Radiology 148:485–488

Itai Y, Moss AA, Ohtomo K (1982) Computed tomography of cystadenoma and cystadenocarcinoma of the pancreas. Radiology 145:419–425

Itai Y, Ohhashi K, Furui S et al (1988) Microcystic adenoma of the pancreas: spectrum of computed tomographic findings. J Comput Assist Tomogr 12:797–803

Johnson CD, Stephens DH, Charboneau JW, Carpenter HA, Welch TJ (1988) Cystic pancreatic tumors: CT and sonographic assessment. AJR Am J Roentgenol 151:1133–1138

King AD, Ko GT, Yeung VT, Chow CC, Griffith J, Cockram CS (1998) Dual phase spiral CT in the detection of small insulinomas of the pancreas. Br J Radiol 71:20–23

Koito K, Namieno T, Nagakawa T, Morita K (1997) Delayed enhancement of islet cell carcinoma on dynamic computed tomography: a sign of its malignancy. Abdom Imaging 22:304–306

Krudy AG, Doppman JL, Jensen RT et al (1984) Localization of islet cell tumors by dynamic CT: comparison with plain CT, arteriography, sonography, and venous sampling. AJR Am J Roentgenol 143:585–589

Lewandrowski K, Warshaw A, Compton C (1992) Macrocystic serous cystadenoma of the pancreas: a morphologic variant differing from microcystic adenoma. Hum Pathol 23:871–875

Loser C, Folsch UR, Peiper HJ, Schuster R, Creutzfeldt W (1990) Cystic neoplasms of the pancreas: a clinical and radiological study of eight cases. Klin Wochenschr 68:780–787

Minami M, Itai Y, Ohtomo K, Yoshida H, Yoshikawa K, Iio M (1989) Cystic neoplasms of the pancreas: comparison of MR imaging with CT. Radiology 171:53–56

Nordback IH, Hruban RH, Boitnott JK, Pitt HA, Cameron JL (1992) Carcinoma of the body and tail of the pancreas. Am J Surg 164:26–31

Patten RM, Byun JY, Freeny PC (1993) CT of hypervascular hepatic tumors: are unenhanced scans necessary for diagnosis? AJR Am J Roentgenol 161:979–984

Rhodes I, Humar A, Lum PA, Yazdi HM, Tao HH, Barron PT (1993) Computed tomographic and cytologic assessment of cystic pancreatic neoplasms: a difficult preoperative diagnosis. Can Assoc Radiol J 44:359–363

Roberts L Jr, Dunnick NR, Foster WL Jr et al (1984) Somatostatinoma of the endocrine pancreas: CT findings. J Comput Assist Tomogr 8:1015–1018

Semelka RC, Cumming MJ, Shoenut JP et al (1993) Islet cell tumors: comparison of dynamic contrast-enhanced CT and MR imaging with dynamic gadolinium enhancement and fat suppression. Radiology 186:799–802

Soyer P, Rabenandrasana A, Van Beers B et al (1994) Cystic tumors of the pancreas: dynamic CT studies. J Comput Assist Tomogr 18:420–426

Stafford-Johnson DB, Francis IR, Eckhauser FE, Knol JA, Chang AE (1998) Dual-phase helical CT of nonfunctioning islet cell tumors. J Comput Assist Tomogr 22:335–339

Stark DD, Moss AA, Goldberg HI, Deveney CW (1984) CT of pancreatic islet cell tumors. Radiology 150:491–494

Thompson GB, van Heerden JA, Grant CS et al (1988) Islet cell carcinomas of the pancreas: a twenty-year experience. Surgery 104:1011

Thomsen HS, Levine E, Meilstrup JW et al (1997) Renal cystic diseases. Eur Radiol 7:1267–1275

Van Hoe L, Gryspeerdt S, Marchal G, Baert AL, Mertens L (1995) Helical CT for the preoperative localization of islet cell tumors of the pancreas: value of arterial and parenchymal phase images. AJR Am J Roentgenol 165:1437–1439

Zirinsky K, Abiri M, Baer JW (1984) Computed tomography demonstration of pancreatic microcystic adenoma. Am J Gastroenterol 79:139–142

Zollinger RM (1985) Gastrinoma: factors influencing prognosis. Surgery 97:49–54

Zollinger RM, Ellison EH (1955) Primary peptic ulcerations of the jejunum associated with islet cell tumors of the pancreas. Ann Surg 142:709

20 Helical CT of Acute and Chronic Pancreatitis

P.C. FREENY

CONTENTS

20.1 Introduction 227
20.2 Techniques of Helical CT of the Pancreas 2227
20.3 Acute Pancreatitis 229
20.3.1 Indications for CT 229
20.3.2 CT Staging of Severity 229
20.3.3 Recommendations for Use of CT 232
20.4 Chronic Pancreatitis 232
20.4.1 Diagnosis 233
20.4.2 Morphologic Staging 233
20.4.3 Approach to Diagnosis and Staging 234
20.4.4 Treatment Alternatives 235
20.5 Complications of Acute
and Chronic Pancreatitis 235
20.5.1 Fluid Collections 236
20.5.2 Percutaneous Catheter Drainage 236
20.5.3 Vascular Complications 236
20.5.4 Biliary Tract Involvement 238
20.5.5 Gastrointestinal Involvement 238
20.5.6 Solid Organ Involvement 239
References 239

20.1
Introduction

It is generally accepted that computed tomography (CT) is the best single imaging modality for the initial evaluation of patients with acute pancreatitis. It can accurately detect the disease, depict complications, assess or stage severity, and guide interventional techniques (BALTHAZAR et al. 1994). The exact role of CT in chronic pancreatitis is less well defined, and competing modalities of endoscopic retrograde cholangiopancreatography (ERCP) and transabdominal and endoscopic sonography also are considered to be important modalities both for diagnosis of the disease and for detection of complications, morphologic staging, and precise definition of ductal anatomy.

This chapter will discuss the current techniques

P. C. FREENY, MD; Department of Radiology, Box 357115, University of Washington School of Medicine, 1959 Pacific Ave., Seattle, WA 98195, USA

and applications of helical CT of the pancreas in patients with acute and chronic pancreatitis.

20.2
Techniques of Helical CT of the Pancreas

Helical CT of the pancreas is performed using 5-mm collimated scans at a pitch of 1:1 to 1.5:1, allowing the examination to be accomplished with a single breathhold. Reconstruction intervals of 5–7 mm can be used for routine evaluation, and thin reconstruction intervals of 1–3 mm can be acquired if fine anatomical detail is needed.

We prefer to use water as the oral contrast agent to distend the stomach and duodenum for the first CT scan in patients with acute or chronic pancreatitis. Water facilitates evaluation of the pancreatic head and periampullary region and can be particularly helpful for evaluation of the distal common bile duct and pancreatic duct for the presence of stones (WINTER et al. 1996) (Fig. 20.1). A positive oral contrast agent is used for subsequent examinations to opacify the gastrointestinal tract so as to facilitate differentiation of pancreatic fluid collections from loops of bowel and detection of involvement of the gastrointestinal tract by the inflammatory process.

A bolus of 150 ml of a 60% contrast agent is injected at a rate of 3 ml/s with a scan delay of 60 s. Normal pancreatic parenchyma will show an increase in attenuation of 40–60 HU above baseline attenuation of normal nonenhanced parenchyma, permitting assessment of parenchymal perfusion. In addition, the peripancreatic vascular structures will show excellent contrast enhancement, allowing detection of vascular complications associated with acute pancreatitis.

Intravenous contrast medium can occasionally mask or obscure the presence of blood, which can be seen as a collection of high-attenuation material. Thus, we usually obtain an initial non-contrast-enhanced scan if acute or active hemorrhage is sus-

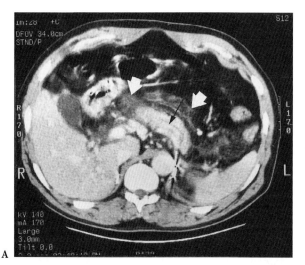

Fig. 20.1A, B. Acute biliary pancreatitis. **A** CT at the level of the pancreatic body-tail shows peripancreatic inflammation (*white arrows*) and mild dilatation of the pancreatic duct (*black arrow*). The patient had undergone unrelated bilateral nephrectomies several years earlier. **B** Scan at the level of the pancreatic head shows a common bile duct stone impacted at the ampulla of Vater (*small black arrow*) causing mild pancreatic duct dilatation (*long black arrow*). The stone is nicely demonstrated with water distension of the duodenum (*white arrow*). Positive oral contrast may well have obscured the stone

Dual helical CT is performed using an initial test bolus of 20 ml of contrast power-injected at 5 ml/s. A cursor is placed on the abdominal aorta at the level of the celiac artery, and ROIs are obtained to determine the time of peak aortic enhancement. Arterial phase scan delay is calculated as time to peak aortic enhancement minus 2 s. A bolus of 180 ml of contrast is then power-injected at a rate of 5 ml/s. The portal venous phase scans are acquired at 60 s post contrast.

Contraindications to the use of intravenous contrast include a previous severe (anaphylactic) allergic reaction to iodinated contrast material and markedly diminished renal function not yet requiring dialysis (if the patient is on dialysis, contrast material usually can be administered). In these two instances, a non-contrast-enhanced scan should be obtained and evaluated for its adequacy (i.e., does the scan provide sufficient information to manage the patient appropriately?). If the scan is considered inadequate, patients with contrast allergies can be premedicated. In the case of diminished renal function, the potential for contrast-induced nephropathy leading to dialysis must be weighed against the potential benefit of a contrast-enhanced CT. If contrast enhancement is believed to be necessary, the patient can be hydrated with intravenous fluids for 3–6 h before and after the scan and given 25–50 g of mannitol

pected (Fig. 20.2). A dual helical CT is subsequently acquired during both the arterial and portal venous phases (Fig. 20.3). The arterial phase scans can be used to detect active arterial bleeding or the presence of an arterial pseudoaneurysm, while the portal venous phase can be used to detect venous involvement, such as splenic, portal, or superior mesenteric vein thrombosis and associated varices.

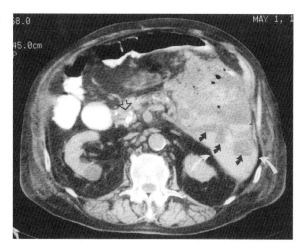

Fig. 20.2. Pancreatic fluid collection with acute hemorrhage. This patient with known chronic calcific pancreatitis and a fluid collection around the tail of the pancreas developed acute abdominal pain. CT scan at the level of the pancreas shows a large heterogeneous fluid collection. The dependent portion of the collection (*white arrows*) shows fluid-fluid levels (*black arrows*) with increased attenuation, consistent with acute hemorrhage. Multiple calcifications are noted in the head and body of the pancreas (*open arrow*)

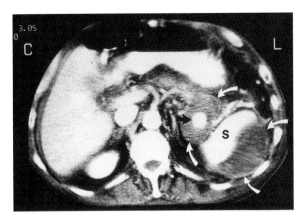

Fig. 20.3. Acute pancreatitis and arterial pseudoaneurysm. This patient had acute pancreatitis with development of a pseudocyst (*white arrows*) involving the tail of the pancreas and the spleen (*S*). CT scan was obtained following a sudden increase in left upper abdominal pain. Scan shows a compact enhancing mass (*black arrow*) within the pseudocyst, indicating a pseudoaneurysm. Subsequent angiography confirmed the presence of the pseudoaneurysm, and successful transcatheter embolization was performed

immediately after the contrast bolus. A low osmolar contrast agent is used at a volume 90–100 ml. If neither of these alternatives is acceptable, contrast-enhanced MR can be performed.

20.3
Acute Pancreatitis

Acute pancreatitis is characterized by a spectrum of inflammatory disease ranging from *mild* (interstitial or edematous pancreatitis) to *severe* (pancreatitis with associated parenchymal and/or peripancreatic fat necrosis, pancreatic abscess, pseudocyst, or other local or systemic complications). In a series of 897 patients with acute pancreatitis reported by BEGER (1991), 76% (679) had acute interstitial pancreatitis, 18% (157) had necrotizing pancreatitis, 5% (41) developed pseudocysts, and 2% (20) developed a pancreatic abscess. As the severity of the inflammatory process increases, the associated morbidity and mortality also increase. In BEGER's series, the mortality rate for patients with acute interstitial pancreatitis was only 0.4%, while it rose to 12% in patients with necrotizing pancreatitis and to 17% if a pancreatic abscess was present. Thus, staging and early detection of complications of acute pancreatitis are important for appropriate patient management (LONDON et al. 1991; BALTHAZAR et al. 1994).

Contrast-enhanced helical CT currently is the most accurate single imaging modality for diagnosis, for staging the severity of the inflammatory process, and for detecting complications of acute pancreatitis (BALTHAZAR et al. 1990; LARVIN et al. 1990; FREENY 1991, 1993). Most importantly, CT has been shown to have a sensitivity of 87% and an overall detection rate of over 90% for pancreatic gland necrosis (KIVISAARI et al. 1983; BLOCK et al. 1986; BALTHAZAR et al. 1990).

20.3.1
Indications for CT for Acute Pancreatitis

CT has two major roles in the evaluation of patients with known or suspected acute pancreatitis: (1) *staging* the severity of the inflammatory process; and (2) *detection of complications*, and particularly the identification and quantification of parenchymal and peripancreatic necrosis. In patients in whom the clinical diagnosis of acute pancreatitis is equivocal, CT also can be used for *diagnosis*.

20.3.2
CT Staging of the Severity of Acute Pancreatitis

The ability to stage the severity of acute pancreatitis accurately may have important implications for prognosis and treatment (BALTHAZAR 1989; BALTHAZAR et al. 1985, 1990; BEGER et al. 1986a, b; LONDON et al. 1991). Several studies have shown that initial clinical evaluation may be able to identify only 35–40% of patients with severe acute pancreatitis, i.e., patients who are likely to have high morbidity (MACMAHON et al. 1980; CORFIELD et al. 1985; WILSON et al. 1990; AGARWAL and PICHUMONI 1991). This is because clinical criteria alone measure only the physiologic or systemic response of the patient. However, recent studies have shown that CT performed early in the course of acute pancreatitis can accurately identify patients with severe pancreatitis (BEGER and BÜCHLER 1986; BALTHAZAR et al. 1990; BÜCHLER 1991). CT can both depict the existing extent of damage to the pancreas, particularly the presence of gland necrosis, and identify other complications prior to clinical manifestation that subsequently may result in major sequelae. These complications include extensive peripancreatic fluid collections, abscess formation, and vascular, biliary, or gastrointestinal tract involvement (BALTHAZAR et al. 1990).

The morphologic severity of acute pancreatitis can be defined precisely using the *CT Severity Index* (CTSI) developed by BALTHAZAR et al. (1990). This index is composed of assessment of the severity of the acute inflammatory process (categorized into stages A through E, corresponding to scores of 0–4, respectively) and assessment of the presence and extent of parenchymal gland necrosis.

20.3.2.1
Assessment of Acute Inflammatory Process

Stage A: Normal Pancreas (Score 0). Patients with acute edematous or interstitial pancreatitis may have a normal pancreatic CT in 20–25% of cases (HILL et al. 1982). This is because the inflammatory process is so mild that fluid collections and peripancreatic soft tissue changes do not occur. The gland may be slightly enlarged, but without a baseline scan performed prior to the onset of the acute attack, this change may be difficult to detect.

Stage B: Intrinsic Pancreatic Changes (Score 1). Stage B acute pancreatitis represents a spectrum of changes, including focal or diffuse gland enlargement, mild heterogeneity of the gland parenchyma, and small intrapancreatic fluid collections caused by rupture of a small lateral side-branch duct or a small zone (<3 cm) of parenchymal necrosis and ductal rupture (Fig. 20.4).

Stage C: Intrinsic and Extrinsic Inflammatory Changes (Score 2). Stage C acute pancreatitis is manifested by intrinsic gland abnormalities as described for stage B, but also includes mild inflammatory changes of the peripancreatic soft tissues (Fig. 20.5).

Stage D: Extrinsic Inflammatory Changes (Score 3). Patients with stage D acute pancreatitis manifest more prominent peripancreatic inflammatory changes, but not more than one pancreatic fluid collection (Fig. 20.6).

Stage E: Multiple or Extensive Extrapancreatic Fluid Collections or Abscess (Score 4). This is the most severe CT stage of acute pancreatitis and is manifested by marked intrapancreatic (fluid collections, necrosis) and peripancreatic (fluid collections, extraglandular fat necrosis) inflammatory changes, or frank pancreatic abscess formation (Fig. 20.7). These patients have a high morbidity owing to systemic complications (respiratory and renal failure,

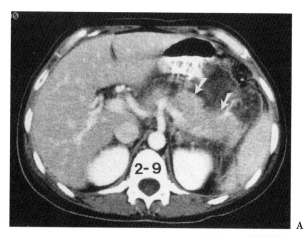

A

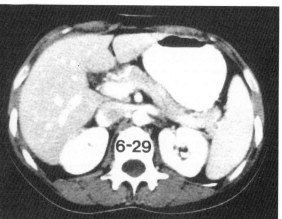

B

Fig. 20.4A, B. Acute pancreatitis: stage B. **A** Initial CT scan on 2-9 shows diffuse enlargement of the pancreatic tail (*arrows*) without significant peripancreatic inflammatory change. **B** Follow-up CT scan 4 months later shows a pancreas with normal appearance

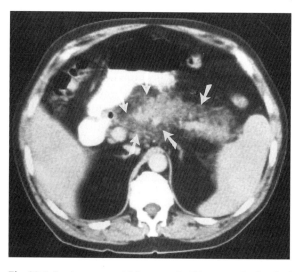

Fig. 20.5. Acute pancreatititis: stage C. CT scan at the level of the body of the pancreas shows peripancreatic inflammatory changes (*arrows*)

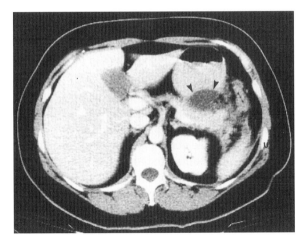

Fig. 20.6. Acute pancreatitis: stage D. CT scan at the level of the pancreatic tail shows a single, small fluid collection anterior to the pancreas (*arrowheads*). No other fluid collections were present

cardiovascular collapse) and a high mortality. Thus, serial CT scans are important for following the progression of the disease and for detecting additional complications.

20.3.2.2
Assessment of Gland Necrosis

The presence and extent or the absence of gland necrosis are assessed and the corresponding score added to produce the CTSI score. If necrosis is present, the extent is estimated as less than one-third, one-half, or greater than one-half on the basis of the area of gland parenchyma involved as demonstrated on axial scans. A score of 0 is given if no necrosis is present, and scores of 2, 4, and 6 for less than one-third, up to one-half, and greater than one-half, respectively.

Necrosis can be detected by CT as a focal or diffuse area of diminished pancreatic parenchymal contrast enhancement (Fig. 20.8) (KIVISAARI et al. 1983; MAIER 1987; LARVIN et al. 1990; JOHNSON et al. 1991). CT has an accuracy of 87% for detection of parenchymal necrosis (MAIER 1987). The false-negative rate is about 20% in patients with minor necrosis, but in cases of major or extended necrosis (>50%), the false-negative rate is less than 10%. False-positive CT scans are rare and specificity approaches 100%. BRADLEY et al. (1989) subsequently confirmed these results and indicated that CT detection of gland necrosis had important prognostic implications.

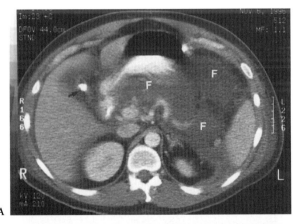

A

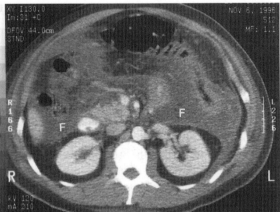

B

Fig. 20.7A, B. Acute pancreatitis: stage E. A CT scan shows multiple fluid collections (*F*) surrounding the pancreas and filling the anterior pararenal space and lesser sac. Gallstone noted incidentally (*black arrow*). B Scan at a lower level shows extensive peripancreatic fluid collections (*F*) with extension into the inferior portion of both anterior pararenal spaces

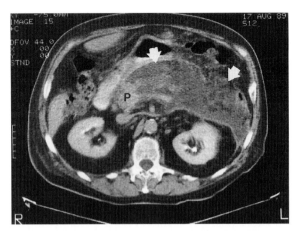

Fig. 20.8. Acute necrotizing pancreatitis. Contrast-enhanced CT scan shows normal enhancement of the pancreatic head (*P*). The body and tail are replaced by a well-circumscribed low-attenuation area. No enhancement of the body and tail of the pancreas was identified, indicating subtotal gland necrosis

The CTSI score thus can range from zero to 10 and shows excellent correlation with the clinical severity of the disease. BALTHAZAR (et al. 1990) showed that patients with a CTSI of 0–1 had no mortality or morbidity, those with an index of 2–3 had an 8% morbidity and a 3% mortality, those with an index of 4–6 had a 35% morbidity and a 6% mortality, and those with an index of 7–10 had a 92% morbidity and a 17% mortality.

The presence of necrosis as an isolated finding also correlated with subsequent patient morbidity and mortality (BALTHAZAR et al. 1990). Patients with no necrosis had no mortality and only a 6% morbidity, while those with one-third necrosis had no mortality and a 40% morbidity, those with 50% necrosis had a 25% mortality and a 75% morbidity, and those with greater than 50% necrosis had an 11% mortality and a 100% morbidity. These figures are similar to those from BEGER's series (BEGER 1991).

It should be noted that most patients with acute pancreatitis who develop necrotizing pancreatitis do so within the first 24 h, and virtually all within the first 72 h following the onset of clinical symptoms (M. Büchler, personal communication). Because the CT findings of necrosis may be equivocal within the first 24– 48 h, the initial CT scan obtained in patients with clinically severe acute pancreatitis should be postponed until 72 h unless the patient is critically ill and in need of emergency surgery.

Secondary infection of necrotic pancreatic tissue also has a significant effect on patient morbidity and mortality. In BEGER's series of 114 patients with pancreatic necrosis, intestinal microorganisms were cultured from the necrotic tissue in 39% of cases (BEGER et al. 1986b). When the necrotic tissue was infected, patients with less than 50% gland necrosis showed an increase in mortality from 13% to 39%, while patients with subtotal necrosis (>50%), showed an increase in mortality from 14% to 67%.

Thus, the most important role of CT in evaluation of patients with clinically severe acute pancreatitis is detection of gland necrosis and identification of the presence of infection. However, about half of all patients with acute pancreatitis who have clinically suspected sepsis on the basis of the presence of fever and leukocytosis are not infected. Thus, because infection of fluid collections or necrotic tissue cannot be determined by CT, patients who manifest clinical signs of sepsis should undergo needle aspiration of the suggestive areas under CT or ultrasound guidance (BANKS and GERZOF 1987; BANKS 1991). In these patients, a positive gram stain and/or culture indicates the need for intervention.

20.3.3
Recommendations for Use of CT in Acute Pancreatitis

The following guidelines are suggested for the use of CT in patients with acute pancreatitis.

Performance of Initial CT Scans. An initial CT scan should be obtained (1) in patients with clinically severe acute pancreatitis (based on Ranson criteria or APACHE II score) at the time of initial evaluation who do not manifest rapid clinical improvement within 72 h of conservative medical treatment; and (2) in patients who demonstrate clinical improvement during medical therapy but then manifest an acute change in clinical status, e.g., fever, pain, inability to tolerate oral intake, hypotension, falling hematocrit, indicating a developing complication, such as a fluid collection, pseudocyst, or secondary infection.

Performance of Follow-up CT Scans. A follow-up CT scan should be obtained
1. In patients whose initial scans show a CTSI score of 3–10. In these patients, follow-up scans are suggested because complications that may require treatment or close observation can develop without becoming clinically evident, such as evolution of a fluid collection into a pseudocyst or development of an arterial pseudoaneurysm. These routine follow-up scans should be obtained 7–10 days after the initial scan and at the time of hospital discharge.
2. In all patients, regardless of CTSI score, who either do not show continued clinical improvement or who show clinical deterioration.

20.4
Chronic Pancreatitis

Chronic pancreatitis comprises a broad spectrum of inflammatory changes in the gland and can be caused by a wide variety of etiologies. Understanding of the morphologic changes produced by the chronic inflammatory process has expanded in the last decade as more sophisticated imaging modalities have been utilized for evaluation.

CT has four primary roles in the evaluation of patients with chronic pancreatitis: diagnosis; staging the severity of the disease; detection of complications; and assistance in choosing treatment alternatives.

20.4.1
Diagnosis

Diagnosis of chronic pancreatitis is based upon *clinical findings*, assessment of endocrine and exocrine pancreatic *function*, and identification of *morphologic* changes in the gland as depicted by imaging studies. Evaluation of all three aspects is essential, since many patients with chronic pancreatitis will have abnormalities of only one or two.

A morphologic diagnosis of chronic pancreatitis can be made with sonography, CT, magnetic resonance pancreatography (MRP), and ERCP. ERCP continues to be the gold standard for diagnosis, but CT is important for its ability to display changes in the parenchyma and to detect complications of the inflammatory process.

The CT findings of chronic pancreatitis consist of a broad spectrum of changes, which depend on the severity of the chronic inflammatory process. These include alterations in size and shape of the gland, changes in parenchymal attenuation, intraductal calculi, pancreatic and bile duct dilatation, fluid collections, and vascular involvement (portal venous obstruction, arterial pseudoaneurysms) (Figs. 20.9, 20.10). LUETMER et al. (1989) reported a false-negative rate of only 7% (4 of 56 patients) in CT detection of chronic pancreatitis. However, the spectrum of clinical and/or functional severity of the disease in their patients was not reported. In mild chronic pancreatitis, the CT findings are often normal.

20.4.2
Morphologic Staging

The severity of chronic pancreatitis can be staged by assessing the degree of exocrine or endocrine dysfunction of the pancreas, the morphologic findings depicted by US, CT, MRCP or ERCP, or by the clinical syndrome manifested by the patient, e.g., persistent pain, endocrine deficiency, and complications related to exocrine dysfunction, such as malabsorption.

The imaging section of the 1983 Cambridge Symposium in 1983 attempted to develop a consistent set of definitions of morphological changes (AXON et al. 1984; SARNER and COTTON 1984). Subsequently, several reports have been published, which have correlated morphology, function, and clinical status in patients with chronic pancreatitis (BRAGANZA et al. 1982; GIRDWOOD et al. 1984; MALFERTHEINER 1986; MALFERTHEINER et al. 1986, 1989).

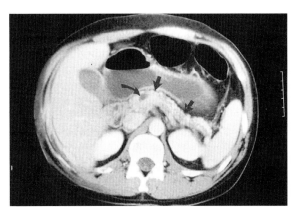

Fig. 20.9. Diffuse chronic calcific pancreatitis. CT scan at the level of the body and tail of the pancreas shows diffuse pancreatic ductal calcifications (*straight arrows*) and segmental dilatation of the main pancreatic duct in the midportion of the body (*curved arrow*). Lower scan (not shown) showed a large stone within the pancreatic head causing pancreatic duct obstruction

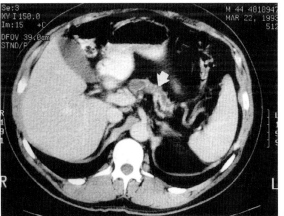

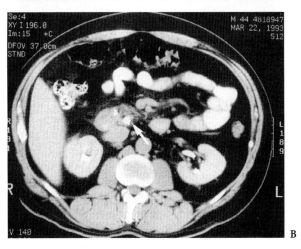

Fig. 20.10A, B. Focal chronic calcific pancreatitis. **A** Scan shows atrophy of the body and tail of the pancreas and dilatation of the pancreatic duct (*arrow*). **B** Scan at the level of the pancreatic head shows an obstructing calculus (*arrow*) in the main pancreatic duct

Morphology and Function. In our experience, comparison of the morphological severity of the disease based on the Cambridge classification with the clinical findings and alterations in endocrine and exocrine function showed that CT and clinical/functional staging agreed in only about 46% of patients. In the 54% where there was disagreement between CT and/or ERCP and clinical/functional staging, CT and ERCP upstaged virtually all patients. Overall correlation of CT/ERCP and clinical staging in patients with mild to moderate disease was only 29%, while in severe disease it was 100%.

Published reports comparing morphology and function can be summarized by saying that in mild or early chronic pancreatitis, the most accurate diagnosis is achieved by the use of both function tests and imaging modalities, primarily CT and ERCP (BRAGANZA et al. 1982; GIRDWOOD et al. 1984; MALFERTHEINER 1986; MALFERTHEINER et al. 1986, 1989). The correlation was excellent in most cases, but there were a few patients with minimal morphological changes and marked functional abnormalities, and some with marked morphologic changes and minimal functional alteration. Thus, while structure and function could not always be directly related, the best correlation was found in patients with more advanced disease.

Pancreatic Duct Calcifications. An important recent observation concerns the relationship of pancreatic ductal calculi and exocrine function. In the past, duct calculi were believed to indicate advanced disease and severe exocrine dysfunction. In LANKISCH's series, however, 50% of patients with calculi had only mild to moderate exocrine dysfunction, while the other half had severe impairment (LANKISCH et al. 1986). In our experience, there is a definite trend toward increasing clinical severity of chronic pancreatitis and the presence of focal or diffuse ductal calculi: 89% of patients with clinically severe chronic pancreatitis had calculi. However, calculi also were present in 55% of patients with only mild to moderate clinical disease severity. Severe abdominal pain was present in 74% of patients with calculi, but was also present in 44% of patients with no calculi. Thus, the presence of pancreatic duct calculi per se is a poor predictor of clinical/functional disease severity.

Morphology, Function, and Clinical Course. If all clinical stages of chronic pancreatitis are considered, the severity of the patient's clinical course (i.e., amount of pain, presence of diabetes mellitus, mal-absorption, and propensity to develop complications, such as pseudocysts and vascular involvement) cannot be predicted from the morphologic changes and vice versa. There also is no significant correlation between the degree of exocrine gland dysfunction and the severity of clinical symptoms, such as pain (MALFERTHEINER et al. 1989). However, if only patients with advanced stages of chronic pancreatitis (defined as >75% reduction of enzyme and/or bicarbonate secretion in the secretin-cerulein test) are considered, a significant correlation is found between the clinical and morphologic severity of the disease in 80% of patients, while patients with mild to moderate stages (defined as <50–75% reduction of enzymes and/or bicarbonate) show poor correlation. Advanced morphologic changes (ERCP, CT) are found in 65% of these patients. The poor morphologic-clinical correlation raises the question of whether the morphologic grading of ERCP and CT has been defined incorrectly, or whether the morphologic changes might precede a more severe clinical course. Prospective studies are needed to evaluate these questions.

20.4.3
Approach to Diagnosis and Staging of Chronic Pancreatitis

The clinical diagnosis of chronic pancreatitis is best confirmed with a combination of the imaging modalities of CT, MRCP, or ERCP. Although some investigators recommend US because of its lower cost, we believe that CT is superior because of the broad spectrum of information it provides and the rarity of a technically unsatisfactory examination. In particular, CT is more useful for differentiating pancreatic cancer from chronic pancreatitis and for detecting the complications of chronic pancreatitis. The value of MRP appears quite promising, but only preliminary studies representing a broad spectrum of the stages of chronic pancreatitis are available (BARISH et al. 1997).

ERCP is more sensitive than CT in detecting chronic pancreatitis, particularly in the mild to moderate forms of the disease, and often provides valuable information if a surgical drainage procedure is contemplated. It may also be useful for the differentiation of chronic pancreatitis and pancreatic carcinoma. The pancreatogram can be analyzed and brush cytology or direct pancreatic intraductal endoscopy or ultrasonography can be performed (STEER et al. 1995).

Pancreatic function tests are not widely utilized in the United States. However, it seems clear from European data that function tests combined with imaging procedures provide the best diagnosis and the most accurate means of staging the severity of chronic pancreatitis. However, if diabetes and steatorrhea (malabsorption) are already present, function tests are probably superfluous.

20.4.4
Treatment Alternatives

Patients with chronic pancreatitis can be treated with conservative medical therapy, surgery, or interventional endoscopic or radiologic techniques. Imaging procedures play a crucial role in selection of the appropriate therapeutic approach.

The primary indications for surgery are persistent pain and treatment of complications of chronic pancreatitis, such as biliary or duodenal obstruction, pseudocysts, and vascular involvement (Fig. 20.11). Imaging studies can be used to detect these complications and possible causes for pain, such as a pseudocyst or obstruction of the pancreatic or bile duct, and thus can be used to select the appropriate operation or treatment (LIPPERT and SCHULZ 1997).

Some complications of chronic pancreatitis, such as fluid collections, biliary obstruction, pancreatic duct calculi and strictures, and acute arterial hemorrhage, can be treated with nonoperative endoscopic or radiologic techniques. These procedures include percutaneous or endoscopic drainage of fluid collections, endoscopic removal of pancreatic duct calculi, endoscopic or transhepatic dilatation of bile duct strictures and placement of stents for decompression, endoscopic pancreatic duct stricture dilatation or stent placement, sclerotherapy for control of variceal hemorrhage, and transcatheter embolotherapy for control of arterial hemorrhage or pseudoaneurysm formation (FREENY et al. 1988; VAN SONNENBERG et al. 1989; VUJIC 1989; KOZAREK et al. 1991; DEVIERE et al. 1994). Radiologic guidance and monitoring can often be crucial for safe and efficacious performance of these techniques.

20.5
Complications of Acute and Chronic Pancreatitis

The complications of acute and chronic pancreatitis are similar and include formation of fluid collec-

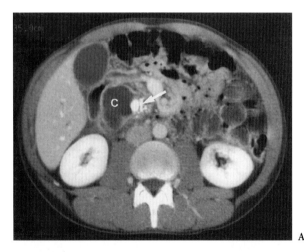

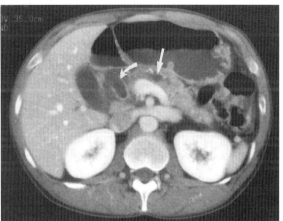

Fig. 20.11A, B. Chronic calcific pancreatitis with pancreatic pseudocyst and biliary duct obstruction. A Scan at the level of the head of the pancreas shows a large calculus in the pancreatic duct (*arrow*) and a pseudocyst (*C*). B Scan at the level of the body of the pancreas shows dilatation of the pancreatic duct with small intraductal calcifications (*straight arrow*). The common bile duct proximal to the pancreatic pseudocyst is dilated (*curved arrow*). Biliary obstruction was subsequently shown to be caused by compression of the common bile duct by the pancreatic pseudocyst. Following pseudocyst drainage, biliary duct obstruction resolved

tions (including pseudocysts and abscesses) and spread of the inflammatory reaction to involve the gastrointestinal tract, bile ducts, and vascular system, and pancreatic ascites. Many of these complications can be detected by CT, and early recognition can be expected to result in reduced morbidity and mortality by leading to early and appropriate surgical, radiologic, or endoscopic treatment.

The association of chronic pancreatitis and pancreatic carcinoma continues to be debated (GOLD and CAMERON 1993; LOWENFELS et al. 1993). It is currently accepted that there is an increased incidence of pancreatic cancer, but it is very small. GOLD estimated that in the U.S. only about 24 cases per year could be explained on the basis of chronic pancreatitis.

20.5.1
Fluid Collections

Fluid collections develop in about 50% of patients with acute pancreatitis (KOURTESIS et al. 1990; YEO et al. 1990). In many cases, the collections resolve spontaneously and never produce clinical symptoms (Fig. 20.12). In other patients, however, the collections can persist, enlarge, become secondarily infected, erode into contiguous structures, or extend

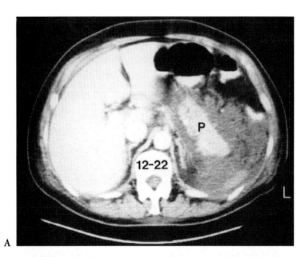

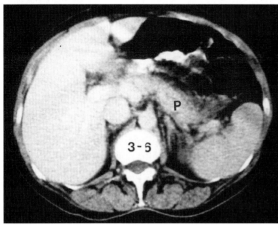

Fig. 20.12A, B. Acute pancreatitis. A CT scan on 12– 22 shows a large fluid collection surrounding the tail of the pancreas (P), indicating stage D acute pancreatitis. B Following conservative therapy, a follow-up CT scan was obtained on 3– 6. The peripancreatic fluid collection has resolved and pancreas (P) is normal

to involve areas distant to the pancreas (Fig. 20.13). These persistent or enlarging collections and their secondary complications can be detected by CT and a decision can then be made on surgical, endoscopic, or percutaneous drainage.

Large peripancreatic fluid collections are often associated with coexisting peripancreatic fat necrosis (Fig. 20.12). It is usually not possible to make this differentiation by CT. However, if the peripancreatic process has low CT attenuation numbers (<15 HU), it is most likely to be a simple peripancreatic fluid collection, while higher numbers (>25 HU) are highly indicative of coexisting fat necrosis. The presence or absence of secondary infection within these peripancreatic collections also cannot be determined accurately on the basis of CT morphology. The presence of gas within a collection may be caused by gas-forming bacteria, but also can be caused by a gastrointestinal fistula in the absence of infection (MENDEZ and ISIKOFF 1979). The presence of infection within a fluid collection can be confirmed with CT-guided fine-needle aspiration. If percutaneous drainage is to be performed, CT should be obtained to define the precise anatomical relationship of the collection to surrounding structures, so that the catheter can be placed safely in the appropriate location (FREENY et al. 1988).

20.5.2
Percutaneous Catheter Drainage

Infected fluid collections can be treated effectively by percutaneous catheter drainage (PCD) (FREENY et al. 1988; VAN SONNENBERG et al. 1989; BALTHAZAR et al. 1994). The initial fine-needle aspiration should be used to determine the presence of infection and the quality of the fluid (i.e., whether it is sufficiently liquid to be drained via catheter).

CT should be obtained prior to PCD to define precisely the location, size, and number of collections and their relationship to surrounding structures, and to identify vascular involvement, such as pseudoaneurysm or venous obstruction with large varices, which could result in major complications during or following PCD (see Fig. 20.3).

20.5.3
Vascular Complications

Involvement of the peripancreatic arteries and veins by the inflammatory process associated with acute

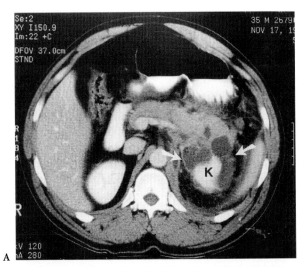

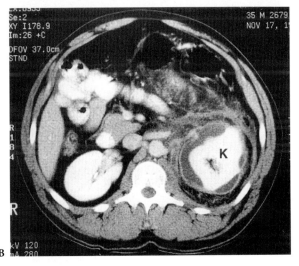

patients, emergency angiography and transcatheter embolotherapy or surgery are required; CT has little to offer and may delay diagnosis and treatment.

Arterial pseudoaneurysms can develop within the pancreatic parenchyma, adjacent to the gland, or within a pseudocyst (see Fig. 20.3). They can be diagnosed by angiography or CT by demonstrating a contrast-enhancing mass. They can be treated surgically, but transcatheter embolotherapy is efficacious and can be performed at the time of diagnostic angiography (FREENY and LAWSON 1982; FREENY 1984; VUJIC et al. 1984; WALTMAN et al. 1986; VUJIC 1989).

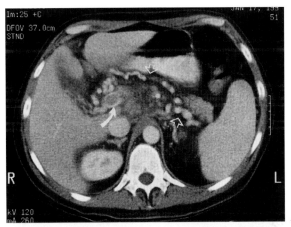

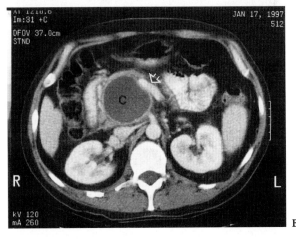

Fig. 20.13A–C. Acute pancreatitis with renal involvement. **A** Initial CT scan shows multiple fluid collections around the tail of the pancreas (*arrows*) involving the left kidney (*K*). **B** Scan at a lower level shows a subcapsular fluid collection involving the left kidney (*K*). Note deformity of the renal margins due to extension of the pancreatic fluid collection beyond the renal capsule

and chronic pancreatitis is common and can be detected accurately by CT. Complications include arterial stenosis or occlusion, erosion of intrapancreatic or peripancreatic arteries with acute hemorrhage (see Fig. 20.2), formation of arterial pseudoaneurysms (see Fig. 20.3), and thrombosis of branches of the portal venous system with formation of varices or acute mesenteric infarction (Fig. 20.14).

Acute pancreatic hemorrhage may be a catastrophic event heralded by pain and shock. In these

Fig. 20.14A, B. Acute pancreatitis with pseudocyst and venous thrombosis. **A** CT scan at the level of the midportion of the body of the pancreas shows thrombus within the main portal vein (*curved arrow*) and peripancreatic and perigastric varices (*open arrows*). **B** Scan at the level of the pancreatic head shows a large pseudocyst (*C*) with adjacent mesenteric varix (*open arrow*) upstream from the portal vein thrombus

20.5.4
Biliary Tract Involvement

CT is quite accurate in detecting involvement or associated abnormalities of the biliary tract. The most common biliary tract abnormality associated with acute pancreatitis is choledocholithiasis (see Fig. 20.1). Biliary tract involvement by the inflammatory process associated with acute and chronic pancreatitis can be manifested by transient dilatation of the suprapancreatic segment of the common bile duct owing to periductal inflammation or to compression by an adjacent pseudocyst or fluid collection (see Fig. 20.11), or chronic obstruction owing to a ductal stricture caused by the surrounding inflammatory process. Pancreatic pseudocysts also can involve the common bile duct directly or they can invade into the liver, producing an intrahepatic biliary fistula (ROHRMANN and BARON 1989).

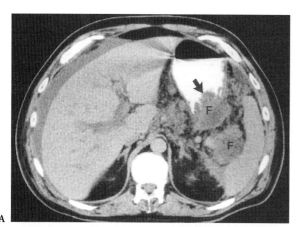

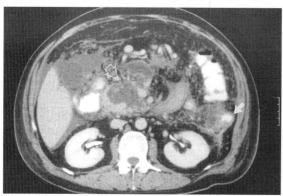

Fig. 20.15A, B. Acute pancreatitis with gastric and colonic involvement. A CT scan through the upper abdomen shows fluid collections (*F*) in the region of the tail of the pancreas with involvement of the stomach and distortion of gastric folds (*arrow*). The patient also has pancreatic ascites. B Scan at a lower level shows extension of the inflammatory process into the root of the small bowel mesentery (*open arrow*) and involvement of the descending colon (*closed arrow*)

20.5.5
Gastrointestinal Tract Involvement

While both CT and barium contrast studies can detect involvement of the gastrointestinal tract by acute and chronic pancreatitis, CT provides the most information concerning the extent of the inflammatory process extrinsic to or surrounding the involved segment of the gastrointestinal tract (Fig. 20.15) (SAFRIT and RICE 1989). The etiology of the involvement usually can be elucidated (e.g., fluid collection, pseudocyst, or direct extension of the inflammatory process) and the appropriate surgical or interventional treatment can be planned (Fig. 20.16).

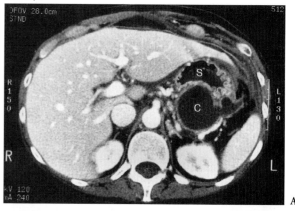

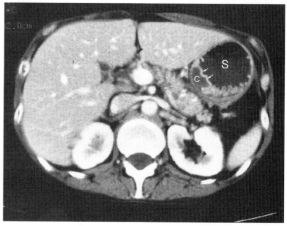

Fig. 20.16A, B. Acute pancreatitis: intramural gastric pseudocyst. A CT scan at the level of the pancreatic tail shows a large pseudocyst (*C*) pressing against the posterior wall of the stomach (*S*). B Scan at a lower level shows dissection of the pseudocyst (*C*) into the wall of the stomach (*S*). Elevation of the gastric mucosa (*small arrows*) is nicely demonstrated with water distension of the stomach

20.5.6
Solid Organ Involvement

The inflammatory process of acute or chronic pancreatitis can extend to involve the solid organs contiguous to the pancreas, particularly the spleen (Figs. 20.3, 20.17), left kidney (see Fig. 20.13), and the liver (see Fig. 20.18) (LILIENFELD and LANDE 1976; FARMAN et al. 1977; FREENY and LAWSON 1982; FISHMAN et al. 1995).

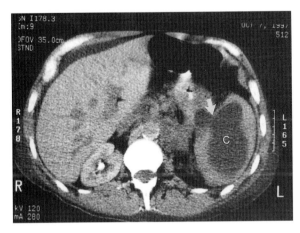

Fig. 20.17. Acute pancreatitis: intrasplenic pseudocyst. CT scan shows dissection of pancreatic fluid collection (*arrow*) into the adjacent spleen, forming an intrasplenic pseudocyst (*C*)

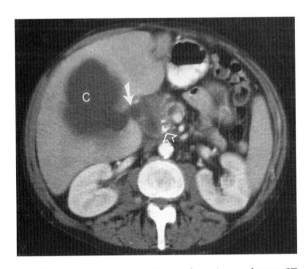

Fig. 20.18. Chronic pancreatitis: intrahepatic pseudocyst. CT scan at the level of the pancreatic head shows multiple small calcifications (*open arrow*). A pancreatic fluid collection extends from the pancreatic head into the liver (*closed arrow*) forming an intrahepatic pseudocyst (*C*)

References

Agarwal N, Pitchumoni C (1991) Assessment of severity in acute pancreatitis. Am J Gastroenterology 86:1385–1391

Axon A, Classen M, Cotton P et al (1984) Pancreatography in chronic pancreatitis: international definitions. Gut 25:1107–1112

Balthazar E (1989) CT diagnosis and staging of acute pancreatitis. Radiol Clin North Am 27:19–37

Balthazar E, Ranson J, Naidich D et al (1985) Acute pancreatitis: prognostic value of CT. Radiology 156:767–772

Balthazar E, Robinson D, Megibow A, Ranson J (1990) Acute pancreatitis: value of CT in establishing prognosis. Radiology 174:331–336

Balthazar E, Freeny P, van Sonnenberg E (1994) Imaging and intervention in acute pancreatitis. Radiology 193:297–306

Banks P (1991) Infected necrosis: morbidity and therapeutic consequences. Hepatogastroenterology 38:116–119

Banks P, Gerzof S (1987) Indications and results of fine needle aspiration of pancreatic exudate. In: Beger H, Büchler M (eds) Acute pancreatitis. Springer, Berlin Heidelberg New York, pp 171–174

Barish M, Soto J, Ferrucci J (1997) Magnetic resonance pancreatography. Endoscopy 29:487–495

Beger H (1991) Surgery in acute pancreatitis. Hepatogastroenterology 38:92–96

Beger H, Büchler M (1986) Outcome of necrotizing pancreatitis in relation to morphological parameters. In: Malfertheiner P, Ditchuneit H (eds) Diagnostic procedures in pancreatic disease. Springer, Berlin Heidelberg New York, pp 130–132

Beger H, Maier W, Block, S, Büchler M (1986a) How do imaging methods influence the surgical strategy in acute pancreatitis? In: Malfertheiner P, Ditchuneit H (eds) Diagnostic procedures in pancreatic disease. Springer, Berlin Heidelberg New York, pp 54–60

Beger H, Bittner R, Block S, Büchler M (1986b) Bacterial contamination of pancreatic necrosis. A prospective study. Gastroenterology 91:433–438

Block S, Maier W, Bittner R et al (1986) Identification of pancreas necrosis in severe acute pancreatitis: imaging procedures versus clinical staging. Gut 27:1035–1042

Bradley E III, Murphy F, Ferguson C (1989) Prediction of pancreatic necrosis by dynamic pancreatography. Ann Surg 210:495–504

Braganza J, Hunt L, Warwick F (1982) Relationship between pancreatic exocrine function and ductal morphology. Gastroenterology 82:1341–1347

Büchler M (1991) Objectification of the severity of acute pancreatitis. Hepatogastroenterology 38:101–108

Corfield A, Williamson R, McMahon M et al (1985) Prediction of severity in acute pancreatitis: prospective comparison of three prognostic indices. Lancet 2:403–406

Deviere z et al (1994) z

Farman J, Dallemand S, Schneider M et al (1977) Pancreatic pseudocysts involving the spleen. Gastrointest Radiol 1:339–343

Fishman E, Soyer P, Bliss D, Bluemke D, Devine N (1995) Splenic involvement in pancreatitis: spectrum of CT findings. AJR 164:631–635

Freeny P (1984) Computed tomography of the pancreas. Clin Gastroenterol 13:791– 818

Freeny P (1991) Angio-CT: diagnosis and detection of complications of acute pancreatitis. Hepatogastroenterology 38:109–115

Freeny P (1993) Incremental dynamic bolus computed tomography of acute pancreatitis state of the art. Int J Pancreatol 13:147–158

Freeny P, Lawson T (1982) Radiology of the pancreas. Springer, Berlin Heidelberg New York

Freeny P, Lewis G, Traverso L, Ryan J (1988) Infected pancreatic fluid collections: percutaneous catheter drainage. Radiology 167:435–441

Girdwood A, Hatfield A, Bornman P et al (1984) Structure and function in noncalcific pancreatitis. Dig Dis Sci 29:721–726

Gold E, Cameron J (1993) Chronic pancreatitis and pancreatic cancer. N Engl J Med 328:1485–1486

Hill M, Barkin J, Isikoff M, Silverstein W, Kalser M (1982) Acute pancreatitis: clinical vs. CT findings. AJR 139:263–269

Johnson C, Stephens D, Sarr M (1991) CT of acute pancreatitis: correlation between lack of contrast enhancement and pancreatic necrosis. AJR 156:93–95

Kivisaari L, Somer K, Standertskjold-Nordenstam C-G et al (1983) Early detection of acute fulminant pancreatitis by contrast-enhanced computed tomography. Scand J Gastroenterol 18:39–41

Kourtesis G, Wilson S, Williams R (1990) The clinical significance of fluid collections in acute pancreatitis. Am Surg 56:796–799

Kozarek R, Ball T, Patterson D et al (1991) Endoscopic transpapillary therapy for disrupted pancreatic duct and peripancreatic fluid collections. Gastroenterology 1362–1370

Lankisch P, Otto J, Erkelenz I, Lembcke B (1986) Pancreatic calcifications: no indicator of severe exocrine pancreatic insufficiency. Gastroenterology 90:617–621

Larvin M, Chalmers A, McMahon M (1990) Dynamic contrast enhanced computed tomography: a precise technique for identifying and localising pancreatic necrosis. Br Med J 300:1425–1428

Lilienfeld R, Lande A (1976) Pancreatic pseudocysts presenting as thick walled renal and perinephric cysts. J Urol 115:123–125

Lippert H, Schulz H (1997) What does the surgeon need in the preoperative evaluation of chronic pancreatitis? In: Malfertheiner P, Dominguez-Munoz J, Schultz H, Lippert H (eds) Diagnostic procedures in pancreatic disease. Springer, Berlin Heidelberg New York, pp 223–230

London N, Leese T, Lavelle J et al (1991) Rapid-bolus contrast-enhanced dynamic computed tomography in acute pancreatitis: a prospective study. Br J Surg 78:1452–1456

Lowenfels A, Maisonneuve P, Calvallini G, Ammann R (1993) Pancreatitis and the risk of pancreatic cancer. N Engl J Med 328:1433–1437

Luetmer P, Stephens D, Ward E (1989) Chronic pancreatitis: reassessment with current CT. Radiology 171:353–357

MacMahon M, Playforth M, Pickford I (1980) A comparative study of methods for the prediction of te severity of attacks of acute pancreatitis. Br J Surg 67:22–25

Maicr W (1987) Early objective diagnosis and staging of acute pancreatitis by contrast enhanced CT. In: Beger H, Büchler M (eds) Acute pancreatitis. Springer, Berlin Heidelberg New York, pp 132–140

Malfertheiner P (1986) Combined functional and morphological diagnostic approach in chronic pancreatitis. In: Malfertheiner P, Ditschuneit H (eds) Diagnostic procedures in pancreatic disease. Springer, Berlin Heidelberg New York, pp 262–267

Malfertheiner P, Büchler M (1989) Correlation of imaging and function in chronic pancreatitis. Radiol Clin North Am 27:51–64

Malfertheiner P, Büchler M, Stanescu A (1986) Correlation of morphological lesions, functional changes, and clinical stages in chronic pancreatitis. In: Malfertheiner P, Ditschuneit H (eds) Diagnostic procedures in pancreatic disease. Springer, Berlin Heidelberg New York, pp 268–273

Mendez G, Isikoff M (1979) Significance of intrapancreatic gas, demonstrated by CT: a review of nine cases. AJR 132:59–62

Rohrmann C, Baron R (1989) Biliary complications of pancreatitis. Radiol Clin North Am 27:93–104

Safrit H, Rice R (1989) Gastrointestinal complications of pancreatitis. Radiol Clin North Am 27:73–79

Sarner M, Cotton P (1984) Definitions of acute and chronic pancreatitis. Clin Gastroenterol 13:865–870

Steer M, Waxman I, Freedman S (1995) Chronic pancreatitis. N Engl J Med 332:1482–1490

van Sonnenberg E, Wittich G, Casola G et al (1989) Percutaneous drainage of infected and noninfected pancreatic pseudocysts: experience in 101 cases. Radiology 170:757–761

Vujic I (1989) Vascular complications of pancreatitis. Radiol Clin North Am 27:81–91

Vujic I, Anderson B, Stanley J, Gobien R (1984) Pancreatic and peripancreatic vessels: embolization for control of bleeding in pancreatitis. Radiology 150:51–55

Waltman A, Luers P, Athanasoulis C, Warshaw A (1986) Massive arterial hemorrhage in patients with pancreatitis. Complementary roles of surgery and transcatheter occlusive techniques. Arch Surg 121:439–443

Wilson C, Heath D, Imrie C (1990) Prediction of outcome in acute pancreatitis: a comparative study of APACHE II, clinical assessment and multiple factor scoring systems. Br J Surg 77:1260–1264

Winter T, Ager J, Nghiem H et al (1996) Upper gastrointestinal tract and abdomen: water as an orally administered contrast agent for CT. Radiology 201:365–370

Yeo C, Bastidas J, Lynch-Nyhan A et al (1990) The natural history of pancreatic pseudocysts documented by computed tomography. Surg Gynecol Obstet 170:411–417

Biliary and Pancreatic Diseases: Role of Spiral CT and Controversies

21 The Case for Ultrasonography

R. Lencioni, F. Donati, G. Granai, C. Bartolozzi

CONTENTS

21.1   Introduction   243
21.2   Acute Pancreatitis   243
21.3   Chronic Pancreatitis   244
21.4   Ductal Adenocarcinoma   245
21.5   Cystic Neoplasms   245
21.6   Endocrine Tumors   246
        References   246

21.1 Introduction

Evaluation of the pancreas is one of the most challenging and troublesome issues in abdominal ultrasonography (US). In fact, comprehensive US examination of the pancreas, especially of the body and the tail, is frequently hampered by bowel gas and may be unsuccessful in some instances. In contrast, spiral CT is currently the single best pancreatic imaging modality available in terms of overall accuracy, reliability, and reproducibility. Nevertheless, in many countries, US is the first imaging examination performed in patients with suspected pancreatic disease. Knowledge of US features of the main pancreatic disorders and of the limitations of US compared with CT is therefore mandatory.

R. Lencioni, MD; Division of Diagnostic and Interventional Radiology, Department of Oncology, University of Pisa, Via Roma 67, I-56125 Pisa, Italy
F. Donati, MD; Division of Diagnostic and Interventional Radiology, Department of Oncology, University of Pisa, Via Roma 67, I-56125 Pisa, Italy
G. Granai, MD; Division of Diagnostic and Interventional Radiology, Department of Oncology, University of Pisa, Via Roma 67, I-56125 Pisa, Italy
C. Bartolozzi, MD; Professor and Chairman, Division of Diagnostic and Interventional Radiology, Department of Oncology, University of Pisa, Via Roma 67, I-56125 Pisa, Italy

21.2 Acute Pancreatitis

Pancreatitis is one of the most complex of all acute abdominal disorders: in many instances there are no pathognomonic clinical or laboratory features to establish the diagnosis unequivocally. Diagnostic imaging is used not only to make the diagnosis itself, but also to clarify the cause of the pancreatitis, to assess the severity of the pancreatic involvement, and to diagnose complications, such as fluid collection, necrosis, phlegmon, and any abscess in or around the pancreas. Noninvasive imaging of the pancreas with US and CT has been a major diagnostic breakthrough (BAERT 1994)

CT is the modality of choice for evaluation of patients with acute pancreatitis, being a long way ahead of all other examination techniques. US may be used as the first-level examination in cases of mild, edematous pancreatitis that responds rapidly to conservative therapy; suspected biliary pancreatitis with a mild clinical course; and follow-up of pancreatic fluid collections (JEFFREY 1989). US may also be used as an additional examination in cases of severe, necrotizing pancreatitis, but only if further assessment of the gallbladder and biliary tree is desirable. Finally, US may help guide diagnostic needle aspiration or drainage of peripancreatic fluid collections.

US examination of pancreas is frequently hampered by bowel gas, and may be completely unsuccessful in 10–20% of patients with acute pancreatitis. Moreover, it has to be emphasized that a normal pancreatic sonogram does not exclude acute pancreatitis: in fact, the ability of US to depict inflammatory changes within the pancreas, including necrotic foci, is low. Nevertheless, characteristic alterations in the size and echogenicity of the pancreas and the peripancreatic compartments may be of clinical value in a number of cases. Abnormal US findings may be diffuse or focal, with the involved region of the pancreas usually hypoechoic or isoechoic.

The variable echogenicity of the pancreas in acute pancreatitis depends on the degree of intrapancreatic fat or hemorrhage, the presence of underlying chronic pancreatitis with calcification, and the degree of extrapancreatic spread of acute pancreatitis. A diffusely enlarged hypoechoic pancreas is seen in about one third of cases (RADECKI et al. 1994). The presence of calcifications and irregular ductal dilatation supports the diagnosis of acute pancreatitis superimposed on chronic pancreatitis. Focal intrapancreatic masses in pancreatitis may be due to an acute fluid collection, phlegmon, or hemorrhage. If a focal hypoechoic region is seen, however, the presence of a pancreatic neoplasm cannot be excluded.

Intrapancreatic changes in size, echogenicity, and ductal dilatation are often reliable evidence of acute pancreatitis, but they are not invariably present. Indeed, the extrapancreatic involvement may be the predominant US feature of acute pancreatitis in a significant percentage of patients (RADECKI et al. 1994). Compared with CT, US is far less precise in defining complex extrapancreatic spread along fascial planes and within retroperitoneal compartments. Moreover, most gastrointestinal and vascular complications of pancreatitis can only be diagnosed with CT.

Recently, endoscopic US was shown to be extremely helpful in a number of circumstances. This technique is as potent as CT for differentiating edematous and necrotizing pancreatitis and for identifying peripancreatic involvement. Moreover, it proved to be as sensitive as endoscopic retrograde cholangiopancreatography (ERCP) for the detection of common bile duct stones. Endoscopic US, however, is limited by poor availability and by its inability to assess the extent of inflammatory spread into the retroperitoneum (SUGIYAMA et al. 1995).

21.3
Chronic Pancreatitis

Chronic pancreatitis is a slowly progressive disease. Initially, only focal changes occur, but diffuse structural abnormalities accompanied by various degrees of functional impairment are seen in the late stage. Morphological abnormalities in chronic pancreatitis can now be detected with high accuracy by several imaging methods.

The diagnostic accuracy of US in chronic pancreatitis is reported to vary between 60% and 80% (RADECKI et al. 1994). Two points must be stressed regarding US imaging for chronic pancreatitis. First,

a high number of false-negative results can occur. This is due to the fact that a number of patients with early chronic pancreatitis can be missed by US because of morphofunctional dissociation. Second, owing to its wide use, there is also considerable risk of false-positive results, especially when too much confidence is placed in nonspecific signs, such as an heterogeneous echogenicity. US findings such as a coarse echo pattern or changes of pancreatic size in the absence of other detectable morphological abnormalities may appropriately be assigned to chronic pancreatitis only when they are accompanied by pancreatic dysfunction.

Signs on US include ductal and parenchymal changes. Ductal changes are (a) dilatation of the main duct (more than 3–4 mm); (b) irregularity of the duct; (c) increased or irregular echogenicity of the wall of the duct; and (d) intraductal stones. Parenchymal changes include: (a) gland enlargement (diffuse or focal) or atrophy; (b) irregular outer contour to the gland with lobulated margins; and (c) focal changes in parenchymal echogenicity, including echogenic foci (calcifications) within the parenchyma.

The most frequent US findings in chronic pancreatitis are the following: (a) characteristic US appearance of the disease, with irregular dilatation of the pancreatic duct, sometimes with clear-cut intraductal stones, associated with changes in parenchyma echogenicity which include calcific foci (50% of the cases); (b) isolated dilatation of the main pancreatic duct (15% of cases); and (c) focal enlargement, usually with a hypoechoic appearance mimicking a mass (5% of cases). In the remaining 30% of cases US is completely normal. In the first case, US findings may be considered, in the appropriate clinical setting, almost pathognomonic for chronic pancreatitis. In the second case, further investigation has to be scheduled: MR cholangiopancreatography may offer advantages over spiral CT as second step in this case. In the instances when focal enlargement, resembling a mass, is depicted, CT or MR imaging should be performed to differentiate focal chronic pancreatitis from adenocarcinoma. Biopsy may also be useful in doubtful cases (LENCIONI et al. 1992; DI STASI et al. 1998).

Exocrine function cannot be reliably predicted on the basis of morphologic alterations on US in most patients (MALFERTHEINER and BUCHLER 1989). US may be useful to detect complications, especially pseudocysts, which are present in about 20% of patients with chronic pancreatitis.

21.4
Ductal Adenocarcinoma

US is often the first imaging examination performed in patients presenting with jaundice. In fact, US is an excellent modality for the initial evaluation of jaundiced patients, as it allows differentiation of obstructive from nonobstructive jaundice and identification of the level of the obstruction. Definition of the cause of the obstruction is less frequently achieved with US. US is also frequently used for the initial evaluation of patients with suspected pancreatic carcinoma (YASSA et al. 1997). However, while US may be valuable in tumors of the head of the pancreas, it is far less accurate in evaluating tumors in the body and the tail because of interference from bowel gas, resulting in incomplete visualization of the gland (ARIYAMA et al. 1998a).

The US findings of pancreatic carcinoma are similar to those at CT: a focal or diffuse hypoechoic mass, enlarging the gland or deforming its contour, and dilatation of the pancreatic or biliary ducts. At this point the tumor is generally at least 2–3 cm in diameter, symptomatic, and frequently unresectable (ARIYAMA et al. 1998b). Occasionally, potentially resectable tumors may be discovered by US as biliary or pancreatic ductal dilatation without any apparent mass.

Ancillary findings suggesting malignancy, such as local spread, vascular invasion, hepatic or lymph node metastases, and ascites, can also be recognized by US (FREENY 1989). Many patients with pancreatic duct cell carcinoma have detectable hepatic metastases at their initial evaluation. However, US is far less accurate than CT in depicting extrapancreatic extension of the primary mass into surrounding fat and vascular encasement (BOLAND et al. 1999).

21.5
Cystic Neoplasms

Cystic neoplasms are an uncommon group among pancreatic tumors. Because of advances in non-invasive diagnostic procedures, these lesions are more frequently detected and surgically treated. Cystic neoplasms are currently divided into microcystic (serous) adenoma and macrocystic (mucinous) adenoma / adenocarcinoma. In addition, the entity called ductectatic mucinous cystadenoma / cystadenocarcinoma has to be considered (BAERT 1994).

The typical most common US pattern of microcystic adenomas is a solid-appearing, mild to moderately echogenic mass. Real cystic areas are rarely detected, since almost all the cysts are less than 2 mm in diameter. Less commonly, a mass with both hypoechoic and hyperechoic regions is seen (LENCIONI et al. 1991). The least common appearance is that of a multiloculated larger cyst (MATHIEU et al. 1989). Radiating septa and central scar are sometimes visible, although better appreciated on CT. Bright central echogenic foci with or without shadowing ave caused by calcification which are also better visualized on CT than on US. The combination of an echogenic solid-appearing mass on US with a hypodense contrast-enhancing honeycombed mass on CT suggests the diagnosis of serous microcystic adenoma (FRIEDMAN 1994).

On US, mucinous cystic tumors are unilocular or more often multilocular cystic masses with good through transmission and posterior wall enhancement (MATHIEU et al. 1989). The most important findings are the demonstration of internal septa separating the different cystic cavities and the possible visualization of nodular or papillary solid excrescences with irregular borders. Occasional shadowing echogenic foci, corresponding to calcification, can be identified in the wall (FRIEDMAN 1994). Contrast-enhanced CT demonstrates enhancement in the wall, septations, and solid excrescences. The proper evaluation of patients with pancreatic cystic neoplasms remains controversial so far as the distinction between mucinous cystadenoma (which, however, has malignant potential) and mucinous cystadenocarcinoma is concerned. The presence of solid excrescences on either sonography or CT correlates with a pathological diagnosis of frank mucinous cystadenocarcinoma. Needle aspiration and biopsy can be helpful in selected patients (CARLSON et al. 1998).

Ductectatic mucinous cystadenoma and cystadenocarcinoma is a recently described entity histologically identical to mucinous cystic neoplasm. It is characterized by cystic dilatation of a side branch of the duct that contains thick mucoid secretions. US and CT typically demonstrate small cystic lesions with lobulated or irregular margins located in the uncinate process. This location is an important clue to the correct diagnosis. Endoscopic or operative US gives a display of internal architecture superior to that obtained transabdominally (TAKI et al. 1997). ERCP is characteristic, showing localized cystic dilatation of a branch duct with grape-like clusters of contrast material pools. Small filling defects caused

by solid tumor nodules or mucin balls may be seen
(FRIEDMAN 1994).

21.6
Endocrine Tumors

Detection and localization of endocrine tumors frequently require the most sophisticated imaging
techniques available. Since the initial diagnosis is
based on the clinical syndrome and the elevated hormone level, the role of diagnostic imaging is to confirm that a functioning islet cell tumor is present,
define its location, judge the extent of its dissemina-
tion, and assist in postoperative follow-up (FRIED-
MAN 1994).

In general, on US examination functional pancreatic islet cell tumors tend to appear as homogeneous,
solid, round or oval well-marginated masses. Central
tumor calcification, central fluid, and large size, in
contrast, suggest malignancy (ZERBEY et al. 1996).
US is capable of showing subtle differences in pancreatic texture and can sometimes image small islet
cell tumors. However, a definite diagnosis requires
further testing with spiral CT in almost every case,
and if this is not satisfactory, with dynamic MR imaging or angiography.

References

Ariyama J, Suyama M, Satoh K, Sai J (1998a) Imaging of small
    pancreatic ductal adenocarcinoma. Pancreas 16:396–401
Ariyama J, Suyama M, Satoh K, Wakabayashi K (1998b) Endo-
    scopic ultrasound and intraductal ultrasound in the diag-
    nosis of small pancreatic tumors. Abdom Imaging 23:380–
    386
Baert AL (1994) Radiology of the pancreas: cystic tumors of
    the pancreas. Springer, Berlin Heidelberg New York, pp
    173–195
Boland GW, O'Malley ME, Saez M, Fernandez-del-Castillo C,
    Warshaw AL, Mueller PR (1999) Pancreatic-phase versus
    portal vein-phase helical CT of the pancreas: optimal tem-
    poral window for evaluation of pancreatic adenocarci-
    noma. AJR Am J Roentgenol 172:605–608
Carlson SK, Johnson CD, Brandt KR, Batts KP, Salomao DR
    (1998) Pancreatic cystic neoplasms: the role and sensitiv-
    ity of needle aspiration and biopsy. Abdom Imaging
    23:387–393
Di Stasi M, Lencioni R, Solmi L, et al (1998) US-guided biopsy
    of pancreatic masses: results of a multicenter study. Am J
    Gastroenterol 93:1329–1333
Freeny PC (1989) Radiologic diagnosis and staging of pan-
    creatic ductal adenocarcinoma. Radiol Clin North Am
    27:121–128
Friedman AC (1994) Pancreatic neoplasms and cysts. In:
    Friedman AC, Dachman AH (eds) Radiology of the liver,
    biliary tract, and pancreas. Mosby, St Louis, pp 807–934
Jeffrey RB Jr (1989) Sonography in acute pancreatitis. Radiol
    Clin North Am 27:5–17
Lencioni R, Bagnolesi P, Palla S, Cioni R (1991) Serous
    microcystic adenoma of the pancreas: a rare case of
    double location. Radiol Med 82:875–877
Lencioni R, Bagnolesi P, Cilotti A, et al (1991) Ultrasound-
    guided fine needle biopsy of the pancreas: smear cytology
    versus microhistology. Eur Radiol 2:252–257
Malfertheiner P, Buchler M (1989) Correlation of imaging
    and function in chronic pancreatitis. Radiol Clin North
    Am 27:51–64
Mathieu D, Guigui B, Valette PJ, et al (1989) Pancreatic cystic
    neoplasms. Radiol Clin North Am 27:163–175
Radecki PD, Friedman AC, Dabezies MA (1994) Pancreatitis.
    In: Friedman AC, Dachman AH (eds) Radiology of the
    liver, biliary tract, and pancreas. Mosby, St Louis, pp 763–
    805
Sugiyama M, Wada N, Atomi Y, Kuroda A, Muto T (1995) Di-
    agnosis of acute pancreatitis: value of endoscopy
    sonography. AJR Am J Roentgenol 165:867–872
Taki T, Goto H, Naitoh Y, Hirooka Y, Furukawa T, Hayakawa T
    (1997) Diagnosis of mucin-producing tumor of the pan-
    creas with an intraductal ultrasonographic system. J Ul-
    trasound Med 16:1–6
Yassa NA, Yang J, Stein S, Johnson M, Ralls P (1997) Gray-scale
    and color flow sonography of pancreatic ductal adenocar-
    cinoma. J Clin Ultrasound 25:473–480
Zerbey AL III, Lee MJ, Brugge WR, Mueller PR (1996) Endo-
    scopic sonography of the upper gastrointestinal tract and
    pancreas. AJR Am J Roentgenol 166:145–150

22 The Case for Spiral CT

V. Raptopoulos

CONTENTS

22.1   Introduction   247
22.2   Use of Spiral CT in Different Segments
        of the Pancreatobiliary System   247
22.2.1 The Liver   247
22.2.2 The Bile Ducts   248
22.2.3 The Gallbladder   248
22.2.4 The Pancreas   248
22.2.5 Lymph Nodes   249
22.2.6 Global Test   249
22.2.7 Vessels   249
22.2.8 Non-invasive Test   250
22.2.9 Interventional Procedures   250
22.3   Cost   250
22.4   Simplicity   250
22.5   Conclusion   250

22.1
Introduction

Advances in imaging have produced a plethora of noninvasive and invasive tests dealing with imaging of the bile ducts and the pancreas. These tests range from plain abdominal films to laparoscopy or endoscopy-guided ultrasound, from intravenous cholangiography to magnetic resonance cholangiopancreatography (MRCP) and virtual endoluminal CT cholangiopancreatoscopy (Table 22.1.) Some provide very specific information only, while others are more global. For example, biliary scintigraphy is a very accurate test for acute cholecystitis, but in contrast to ultrasound it does not provide images of the liver or other abdominal organs. Although most tests provide anatomic information, functional data can be provided as well. Oral cholecystography, for instance, indirectly reflects the integrity of the enterohepatic circulation of the bile, while cholecystokinin (CCK) biliary scintigraphy may give some information about sphincter of Oddi dyskinesia. Finally, when considering a test, the availability or

V. Raptopoulos, MD; Department of Radiology, Beth Israel Deaconess Medical Center and Harvard Medical School, 330 Brookline Ave., Boston, MA 02215, USA

variability of technology, the individual patient concerned, the cost and the local expertise available should be considered. For example, the latest multidetector CT platform is capable of obtaining high-resolution volumetric images of the abdomen in various vascular phases, while patients with pacemakers cannot undergo MRI. 3D volume renderings and endoluminal navigation require advanced workstations equipped with high-power computers and specialized software. Similarly, endoscopic ultrasound (EUS) may be extremely accurate in the evaluation of pancreatic head carcinoma, but requires both special equipment and high operator dexterity.

What, then, is the case for CT in diseases of the pancreas and bile ducts? In Table 22.1, the relative value of various tests is ranked on the basis of the author's experience, assessment of literature and biases: 14 modalities are ranked as to their value in assessing 12 components comprising imaging evaluation of the bile ducts and pancreas. Compared with other modalities, CT receives the highest overall rank, making it the preferred general imaging modality for the hepatobiliary and pancreatic complex.

As a general test, CT is the most inclusive modality available. It is extremely accurate in evaluating most of the components constituting pancreatobiliary investigation, and in many cases the only modality or the modality of choice. What is expected from a routine general use scanner and from the most advanced equipment is summarized in Table 22.2.

22.2
Use of Spiral CT in Different Segments of the Pancreatobiliary System

22.2.1
The Liver

Assessment of the size and shape and attenuation provides information about parenchymal abnor-

Table 22.1. Relative value and relative feasibility of diagnostic tests for hepatobiliary and pancreatic imaging (*XR* X-rays, plain radiography, *OCG* oral cholangiography, *IVC* intravenous cholangiography, *Nuc.* nuclear medicine, *US* ultrasound, *CT* computed tomography, *MRI* magnetic resonance imaging, *ERCP* endoscopic retrograde pancreatocholangiography, *EUS* endoscopic ultrasound, *PTC* percutaneous cholangiography, *Ang.* angiography, *Lap.* laparoscopy, *LUS* laparoscopic ultrasound, *Op.* operation, laparotomy)

Location	Test Noninvasive							Invasive						
	XR	OCG	IVC	Nuc.	US	CT	MRI	ERCP	EUS	PTC	Ang.	Lap.	LUS	Op.
Liver	2	2	2	2	7	8	9	2	6	2	6	7	9	8
Gallbladder	2	6	6	7	9	6	4	6	10	6	4	10	10	10
Bile ducts	2	2	6	6	7	7	9	9	8	8	2	10	9	10
Pancreas	2	0	0	4	7	9	7	6	8	0	7	6	10	10
Pancreatic duct	0	0	0	0	6	7	9	10	6	0	0	0	10	0
Lymph nodes	0	0	0	0	6	8	6	0	9	0	0	10	10	10
Global	2	0	0	0	7	10	8	4	4	0	6	9	10	10
Vessels	0	0	0	0	7	8	8	8	0	0	10	6	8	10
Noninvasive	8	8	6	8	10	8	9	6	6	4	6	2	2	0
Interventional	0	0	0	0	7	9	4	5	8	6	4	9	9	10
Low expense	10	9	9	7	8	7	6	4	3	4	3	2	1	0
Simplicity	10	10	10	8	4	10	5	2	2	2	2	0	0	0
Total	38	37	39	42	85	97	84	62	70	32	50	71	88	78

malities such as fatty infiltration (low attenuation of <35 HU) or cirrhosis (enlarged caudate and left lobes, shrunken right lobe, lobular surface). Primary or metastatic liver neoplasms are seen and characterized, as are infection and abscess.

22.2.2
The Bile Ducts

CT is accurate in the detection of intra- or extrahepatic dilatation, and in identification of the location of an obstruction. Although obstructing tumors are seen, CT is less accurate in identifying strictures, bile duct wall thickening resulting from sclerosing cholangitis or cholangiocarcinoma, and stones. Advanced imaging and image processing with CT cholangiopancreatography (CTCP) using minimum-intensity projections and virtual endoluminal CT cholangiopancreatoscopy can improve bile duct assessment, especially for strictures and intraluminal abnormalities. However, MRCP is a more accurate and straightforward test. Noncontrast thin (5 mm)-section CT can detect over 85% of bile duct stones.

Intravenous CT cholangiography with nonionic agents (popular in Europe but not available in the US) is a feasible special technique to assess biliary anatomy, but requires normal or near-normal liver function. Conversely, MRCP is not dependent on liver function and can be used in patients with obstruction. Intravenous CT cholangiography could be used before laparoscopic cholecystectomy or in live liver transplant donor candidates.

22.2.3
The Gallbladder

CT is considerably less accurate than ultrasound in detecting gallstones, the most common abnormality. Nevertheless, on a routine CT examination, at least 70% of stones should be detected, while CT is very accurate in assessing acute cholecystitis and tumors.

22.2.4
The Pancreas

CT allows accurate assessment of acute pancreatitis and its complications. It can also be used to assess

Table 22.2. Expectations of CT in the evaluation of bile ducts and pancreas

	Routine examinations	Advanced imaging
Liver	Attenuation (fat, edema, calcium, iron), cirrhosis, tumors and metastases	Biphasic techniques improve tumor detection and characterization
Bile ducts	Dilatation (less for strictures, stones)	CTCP and endoluminal cholangioscopy improves stricture, stone detection
Gallbladder	Inflammation, tumors (less for stones, chronic cholecystitis)	Intravenous CT cholangiography for normal anatomy
Pancreas	Acute and chronic pancreatitis, Pancreatic tumors (assess unresectability)	Biphasic improves carcinoma and islet cell tumor detection. CTA improves resectability assessment
Pancreatic duct	Dilatation, cause of obstruction	CTCP and virtual endoscopy may provide additional details
Lymphadenopathy	Lymph node enlargement	
Abdomen and retroperitoneum	Global information	
Vessels	Aorta, portal and hepatic veins, SMV and SMA	Spiral CT and CT-angiography provides small vessel detail, improves operative staging pancreatic carcinoma
Interventional	Biopsy, drains, ablations	CT fluoroscopy

the severity of disease and to predict outcome. CT-guided procedures are used to biopsy tumors, sample fluid collections and drain abscesses. In the case of an unresectable tumor, percutaneous biopsies can confirm the unfortunate state of affairs without adding to patient discomfort.

Pancreatic duct dilatation is shown accurately, but fine details of pancreatic duct anomalies, such as pancreas divisum, are better seen on MRCP. CTCP with minimum-intensity projections or virtual pancreatoscopy can provide some additional information, especially on the nature of strictures or cystic dilatation. This may hinder the need for additional tests if CT has to be done regardless.

22.2.5
Lymph Nodes

Routine CT examination detects peripancreatic and porta hepatic nodes. Although EUS may be more accurate for the detection of peripancreatic lymphadenopathy, CT remains the best test for detecting lymph node enlargement beyond the liver and pancreas, in the abdomen, pelvis and retroperitoneum.

22.2.6
Global Test

Other abnormalities in the abdomen are readily detected, since CT provides global regional information. For example, during scanning through the pancreas, the liver, spleen, great vessels, kidneys, spine, body wall are visualized at the same time. With ultrasound special effort is needed, while MRI may need special sequences for different organs. Most other tests are organ or abnormality specific.

22.2.7
Vessels

The acquisition of major vessel information is an integral part of contrast-enhanced CT. The patency of portal and hepatic veins is assessed, and the diagnosis of portal vein thrombosis or Budd-Chiari is easy. In addition, varices, splenic infarctions, and major vessel occlusion or dissection require no specific protocols. CT angiography provides exquisite anatomic detail that may help in vessel evaluation, tumor staging and preoperative planning.

22.2.8
Noninvasive Test

Except for exposure to nonionizing radiation and the risks associated with the use of intravenous contrast material, CT is a noninvasive test. It is very well tolerated by the patients. With modern spiral scans, the upper abdomen can be scanned during one or two breath-holds. Usual examination times have been reduced to approximately 10 min on the CT table, including data acquisition for sophisticated image processing. Similarly, advancements in computer software and improved hardware allow for quick volume rendering techniques in a fraction of the time required in early image post-processing programs. Experimental programs for direct 3D viewing are under way, which add substantially to the time available for interpretation while providing exquisite anatomic detail.

22.2.9
Interventional Procedures

A number of percutaneous interventional procedures are now available, including fine-needle aspiration (FNA) and core biopsies. Catheter drain placements and the use of taps or needle drains are everyday practice in dealing with tumors, abscesses or pancreatitis. CT Fluoroscopy has facilitated more accurate localization, and bolder techniques requiring lesser operator dexterity or less training procedures. CT can guide and monitor tumor ablation, be it with alcohol, radiofrequency or other techniques.

22.3
Cost

Although it is an expensive test, the notion that CT is substantially more expensive than US may be oversimplified. It is true that a CT scanner costs 3–4 times as much as an ultrasound machine. This may be why our institution currently houses four times as many ultrasound machines as we have CT rooms. However, we perform comparable total numbers of CT and US examinations. In contrast, while we have four fifths as many MRI machines as CT rooms, the ratio of CT to MR exams is 2:1. Thus the speed of current CT examinations and improved utilization markedly reduces the overall cost of the examinations. Furthermore, the global information provided decreases the need for many additional tests. Outcome studies are needed to study whether high utilization of the equipment and the value of the diagnoses obtained make CT more cost effective than other modalities.

22.4
Simplicity

Operating a CT scanner is simpler than operating an US machine, and much simpler than performing MRI. Modern scanners have in-programmed protocols and a number of automated tasks, including starting scanning in relationship to injection timing, or fine-tuning the mA for the patient's body habitus, which results in a decrease in the radiation exposure. In addition, CT is a simple test for the patients. Finally, the clinicians are most familiar with the highly detailed and high-resolution images, which closely resemble the actual anatomy.

22.5
Conclusion

CT provides global information on the upper abdomen. It is an accurate, informative and versatile test. The information obtained by an average image and overall study quality study far surpasses the information provided by other modalities.

23 The case for MRI

P. Pavone, A. Laghi, V. Panebianco, C. Catalano, F. Fraioli, R. Passariello

CONTENTS

23.1   Introduction *251*
23.2   Technical Improvements in MRI *251*
23.2.1 Fast Imaging *251*
23.2.2 Contrast Agents *252*
23.2.3 Magnetic Resonance
        Cholangiopancreatography *252*
23.3   Clinical Indications for MRI
        (Present and Future) *252*
23.3.1 Biliary System *252*
23.3.2 Pancreas *253*

23.1
Introduction

MR imaging (MRI) was used in the early phase mostly for applications in neuroradiology and musculoskeletal radiology. In the 1980s and early 1990s a large number of papers were published on the potential use of MRI in the upper abdomen, including the pancreas. However, no true outcome study was generated: in fact, pancreatic MRI was considered mostly useless, and CT remained the procedure of choice for evaluation of diseases of this organ. Furthermore, no potential application concerning the biliary tree was identified, and that field was considered outside the scope of MRI.

Things have changed completely in the past 5 years, owing to new technical advances. Nowadays we can image the pancreas with a spatial resolution rivaling that of spiral CT and with a definitely higher contrast resolution. Newer contrast media are being produced that are able to improve the contrast resolution of MRI in the detection of small lesions within

P. Pavone, MD; Professor, Department of Radiology, University of Parma, Via Antonio Gramsci, 14, 43100 Parma, Italy
A. Laghi, MD; V. Panebianco, MD; C. Catalano, MD; F. Fraioli, MD; R. Passariello, MD; Istituto di Radiologia – Cattedra II, Università Degli Studi di Roma "La Sapienza", Policlinico Umberto I, Viale Regina Elena, 324, I-00161 Roma, Italy

the pancreas and the liver. Moreover, the biliary tree and the pancreatic duct can be imaged with magnetic resonance cholangiopancreatography (MRCP), the only noninvasive technique that can compete with ERCP.

In this brief overview we will summarize the technical achievements that have allowed these improvements, enabling MRI to be considered as an efficient imaging modality for the diagnosis of pancreato-biliary diseases. We will outline the areas in which, in our opinion, MRI can already be proposed as a valid substitute for spiral CT.

23.2
Technical Improvements in MRI

23.2.1
Fast Imaging

The pancreas is an abdominal organ and, as such, is subject to respiratory movement. With older MRI equipment, respiratory gating procedures were used to optimize image quality. However, this resulted in blurring of anatomical contours due to signal averaging.

Currently, with high-field MRI equipment (field strength over 1 T) optimized sequences are available that allow coverage of the whole upper abdomen in a few seconds, so that imaging in one breath-hold is feasible. The spatial resolution of these images is comparable to that of spiral CT.

Moreover, one of the major advantages of MRI is its very high contrast resolution. In the pancreas even small neoplastic lesions can thus be detected because of the strong differences in signal intensity compared with the normal surrounding parenchyma. In particular, the T1 relaxation time is much longer in neoplastic tissue than in normal pancreas, so that tumors are usually well seen as hypointense lesions on T1-weighted images.

23.2.2
Contrast Agents

Despite the high intrinsic contrast, much research has been devoted to the evaluation of contrast media that are able to improve conspicuity of pancreatic tumors. Gadolinium chelates influence signal intensity in areas where the contrast medium is distributed through vascular diffusion. Carcinomas of the exocrine pancreas can be better visualized in dynamic studies, using images acquired immediately after the injection of contrast medium. They appear hypovascular compared with the normal pancreas.

Another approach is to use specific contrast media with a special tropism toward the pancreatic cells. In particular, a manganese compound (Mn-DPDP, Teslascan Nycomed), initially proposed as a hepato-biliary contrast medium, has been observed to provide high enhancement of normal pancreatic parenchyma. Further studies are needed to show that this agent really improves the diagnosis of pancreatic tumors. However, this approach seems very promising.

23.2.3
Magnetic Resonance Cholangiopancreatography

MRCP is a major breakthrough in upper abdominal MRI. This technique makes it possible to image the biliary tree and the pancreatic duct noninvasively and without the need for a contrast medium.

MRCP has become possible only recently, thanks to major advances in gradient technology. Thus, using gradient higher than 15 mT/m (versus 3–10 mT/m with earlier equipment), it has been possible to develop turbo-spin echo (consisting in a rapid repetition of 180° pulses), with very long echo times and without signal degradation. Thus, it is possible to register the high signal of fluids with prolonged T2 values (specifically bile and pancreatic juice) while completely canceling the signals from solid organs.

Using this technique, images in the upper abdomen can be obtained which demonstrate only the biliary tree and the pancreatic duct. The more the ducts are dilated, the higher is the signal obtained, leading to images of very high quality.

23.3
Clinical Indications for MRI (Present and Future)

Despite the recent technical improvements, MRI has yet to confirm its position against spiral CT. In fact, in most centers MR systems are overwhelmed by neurological and musculoskeletal examinations. The awareness of newer MR techniques takes time to reach the referring clinicians, leading to limited requests for MR examination of the biliary tree and the pancreas. Furthermore, the advantages over spiral CT are not always obvious, and radiologists prefer to stay with a technique that they feel more confident with.

The indications we propose in this chapter reflect the results of studies that have been carried out personally in our department or have been published in the literature.

23.3.1
Biliary System

Spiral CT has a relevant role in the evaluation of the biliary tree only for the diagnosis and staging of neoplastic diseases, whether intrinsic or extrinsic. MRI may substitute spiral CT in this indication, but it can also be proposed in a number of other indications in which ERCP, but not spiral CT, is of value. Thus, MRI also rivals ERCP in usefulness.

The largest area of possible indications for MRCP of the biliary tract includes benign biliary diseases. Most common benign biliary diseases are usually accompanied by mild symptoms, and the use of an invasive imaging modality such as ERCP is problematic. The first, and probably most frequent, reason for which patients are referred is evaluation for suspected stones in the common bile duct. Biliary stones are not detected on US in over 50% of cases, and the diagnosis is mostly made by ERCP. We have studied a series of patients presenting with symptoms suggestive of choledocholithiasis in whom US was negative and who were considered as candidates for ERCP. In these patients MRCP had an accuracy of over 90%, but the most interest aspect of this is that there was a prevalence of disease in only 28%. It means that only in 28% was the clinical diagnosis correct and the patient really had a bile duct stone. In the other patients there was either some other disease or no biliary involvement at all. The routine use of MRCP in this group of patients would lead to a reduction in the frequency of diagnostic ERCPs and to more accurate selection of patients for the different therapeutic approaches available.

MRCP is also very well suited to the evaluation of biliary-enteric anastomosis. In this group of patient complications occur quite frequently, and ERCP cannot be performed for anatomical reasons. MRCP can provide a complete overview of the bile ducts, showing alterations of the peripheral ducts (signs of cholangitis), stenosis of the anastomosis or the presence of stones. Only after one of these conditions has been established can therapeutic measures be undertaken.

MRCP has a highly relevant part to play in the evaluation of symptomatic patients following laparoscopic cholecystectomy. In fact, surgeons are reluctant to submit these patients to invasive imaging modalities, but at the same time they need to know what is causing the symptoms. In our series, in a selected group of patients we were able to show that in about a third of cases there were no morphological changes of the biliary tree; in another third there were residual stones in the common bile duct; whereas in the last third of patients the cause of the symptoms was a iatrogenic stenosis of the bile duct. In this group of patients the information provided by MRCP allowed us to assess the level of stenosis, providing an important clue as to what type of approach to use to dilate the stenosis (ERCP or a transhepatic approach).

MRCP has also proven to be helpful in liver transplant patients. Biliary complications may occur in such patients, but they cause symptoms or laboratory changes that are similar to those observed in chronic rejection or drug overload. In these patients either liver biopsy or biliary imaging has to be performed. With MRCP, we are now able to assess the patency of the biliary tree, especially at the level of the anastomosis. Stenosis is readily demonstrated at that level. Moreover, in our series we were able also to detect stenosis of the intrahepatic bile ducts, which was probably related to ischemic damage to the donor organ before transplantation.

Finally, another rare condition that benefits from MRCP is primary sclerosing cholangitis. In these patients ERCP or PTC (percutaneous transhepatic cholangiography) is needed to establish the diagnosis and to define the extent of biliary involvement. However, MRCP can be used to evaluate the progression of the disease in follow-up studies, thus limiting the need for repeated invasive procedures.

Neoplastic involvement of biliary disease can also be assessed consistently using MRCP. In these cases MRCP must always be performed in combination with standard MR images, providing a complete ana-tomical overview of the liver, porta hepatis, biliary tree and pancreas. Clinically, patients present with obstructive jaundice, and MRCP is performed to define the cause of the biliary obstruction. In our series MRCP had an accuracy of 94% in assessing the cause of obstructive jaundice, making it possible to differentiate benign from malignant diseases. Furthermore, MRI is useful for the staging of the neoplastic disease, providing information on local extent and liver involvement. The advantage of MRI over spiral CT consists in the fact that MRI yields images of the obstructing lesion, as CT does, and of the biliary tree, as ERCP does, but both at the same time ("one-stop shopping"). Thus, one single noninvasive examination can replace two examinations, one of which is an invasive procedure.

23.3.2
Pancreas

While the use of MRCP can easily be justified for the evaluation of the biliary tree, its routine application in pancreatic diseases may appear less straightforward at first glance. However, we are convinced that MRI and MRCP may have an important role in this sector too.

Obviously there is no role for MRI in acute pancreatitis. The data offered by contrast-enhanced spiral CT are superior in terms of evaluation of pancreatic perfusion and demonstration of complications. The same negative statement was also true until recently for chronic pancreatitis. In fact, CT allows better morphological evaluation of the pancreatic parenchyma and is very sensitive in demonstration of the presence of pancreatic calcifications, an important clue to the diagnosis of chronic pancreatitis. However, recently, thanks to the images of the pancreatic duct offered by MRCP, the role of MRI in this condition has been redefined.

With MRCP, the dilatation of the pancreatic duct is easily demonstrated and primary chronic pancreatitis can be distinguished from secondary chronic pancreatitis. Thus, pancreas divisum, duct stones, or tumors can be recognized as the cause of the pancreatic duct dilatation. Furthermore, complications related to pancreatic duct dilatation, such as pseudocysts are evident. Finally, it is possible to study the involvement of the pancreatic parenchyma, with evidence of atrophy and calcifications (spots of marked hypointensity).

All these findings allow to correctly establish the cause of chronic pancreatitis and to assess the severity of the pancreatic parenchymal involvement, in order to decide on an appropriate treatment.

Even more information can be obtained with the use of secretin. This drug stimulates pancreatic secretion, and has been used during dynamic MRCP. In the early stages of chronic pancreatitis, secretin allows demonstration of stasis of pancreatic secretion, improving the sensitivity of this technique.

In pancreatic adenocarcinoma, MRI is seldom performed as an alternative to spiral CT. However, current techniques provide a spatial resolution similar to that of spiral CT and the contrast resolution is higher. The association of MRCP images with those of MRI provides the same information as CT and ERCP in a single examination. It can be forecast that as MRI systems become more widely accessible this technique will become the standard initial procedure for the detection of pancreatic carcinoma.

MRI already has an important part to play in the detection of pancreatic islet cell tumors. These small lesions (less that 2 cm in diameter in over 80% of cases) are difficult to detect with all other imaging modalities. However, because of their long T2 relaxation times, there are much brighter than normal pancreatic tissue and thus easily recognized even without the use of contrast media on T2-weighted images. After injection of gadolinium chelates the hypervascularity characteristic of these tumors can be demonstrated. Since these tumors are rare, we believe that in patients with clinical and laboratory findings strongly suggesting the presence of such a tumor of the pancreas, MRI should be the first procedure to be performed.

24 Synthesis

C. D. Becker

CONTENTS

24.1 Introduction   255
24.2 Advantages of Spiral CT   255
24.3 Drawbacks of Spiral CT   256
24.4 Conclusions   256
References   256

24.1
Introduction

The increased speed of spiral acquisition, and particularly the ability to obtain high quality 3-D reconstructions of arteries, veins, and the biliary and pancreatic ductal system, has unquestionably enhanced the performance of CT in the evaluation of patients with suspected disorders of the bile ducts and pancreas. In order to assess the current role of CT in clinical hepatobiliary imaging in comparison with magnetic resonance imaging (MRI) and ultrasonography (US), besides technical performance we have to assess the suitability, answer some specific diagnostic questions, and consider some more general practical and economic aspects. The diagnostic key elements for the biliary system and pancreas are summarized in Table 24.1. Some controversy is inevitable, and the choice of the most appropriate imaging technique in a given situation will often depend on the clinical context, local expertise and availability of the different modalities. Nonetheless, each imaging technique has some inherent characteristics that determine its suitability in certain clinical settings. These points are addressed below.

C.D. BECKER, MD; Department of Radiology, Division of Diagnostic and Interventional Radiology, Geneva University Hospital, 24, Rue Micheli-du-Crest, CH-1211 Geneva 14, Switzerland

24.2
Advantages of Spiral CT

In any comparison of spiral CT for diagnostic imaging of the pancreas and biliary system with MRI and US, some important general features must be considered. From a practical and clinical point of view, it is an advantage of spiral CT that the diagnostic information obtained in a standard abdominal study is usually not limited to the bile ducts, pancreas, and surrounding vessels, but also covers the other intraabdominal organs. Spiral CT therefore also fulfills the role of a rapid overall screening test in patients with unexplained abdominal pain. In contrast, MRI is usually done to evaluate an organ or a limited region of the abdomen for specific pathologies by means of dedicated sequences. Compared with MRI,

Table 24.1. Diagnostic key elements

Biliary system
 Cholecystolithiasis/gallbladder disease
 Choledocholithiasis
 Presence, level and cause of bile duct dilatation
 Morphology of stenoses
 Solid masses and cysts
 Pneumobilia

Pancreas
 Pancreatic parenchyma: solid, cystic or
  hypervascular mass, lack of perfusion,
  fatty infiltration, calcifications
 Peripancreatic fatty tissue: infiltration
 Pancreatic duct: congenital abnormality, dilatation,
  stenosis, filling defects, fistula

Visceral arteries and portal vessels
 Stenosis, thrombosis, external compression of portal
 vessels, venous collaterals, arterial encasement

Duodenum
 Infiltration of duodenal wall, mass protruding into
 duodenal lumen, compression

Other
 Lymph nodes
 Other intraabdominal pathologies

---

spiral CT is much less limited by the patient's general condition and ability to cooperate. In the vast majority of institutions a spiral CT study is easier to obtain and less costly than an abdominal MRI study. Because examination protocols for spiral CT are relatively easy to standardize, the quality of studies is quite consistent, whereas technical MRI parameters of the pancreas and bile ducts vary considerably among institutions, thus leading to major variation in the quality of studies.

Ultrasonography, the most economical, most widespread and least invasive cross-sectional imaging modality, is unchallenged as the method of choice for imaging of the gallbladder and is also the most commonly used initial noninvasive imaging test for the biliary tract and pancreas. Although in principle US enables an evaluation of many elements listed in Table 24.1, its value may vary considerably depending on the operator's expertise and on patient- related technical limitations, particularly intraabdominal gas collections and obesity. Even in experienced hands, the diagnostic information provided by US will often remain incomplete.

Spiral CT is very well suited to determining the presence, level and cause of bile duct dilatation and to the demonstration of solid and cystic mass lesions. CT may also be considered as the technique of choice for pancreatic imaging in the majority of situations. CT not only provides complete demonstration of the gland regardless of bowel gas or patient habitus, but it is also very well suited to delineation of intra-and extrapancreatic masses, perfusion abnormalities and calcifications of the pancreatic parenchyma, infiltration of the peripancreatic fatty tissue, ductal dilatation and vascular involvement due to tumors and pancreatitis (RAPTOPOULOS et al. 1997). The advantages of CT angiography are discussed in a separate chapter.

24.3
Drawbacks of Spiral CT

Besides radiation exposure and side-effects and contraindications for contrast materials, some diagnostic shortcomings need to be mentioned.

Despite the excellent overall diagnostic performance of spiral CT, certain questions cannot be answered by spiral CT with sufficient accuracy. Because 15–25% of gallstones are isoattenuating with bile, the sensitivity of CT for detecting gallstones is suboptimal (BARON 1997). It is therefore generally ac-

cepted that US remains indispensable to rule out gallbladder calculi. The best sensitivity with CT for the detection of bile duct calculi has been obtained in a recent study using unenhanced spiral CT and a meticulous, dedicated protocol for scanning and image interpretation: it was reported to be 88% (NEITLICH et al. 1997). CT cholangiography may make it possible to increase the sensitivity but requires special patient preparation, and it is of limited value in patients with impaired hepatic function tests (STOCKBERGER et al. 1994). MR cholangiopancreatography (MRCP) has been shown in several recent studies to yield a sensitivity of 90–100% for bile duct stones (BECKER et al. 1997a; FULCHER et al. 1998; HOLZKNECHT et al. 1998; REINHOLD et al. 1998;). Because MRCP is independent of the excretory function and uses no contrast material, it is now considered superior to spiral CT for the detection of choledocholithiasis. MRCP may also be considered superior for delineation of the morphology of the biliary and pancreatic ducts in the presence of stenoses. Therefore, MRCP is the noninvasive imaging modality of choice for these specific indications (BECKER et al. 1997a, b; FULCHER et al. 1998). The ability to evaluate, the parenchymal organs, ductal structures and vessels at the same examination has greatly enhanced the completiveness of MR imaging in this area.

24.4
Conclusions

Spiral CT is currently the single most comprehensive and consistent imaging technique for the work-up of patients with suspected pancreatic and biliary disorders. In the vast majority of cases, the inherent drawbacks of CT, namely the need for relatively large doses of iodinated contrast material and the associated risk of side effects, will be outweighed by the benefit of the comprehensive diagnostic information obtained with CT. If gallbladder stones are suspected and CT is negative, US is indispensable as a complementary examination. MRCP is the method of choice for evaluation of bile duct stones choledocholithiasis and stenosis of the biliary and pancreatic ducts.

References

Baron RL (1997) Diagnosing choledocholithiasis: how far can we push helical CT? Radiology 203:601–603

Becker CD, Grossholz M, Mentha G, de Peyer R, Terrier F (1997a) Choledocholithiasis and bile duct stenosis: diagnostic accuracy of MR cholangiopancreatography. Radiology 205:523–530

Becker CD, Grossholz M, Mentha G, de Peyer R, Terrier F (1997b) MR cholangiopancreatography: technique, potential indications, and diagnostic features of benign, postoperative, and malignant conditions. Eur Radiol 7:865–874

Fulcher AS, Turner MA, Capps GW, Zfass AM, Baker KM (1998) Half-Fourier RARE MR cholangiopancreatography: experience in 300 subjects. Radiology 207:21–32

Holzknecht N, Gauger J, Sackmann M, et al (1998) Breath-hold MR cholangiography with snapshot techniques: prospective comparison with endoscopic retrograde cholangiography. Radiology 206:657–664

Neitlich JD, Topazian M, Smith RC, Gupta A, Burrell MI, Rosenfield AT (1997) Detection of choledocholithiasis: comparison of unenhanced helical CT and endoscopic retrograde cholangiopancreatography. Radiology 203:753–757

Raptopoulos V, Steer ML, Sheiman RG, Vrachliotis TG, Gougoutas CA, Movson JS (1997) The use of helical CT and CT angiography to predict vascular involvement from pancreatic cancer : correlation with findings at surgery. AJR Am J Roentgenol 168:871–977

Reinhold C, Taourel P, Bret PM, et al (1998) Choledocholithiasis: evaluation of MR cholangiography for diagnosis. Radiology 209:435–442

Urinary Tract

25 Tailoring the Imaging Protocol

H. Genghis Khan, F. Terrier

CONTENTS

25.1 Introduction 261
25.2 Technique for Image Acquisition
and Scanning Parameters 263
25.3 The Tailored Renal Scan 264
25.3.1 Detection, Characterization and Staging
of a Renal Mass 264
25.3.2 Acute Flank Pain 264
25.3.3 Diseases of the Urinary Tract 266
25.3.4 CT Angiography 266
References 267

25.1 Introduction

Spiral computed tomography (CT) of the kidneys is becoming the state of the art for evaluation of renal diseases (Holmes et al.1997; Kauczor 1994a, b; Rubin 1996a, b; Rubin and Silverman 1995; Smith et al. 1998; Wyatt et al. 1995a, b). Conventional CT has certain limitations. Variable patient respiration causes motion artifacts, which degrade image quality, and gaps in scanning, which may lead to failure in imaging portions of the kidneys. Partial volume can result in inaccurate attenuation measurements and hinder the evaluation of subtle features. Owing to the slow speed of the scanning sequence, studies are not possible during the early phase of renal enhancement (cortical phase), and long acquisition times do not allow multiphasic renal imaging. With spiral CT, data are continuously acquired from a volume during a single breath-hold, providing excellent quality images without respiratory misregistration and partial volume effects. A recent study comparing low-mA, 1.5 pitch helical CT and conventional CT showed that the radiation dose saving to the patient is significant in the former and there appears to be little degradation of image quality (Hopper et

H. Genghis Khan, MD; Department of Radiology, University Hospital of Geneva, CH-1211 Geneva 14, Switzerland
F. Terrier, MD; Department of Radiology, University Hospital of Geneva, CH-1211 Geneva 14, Switzerland

al.1998). With a pitch of 1.5, a radiation saving of 34% can be achieved (King and Miller 1993). Using high-speed spiral CT, the kidneys can be studied at different phases of contrast enhancement after bolus injection of contrast medium. Four distinct phases can be defined (Yuh 1997). Baseline precontrast images are obtained before intravenous injection of contrast media. Density measurements of renal masses or cysts, urolithiasis, and renal calcifications are performed.

The arterial or cortical phase (CP) occurs approximately between 25 and 80 s after the initiation of intravenous contrast medium administration (Yuh and Cohan, 1997). Contrast medium fills the cortical capillaries and the proximal convoluted tubules. During this phase the corticomedullary differentiation is excellent because of the significant difference in attenuation between the renal cortex, where enhancement is intense, and the medulla, which enhances to a lesser degree (Fig. 25.1A). The difference in attenuation approaches 100 HU (Cohan et al. 1995). According to the literature this phase does not allow accurate detection of small renal masses(<3 cm) (Yuh 1997). Asymmetry in enhancement helps in the diagnosis of renal artery stenosis, renal vein thrombosis, and renal obstruction (Wyatt et al. 1995a). Vascular anomalies such as arteriovenous malformations and renal artery aneurysms can be diagnosed. The CP images demonstrate the location and number of renal arteries and renal vein patency. Moreover, this phase is useful for creating 3D images of the renal vasculature. CT angiography (CTA) is evolving rapidly into a clinically useful tool for vascular imaging (Bluemke and Chambers 1995; Chernoff et al. 1994; Dorffner et al. 1998; Galanski et al. 1993; Lin et al. 1998; Michel et al. 1996; Quillin et al. 1996; Rubin 1996; Rubin et al.1994; Smith et al. 1998a, b; Urban and Fishman 1998). The generated dataset can be reformatted into multiplanar reconstructions or rendered into three-dimensional (3D) images of the vasculature. Such 3D images are useful in the diagnosis of renal artery stenosis (RAS) and for better

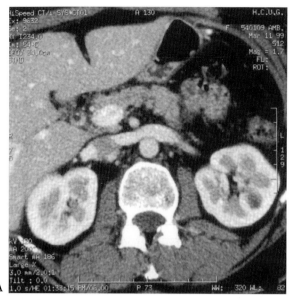 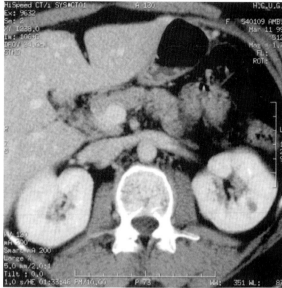

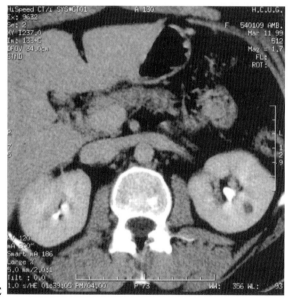

Fig. 25.1A–C. Normal contrast enhanced renal spiral CT showing different phases of enhancement. A Cortical phase (CP.) Note the excellent differentiation between the cortex and medulla. A simple renal cyst is also seen. B Nephrographic phase (NP). Homogeneous enhancement of the renal parenchyma. C Excretory phase (EP). Contrast medium is present in the infundibula and calices

definition of the extent of renal masses and for planning nephron-sparing surgery. They also facilitate the transmission of information to the clinicians and improve the demonstration of key anatomic relationships (BLUEMKE and CHAMBERS 1995).

The nephrographic phase (NP) occurs approximately between 80–120 s after contrast medium injection (YUH and COHAN, 1997) and is characterized by an increase in the attenuation of the medulla and a decrease in the attenuation of the cortex. The difference in attenuation between the cortex and the medulla is minimal, usually less than 10 HU (COHAN et al. 1995), and the entire renal parenchyma is homogeneously enhanced (Fig. 25.1B). Several studies

have shown that this phase is the most accurate for identifying small renal masses (CHERNOFF et al. 1994; KAUCZOR et al. 1994; MIELE et al. 1998; WILDBERGER et al. 1997; WYATT et al. 1995a, b).

The NP is an important indicator of functional and structural renal disease. The anomalies of the nephrogram can be readily seen by CT. Unilateral global absence of enhancement is seen in cases of blunt trauma with renal pedicle injury. Segmental absence of enhancement is seen with infarction and is most often due to arterial emboli. Global persistence of the nephrogram may be unilateral (in cases of renal artery stenosis, renal vein thrombosis, or urinary tract obstruction) or bilateral (systemic hypotension, intratubular obstruction, or abnormalities in tubular function). The striated nephrogram (unilateral or bilateral) may be the result of acute renal obstruction, acute pyelonephritis, hypotension, contusion, renal vein thrombosis, and autosomal recessive polycystic kidney disease. The cortical rim sign is seen with renal infarction and occasionally with acute tubular necrosis, and renal vein thrombosis (SAUNDERS et al. 1995).

The excretory phase (EP) begins within 2–5 min of contrast medium administration (YUH and COHAN, 1997). The calyces, infundibula and the renal pelvis are opacified by the excreted contrast medium (Fig. 25.1C). The nephrogram is homogenous but the attenuation of the parenchyma is lower than during the NP. Filling defects within the collecting system, such as calculi and tumors, can readily be detected during this phase.

The changes with time in renal parenchymal and vascular enhancement (Fig. 25.2) can be exploited to study renal physiology as shown by time–density curve. Both global and regional function and urinary filtration can be evaluated by CT (BLOMELY 1996).

During the routine evaluation of the abdomen the contrast-enhanced images of the kidneys are usually obtained during the late cortical phase or at an intermediate point between the CP and NP, which can create problems in scan interpretation. In such cases it is preferable to refer the patient for a dedicated renal CT at a future date. Not all phases are required in the routine evaluation of the kidneys. The examination has to be tailored to the diagnostic clinical problem.

25.2
Technique for Image Acquisition and Scanning Parameters

For helical renal CT thin collimation (equivalent to slice thickness) combined with slow table translation and thin reconstruction intervals produce images with the lowest degree of volume-averaging artifacts (SMITH et al. 1998a). Collimator width varies between 3 mm and 5 mm, table speed between 3 and 5 mm/s, and the reconstruction increment between 2 mm and 5 mm. The section sensitivity profile is slightly larger than for nonhelical sections but the slice broadening appears insignificant when using 180° linear interpolation (POLACIN and MARCHAL 1992b).

A nonenhanced scan is obtained with 5-mm collimated images obtained at a pitch of 1:1 using 120 kV and 220 mA. For an enhanced CT study, the kidneys are scanned with a pitch of 1.5–1.6. Certain investigators inject a mini-test bolus of 20 ml at a rate of 3–4 ml/s in order to optimize selection of the sequence timing. Then approximately 150 ml(2–3 ml/kg) of 240–300 mgI/ml of nonionic contrast is administered through an antecubital vein via a power injector at rates varying between 3 and 5 ml/s. The injection is monophasic. Oral contrast medium (or water) is administered in cases of staging of renal cell carcinoma, in order to differentiate bowel loops from retroperitoneal adenopathies.

Patient cooperation is essential to generate good-quality reconstructions, because patient motion de-

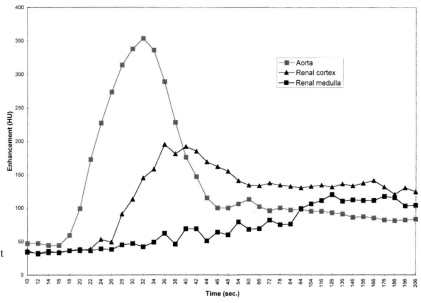

Fig. 25.2. Tissue–density curve after injection of 60 ml of Ultravist 300 (Schering, Berlin) at a rate of 3 ml/s. Note typical aortic, renal cortical and renal medullary curves

grades reconstructed images. The patient is encouraged to hyperventilate prior to the study in order to obtain proper breath-hold during the study. Usually a 20- to 30-s breath-hold is required to obtain motion-free images.

The acquired data can be sent to a freestanding workstation for interactive review and for multiplanar reconstructions in the coronal, sagittal, and oblique planes. Editing is performed to eliminate unwanted soft tissue and bony structures. This permits a clear depiction of the vascular anatomy. Generation of the multiplanar volume reconstructions takes little longer than axial imaging. Images in an oblique or curved coronal plane are useful in defining normal vascular anatomy and detecting vascular involvement by tumor. The data can also be analyzed in cine mode, which is a sensitive way of distinguishing small vessels and following their course (GARTENSCHLAGER et al. 1996). The multiplanar reconstructions are rendered in several forms. Algorithms such as Surface Shaded Display (SSD) or Maximum Intensity Projection (MIP) can be used to create a 3D display. SSD renders structures with attenuation in an arbitrary threshold range, in which the gray scale encodes surface reflections from an imaginary source of illumination (RUBIN et al. 1994). In the MIP rendering, the gray scale reflects CT attenuation, and materials of different attenuation can thus be differentiated. One can thus distinguish between intraarterial contrast medium, vascular calcification and perfused renal parenchyma. Although most radiologists read axial images and use planar images to confirm anomalies or to display them better, several recent studies show that the reformatted images yield important additional information in some cases (MCNICHOLAS et al. 1998; URBAN 1998).

A supine kidney-urinary bladder (KUB) film is obtained systematically after each contrast-enhanced study. It allows examination of the intrarenal collecting system and the entire length of the ureters.

25.3
The Tailored Renal Scan

As described before, a dedicated renal CT is conducted differently than a routine abdominal scan. Moreover, the typical scanning parameters vary according to the clinical question. Helical scanning of renal trauma will not be addressed, as it will be discussed elsewhere.

25.3.1
Detection, Characterization and Staging of a Renal Mass

CT is the modality of choice for the diagnosis and staging of renal tumors. Spiral CT is also useful for assessment of treatment results and in detecting recurrence (YUH 1997). The CT scans are obtained as part of a triphasic CT renal protocol that includes unenhanced imaging, and imaging in both nephrographic and excretory phases.

The study begins with a nonenhanced scan. If density measurements are between 0 and 20 HU and if after administration of contrast medium the enhancement noted is less than 12 HU, then the diagnosis of a cyst can be made confidently. A mass with attenuation values that increase more than 12 HU after contrast is suspicious for renal cell carcinoma (RCC) (SMITH et al, 1998). Spiral CT shows extension of the tumor to the renal vein and the inferior vena cava as well as the development of collateral vasculature. Locoregional nodal metastases as well as secondary lesions of liver, bone and lung can be detected by CT.

Spiral CT provides many advantages in the study of renal cysts, especially in the differential diagnosis between benign complicated cyst and cystic renal cell carcinoma. It can visualize the margins or walls of cystic lesions with great precision. Malignancy should be suspected when the wall and the septations are thick (>1 mm), and are associated with solid and enhancing elements (WYATT et al. 1995a, b).

The complications of polycystic kidney disease such as cyst hemorrhage, and calculi can be readily detected by spiral CT.

For the contrast-enhanced CT the field of view is centered on the kidneys (approx. 15 cm) but can be extended to the liver if a renal mass is discovered. The images are acquired in the nephrographic phase(90 s), and in the excretory phase (180 s) (It should ne noted that the cortical phase is less sensitive than the nephrographic phase for detection of a renal mass, so that it is not routinely performed). The images are reconstructed at 1.5- to 3-mm intervals when small renal masses are being assessed (10 mm or less in diameter). Multiplanar reconstructions can be performed if needed. These help in differentiating an adrenal mass from a renal mass.

25.3.2
Acute Flank Pain

The nonenhanced CT or Uro-CT plays an important role in patients suspected of having renal colic (Gaucher et al. 1998; Hubert et al. 1997; Katz et al. 1997; Liberman et al. 1997; Preminger et al. 1998; Yilmaz et al. 1998). The site and cause of urinary obstruction can be diagnosed without injection of intravenous contrast medium Thus, patients with allergy to iodinated contrast media, those in renal failure or with nonfunctioning kidneys are examined rapidly by spiral CT. In cases of suspected renal colic, spiral CT is more effective than intravenous urography (IVU) in identifying intra-ureteric stone and as effective as intravenous urography (IVU) in determining whether there is renal obstruction (Fielding et al. 1997; Fink et al. 1994; Katz et al. 1997; Liberman et al. 1997; Yilmaz et al. 1998). Small calculi can be detected with improved sensitivity. Even stones that are radiolucent on radiographs are readily identified on CT. According to an in-vitro study by Olcott and Napel (1997), 3D spiral CT enables highly accurate determination of the volume and dimensions of renal calculi and provide valuable information for planning treatment in patients with nephrolithiasis.

The field of view is centered on the kidneys and retroperitoneum (approx. 30 cm). The reconstruction increment varies between 4 and 5 mm. A calculus, because of its high density, is well defined against the nonopacified collecting system and ureter. Residual calculi after shock-wave lithotripsy are readily assessed (Figs. 25.3, 25.4).

An enhanced CT is done in cases of renal colic when causes other than lithiasis are suspected. Images are acquired in the nephrographic phase 100 seconds after the injection or in the excretory phase 180 s after the injection. For some authors early signs of acute pyelonephritis can be seen during the CP with loss of normal corticomedullary differentiation and delayed appearance of the cortical nephrogram (Wyatt et al. 1995a). In our institution we prefer NP or EP images which demonstrate focal areas of striated or wedge-shaped perfusion abnormalities, which result in a patchy nephrogram. Small foci of abscesses can be demonstrated and their thickened irregular enhancing wall characterized by spiral CT. The CP is useful sometimes for characterization of renal pseudotumors which can resemble a renal mass on sonography (dromedary hump, sequelae of pyelonephritis with associated cortical scarring and hyperplasia). Multiplanar reconstructions help dis-

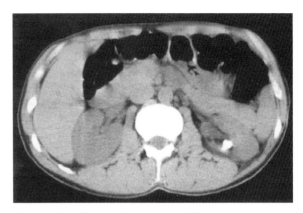

Fig. 25.3. Uro-CT (unenhanced renal CT). Residual calculi after short-wave lithotripsy are seen in the middle left renal calyx

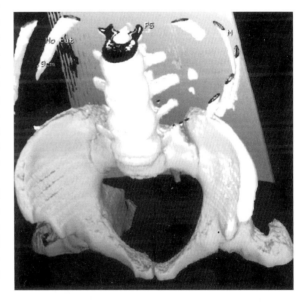

Fig. 25.4. Same patient as in Fig. 25.5. 3D coronal oblique projection revealing residual stones in the left middle and inferior renal calyx

criminate normal variants such as a prominent column of Bertin or dromedary hump from a renal mass.

25.3.3
Diseases of the Urinary Tract

Abnormalities of the ureter and periureteral area are often visible on CT in many different disease processes that affect the ureter primarily or secondarily (Berchtold et al. 1998).

Transitional-cell carcinomas of the ureters are usually suspected on an IVU study. A dedicated spiral CT confirms the diagnosis and allows local staging (Figs. 25.5, 25.6). The sensitivity of CT is similar to that of retrograde pyelography. Most often the tumor presents as sessile intraluminal filling defects. Besides, CT reveals the extraureteral soft-tissue extension and nodal involvement (WINALSKI and TUMEH 1990). Fungus balls and blood clots do not show any change in density after injection of contrast medium.

The CT examination is biphasic and begins with a nonenhanced study. Then a contrast-enhanced study with a narrow collimation of 3 mm and images in the EP with a time delay of 4 min to several hours are acquired if obstruction is present. The field of view is of approximately 40 cm covering the kidneys, the retroperitoneum, and pelvis.

The reconstruction increment varies between 2 and 3 mm. If the contrast medium in the urinary tract is too dense, the images have to be displayed at a wider window setting than that used for routine scans. Multiplanar reconstructions are extremely useful in showing the site of obstruction and the repercussion on the urinary tract. The collecting system can be displayed in a planar format similar to that of the IVU (Fig. 25.7). 3D display of helical CT data provides a noninvasive method for evaluating bladder cancer. It is complementary to cystoscopy for evaluating the bladder base, tumor mapping before transurethral resection and post-chemotherapy evaluation (NARUMI et al.1996).

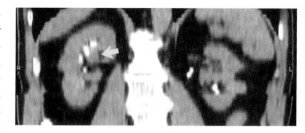

Fig. 25.6. Transitional cell carcinoma. Coronal reformatted image of Fig. 25.7, showing a filling defect (*arrow*) in the pelvis and infundibula of the upper group calices of the right kidney

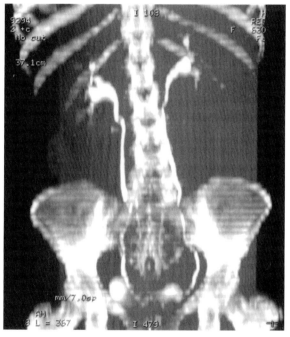

Fig. 25.7. Contrast enhanced 3D coronal reconstruction. Note perfect visualization of normal pelvi-calical and ureteral anatomy

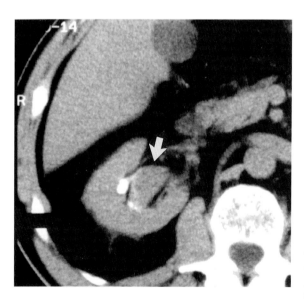

Fig. 25.5. Transitional cell carcinoma. EP CT, revealing a filling defect (*arrow*) in the renal pelvis

25.3.4
CT Angiography

CT Angiography (CTA) has emerged as a minimally invasive tool for exploring the aorta and its branches. CTA is replacing conventional angiography in many applications in the abdomen (POZNIAK 1998). It is particularly useful for the detection of renal artery stenosis, tumor involvement of major vessels, and extent of abdominal aortic aneurysm. The advantages of CTA relative to that of angiography are that it allows an evaluation of the arterial lumen and wall, depicts the parenchyma, and does not need an arterial puncture which can be a source of morbidity. CTA reduces the duration of work-up to one day and results in substantial cost reduction. The spiral CT dataset provides a reliable, non-invasive screening method for detecting renal artery stenosis (RAS) (BLUEMKE and CHAMBERS 1995; BRINK 1997; DORFFNER et al. 1998; GALANSKI et al. 1993; LIN et al. 1998). It accurately depicts normal and accessory renal arteries. The diagnostic accuracy of CTA is similar to that of angiography (OLBRICHT et al. 1995). Both axially displayed images and 3D views allow accurate diagnosis of RAS. MIP is more accurate than SSD in grading RAS with respect to conventional angiography (RUBIN 1996; RUBIN et al. 1994; GALANSKI et al. 1993; SMITH et al. 1998b).

Proper surgical planning in ureteropelvic junction disease requires a search for anatomic variants in renal blood supply such as crossing vessels. CTA has a similar accuracy to arteriography in this regard, although moreover it is a less invasive and less expensive alternative (QUILLIN et al. 1996; PFISTER et al. 1997; WOLF et al. 1996). The sensitivity and specificity of CTA in the preoperative evaluation of potential living related donors regarding normal anatomy is comparable to digital subtraction angiography (DSA) (POZNIAK et al. 1998).

CTA is useful in planning nephron-sparing surgery, because it shows the resectability of the latter in evaluating its relationship to the parenchyma and the hilum (CHERNOFF et al. 1994].

The study protocol is triphasic and begins with unenhanced scout images from the top of the L1 vertebral body to the bottom of the L3 vertebral body with 8 mm collimation in order to localize the area to be covered. A test bolus is used to define the scanning delay. It is obtained at a single location above the target site and a time-density curve is generated. The time to peak attenuation in the aorta determines the scanning delay. The time delay from the start of contrast medium injection to initiation of image acquisition ranges from 12 s to 25 s with a mean of 18 s (RUBIN et al.1994).

Breath-hold contrast-enhanced CT is performed during the cortical phase. To produce high quality 3D display and 3D datasets, a 3-mm collimation, minimal table speed and reconstruction increment of 2 mm are required (RUBIN 1996; POZNIAK et al. 1998). The field of view is about 30 cm, beginning at the level of the superior mesenteric artery and covering the kidneys and the retroperitoneum up to the aortic bifurcation. Multiplanar reconstruction and 3D reformatting are an essential part of the study. Many authors believe that 3D images demonstrate complex extrahilar renal vascular anatomy better than the 2D images (SMITH et al. 1998a; RUBIN 1996; POZNIAK et al. 1998).

At the end of the arterial phase delayed images are obtained during the nephrographic phase covering the area between the diaphragm and the iliac crests with a 10-mm collimation and a 1:1 pitch. They are needed to study the renal parenchyma and if necessary the collecting system.

References

Berchtold RB, Chen MY, Dyer RB, Zagoria RJ (1998) CT of the ureteral wall. AJR Am J Roentgenol 170:1283–1289

Blomely MJ, Dawson P (1996) The quantification of renal function with enhanced computed tomography (review). Br J Radiol 69:989–995

Bluemke DA, Chambers TP (1995) Spiral CT angiography: an alternative to conventional angiography (editorial comment). Radiology 195:317–319

Brink JA (1997) Spiral CT angiography of the abdomen and pelvis: interventional applications. Abdom Imaging 22:365–372

Chernoff DM, Silverman SG, Kidinis R, et al (1994) Three-dimensional imaging and display of renal tumors using spiral CT: a potential aid to partial nephrectomy. Urology 43:125–129

Cohan RH , Sherman LS, Korobkin M, Bass JC, et al (1995) Renal masses: assessment of corticomedullary phase and nephrographic phase CT scans. Radiology 196:445–451

Dorffner R, Thurner S, Prokesch R, Youssefzadeh S, Holzenbein T, Lammer J (1998) Spiral CT during selective accessory renal artery angiography: assessment of vascular territory before aortic stent-grafting. Cardiovasc Intervent Radiol 27:179–182

Fielding JR, Steele G, Fox LA, Heller H, Loughlin KR (1997) Spiral computerized tomography in the evaluation of acute flank pain: a replacement for excretory urography. J. Urol 157:2071–2073

Fink BK, Fink U, Pentenrieder M, Kohz P, Englmeier HK, Schmeller N (1994) The technic and value of the 3-dimensional imaging of renal calyx staghorn calculi with spiral CT. Rofo Fortschr Geb Rontgenstr Neuen Bildgeb Verfahr 16:66–94

Galanski M, Prokop M, Chavan A, Schaefer CM, Jandeleit K, Nischelsky JE (1993) Renal arterial stenoses: spiral CT angiography. Radiology 189:185–192

Gartenschlager M, Anders M, Schweden F, Neufang A, Leissner J, Thelen M (1996) Infarct of the lower renal artery segment: diagnosis with CT-angiography and 3-dimensional spatial representation. Aktuelle Radiol 6:334–337

Gaucher O, Hubert J, Blum A, Regent D, Mangin P (1998) Evaluation of spiral computed tomography in the demonstration of kidney stones. Ex vivo study. Prog Urol 8:347–351

Holmes NM, McBroom S, Puckett ML, Kane CJ (1997) Renal imaging with spiral CT scan: clinical applications. Techn Urol 3:202–208

Hopper KD, Kasales CJ, Mahraj R, et al (1998) Utility of low mA 1.5 pitch helical CT versus conventional high mA abdominal CT. Clin Imaging 22:54–59

Hubert J, Blum A, Cormier L, Claudon M, Regent D, Mangin P (1997) Three-dimensional CT-scan reconstruction of renal calculi. A new tool for mapping-out staghorn calculi and follow-up of radiolucent stones. Eur Urol 31:297–301

Katz DS, Lane MJ, Sommer FG (1997) Non-contrast spiral CT for patients with suspected renal colic. Eur Radiol 7:680–685

Kauczor HU, Schwickert HC, Albers P, Voges G, Schweden F (1994) Possibilities and limitations of spiral-CT in the study of cancer of the kidney pelvis. Rofo Fortschr Geb Rontgenstr Neuen Bildgeb Verfahr 160:329–333

Kauczor HU, Schwickert HC, Schweden F, Schild HH, Thelen M (1994) Bolus-enhanced renal spiral CT: technique, diagnostic value and drawbacks. Eur J Radiol 18:153–157

King SH, Reynolds MD, Miller KL (1993) Surface dose comparison for spiral and axial scanning with use of a fourth-generation CT system. Radiology 189[P]:356

Liberman SN, Halpern EJ, Sullivan K, Bagley DH (1997) Spiral computed tomography for staghorn calculi. Urology 50:519–524

Lin YP, Wu MH, Ng YY, et al (1998) Spiral computed tomographic angiography – a new technique for evaluation of vascular access in hemodialysis patients. Am J Nephrol 18:117–122

McNicholas MM, Rastopoulos VD, Schwartz RK, Sheiman RG, et al (1998) Excretory phase CT urography for opacification of the urinary collecting system. AJR Am J Roentgenol 170:1261–1267

Michel LA, Lacrosse M, Decanniere L, et al (1996)Blunt renal traumas: contribution of spiral CT with three dimensional reconstruction to the surgical decision process? Int Surg 81:377–381

Miele V, Galluzzo M, Bellussi A, Valenti M (1998) Spiral computerized tomography in the study of renal neoplasms in children. Radiol Med (Torino) 95:486–492

Narumi YK, Sawai Y, Kuroda C, et al (1996) The bladder and bladder tumors: imaging with three dimensional display of helical CT data. AJR Am J Roentgenol 167:1134–1135

Olbricht CJ PK, Prokop M, Chavan A, et al (1995) Minimally invasive diagnosis of renal artery stenosis by spiral computed tomography angiography. Kidney Int 48:1332–1337

Olcott EW SF, Napel S (1997) Accuracy of detection and measurement of renal calculi: in vitro comparison of three-dimensional spiral CT, radiography, and nephrotomography. Radiology 204:19–25

Pfister C, Thoumas D, Simon I, Benozio M, Grise P (1997) Value of helical CT scan in the preoperative assessment of the ureteropelvic junction syndrome. Prog Urol 7:594–599

Polacin AK, Kalendar WA (1994) Evaluation of spiral resolution and noise in spiral CT. Radiology 193:170

Polacin AKW, Marchal G (1992) Evaluation of section sensi-

tivity profiles and image noise in spiral CT. Radiology 185:29–35

Pozniak MA, Balison DJ, Lee FT, Tambeaux RH, et al (1998) CT angiography of potential renal transplant donors. Radiographics 18:565–587

Preminger GM, Vieweg J, Leder RA, Nelson RC (1998) Urolithiasis: detection and management with unenhanced spiral CT – a urologic perspective (editorial). Radiology 207:308–309

Quillin SP, Brink JA, Heiken JP, Siegel CL, McClennan BL, Clayman RV (1996) Helical (spiral) CT angiography for identification of crossing vessels at the ureteropelvic junction. AJR Am J Roentgenol 166:1125–1130

Rubin GD (1996) Spiral (helical) CT of the renal vasculature. Semin Ultrasound CT MR 17:374–397

Rubin GD, Silverman SG (1995) Helical CT of the retroperitoneum. Radiol Cin North Am 33:302–332

Rubin GD, Dake MD, Napel S, et al (1994) Spiral CT of renal artery stenosis: comparison of three-dimensional rendering techniques. Radiology 190:181--189

Saunders HS, Dyer RB, Shifrin RY, Scharling ES, et al (1995) The CT nephrogram: implications for evaluation of urinary tract disease; Discussion. Radiographics 15:1069–1085; 1086–1088

Smith PA, Marshall FF, Fishman EK (1998) Spiral computed tomography evaluation of the kidneys: state of the art. Urology 51:3–11

Smith PA, Ratner LE, Lynch FC, Corl FM, Fishman EK (1998) Role of CT angiography in the preoperative evaluation for laparoscopic nephrectomy. Radiographics 51:3–11

Urban BA, Fishman EK (1998) Helical CT with multiplanar display: role in evaluation and clarification of complex renal pathology. J Comput Assist Tomogr 22:548–554

Wildberger JE, Adam G, Boeckmann W, et al (1997) Computed tomography characterization of renal cell tumors in correlation with histopathology. Invest Radiol 32:596–601

Winalski CS, L J, Tumeh SS (1990) Ureteral neoplasms. Radiographics 10:271–283

Wolf JS Jr, Siegel CL, Brink JA, Clayman RV (1996) Imaging for ureteropelvic junction obstruction in adults. J Endourol 10:93–104

Wyatt SH, Urban BA, Fishman EK (1995) Spiral CT of the kidneys: role in characterization of renal disease. I. Non-neoplastic disease. Crit Rev Diagn Imaging 36:1–37

Wyatt SH, Urban BA, Fishman EK (1995) Spiral CT of the kidneys: role in characterization of renal disease. II. Neoplastic disease. Crit Rev Diagn Imaging 36:39–72

Yilmaz S, Sindel T, Arslan G, et al (1998) Renal colic: comparison of spiral CT, US and IVU in the detection of ureteral calculi. Eur Radiol 8:212–217

Yuh BI, Cohan RH (1997) Helical CT for detection and characterization of renal masses. Semin Ultrasound CT MR 18:82–90

26 Spiral CT of Renal Perfusion Abnormalities

M.J. Lane, R. Brooke Jeffrey

CONTENTS

26.1   Introduction   269
26.2   Spiral CT Technique for Evaluation
        of Renal Perfusion   269
26.3   Normal Patterns of Renal Contrast
        Enhancement   270
26.4   Spiral CT Diagnosis of Abnormal Arterial
        Inflow   270
26.5   Renal Parenchymal Perfusion Disorders   273
26.6   Perfusion Abnormalities Secondary
        to Renal Vein Thrombosis   274
26.7   Perfusion Defects Secondary to Renal
        Obstruction   275
        References   276

26.1
Introduction

Contrast-enhanced spiral CT is an ideal method for the evaluation of renal perfusion. The ability to visualize the kidney during multiple phases of contrast enhancement facilitates the diagnosis of abnormalities of major arterial inflow, segmental perfusion and global excretion. This chapter will focus on the spiral CT technique and interpretation of disorders of renal perfusion. Specific emphasis will be directed at understanding of the temporal progression of renal contrast enhancement as an aid to the evaluation of renovascular and parenchymal perfusion disorders.

M.J. Lane, MD; Department of Radiology, Stanford University Medical Center, 300 Pasteur Drive, H-1307, Stanford, CA 94305–5105, USA
R. Brooke Jeffrey, Jr., MD; Department of Radiology, Stanford University Medical Center, 300 Pasteur Drive, H-1307, Stanford, CA 94305–5105, USA

26.2
Spiral CT Technique for Evaluation of Renal Perfusion

Optimal evaluation of renal perfusion with spiral CT requires careful attention to intravenous contrast injection and technical scanning parameters. Important factors affecting image quality include: the rate and volume of intravenous contrast, scan collimation, pitch and breath-held scan acquisition (Rubin and Napel 1995). It is equally important to obtain images routinely during early (corticomedullary or nephrographic) and late (excretory) phases of contrast enhancement.

Renal abnormalities are often visualized incidentally as part of a routine survey evaluation of the upper abdomen. Therefore, a specific renal protocol is not often utilized for these screening studies. The standard spiral CT technique for imaging the upper abdomen is typically performed only with intravenous contrast material. Preliminary noncontrast scans, which are essential for accurate diagnosis of renal stones and masses, are not obtained with this scanning protocol. Furthermore, the typical scan collimation of 7–8 mm may not be optimal to evaluate small (<2 cm) renal lesions.

Most survey spiral CT examinations of the upper abdomen are performed during the portal venous phase to maximize hepatic enhancement. Scans are obtained 60–70 s after initiation of the contrast bolus. The renal parenchyma is imaged in the corticomedullary phase during these survey examinations. Both renal masses and segmental perfusion abnormalities are suboptimally evaluated in the corticomedullary phase. Therefore, it is mandatory in all patients that delayed images be routinely obtained 3–4 min after contrast injection to evaluate renal perfusion and excretion with a second spiral acquisition through the kidneys. Seven-millimeter collimation is usually sufficient for the delayed spiral scan unless a small renal mass is suspected. In this instance 3- to 5-mm scans should be obtained.

For patients with known or suspected renal parenchymal pathology, a dedicated renal "triple phase" examination with narrow collimation is optimal. Preliminary noncontrast scans are performed with a breath-held spiral acquisition using 5-mm collimation and a pitch of 1:1. Noncontrast scans are essential for identification of renal calcifications and to define a baseline attenuation for evaluation of renal masses. Following a 60-s delay from the start of a bolus injection (150 ml of 60% nonionic contrast material injected at 2.5 ml per s) a 30-s breath-held spiral acquisition is performed during the late corticomedullary phase and early nephrographic phase. Delayed images with a 5-mm spiral acquisition are then performed at 3–4 min after contrast injection during the excretory phase.

26.3
Normal Patterns of Renal Contrast Enhancement

The appearance of normal renal perfusion on spiral CT is dependent upon the timing of image acquisition following administration of the contrast bolus. The CT appearance of the nephrogram is based upon the distinct phases after intravenous administration of contrast material. These phases include: the cortical arteriogram (vascular phase), the cortical nephrogram (corticomedullary phase), the tubular nephrogram (nephrographic phase) and the excretory phase (BOIJSEN 1983). The majority of routine spiral CT scans are taken during the corticomedullary nephrogram phase of renal enhancement. This phase begins 30–45 s after intravenous contrast injection (BOIJSEN 1983; HATTERY et al. 1988; ISHIKAWA et al. 1981). The corticomedullary nephrogram occurs when contrast material enters the cortical capillaries and peritubular spaces and filters into the proximal convoluted tubules. This phase allows for excellent corticomedullary differentiation (BIRNBAUM et al. 1991; BOIJSEN 1983; ISHIKAWA et al. 1981). The tubular or nephrogram phase of the nephrogram appears (45–120 s) as the contrast material exits the cortical vasculature, is filtered in the glomeruli and enters the loops of Henle and the collecting tubules. It is at this point that the corticomedullary attenuation differentiation is lost, resulting in a homogeneous tubular nephrogram (BOIJSEN 1983; NEWHOUSE and PFISTER 1979). Both the corticomedullary and the tubular phase of renal enhancement may be useful in evaluation of renal vascular and parenchymal pathology. The corticomedullary phase may allow differentiation of normal cortical tissue (dromedary humps or columns of Bertin) from a renal mass. The nephrogram phase has been shown to improve detection of small renal lesions that are isointense to the medullary parenchyma during the corticomedullary phase (COHAN et al. 1995).

The density of the cortical nephrogram during the corticomedullary phase and the time delay to the tubular nephrogram may be affected by factors intrinsic to the patient. Low cardiac output, renal insufficiency or vascular diseases involving the renal artery or vein may all lead to renal hypoperfusion and therefore decrease renal attenuation during the nephrographic phase. When the appearance of the nephrogram is diminished, delayed images through the kidneys may be of great value. As previously noted, it is important to obtain images routinely during the excretory phase of renal enhancement, which typically occurs 3–4 min after injection. Contrast filling the renal pelvis can help differentiate peripelvic cysts from a dilated renal pelvis. The excretory phase is also helpful for diagnosis of the level of ureteral obstruction.

The normal CT nephrograms should be bilaterally symmetrical in the progression from the corticomedullary to the excretory phase. The demonstration of an asymmetrical hypodense nephrogram or a unilaterally prolonged nephrogram is a reliable indicator of underlying pathology (BIRNBAUM et al. 1991). The pathogenesis of the abnormal nephrogram typically falls into four distinct categories: disorders of renal arterial inflow, renal parenchyma perfusion disorders, venous outflow impairment and ureteral obstruction.

The appearance of a unilateral delayed nephrogram is usually due to alterations in normal hemodynamics resulting from diminished glomerular filtration or reduced contrast perfusion. Furthermore, the delayed or abnormal nephrogram can be global or segmental, depending upon the anatomic cause of the abnormality.

26.4
Spiral CT Diagnosis of Abnormal Arterial Inflow

Both global and segmental arterial perfusion abnormalities can be readily diagnosed with contrast-enhanced spiral CT. Acute renal artery occlusion may be due to atherosclerosis, thromboembolic disease, or renal artery dissection, whether iatrogenic or secondary to blunt trauma (WONG et al. 1984). Rapid deceleration injuries to the kidney may result in a traumatic intimal dissection of the main renal artery. This may lead to either partial or complete occlusion of arterial inflow. The characteristic CT findings of traumatic renal artery occlusion are lack of renal parenchymal enhancement and renal excretion. These findings are so specific that immediate surgery should be performed to revascularize the kidney. Delay in performing arteriography to confirm the CT findings is unwarranted (Fig. 26.1). Because the injury is purely to the main renal artery and not to the renal parenchyma, there is typically little or no perinephric blood. Patients with complete avulsion of the renal pedicle rarely undergo CT examination owing to hypotension from extensive blood loss. In the case of a laceration to the renal artery a "sentinel hematoma" may be noted on CT adjacent to the renal hilum. In patients with partial occlusion of the main renal artery, diminished but detectable renal perfusion and excretion can be observed. Selective arteriography is often helpful in the planning of arterial reconstruction for these patients (Fig. 26.2).

Segmented renal infarcts are a common cause of focal perfusion defects in the kidney. Cardiac emboli are the leading cause of segmental renal infarction (Fig. 26.3). Other etiologies include vasculitis, extension of aortic dissection and segmental venous occlusion (WONG et al. 1984). Segmental renal infarcts have a classic CT appearance of a discrete wedge-shaped peripheral low-attenuation zone. A "cortical rim sign" may be present, which represents a thin

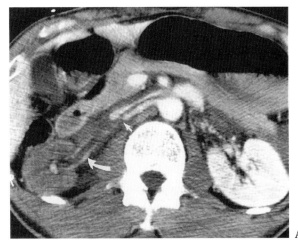

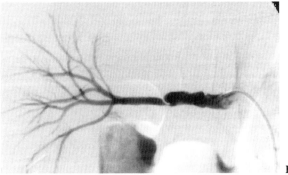

Fig. 26.2 A, B. Traumatic renal artery dissection. Contrast-enhanced spiral CT in a 41-year-old man following a motorcycle accident. The small right kidney demonstrates markedly diminished contrast enhancement. A Note the abrupt change in caliber of the right renal artery (*arrow*) at the site of arterial obstruction by the dissection. The distal right renal artery is still patent (*curved arrow*). B Selective arteriogram reveals high-grade obstruction of midportion of right renal artery attributable to intimal dissection

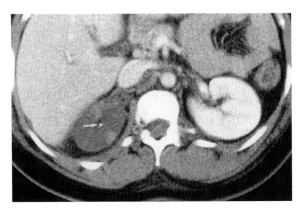

Fig. 26.1. Traumatic renal artery occlusion. Contrast-enhanced spiral CT in a 35-year-old woman following a motor vehicle accident. Note the global lack of contrast enhancement of the right kidney owing to renal artery occlusion. An incidental stone is noted within the renal pelvis (*arrow*)

rim of enhancement of the outer layers of the renal cortex owing to the blood supply from capsular collaterals. This sign is an important feature that can be helpful in differentiating a segmental infarct from a segmental area of hypoperfusion due to pyelonephritis (Fig. 26.4). Delayed images obtained during the excretory phase (3–4 min after contrast injection) will demonstrate no significant contrast enhancement in an area of segmental infarction. Delayed images in an area of pyelonephritis, however, will demonstrate enhancement due to a slow filling-in with contrast (Fig. 26.5).

Global or segmental renal infarction may be due to aortic dissection that involves the renal artery. Spiral CT can often give clear visualization of the true and false lumens diagnostic for dissection. Identification of the intimal flap and its potential ex-

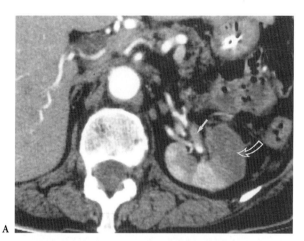

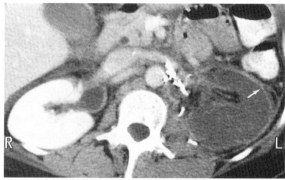

Fig. 26.4. Cortical rim sign of renal infarction. Contrast-enhanced CT in a 50-year-old woman following retroperitoneal lymph node dissection for ovarian cancer. Note the multiple surgical clips in the left retroperitoneum. There is global lack of contrast enhancement of the left kidney as a result of inadvertent clipping of the left renal artery. The cortical rim sign (*arrow*) is evident as capsular collaterals perfuse the peripheral margin of the cortex

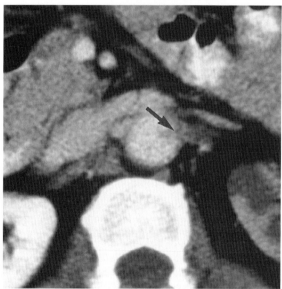

Fig. 26.3A, B. Embolic renal infarct in two patients. **A** Contrast-enhanced spiral CT in an 82-year-old woman with atrial fibrillation. Note low-density thrombus in the anterior segmental renal artery (*arrow*). Perfusion of the anterior segment of the left kidney is diminished (*curved arrow*). **B** In another patient, note the proximal left renal artery filling defect caused by an acute embolus. (By permission from JEFFREY and RALLS 1996)

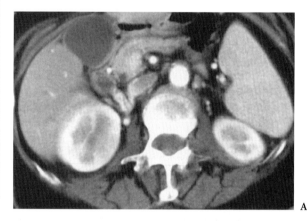

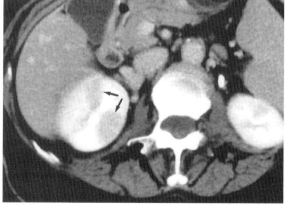

Fig. 26.5A, B. Multifocal pyelonephritis better depicted on delayed images in an 81-year-old woman with recurrent episodes of flank pain and fever. A biphasic spiral CT was obtained to exclude abscess. **A** Corticomedullary images of right kidney are unremarkable. **B** Delayed images taken during nephrographic phase (*arrow*) reveal clearly defined areas

tension into the renal arteries is of great significance for either angiographic intervention or preoperative planning (Fig. 26.6). This is of critical importance in the assessment of the renal arteries, particularly in patients with diminished renal function and delayed or asymmetrical nephrograms. The nephrogram of the affected kidney may be delayed if its blood supply arises from the false lumen. A delayed nephrogram does not necessarily imply a diminished renal function (RUBIN 1996).

Multiple subsegmental cortical infarcts are characteristic of vasculitis and may be noted in pol-

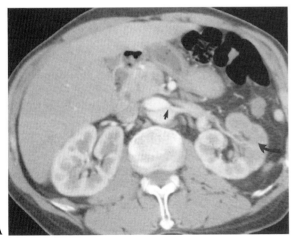

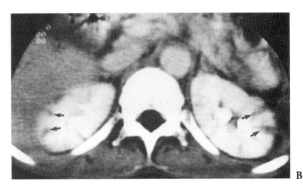

A

Fig. 26.6. Aortic dissection extending into renal artery. Spiral CT angiogram of the abdominal aorta in a 67-year-old man with a known aortic dissection shows the dissection flap extending into the left renal artery (*arrow*). Note the diminished perfusion of the anterior segment of the left kidney (*curved arrows*)

yarteritis nodosa or vasculitis associated with amphetamine abuse (Fig. 26.7). Arteriography may be required to demonstrate the small microaneurysms diagnostic of vasculitis as they are not well visualized by CT.

26.5
Renal Parenchymal Perfusion Disorders

Acute pyelonephritis is the most common disorder resulting in segmental renal hypoperfusion. In most instances, the diagnosis is established on the basis of clinical findings of flank pain, fever and pyuria. Imaging is performed only if the clinical diagnosis is uncertain, if a medical therapy has failed or when a renal abscess is suspected. Most cases of pyelonephritis are due to ascending gram-negative infections from the bladder. Hematogenous infection is generally caused by fungal or gram-positive organisms. Unless promptly treated, acute uncomplicated pyelonephritis may evolve over a period of days to weeks into a frank abscess. Renal parenchymal infections are more severe in diabetic patients, who are prone to develop virulent gram-negative infections, such as emphysematous pyelonephritis. The role of CT is to determine the extent of the disease process and distinguish pyelonephritis from renal or perirenal abscesses and to guide percutaneous intervention when appropriate.

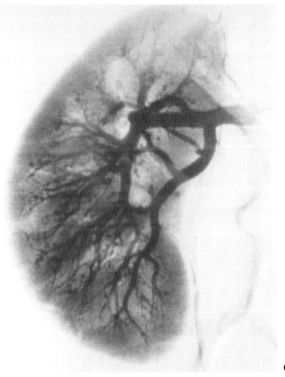

C

Fig. 26.7A, B. Multiple small cortical infarcts resulting from vasculitis. **A** Note the small peripheral subsegmental infarcts (*arrows*). **B** Arteriogram reveals microaneurysms characteristic of polyarteritis nodosa. (By permission from JEFFREY and RALLS 1996)

The findings of pyelonephritis on contrast-enhanced spiral CT include an enlarged kidney, a striated nephrogram and delayed appearance of the nephrographic phase of perfusion (Fig. 26.8) (GOLD et al. 1983, 1990; HILL and CLARK 1972; SOULEN et al. 1989). Involvement of the kidney may be patchy, segmental or diffuse, varying with the severity of the disease and the temporal relationship of the imaging and contrast bolus. Early corticomedullary imaging (typically with spiral CT) may show low-attenuation areas of hypoperfusion and poor corticomedullary differentiation (HILL and CLARK 1972). Imaging

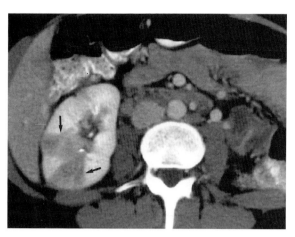

Fig. 26.8. Acute pyelonephritis. Contrast-enhanced spiral CT in a 31-year-old woman with right flank pain and fever demonstrates an enlarged right kidney with multiple wedge-shaped areas of low attenuation (*arrows*) consistent with pyelonephritis. Note the lobar distribution radiating from the renal hilum

during the excretory phase of renal perfusion may show a striated nephrogram thought of as a classic appearance on conventional CT.

The striated nephrogram in pyelonephritis is secondary to obstruction of the tubules by cellular debris, pus and edema (HOFFMAN et al. 1980; SILVER et al. 1976). This results in delayed flow of contrast material through the tubules with continued absorption of water. Subsequently, hyperconcentration of the contrast material occurs allowing for the striated appearance (GADE and GADE 1978; RUBIN and SCHLIFTMAN 1979). This pathologic process may ultimately lead to microvascular occlusion of tiny cortical branches from either vascular spasm, microvascular sludging or extrinsic compression. This accounts for the low attenuation in areas of pyelonephritis seen during the corticomedullary phase. Larger cortical vessels remain patent, however, which is a feature allowing discrimination from segmental renal infarction.

Because the poorly enhanced areas of infection can be focal, the early appearance of acute pyelonephritis may mimic a parenchymal mass, such as a renal cell carcinoma, during the corticomedullary phase of spiral CT. Subsequent spiral CT imaging during the excretory phase is of critical importance for the differential diagnosis. Segmental infarcts will demonstrate no delayed enhancement and a cortical rim sign. Uncomplicated pyelonephritis may demonstrate a striated nephrogram in a wedge-shaped configuration. The cortical rim sign is not a feature of pyelonephritis.

26.6
Perfusion Abnormalities Secondary to Renal Vein Thrombosis

Obstruction of the renal vein can also result in abnormal perfusion of the kidney. Similar to pyelonephritis, renal vein thrombosis may cause a striated nephrogram as a result of interstitial edema. Venous outflow obstruction leads to decreased glomerular filtration and delayed transit of contrast material through the tubules. The CT findings associated with renal vein thrombosis include an enlarged kidney, an enlarged renal vein, perinephric stranding, thickening of the anterior interfascial compartment/ Gerota's fascia and direct visualization of the venous thrombus (Fig. 26.9) (ADLER et al. 1981; GOLD et al. 1983). Several disease states can result in occlusion of the renal vein, including hypercoagulable states, nephrotic syndrome, dehydration, extrinsic compression and tumor thrombus.

Unlike conventional CT, typical spiral CT techniques allow for imaging of the renal vein prior to the excretory phase of contrast enhancement. Visualization of the renal veins during peak enhancement occurs during the corticomedullary phase of renal perfusion, which is the optimal time for identification of intraluminal filling defects. Corticomedullary imaging of the renal vein has been shown to improve staging of renal cell carcinoma with spiral CT. WELCH and LEROY (1997) demonstrated an accuracy of 96% for the absence or presence of tumor thrombus within the renal vein. In their series of 73 patients with renal cell carcinoma, corticomedullary phase imaging detected tumor thrombus in the renal vein in 11 true-positive patients, whereas

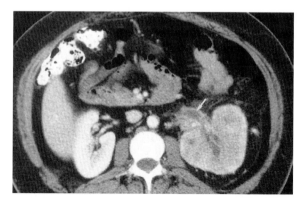

Fig. 26.9. Renal vein thrombosis from renal cell carcinoma. Contrast-enhanced spiral CT in a 54-year-old man with a large left renal cell carcinoma. Note the low-attenuation tumor thrombus in the left renal vein (*arrow*)

only 8 of the same 11 patients showed tumor thrombus in the renal veins on delayed images.

Venous outflow obstruction may be caused by extrinsic compression of the renal vein from adjacent masses. Retroperitoneal lymphadenopathy or direct tumor extension can result in significant renal vein compression or even occlusion (Fig. 26.10).

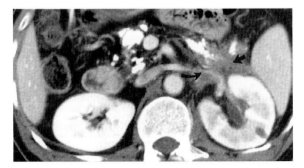

Fig. 26.10. Extrinsic renal vein compression resulting from pancreatitis carcinoma. Contrast-enhanced spiral CT in a 67-year-old woman with chronic pancreatitis and carcinoma involving the pancreatic tail (*arrow*). Note the extrinsic compression of the left renal vein (*curved arrow*) by the infiltrating pancreatic neoplasm. The left kidney remains in the corticomedullary phase owing to venous outflow compression, while the right unobstructed kidney has progressed into the nephrographic phase

26.7
Perfusion Defects Secondary to Renal Obstruction

The classic findings of acute obstructive uropathy on intravenous urography are delayed onset and progressive increased density of the nephrogram (Fig. 26.11) (ELKIN 1963; ELKIN et al. 1964). These findings can also be appreciated on spiral CT. The asymmetry of the corticomedullary nephrogram is a manifestation of the marked delay in transit of contrast material due to increased interstitial pressure (Fig. 26.12). Therefore, obtaining delayed images during the excretory phase is mandatory to visualize the level of obstruction. Whenever obstruction by a ureteral calculus is suspected preliminary non-contrast scans should be performed routinely.

Another cause of bilateral persistent dense nephrograms on CT is severe life-threatening hypotension (KOROBKIN et al. 1971). As in the case of other etiologies of diminished glomerular filtration, tubular stasis and increased water resorption occur in the setting of hypotension (FRY and CATTELL 1972; RUBIN 1996).

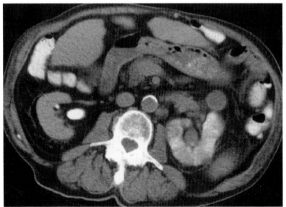

A

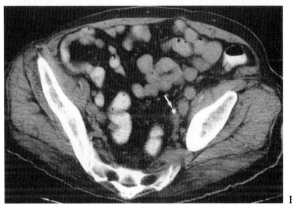

B

Fig. 26.11A, B. Acute ureteral obstruction causing striated nephrogram. A Contrast-enhanced CT during the excretory phase reveals a striated dense nephrogram on the left with a dilated collecting system. B Note a distal left ureteral calculus causing obstruction (*arrow*)

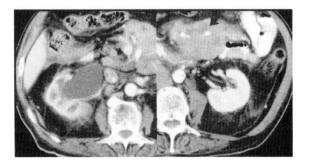

Fig. 26.12. Delayed nephrogram due to obstruction. Contrast-enhanced spiral CT demonstrates a markedly dilated right renal collecting system in the corticomedullary phase. The unobstructed left kidney is visualized during the nephrographic phase of excretion. Note the large lymphomatous mass within the small bowel mesentery (*arrow*). A distal retroperitoneal mass (not shown) resulted in occlusion of the distal right ureter

Finally, bilateral persistent dense nephrograms may be the only clue to contrast-induced nephropathy. Plain films or CT scans obtained one to several days after contrast material administration may suggest acute tubular necrosis or contrast-induced nephropathy (CATTELL et al. 1980; LOVE and OLSON 1991). Similarly, contrast-induced renal failure is probably a manifestation of either tubular obstruction from precipitation of proteins or decreased renal perfusion from toxic effects on erythrocytes leading to sluggish blood flow in capillaries.

References

Adler J, Greweldinger J, Hallac R, Frier S (1981) Computed tomographic findings in a case of renal vein thrombosis with nephrotic syndrome. Urol Radiol 3:181–183

Birnbaum BA, Bosniak MA, Megibow AJ (1991) Asymmetry of the renal nephrogram of CT: significance of the unilateral prolonged cortical nephrogram. Urol Radiol 12:173–177

Boijsen E (1983) Anatomic and physiologic considerations. In: Abrams HL (ed) Abrams angiography: vascular and interventional radiology, 3rd edn, vol 2. Little Brown, Boston, pp 1107–1122

Cattell WR, Sensi M, Ackrill P, Fry IK (1980) The functional basis for nephrographic patterns in acute tubular necrosis. Invest Radiol 15 [Suppl 6]:S79–83

Cohan RH, Sherman LS, Korobkin M, Bass JC, Francis IR (1995) Renal masses: assessment of corticomedullary-phase and nephrographic-phase CT scans. Radiology 196:445–451

Elkin M (1963) Radiological observations in acute ureteral obstruction. Radiology 81:484–491

Elkin M, Boyarsky S, Martinez J, Kaplan N (1964) Physiology of ureteral obstruction as determined by roentgenologic studies. AJR Am J Roentgenol 92:291–301

Fry IK, Cattell WR (1972) The nephrographic pattern during excretion urography. Br Med Bull 28:227–232

Gade R, Gade MF (1978) Microradiography of the collecting ducts in the perfusion fixed rabbit kidney: suggestions for the anatomic basis for the radiographic appearance of cortical striations and intrarenal reflux. Invest Radiol 13:318–324

Gold RP, McClennan BL, Rottenberg RR (1983) CT appearance of acute inflammatory disease of the renal interstitium. AJR Am J Roentgenol 141:343–349

Gold RP, McClennan BL, Kenney PJ, Breatnach ES, Stanley RJ, Lebowitz RL (1990) Acute infections of the renal parenchyma. In: Pollack HM (ed) Clinical urography. Saunders, Philadelphia, pp 79–82

Hattery RR, Williamson B Jr, Hartman GW, LeRoy AJ, Witten DM (1988) Intravenous urographic technique. Radiology 167:593–599

Heneghan M (1978) Contrast-induced acute renal failure (editorial). AJR Am J Roentgenol 131:1113–1115

Hill GS, Clark RL (1972) A comparative angiographic, microangiographic, and histologic study of experimental pyelonephritis. Invest Radiol 7:33–47

Hoffman EP, Mindelzun RE, Anderson RU (1980) Computed tomography in acute pyelonephritis associated with diabetes. Radiology 135:691–695

Ishikawa I, Onouchi Z, Saito Y et al (1981) Renal cortex visualization and analysis of dynamic CT curves of the kidney. J Comput Assist Tomogr 5:695–701

Jeffrey RB Jr, Ralls PW (eds) (1996) CT and sonography of the acute abdomen, 2nd edn. Lippincott-Raven, Philadephia

Korobkin MT, Kirkwood R, Minagi H (1971) The nephrogram of hypotension. Radiology 98:129–133

Love L, Olson MC (1991) Persistent CT nephrogram: significance in the diagnosis of contrast nephropathology – an update. Urol Radiol 12:206–208

Newhouse JH, Pfister RC (1979) The nephrogram. Radiol Clin North Am 17:213–226

Rubin GD (1996) Spiral (helical) CT of the renal vasculature. Semin Ultrasound CT MRI 17:374–397

Rubin GD, Napel S (1995) Increased scan pitch for vascular and thoracic spiral CT. Radiology 197:316–317

Rubin BE, Schliftman R (1979) The striated nephrogram in renal contusion. Urol Radiol 1:119–121

Silver TM, Kass EJ, Thornbury JR, Konnak JW, Wolfman MG (1976) The radiological spectrum in acute pyelonephritis in adults and adolescents. Radiology 118:65–71

Soulen MC, Fishman EK, Goldman SM, Gatewood OMB (1989) Bacterial renal infection: role of CT. Radiology 171:703–707

Welch TJ, LeRoy AJ (1997) Helical and electron beam CT scanning in the evaluation of renal vein involvement in patients with renal cell carcinoma. J Comp Assist Tomogr 21:467–471

Wong WS, Moss AA, Federle MP, Cochran ST, London SS (1984) Renal infarction: CT diagnosis and correlation between CT findings and etiologies. Radiology 150:201–205

27 Retroperitoneum and Ureters

L.Lemaître, C. Ala Edine, F. Dubrulle, L. Masquillier, J. Marecaux

CONTENTS

27.1   General Considerations on Spiral CT
        of the Retroperitoneum and the Ureters   *277*
27.1.1 Technical Parameters   *277*
27.1.2 Contrast Medium Administration   *277*
27.1.3 Protocol for Imaging the Retroperitoneum   *278*
27.1.4 Reconstruction Algorithms   *282*
27.2   Retroperitoneum   *283*
27.2.1 Retroperitoneal Fibrosis   *283*
27.2.2 Lymphadenopathy   *288*
27.2.3 Primary Retroperitoneal Tumors   *291*
27.2.4 Malignant Lymphoma   *296*
27.2.5 Retroperitoneal Hematoma   *296*
27.2.6 Excessive Normal Retroperitoneal Fat
        and Pelvic Lipomatosis   *298*
27.3   Ureter   *300*
27.3.1 Primary Ureteral Tumors   *300*
27.3.2 Metastatic Involvement of the Ureter   *302*
27.3.3 Urolithiasis   *303*
27.3.4 Inflammatory Conditions of the Ureter   *304*
27.3.5 Endometriosis   *309*
27.3.6 Postradiation and Postoperative Ureteritis   *310*
27.3.7 Congenital Anomalies of the Ureter   *312*
27.4   CT-guided Interventions   *312*
27.5   Conclusion   *315*
        References   *316*

27.1
General Considerations on Spiral CT of the Retroperitoneum and the Ureters

27.1.1
Technical Parameters:

Dual-slice CT has been designed to achieve faster scanning. In scanners used for this type of investigation, a wide-fan X-ray beam strikes two side-by-side parallel arcs of detectors producing a double spiral of spatial information. Compared with single-slice CT, dual-slice CT makes it possible to scan the same volume in half the time with no degradation of image quality. Thus, the entire urinary tract can be imaged completely from the upper pole of the kidney to the pelvic floor in less than 25 s during a single breath-hold (30-cm spiral length, pitch 1.5, 5.5-mm slice thickness).

The effect on noise, relative to that of the standard step-by-step CT using the same scanning parameters, depends solely on the reconstruction algorithm. Using the 180° linear interpolation (LI) algorithm, noise is increased by a factor of 1.15, independently of pitch values. For pitches less than 2, the 360° LI algorithm results in good image quality and generates less noise than the 180° LI algorithm. Table speed and scanner geometry (either dual-slice or single-slice) have no effect on noise level (Liang and Kruger 1996).

Dual-slice CT is advantageous in maintaining longitudinal resolution even at a higher scanning rate, particularly at pitches greater than 2.

27.1.2
Contrast Medium Administration

The delivery of contrast medium to the tissues is influenced by numerous factors, such as body weight, cardiac input, injection rate, injection duration and contrast medium concentration. The optimal contrast medium concentration depends mainly on the purpose of the CT examination. For maximal peak enhancement allowing good quality 2D and 3D reconstructions of the arterial system, both a high dose and a high concentration are justified.

Dose (iodine load per kilogram of body weight) is the determinant factor affecting the quality of nephrographic enhancement. Despite experimental data indicating an inverse relationship between parenchyma contrast enhancement on CT and patient's weight, most radiologists administer a uniform dose

L. Lemaître, MD; C. Ala Edine, MD; F. Dubrulle, MD; L. Masquillier, MD; J. Marecaux, MD; Department of Radiology, Hôpital Huriez, Centre Hospitalier Regional Universitaire de Lille, rue Michel Polonovski, F-59037 Lille Cedex, France

of intravenous contrast medium to all patients undergoing abdominal CT, regardless of their weight. It is more suitable to calculate the volume of contrast medium as a percentage of the patient's weight. The dose proposed is 400 mg I/kg for routine CT examination of the kidney, but it can be higher for specific evaluation of the arteries.

Contrast medium concentration has no effect on time to peak enhancement when the same volume and the same injection rate are used. The effect of the injection rate on hepatic enhancement at CT has been studied by CHAMBERS et al. (1994) using an injection of 150 ml at rates of 2 ml/s and 3 ml/s. The higher injection rate shortened the time to peak enhancement of the liver and increased its maximum peak enhancement by 10 HU.

Knowing the time to peak enhancement of the arterial and venous systems and of the cortex, medulla and collecting system is helpful for choosing the optimal timing of the spiral CT sequences. The time-density curves shown in Fig. 27.1 summarize the results obtained in 60 patients after administration of non-ionic iobitridol at a dose of 90 ml and a rate of 3 ml/s.

27.1.3
Protocol for Imaging the Retroperitoneum

Because of the mobility of the kidneys and the surrounding retroperitoneal structures, the acquisition of volumetric data using a single continuous X-ray exposure allowing imaging of the entire urinary tract within a single breath-hold is a great help in eliminating respiratory misregistration (SMITH et al. 1998). Such a spiral acquisition can be performed by

using the following protocol: slice thickness 5 or 5.5 mm, pitch 1.5, 20- to 25-s data acquisition time, tube voltage 140 kVp, and mA high enough to minimize image noise.

For dedicated renal imaging, the following protocol makes it possible to cover both kidneys in their entirety with thin slices: 2.7- or 3.2-mm slice thickness, a pitch of 1 or 1.5, 15- to 30-s data acquisition time (ZEMAN et al. 1996).

The 360° LI algorithm minimizes image noise except in patients whose weight is less than 60–70 kg.

Four spiral acquisitions are routinely performed:
- Native, to visualize calcifications and stones as well as fat in case of a fat-containing lesion,
- At the vascular (cortical) time, to study vascularity of the lesion and its relationship to vessels and kidney,
- At the tubular (nephrographic) time, to study kidneys, ureteral wall and surrounding structures,
- At the excretory time, to study the collecting system.

One additional delayed spiral may be performed in the presence of an obstructed collecting system causing late contrast medium excretion.
- For specific study of the arteries, the spiral needs to be started 20 s after the beginning of the contrast medium injection, and the full capabilities of dual-slice CT have to be used to cover the entire retroperitoneum during the maximal enhancement of the vessels.
- For specific analysis of the venous system, direct opacification of the iliac veins and the inferior vena cava through a bipedal intravenous contrast medium injection may be required. Simultaneous opacification of the retroperitoneal great vessels (inferior vena cava, aorta and its major branches) can be obtained by bipedal injection of 60 ml of 120 mg I/ml in each foot vein and brachial injection of 90 ml of 300 mg I/ml. The spiral is started at the end of the administration of 60 ml at a rate of 3 ml/s, and scanning is performed from the level of femoral or iliac veins to the upper part of the inferior vena cava (Figs. 27.2–27.5).
- For specific analysis of the collecting system, CT urography can be performed (PERLMAN et al. 1996) (Figs. 27.6–27.9). Caution is required to avoid pitfalls related to peristalsis (Figs. 27.10, 27.11), variable urine output rate (Figs. 27.12, 27.13) and vesicoureteral reflux. Nonionic contrast medium at the usual concentration (300 mg I/ml) may lead to insufficient diuresis. Conse-

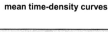

mean time-density curves

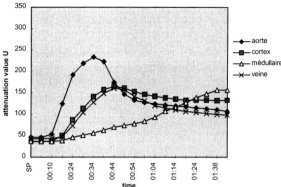

Fig. 27.1. Time–density curves summarizing results obtained in 60 patients after administration of non-ionic Iobitridol in a dose of 90 ml and at a rate of 3 ml/s

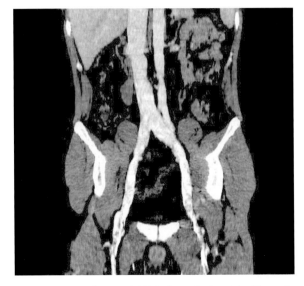

Fig. 27.2. Coronal curved MPR through the right iliac vein and inferior vena cava. This examination was performed in 20 s within a single breath-hold. Sixty milliliters of contrast medium (120 mgI/ml) was injected into each pedal vein at 2 m/s. Acquisition was initiated at the end of the injection. Simultaneous brachial injection of 90 ml of contrast medium (300 mgI/ml) at 3 ml/s allows visualization of the aorta. In this example, coronal curved MPR demonstrates both iliac veins situated in the same curved plane. However, it is usually necessary to study each iliac vein separately

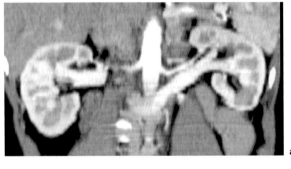

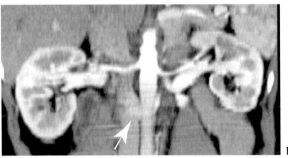

Fig. 27.5a, b. Anomaly of the renal segment of the inferior vena cava results in an retroaortic renal vein or persistent renal collar. a The retroaortic component courses caudally compared to the anterior component. b It explains the flux phenomenon (arrow) inside the inferior vena cava lumen at the level of the third lumbar vertebra

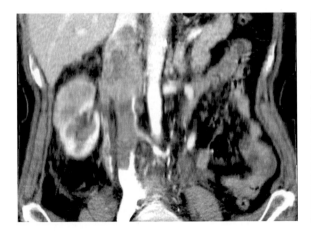

Fig. 27.3. Tumor extension into the inferior vena cava from right renal cell carcinoma – coronal curved MPR through the inferior vena cava clearly displays both tumor extension and crural thrombus below the inferior vena cava obstruction. Opacification of the inferior vena cava along the thrombus through collateral left lumbar vein

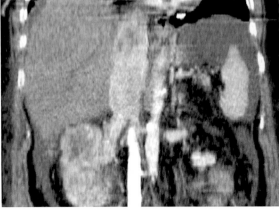

Fig. 27.4. Tumor extension into the inferior vena cava from right renal cell carcinoma – coronal curved MPR through the inferior vena cava clearly displays tumor extension from renal vein into the inferior vena cava up to the level of heart. Note the good opacification of the inferior vena cava below the tumor clot

quently, with early data acquisition at the excretory phase dilatation of the collecting system may be underestimated, and mild dilatation may therefore remain unrecognized. Abdominal compression can be used to obtain better opacification of the collecting system (McNicholas et al. 1998). Personally, we do not advocate such a technique and prefer to use ionic contrast medium to obtain better filling of the collecting system thanks to the diuretic effect.

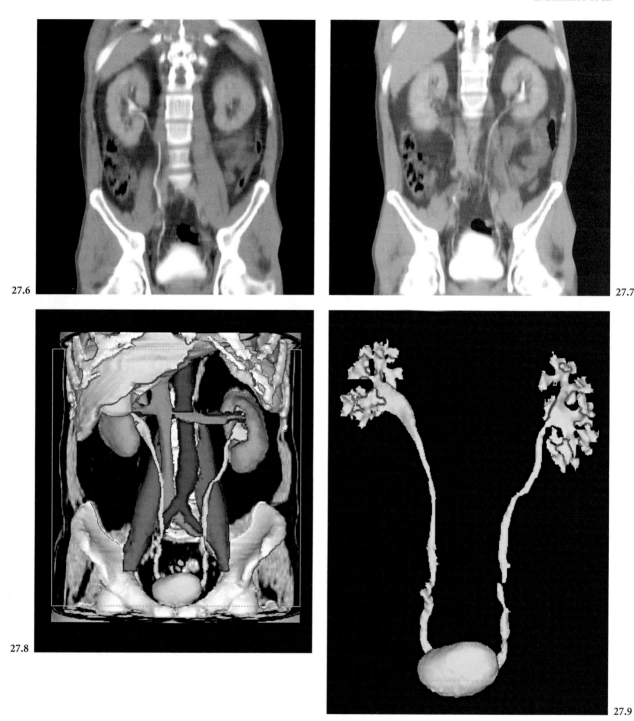

Figs. 27.6–27.9. Spiral CT reconstruction clearly displays the anatomy of the ureter and the retroperitoneum: acquisition with thin slices in one breath-hold (20-s acquisition time) allows good-quality reconstruction of the entire ureters. **Fig. 27.6.** Coronal curved MPR through the normal right ureter. **Fig. 27.7.** Coronal curved MPR through the normal left ureter. **Fig. 27.8.** 3D display of the main retroperitoneal structures. **Fig. 27.9.** 3D anatomy of the collecting systems and ureters

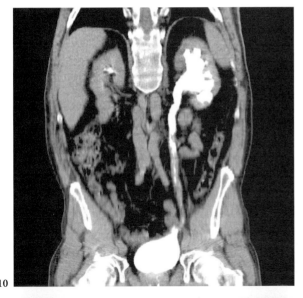

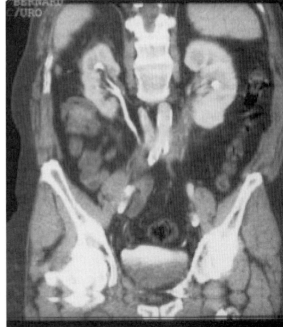

27.10

27.11

27.12

Figs. 27.10, 27.11. A 50-year-old man with psoas hitch: the bladder is fixed with a suture to the psoas muscle and assumes a tent-like appearance on the left side. Coronal curved MPR through the left ureter. **Fig. 27.10.** On the initial spiral CT thickening of the ureter wall is seen. **Fig. 27.11.** The next spiral CT shows dilatation of the collecting system and ureter. Pitfalls in the interpretation may arise from variable urine output rate, peristalsis or vesicoureteral reflux

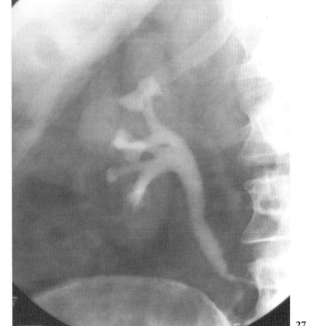

27.13

Fig. 27.12, 27.13. Injection of 30 ml of ionic contrast medium 10 min preceded this CT study. Spiral CT study performed with synchronous pedal and brachial injection (60 ml of 120 mg I/ml into each foot at 2 ml/s and 40 ml of 300 mg I/ml into an arm at 3 ml/s). **Fig. 27.12.** Coronal curved MPR through the right ureter: no dilatation of the collecting system and ureter. **Fig. 27.13.** Post-CT urogram performed 30 min after administration of contrast medium: dilatation of collecting system and medial attraction of the right ureter

27.1.4
Reconstruction Algorithms

Several types of reconstruction algorithms are used to display the urinary tract (Figs. 27.14–27.17). Shaded surface display (SSD) uses multiple threshold levels and colors for segmentation of structures with different attenuation values. 3D rendering techniques have been applied to the study of the lower urinary tract after surgery and are helpful as they increase understanding of the complex postoperative anatomy (FRANK et al. 1998).

The maximum intensity projection (MIP) algorithm is also applied to the collecting system and the ureters. The maximum attenuation value encountered by each ray is encoded in a two-dimensional projectional display. MIP gray scale thus reflects relative X-ray attenuation. It makes it possible to differentiate ureteral stone from intraluminal contrast medium. Because MIP selects only the brightest

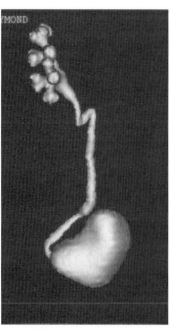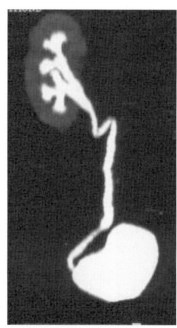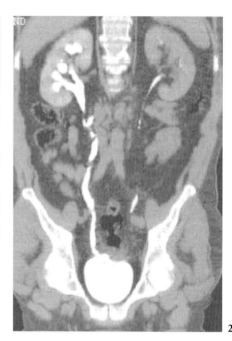

27.14,15   27.1

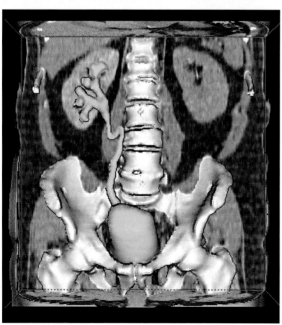

27.17

Figs. 27.14–27.17. Reconstruction techniques. Dilatation of the right collecting system. **Fig. 27.14.** 3D anatomy of the collecting system and ureter (SSD). **Fig. 27.15.** MIP of the dilated collecting system and ureter. **Fig. 27.16.** Coronal curved MPR through the right collecting system and ureter. **Fig. 27.17.** 3D and MPR representation through the right collecting system and ureter

pixel along the X-ray path, a high-attenuation structure anywhere along this path will dominate and thus mask a structure of lower attenuation. Therefore, a stone of lower attenuation than contrast medium may be missed if it is surrounded by intraluminal contrast medium.

Curved multiplanar reformations (MPRs) are also useful for the study of the collecting system and the ureters. They are excellent for displaying anatomic relationships that are not included in a single imaging plane. Thus, the tortuous ureter can be visualized on a single image. However, such images do not incorporate information from adjacent voxels, and inaccurate plane selection may therefore simulate lesions that do not exist or exclude true lesions from the display. Distances should never be measured on curved images, and caution is needed when assessing the relative positions of structures.

Volume rendering (VR) is the newest algorithm applied to the display of CT data. A histogram of the pixel values in the volume of interest (VOI) is obtained and the tissues are then assigned color, transparency and refractive index values depending on the information that is to be stressed in the data set (RUBIN and SILVERMAN 1995).

The images obtained with all these reconstruction algorithms or 3D rendering techniques must be interpreted in association with the axial source images so as to avoid errors that might otherwise result

from segmentation (RUBIN and SILVERMAN 1995). A comparison of SSD, MIP and MPR is summarized in Table 27.1.

27.2
Retroperitoneum

27.2.1
Retroperitoneal Fibrosis

27.2.1.1
Primitive Retroperitoneal Fibrosis

Etiology. This is an idiopathic condition or can be caused by drugs (methysergide).

Pathology. The process usually begins in the area of the aortic and inferior vena cava bifurcation. In the more common limited form of the disease, the fibrous mass is centered over the fourth or fifth lumbar vertebra. In the rarer, extensive, form, the fibrosis extends proximally to the renal pedicles, distally around the common iliac vessels, and laterally beyond the outer edge of the psoas muscles. The fibrotic tissue may encompass and obstruct the inferior vena cava, aorta and ureters.

Table 27.1. Comparison of curved multiplanar reformation (*MPR*), maximum intensity projection (*MIP*), and shaded surface display (*SSD*) with post-Ct radiographic urogram

Ureter	Curved MPR	MIP	SSD	Urogram (radiography)
Advantages	"Slices" through the center of the ureter to show the lumen	Differentiates high attenuating stone from intraureteral contrast medium column	Displays complex anatomy in regions of ureter kinking	Peristalsis, spatial resolution
Disadvantages	Inaccurate curve drawing can falsely mimic lesions not present; peristalsis of the ureter	Confusing in regions of ureter kinking; cannot differentiate low attenuating stone from intraureteral contrast medium column; cannot analyze the distal segment of the ureter without sufficient contrast	Cannot differentiate stone from intra-ureteral contrast medium column; incorrect threshold selection can falsely mimic or miss lesions	Delay between CT scanning and urogram
Prerendering editing	None	Minimum: removal of bones; preferred: removal of all structures other than the ureter	Minimum: none; preferred: removal of all structures other than the ureter	None
Time required	2–5 min	10–20 min	5–30 min	10 min

Histopathology. Histopathological findings range from a marked chronic inflammatory infiltrate to collagenous fibrous tissue with few inflammatory cells.

Findings on Spiral CT

Technical Procedure. Caution is indicated when contrast medium is injected to patients with renal failure.

Contrast medium injection is required to make it possible for CT to depict the great vessels within the mass and to give information on the location and extent of ureter obstruction and its effect on the renal function. The urographic phase can be demonstrated either by a delayed spiral or by radiographic films taken following the CT examination. CT multiplanar reconstructions offer a good view of the collecting system and the ureters. Simultaneous opacification of all great vessels (inferior vena cava, aorta and its major branches) can be obtained by bipedal injection of 60 ml of 120 mg I/ml in each foot vein and brachial injection of 90 ml of 300 mg I/ml.

The CT findings have been described by DEGESYS et al. (1986) and are shown in Figs. 27.18 and 27.19.

CT provides excellent visualization of both retroperitoneal fibrosis and its effects on surrounding structures (KOTTRA and DUNNICK 1996):

- The fibrous plaque appears as a centrally located, soft-tissue mass of variable thickness around the aortoiliac bifurcation. It usually covers the anterior part of the great vessels and extends to the lateral wall of the vena cava and aorta. In the idiopathic form, the posterior wall of the aorta is preserved. On native CT images, its attenuation values are similar to those of muscle tissue. On postcontrast CT images, enhancement varies depending upon the maturity of the fibrous tissue, being strong in areas of active inflammatory fibrosis and weak in dense, organized fibrous tissue. The extent of the fibrous process ranges from a well-confined, symmetrical plaque to a more extensive mass with asymmetrical and not well-defined borders.
- The classic signs of retroperitoneal fibrosis described for the ureters on excretory urography are also found on delayed spiral CT: dilatation of the ureters in their upper part, medial deviation and extrinsic compression with a tapered aspect at the site of obstruction. The dilatation of the upper urinary tract is not a constant finding in the moderate form of the disease, especially on CT images obtained early in the excretory phase, in contrast

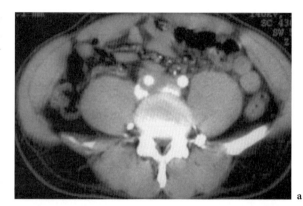
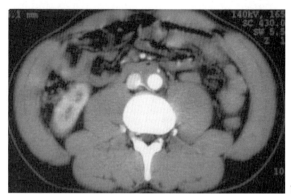
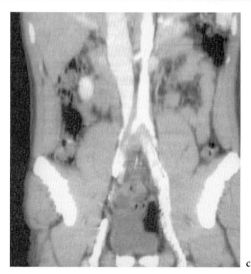

Fig. 27.18a–c. Idiopathic retroperitoneal fibrosis: Initial work-up. Spiral CT study performed with synchronous injection (60 ml of 120 mg I/ml into each foot at 2 ml/s and 40 ml of 300 mg I/ml into one arm at 3 ml/s), 20-s acquisition time, 5-mm slice thickness, table feed of 5 mm/s. **a** At the level of the aortic bifurcation: the process usually begins in the area of the bifurcation and spreads cephalad. Spiral CT with simultaneous opacification of the arterial and venous system nicely displays the relationship of the fibrotic process to the vessels and its effects on them. **b** At the level of inferior mesenteric artery: the inflammatory and fibrous tissue covers the anterior side of the great vessels and preserves their posterior side. **c** Coronal curved MPR along the axis of the inferior vena cava

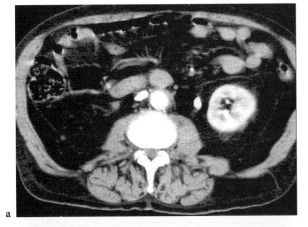

a

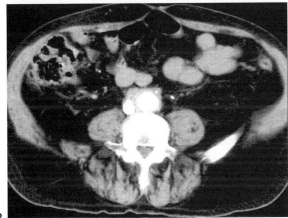

b

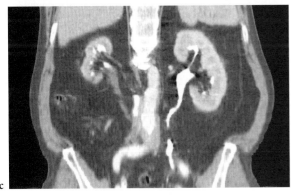

c

Fig. 27.19a–c. Idiopathic retroperitoneal fibrosis : follow-up. Injection of 30 ml of ionic contrast medium had been given 10 min before the CT study. Spiral CT study performed with synchronous arm and pedal injection (60 ml of 120 mg I/ml into each foot at 2 ml/s and 40 ml of 300 mg I/ml at 3 ml/s into one arm); 20-s acquisition time, 5-mm slice thickness, 5-mm/s table feed **a** CT image at the level of lower pole of the left kidney: both ureters are dilated with late opacification of the right collecting system. **b** CT image at the level of inferior mesenteric artery: fibrous tissue covers the anterior side of the aorta and inferior vena cava and surrounds the inferior mesenteric artery; the right ureter is encompassed within the soft-tissue mass. **c** MPR along the axis of the ureter : loss of renal function with late excretion and reduced size of right kidney. Attraction of right ureter towards the fibrous tissue

to delayed images, when the diuretic effect elicited by the contrast medium becomes apparent. Compression of the inferior vena cava is usually found around the confluence, but signs of obstruction are rare. They can be demonstrated very clearly by a spiral performed following bipedal contrast medium injection (CT cavography).

Place of Spiral CT Among the Imaging Techniques. Spiral CT and MRI are the two imaging techniques that provide the most complete information for diagnosis and staging of retroperitoneal fibrosis. However, MRI is emerging as a strong challenge to spiral CT in the work-up of patients with retroperitoneal fibrosis, for various reasons:

- MRI avoids the risks of contrast medium nephrotoxicity.
- MRI offers a useful distinction on T2-weighted sequences between inflammatory tissue, which has a high signal intensity, and mature fibrous tissue, which has a low signal intensity.

27.2.1.2
Periaortic Fibrosis (Inflammatory Aortic Aneurysm)

Etiology. The prevalence of this condition may be as high as 5–23% of all abdominal aortic aneurysms. Fibrosis can also develop around arteriosclerotic aorta and iliac arteries without aneurysmal dilatation. The disease is also known as inflammatory aortic aneurysm or periaortic inflammatory fibrosis (CULLENWARD et al. 1986).

Pathology. The thickened aortic wall is surrounded by a dense fibrotic mass infiltrated with lymphocytes, plasma cells and histiocytes. Ureters, duodenum, inferior vena cava, and renal veins may become incorporated into and adherent to the inflammatory mass. The latter may also encompass the aortic branches.

Findings on Spiral CT. The technical requirements are similar to those described above for idiopathic retroperitoneal fibrosis.

Native CT images are needed for optimal depiction of the calcified aortic wall. Dual-slice spiral CT is useful for determination of the degree of patency of the vessels in the early phase after contrast medium injection and for best visualization of the thickening of the vessel wall. An inflammatory/fibrotic mass surrounds the aorta, but usually spares the posterior aortic wall (Fig. 27.20).

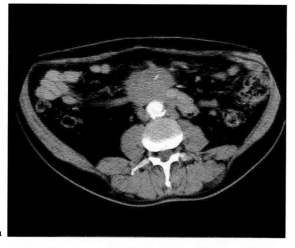

a

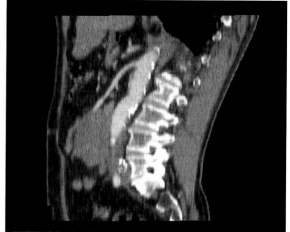

b

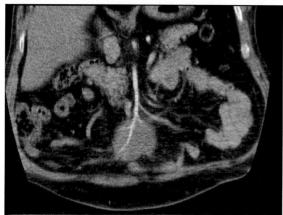

c

Fig. 27.20a–c. Perivascular fibrosis: atypical presentation. Aortic aneurysm treated by prosthesis: prominent fibrous tissue is localized in front of the prosthesis, around the superior mesenteric artery trunk and its branches. **a** Axial spiral CT. **b** Sagittal reconstruction. **c** Coronal reconstruction

The inferior vena cava is attracted towards the aorta, but in most cases the fibrotic process does not extend beyond the lateral aspect of the inferior vena cava.

Place of Spiral CT Among the Imaging Techniques. The comments made above in the section on idiopathic retroperitoneal fibrosis also apply in this case. The refinements of MRI, particularly MR angiography, make this technique very promising for imaging periaortic fibrosis and its effects on the vessels. However, calcifications of the aortic wall are not visible on MRI, whereas they are superbly depicted by spiral CT.

27.2.1.3
Malignant Retroperitoneal Fibrosis

Etiology. Malignant retroperitoneal fibrosis is caused by infiltration of the retroperitoneum by malignant cells.

Pathology. Metastases in the retroperitoneal fat tissue from breast, stomach, colon and lung cancer invoke a desmoplastic reaction and sclerosis in the retroperitoneum. The tumors that most frequently cause this type of desmoplastic response include Hodgkin's disease and other lymphomas (WALDRON et al. 1983), carcinoid, and some sarcomas.

Findings on Spiral CT. Differentiation from idiopathic retroperitoneal fibrosis is often impossible on the basis of morphological changes alone. Neither enhancement of the mass nor asymmetrical or prominent extension is helpful for the differential diagnosis. The most valuable sign is an extension around the posterior wall of the aorta, with anterior displacement of the latter in the case of malignant retroperitoneal fibrosis (Figs. 27.21, 27.22). Spiral CT can help to detect occult cancer in the abdomen or in the chest. Exploratory surgery or percutaneous biopsy is often required to establish the diagnosis.

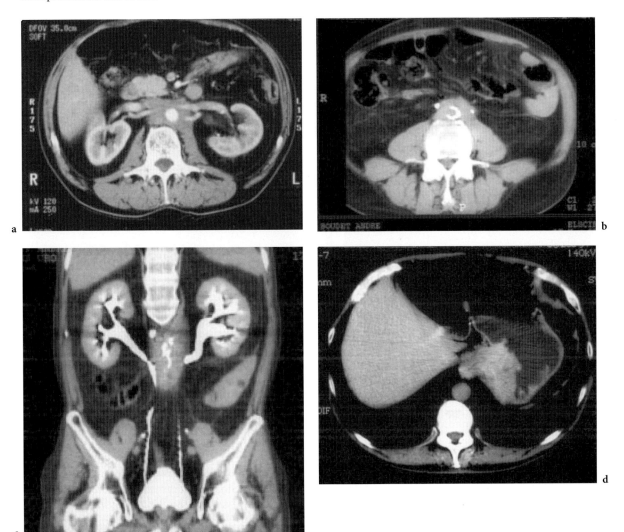

Fig. 27.21a–d. Malignant fibrosis: 60-year old man presenting with weight loss; malignant fibrosis secondary to gastric cancer. **a** At the level of renal pedicle: the soft-tissue infiltration covers both the anterior and posterior side of the aorta, which is anteriorly displaced. **b** Attraction of both ureters towards the soft tissue infiltration. **c** Coronal curved MPR through the ureters: medial attraction of both ureters with mild bilateral dilatation of collecting system. **d** Upper abdominal examination at venous phase demonstrates the cause of the malignant fibrosis: proximal gastric carcinoma, unknown before the work-up

However, the severity of the desmoplastic reaction makes the identification of malignant cells at histology difficult.

Place of Spiral CT Among the Imaging Techniques. The reader is referred to the sections above on idiopathic fibrosis and periaortic fibrosis.

27.2.1.4
Retroperitoneal Fibrosis Due to Vasculitis

The ureters may exhibit functional and morphological abnormalities as the result of systemic vasculitis.

Ureteral dilatation is presumably caused by impaired peristalsis, while the nodular irregularity of the opacified ureter is attributable to a combination of vascular and perivascular inflammation with edema and granulation tissue in the ureteral wall as well as the periureteral and perirenal fatty tissue. Few descriptions have been reported in the literature, and none with CT findings. Periureteral and perirenal involvement are clearly depicted on spiral CT: bilaterality and multifocality are characteristic (GLANZ and GRÜNEBAUM 1976) (Fig. 27.23).

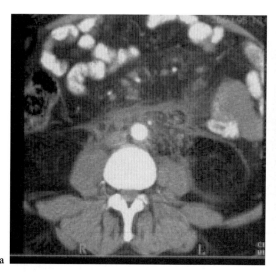
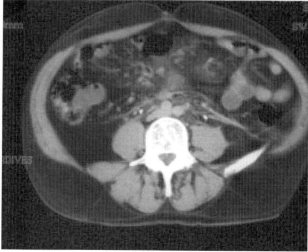

a

b

Fig. 27.22a, b. Infiltration of the retroperitoneum by lymphoma. **a** Infiltration of the fat tissue surrounding the great vessels and causing thickening of the renal fasciae. **b** At the level of aortic bifurcation: periureteral infiltration without dilatation of the ureters

27.2.2
Lymphadenopathy

Pathology. Retroperitoneal and pelvic lymph nodes may be involved with metastatic disease (Fig. 27.24), reactive hyperplasia, lymphoma (Fig. 27.25) or, occasionally, lipomatous replacement.

Metastatic disease can originate from a variety of primary neoplasms, e.g., carcinoma of the uterine cervix, uterine corpus, urinary bladder, prostate, rectum, kidney, testis (Fig. 27.24) and occasionally carcinoma of the breast or the lung.

Findings at Spiral CT. Normal para-aortic and paracaval lymph nodes are frequently visualized as small, round or oval structures in the fat adjacent to the aorta or the inferior vena cava. There is, however, some controversy concerning the dimensions above which abdominal lymph nodes should be considered definitely abnormal.

The diagnosis of lymph node abnormality at CT is based mainly on size criteria (SOM 1992; DORFMAN et al. 1991):

– The criteria based on lymph node size can be used when the nodes are homogeneous and clearly delineated. The most accurate size criterion is the minimal (shortest) axial node diameter. The upper limits of normality according to the location are as follows: retrocrural space, 6 mm; gastrohepatic ligament, 8 mm; upper para-aortic region, 9 mm; portocaval space, 10 mm; lower para-aortic region, 11 mm (DORFMAN et al. 1991; FUKUYA et al. 1995).

– A criterion taking into account the lymph node shape has been introduced by Vassallo et al. (1992) on the basis of longitudinal and axial diameters measured on US in the neck. Metastatic lymph nodes tend to have a more globular shape than hyperplastic ones. This criterion has been referred to as the ratio of maximal longitudinal to maximal transverse diameter (L/T). Its validity has been confirmed on US and spiral CT for enlarged cervical lymph nodes (Steinkamp et al. 1994), but has not been assessed for the retroperitoneal space. The long axis of retroperitoneal lymph nodes follows the axis of the great vessels. The ratio L/T at spiral CT measured on reconstructed slices may provide the most accurate assessment of reactive versus malignant lymph node enlargement (Fig. 27.26). In the study of Steinkamp et al., the performance of spiral CT was superior to that reported for conventional CT in the detection of lymph node metastases. Spiral CT performed during a single breath-hold has no interslice gap. Furthermore, greater vascular enhancement can be achieved because of the shorter scanning time, allowing better differentiation between vessels and small lymp nodes. Volumetric data can be obtained from multiplanar reconstruction (Fig. 27.27).

– The attenuation of lymph nodes at CT is an additional criterion. High attenuation values are more common in metastasis-positive lymph nodes, whereas low attenuation values are more common in metastasis-negative ones. Extranodal spread and nodal ring enhancement are findings observed in large lymph node metastases.

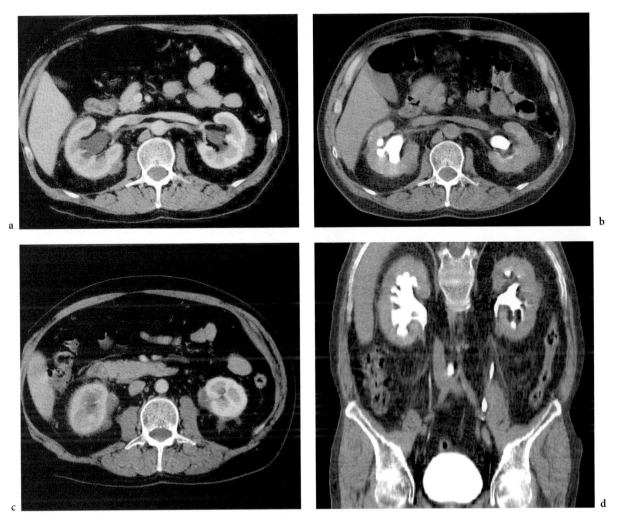

Fig. 27.23a–e. Retroperitoneal fibrosis in a 48-year-old man with Wegener disease and bilateral hydronephrosis. **a, b** Spiral CT at the cortical and the excretory phase at the level of the hilus: soft-tissue infiltration at the outer side of the left kidney and the inner side of the right kidney. **c** Spiral CT at the cortical phase at the level of the lower pole of the kidneys: soft-tissue infiltration around the pyeloureteral junction. **d** MPR along the axis of the right ureter displays the relationship between the collecting system and the perirenal infiltration. A CT-guided core biopsy confirmed the diagnosis of Wegener disease

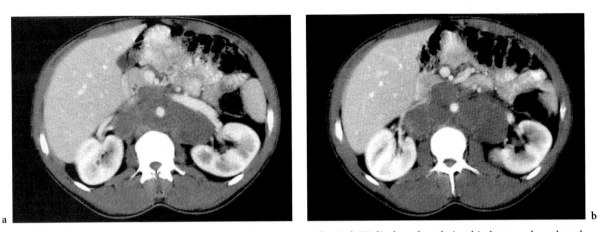

Fig. 27.24a, b. Lymph node metastasis from testicular cancer: axial spiral CT displays the relationship between huge lymph nodes and surrounding structures (pancreas, great vessels, etc.). **a** At the level of superior mesenteric vessels. **b** At the level of left renal vein

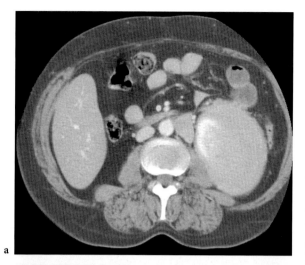

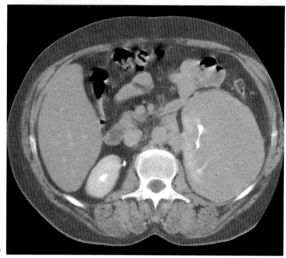

Fig. 27.25a, b. Retroperitoneal and renal lymphoma: axial spiral CT displays the relationship between lymphoma proliferation and surrounding structures. **a** At the level of the lower pole of the left kidney at the early phase: retroperitoneal para-aortic lymphadenopathy and soft-tissue infiltration encompassing the left kidney. **b** At the level of lower pole of the left kidney at the excretory phase: the collecting system is entrapped by the infiltration of the renal parenchyma

Place of Spiral CT Among Imaging Techniques. At present, CT is the method of choice for the detection of retroperitoneal lymphadenopathy. Percutaneous CT-guided fine-needle aspiration or biopsy provides valuable information in 85% of cases of lymph-node invasion by epithelial carcinomas.

CT is limited by its inability to detect abnormality in normal-sized lymph nodes and its low sensitivity in very thin patients due to the lack of contrast-providing retroperitoneal fat.

MRI has a better contrast resolution on enhanced T1-weighted sequences and is more sensitive than CT in demonstrating ring enhancement in the early phase after contrast medium (gadolinium chelate) injection.

Specific Aspects. The value of CT in assessing lymph-node metastases is greater for testicular cancer than for other genitourinary neoplasms. The lymphatic drainage of the testes follows the gonadal veins. Attenuation values of testicular cancer can show a density close to that of water. Most of these patients will undergo either radiation therapy or chemotherapy. The growing teratoma syndrome is related to the cystic transformation of teratoma under therapy. Immature metastatic deposits change to mature teratoma after radiation therapy or chemotherapy and continue to grow. However, only complete histo-

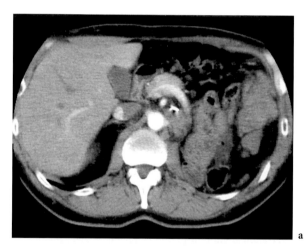

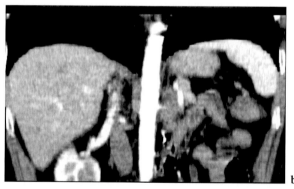

Fig. 27.26a, b. Enlarged retroperitoneal lymph nodes at spiral CT: lymph node metastasis of renal adenocarcinoma in a 50-year-old man being followed up after nephrectomy for renal cell carcinoma. Enlarged lymph node with L/T of 25/16, which is compatible with malignant adenopathy. **a** Axial CT shows lymph node near the previous ostium of the left renal artery. **b** Coronal reconstruction displays a large lymph node

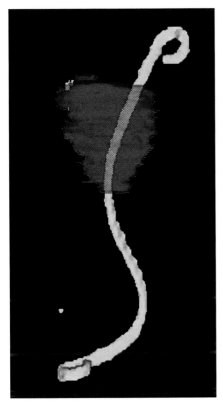

Fig. 27.27. Spiral CT allows estimation of the volume of the lymphoma proliferation (marked in *red*): 70 ml. Ureteral stent was placed to divert urine flow

malignant schwannomas) (Fig. 27.29), heterotopic chromaffin tissue (paragangliomas, ectopic pheochromocytomas) and embryonic remnants (benign and malignant teratomas).

Findings on Spiral CT. Because retroperitoneal fat is usually abundant, CT is the procedure of choice for imaging tumors in this region. It provides useful information on presence, size, composition and extent of a retroperitoneal tumor and its effect on adjacent structures.

– Composition: native CT images are required to demonstrate intratumor calcification and fatty areas. In order to study the vascular architecture, data acquisition has to be performed during the phase of vascular enhancement.

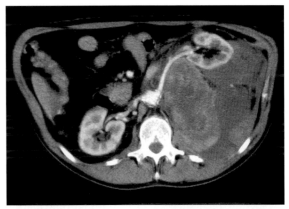

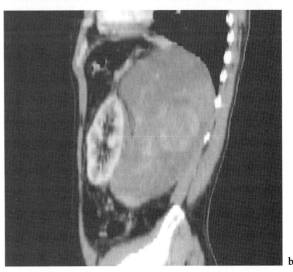

pathological examination of cystic lymph nodes gives information on the presence or absence of immature microscopic components.

27.2.3
Primary Retroperitoneal Tumors

Pathology. Because of their deep location in the body, retroperitoneal tumors are rarely diagnosed until they reach a size sufficient to produce symptoms, either by virtue of their own bulk or by compression of adjacent organs. The origins of such tumors are muscle bundles (leiomyomas, leiomyosarcomas, rhabdomyomas, rhabdomyosarcomas), fasciae and loose areolar connective tissue (myxomas, myxosarcomas, fibromas, fibrosarcomas) (Fig. 27.28), fatty tissue (lipomas, liposarcomas), blood vessels (hemangiomas, angiosarcomas, hemangiopericytomas) and lymphatic vessels (lymphangiomas), sympathetic nerve trunks (ganglioneuromas, neuroblastomas), nerve sheaths (neurofibromas,

Fig. 27.28a, b. Retroperitoneal fibrosarcoma: initial work-up of retroperitoneal tumor. a Axial spiral CT at the arterial phase demonstrate the relationship to the kidney and renal vessels. The renal cortex is regular, so that a pedunculated renal tumor can be excluded. b Coronal MPR displays relationship to the kidney and the diaphragm for preoperative work-up

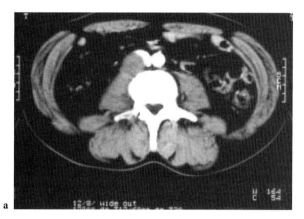
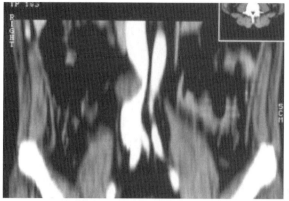

a   b

Fig. 27.29a, b. Retroperitoneal malignant schwannoma: retroperitoneal spiral CT for chronic flank pain. **a** Axial plane at the arterial phase with simultaneous opacification of inferior vena cava (bipedal injection of 60 ml of 120 mg I/ml at 2 ml/s, and brachial injection of 90 ml of 300 mg I/ml at 3 ml/s). The mass is enhanced. It is located behind the inferior vena cava and in front of the psoas muscle. No extension into the inferior vena cava. **b** MPR along the axis of the inferior vena cava demonstrates the well-marginated mass compressing the inferior vena cava

– Origin: demonstrating the relationship to the kidney is a key finding in differentiating a retroperitoneal tumor from an exophytic renal tumor (Figs. 27.28, 27.30), a pedunculated hepatic tumor, or a huge adrenal mass. Multiplanar reconstructions with an increment of 2–2.5 mm are more useful than 3D displays in order to ascertain the epicenter of the lesion precisely and also its relationships to adjacent organs (fat line, spur sign).

– Staging: dual-slice CT gives optimal information about the inferior vena cava. During the arterial phase, only the suprarenal part of the inferior vena cava is well opacified. On images obtained 30–40 s later (equivalent to the tubular phase for kidney or the portal phase for liver), the entire inferior vena cava is homogeneously and densely opacified. However, this technique requires a high dose of contrast medium, namely 150 ml of 300 mg I/ml injected at a rate of 3–4 ml/s. Arterial phase images allow analysis of the lesion and demonstration of the presence of parasitic vessels in malignant tumors invading adjacent structures. Delayed excretory phase images provide information regarding the relationship of the tumor to the ureters.

Place of Spiral CT Among the Imaging Techniques. CT is the procedure of choice to cover the entire abdomen and pelvis. The ability of MRI to provide pictures in axial, coronal and sagittal planes and to delineate blood vessels without the use of contrast medium are distinct advantages over CT. In addition, the characteristic T1 (long) and T2 (short) re-

laxation times of the fibrous tissue make it possible to obtain information on the fibrous composition of some neoplasms.

Specific Aspects.

– Lipomas, liposarcomas: in mature liposarcomas (Fig. 27.31) fat is the main component of the tumor. Areas of solid component must be looked for carefully in order to differentiate lipomas from liposarcomas. More difficult is the distinction between extrarenal angiomyolipomas (AMLs) and liposarcomas of the retroperitoneum (DITONNO et al. 1992) (Figs. 27.32, 27.33). At an early stage, liposarcomas are usually confined outside the perirenal fascia, whereas angiomyolipomas grow in the perirenal fat. However, both AMLs and liposarcomas can become very large, and then the primarily renal or extrarenal origin is difficult to assess. A fat line between the mass and the kidney, compression of the renal surface in a large area, and preservation of renal cortex suggest the diagnosis of liposarcoma. Conversely, discontinuity of the renal cortex and a spur sign (acute angle between the mass and the kidney) are features strongly in favor of a AML.

– Paragangliomas (extra-adrenal pheochromocytomas) (Figs. 27.34, 27.35): paragangliomas are widely dispersed collections of specialized neural crest cells that arise in association with the segmental or collateral autonomic ganglia throughout the body. Extra-adrenal pheochromocytomas represent approximately 10% of all pheochromocytomas. They are often multicentric (15–

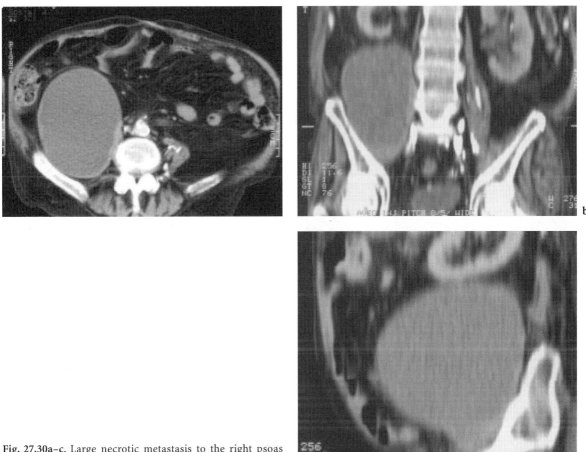

Fig. 27.30a–c. Large necrotic metastasis to the right psoas from urothelial bladder carcinoma. **a** Axial spiral CT: "cystic" mass with thickened wall. **b** Coronal reconstruction. **c** Sagittal reconstruction. The mass is clearly separated from the right kidney

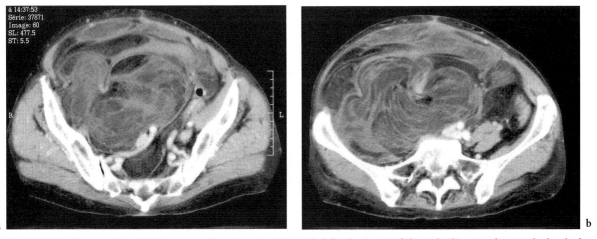

Fig. 27.31a, b. Retroperitoneal liposarcoma: huge tumor with medial displacement of the right iliac vessels. **a** At the level of external iliac vessels. **b** At the level of iliac bifurcation

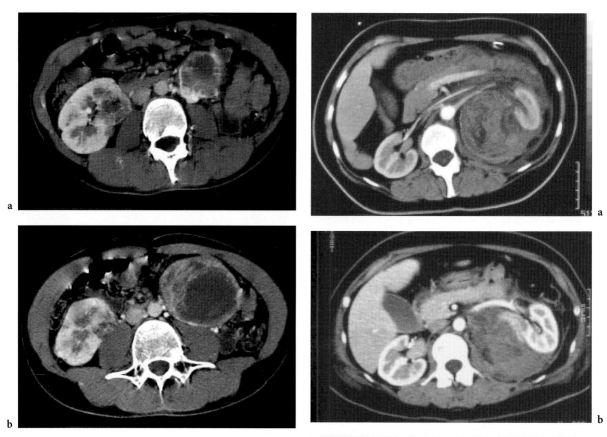

Fig. 27.32a, b. Retroperitoneal angiomyolipoma: tuberous sclerosis in a 14-year-old boy; left radical nephrectomy 3 years before. Retroperitoneal recurrence from retroperitoneal tissue. **a** Well-limited para-aortic mass with strong peripheral enhancement. **b** Numerous dilated retroperitoneal vessels close to the lesion

24%). Ninety-eight percent of all pheochromocytomas are found below the diaphragm. Paragangliomas in the inferior para-aortic area, particularly in the location corresponding to the organ of Zuckerkandl (near the origin of the inferior mesenteric artery), represent 29% of all extra-adrenal tumors. The bladder is involved in 10% of these cases (WHALEN et al. 1992). Spiral CT has become the imaging procedure of choice for the localization of extra-adrenal pheochromocytomas. First, native images are obtained using thin slices (2–3 mm) in order to cover the adrenal glands. Then, post-contrast images of the entire abdomen (including the bladder area) are acquired at the vascular phase using the following protocol: 5.5-mm slice thickness, pitch of 1.5, reconstruction increment of 2.5 mm, 20- to 25-s acquisition time, bolus injection of 120–150 ml of intravenous contrast at a rate of 3–5 ml/s using a

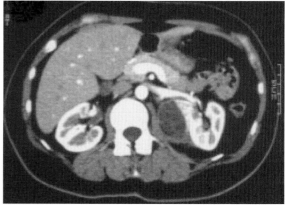

Fig. 27.33a–c. Extrarenal angiomyolipoma with retroperitoneal hemorrhage: spiral CT at 1 day, 15 days and 2 months. **a** First work-up: large hematoma with displacement of the left kidney. The origin of the hemorrhage is difficult to assess in the absence of a nephrogram defect or a renal mass. **b** The regression of the hematoma allows visualization of strong enhancement close to the renal outline, suggesting the presence of a tumor. **c** The hematoma has kept decreasing: surgical exploration confirmed the diagnosis of "extrarenal" angiomyolipoma

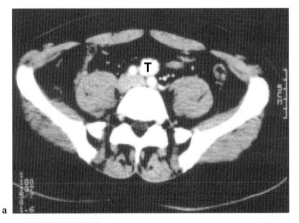

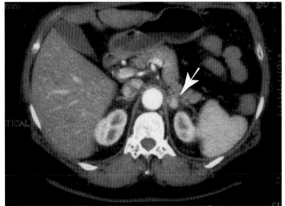

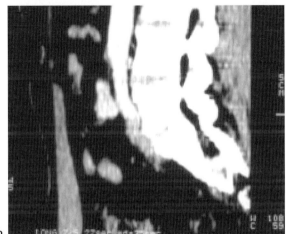

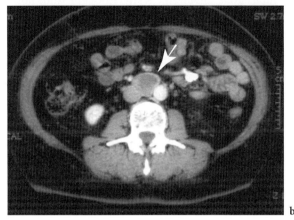

Fig. 27.35a, b. Retroperitoneal paraganglioma in a 53-year-old woman with polycythemia. a Axial spiral CT at the arterial phase demonstrates a strongly enhancing mass (*arrow*) of the left adrenal (pheochromocytoma). b Axial spiral CT at the arterial phase shows another tumor (*arrow*) in the inferior para-aortic region with a rim sign (paraganglioma)

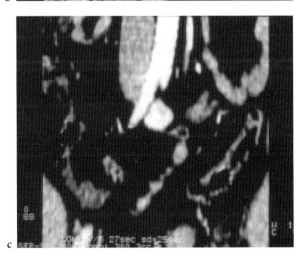

Fig. 27.34a–c. Extra-adrenal pheochromocytoma. a Axial spiral CT at the arterial phase covering the entire abdomen and pelvis: the pheochromocytoma appears as a well-demarcated mass T with homogeneous intense enhancement (blush). b Reconstructed image displays the relationship to the aortic bifurcation. c Reconstructed image (coronal view) displays the relationship to the aortic bifurcation in the coronal plane

power injector. Multiplanar reconstructions provide valuable preoperative information regarding involvement of major vessels. Spiral CT reveals the highly vascular nature of these tumors. Covering the entire abdomen and the pelvis in a single breath-hold is an advantage of spiral CT over MRI.

– Retroperitoneal cystic lymphangiomas: lymphangiomas represent rather hamartomas than true neoplasms and are always benign. They usually present as a large mass in the flank or the abdomen. They often cause superior displacement of the kidney and medial displacement of the ureter. US and CT demonstrate the predominantly cystic nature of the mass. Cystic lymphangiomas may appear as a unilocular cyst without any wall abnormality (MUNECHIKA et al. 1987). However, they also can contain a considerable amount of fibrous component. The multilocular structure is clearly demonstrated on enhanced spiral CT, showing thickened walls. Retroperitoneal lymphangiomyomatosis has been described in association with pulmonary lymphangiomyomatosis (NAEGELI et al. 1990). Underlying abnormalities were dilated lymphatic vessels, thickened lymphatic walls, and muscular proliferation of leiomyomatous origin.

27.2.4
Malignant Lymphoma

Pathology. Abdominal CT is essential to evaluate lymph node involvement in Hodgkin and non-Hodgkin lymphomas. Various sites of extranodal involvement in the abdomen have been described, particularly in non-Hodgkin lymphomas. Extranodal lymphomas can occur at any site in the retroperitoneum, including kidneys, muscles, retroperitoneal conjunctive tissue or even ureteral wall. Extranodal lymphomas (Fig. 27.25) grow either by continuity from involved adjacent lymph nodes or primarily in nonlymphatic organs. The sclerosing variant of follicle center cell lymphomas may be confused histologically with idiopathic retroperitoneal fibrosis, particularly in cases in which biopsy material does not contain lymph node tissue.

Spiral CT. Spiral CT can be performed in a single breath-hold with coverage of the entire abdomen. The organ parenchyma phase is the best sequence to delineate both nodal and extranodal lesions, because lymphomas present as hypodense nodes or masses. The CT appearance of an isolated soft tissue mass of the ureter wall is nonspecific for lymphoma (CHEN et al. 1988). However, the fact that the usually large mass paradoxically does not obstruct the ureters should suggest the diagnosis.

27.2.5
Retroperitoneal Hematoma

Trauma of the kidney is the main cause of retroperitoneal hemorrhage (PODE and CAINE 1992). Spiral CT has been largely accepted as the gold standard for patients with blunt or penetrating abdominal trauma. The speed of spiral CT is particularly advantageous in the evaluation of the acutely traumatized patient. The entire abdomen is surveyed from the dome of the diaphragm to the pubis. Three spirals are required in the protocol: (1) a native spiral,

which covers the entire abdomen and detects hematomas, due to their high density; (2) a spiral in the early vascular phase, for the study of the submesocolic abdomen, including liver, spleen, kidneys, pancreas and great vessels and which shows contrast medium extravasation, pseudoaneurysms, and arterial injury; (3) a delayed spiral CT during the excretory phase, which demonstrates contrast medium leakage from the collecting system, including the bladder.

Spontaneous retroperitoneal or pelvic hemorrhage in the adult is most commonly due to rupture of an abdominal aortic or iliac aneurysm. However, spontaneous retroperitoneal hemorrhage can be due to numerous other causes.

- Benign and malignant tumors: angiomyolipomas (Figs. 27.33, 27.36–27.38), renal cell carcinomas, and adrenal tumors;
- Vascular lesions: renal artery aneurysms, congenital arteriovenous malformations, infarctions and renal venous thrombosis, ruptured gonadal artery (pregnancy);
- Systemic etiologies: polyarteritis nodosa (27.39), anticoagulation therapy, fibrinolytic agents and blood dyscrasia.

Spiral CT is the method of choice for the diagnosis of retroperitoneal abnormalities. The native spiral sequence allows precise determination of the localization, epicenter, and extent of the hematoma. It is helpful for selecting the right level of the spiral sequence performed during the vascular phase. The goal is to depict vascular abnormalities and the presence of a tumor. The thinner the slices, the more sensitive the detection of small vascular lesions or tumor. A slice thickness of 3 mm probably represents the best compromise if the entire hematoma volume can be covered by a single breath-hold sequence. A dose of 120–150 ml of nonionic contrast media containing 300 or 350 mg I/ml is injected via a 18-G angiocatheter in an antecubital vein at a rate of 3–5 ml/s. Scanning begins 20 s after the start of the injection for most applications. Delayed images are often useful to identify extravasation.

Angiography is indicated if no abnormality has been detected by spiral CT, because its resolution is superior to that of spiral CT for the detection of small aneurysms inferior to 2–3 mm in diameter.

Specific Aspects.
- Polyarteritis nodosa: the challenge for spiral CT is the detection of microaneurysms in the small intrarenal arteries. Comparing arteriography and

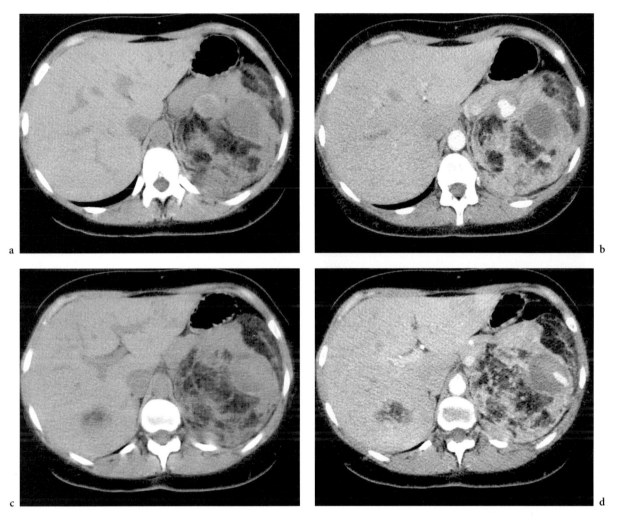

Fig. 27.36a–d. Tuberous sclerosis with angiomyolipoma. Spiral CT with native and early arterial phase: 20-s acquisition time, 5-mm slice thickness, pitch of 1.5, table feed of 5-mm/s. Nonionic contrast medium injection: 120 ml of 300 mg I/ml at 3 ml/ s. **a, b** Native and enhanced spiral CT at the level of the left kidney upper pole: a hematoma surrounds the aneurysmal dilatation of a small intrarenal artery, well identified at the early arterial phase. **c, d** Native and enhanced spiral CT at the left kidney's upper pole, 1 cm below the previous slice: a liquefying hematoma surrounds another aneurysm

spiral CT, we have seen that the latter is capable of detecting 2-mm microaneurysms as strongly enhancing small nodular structures on the faintly nephrographic background. However, in one patient, 20 microaneurysms were identified on angiography, versus only 5 at spiral CT. The microaneurysms can also arise from other aortic branches (adrenal, celiac, hepatic, superior mesentery) (Wilms et al. 1986) (Fig. 27.39).

– Anticoagulation therapy: the incidence of retroperitoneal bleeding in patients receiving intravenous heparin has been reported to be 4.3–6.6%, whereas it was 0.1–0.6% in patients who received oral anticoagulation therapy. It is important to stress that in some cases of spontaneous retroperitoneal hemorrhage occurring during an anticoagulation therapy, a local additional cause has been demonstrated. Hemorrhage in parapyelic and simple renal cysts has been observed among other causes.

– Angiomyolipomas (AMLs) are a common cause of spontaneous retroperitoneal hemorrhages (Randazzo et al. 1987). Large hematomas may obliterate the presence of fat. Differentiation between normal retroperitoneal fat impregnated by blood and angiomyolipomatous proliferation infiltrated by the hematoma can be very difficult (Fig. 27.38). The goal of spiral CT is to delineate

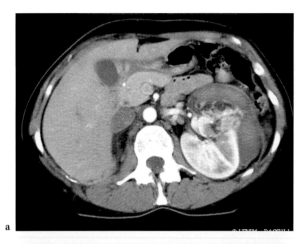

a

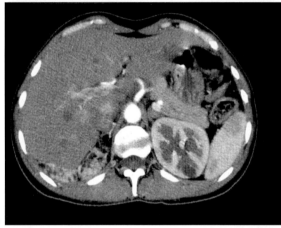

b

Fig. 27.37a, b. Retroperitoneal angiomyolipomatosis (tuberous sclerosis): right radical nephrectomy for renal angiomyolipoma 5 years before; sudden onset of left lumbar pain. **a** Axial spiral CT at the arterial phase: left kidney AML with retroperitoneal hemorrhage. **b** Axial spiral CT at the arterial phase : intense and heterogeneous enhancement of right retroperitoneal tissue, compatible with diffuse angiomyolipomatosis

the contours of the lesion at the early vascular phase thanks to the highly vascular component of AMLs, to detect aneurysmal dilatation of intratumoral "hamartomatous" arteries, and, of course, to demonstrate the lipomatous nature of the tumor.
- Both large and small malignant tumors can arise from the kidneys or the adrenals.
- Ruptured aortic aneurysms (atheromatous, mycotic): the hemorrhage diffuses along the retroperitoneal and extraperitoneal space towards the inguinal canal.
- Hemorrhagic complications of pancreatitis: spiral CT has increased the detection of pseudo-

aneurysms due to erosion of branches of the celiac trunk and superior mesenteric artery before they become symptomatic. Rarely erosion may concern other arteries such as the renal arteries. All patients with hemorrhagic complications of pancreatitis should undergo angiospiral CT to detect these pseudoaneurysms. High attenuation values detected in the inflammatory process on native spiral CT are highly suggestive of such a complication.

27.2.6
Excessive Normal Retroperitoneal Fat and Pelvic Lipomatosis

Pathology. Abundant retroperitoneal fat may displace retroperitoneal organs, but without obstruction or dilatation of the collecting system. Pelvic lipomatosis (or fibrolipomatosis) must be distinguished from retroperitoneal fibrosis. It is characterized by nonneoplastic overgrowth of normal fatty tissue in the perirectal and perivesical space. At laparotomy, a large amount of fat is found but fibrous adhesions are also noted. Inflammatory changes are present in 10%. Pelvic lipomatosis differs from simple lipomas in that it is not encapsulated.

Findings on Spiral CT. CT provides diagnostic proof of pelvic lipomatosis, which obviates the need for other imaging modalities, and shows elevation of the trigone without a prostatic indentation, cephalad displacement and narrowing of the bladder base (pear shape), elongation, straightening and fusiform narrowing of the rectum, elevation of the distal sigmoid colon, symmetric and medial, or less commonly lateral, displacement of the ureters, ureterectasis and often mild dilatation of the upper urinary tract. Fatty tissue is particularly well seen on CT imaging, but the fibrous and inflammatory component is usually not recognized. Pelvic lipomatosis may be associated with cystitis glandularis or cystitis cystica. Recurrent urinary infections, urinary complaints (frequency, dysuria, urgency) and hematuria are the most common clinical symptoms. Multiple small intraluminal defects may be seen in the bladder and the distal ureter. An increased incidence of bladder carcinoma has been suggested, but this is very rare.

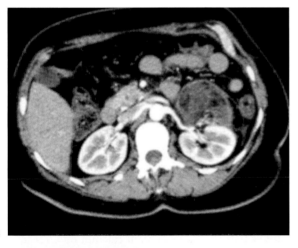

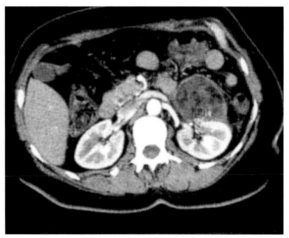

a

b

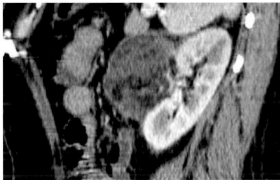

c

Fig. 27.38a–c. Angiomyolipoma with extrarenal extension. Large anterior retroperitoneal mass: on a previous CT examination, the origin of the mass was not identified: fat attenuation suggested liposarcoma or angiomyolipoma with extrarenal extension. **a** Spiral CT at the arterial phase displays small tortuous arterial vessels in the region of the renal hilus, proving renal origin of the mass. **b** Tiny strongly enhancing structures represent the vascular component of the angiomyolipoma and are detected at the early arterial phase. **c** Sagittal reconstruction displays the relationship between tumor and kidney

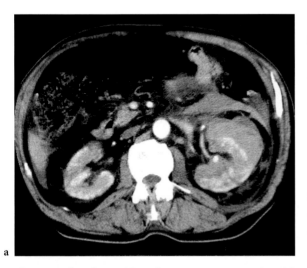

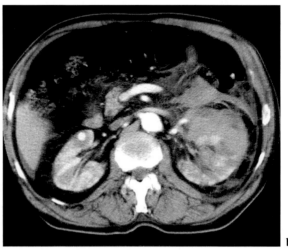

a

b

Fig. 27.39a, b. Polyarteritis nodosa: spontaneous perirenal hematoma due to rupture of small interlobar artery aneurysms. Spiral CT clearly displays small aneurysms with a diameter greater than 4–5mm. Other microaneurysms less than 3 mm in diameter were not visualized on spiral CT but only on selective arteriography. **a** Spiral CT at the arterial phase: perirenal and pararenal hematoma; a aneurysm in the left kidney; multiple nephrographic defects. **b** Spiral CT at the arterial phase: another 10-mm aneurysm in the right kidney

27.3
Ureter

The normal ureter is 24–30 cm long. Its proximal two thirds are situated in the perirenal space. Near the lower pole of the kidney, the ureter moves medially to a position anterior to the psoas muscle. Within the extraperitoneal space of the pelvis, the ureter passes anterior to the common iliac artery in the region of the inferior margin of the sacroiliac joint. From this point, the ureter usually curves laterally in a broad arc that extends to a point near the ischial spine and then medially to the ureterovesical junction.

Sequential CT scanning gives incomplete information on the ureters because of their length, course and dynamics. Spiral CT is advantageous in this matter, because it allows the kidneys, upper urinary tract and bladder to be covered within one acquisition during a single breath-hold with slice thickness of about 5 mm in as little as 20–25 s. Multiplanar reconstructions can be performed along the axis of the ureters, providing a CT urogram. The main limitation of this technique remains the absence of data on peristalsis and dynamics of the ureters.

Native images are required for detection of stones and calcifications, and for demonstrating thickening of the ureter wall. Images obtained early after contrast medium injection provide information on tumor infiltration, diffuse inflammatory thickening of the ureter wall, and presence of postradiation changes.

Delayed images allow to determine the location, extent, and type of ureter obstruction. Both ureters in their entire course and the retroperitoneal and extraperitoneal space are well visualized by CT. However, intraluminal abnormalities are more difficult to identify if the contrast medium concentration in the collecting system is too high. The windows settings can be modified to improve visualization of the ureter content. The timing of the delayed spiral CT must be chosen with care (up to 3 h after contrast medium injection), so that complete filling of the obstructed segment is achieved. In renal failure, contrast medium concentration in the dilated ureter segment proximal to the obstacle may be too low to be recognized on excretory urography but still sufficient for CT. In severe obstruction, opacification of the ureter beyond the obstacle is not always possible.

27.3.1
Primary Ureteral Tumors

Pathology. The most common malignant tumor of the ureter is transitional cell carcinoma. Eighty-five percent of these tumors are broad-based. Pedunculated or diffusely infiltrating tumors are less common. Sessile and infiltrating lesions behave more aggressively and are more advanced at the time of diagnosis. Infiltrating tumors are characterized by thickening and induration of the ureter wall (WONG-YOU-CHEONG et al. 1998).

Spiral CT. CT is useful in distinguishing radiolucent stones (which always contain calcium on CT!) from soft tissue filling defects (BOSNIAK et al. 1982). It is particularly helpful when the ureter is incompletely visualized at excretory urography, either because the kidney is nonfunctioning or because severe stricture of the ureter prevents opacification of the distal segment (KENNEY and STANLEY 1987).

CT is indicated in the work-up of patients with transitional cell carcinoma. Information provided on periureteral invasion and regional lymphadenopathy are important elements in planning therapy (BARON et al. 1982).

Technical Procedures. Native CT images are required to differentiate a tumor mass from a hyperattenuating calculus.

Early CT images after contrast medium injection show enhancement of the tumor which is either a bulky mass or an infiltrating process. They demonstrate its relationship to adjacent structures.

Delayed images after filling of the collecting system precise the location and extent of the tumor.

Findings on Spiral CT. Ureteral carcinomas result in an intraluminal soft-tissue mass (papillary tumor) or in thickening of the ureter wall (infiltrating tumor). Such thickening may be eccentric or circumferential. CT is particularly useful to distinguish a distal pedunculated ureteral tumor protruding through the ureterovesical junction from a bladder cancer infiltrating the ureteral orifice (Figs. 27.40–27.45).

Place of Spiral CT Among Imaging Techniques. Excretory urography is the examination of choice. When the kidney is well functioning, the good opacification of the collecting system and the ureter allows demonstration of the diagnostic features of ureteral carcinoma:

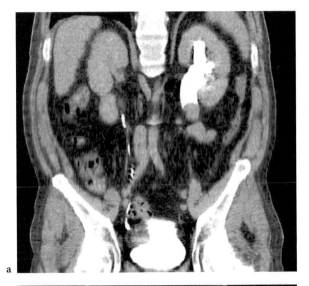

a

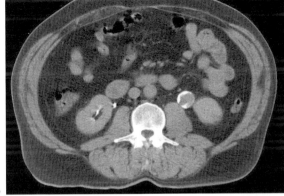

b

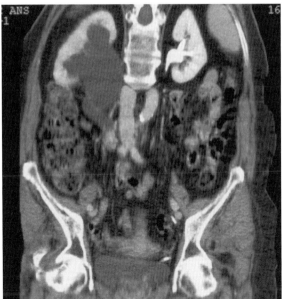

a

Fig. 27.40a, b. Macroscopic hematuria; dilatation of left collecting system with two small calculi at the level of the inferior calix detected on sonography. At excretory urography: large filling defect in the proximal ureter. Spiral CT performed at the late phase of excretory urography shows dilatation of the collecting system above of soft-tissue mass of the proximal ureter. a Reconstructed image from late-phase spiral CT. b Axial spiral CT at the level of obstruction

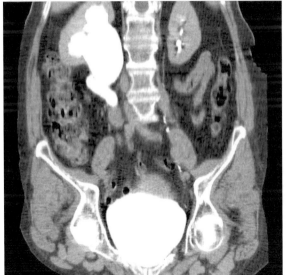

b

Fig. 27.42a, b. Transitional cell carcinoma of the proximal ureter: 65-year-old woman with right flank pain without macroscopic hematuria. a MPR along the axis of the right ureter at the early excretory phase. b MPR along the axis of the right ureter at the late excretory phase: an infiltrating tumor is located in the proximal ureter

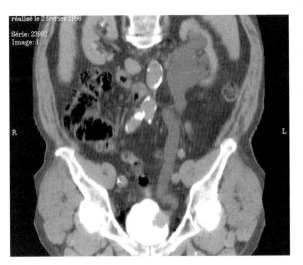

Fig. 27.41. Transitional cell carcinoma of the bladder: dilatation of left collecting system with nonfunctioning kidney; spiral CT is particularly useful for evaluation of the ureter. Reconstructed image from late-phase spiral CT. The tumor is located at the ureterovesical junction

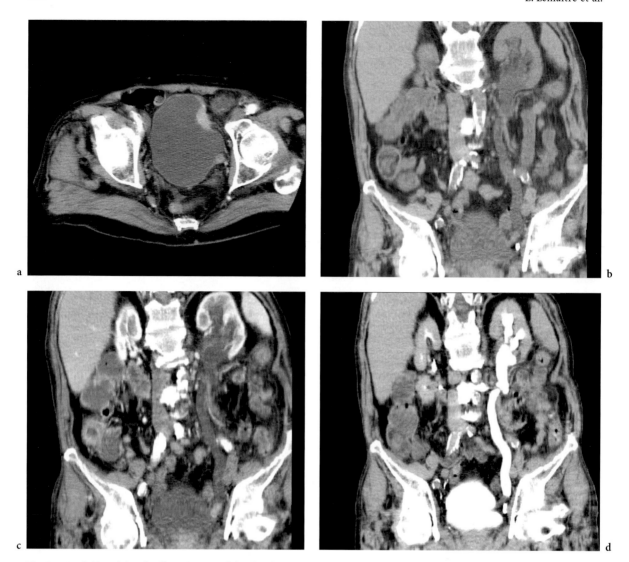

Fig. 27.43a–d. Transitional cell carcinoma of the distal ureter and the bladder in a 65-year-old man with a history of bladder carcinoma. **a** Axial spiral CT at the early phase after contrast-medium injection: thickening of the anterior left bladder wall with enhancement; another tumor is located at the ureterovesical junction. **b** Reconstructed native CT scan: tumor located in the distal ureter. **c** Reconstructed early contrast-enhanced CT scan : enhancement of the tumor. **d** Reconstructed late contrast-enhanced CT scan

- Intraluminal filling defect with cupping immediately above and below the lesion.
- Eccentric or circumferential thickening of the ureter wall.

Limitations of CT include its failure to detect small tumors along the urothelium and microscopic invasion of periureteral tissue.

MR urography is useful in case of a nonfunctioning kidney, because it does not require contrast medium injection.

27.3.2
Metastatic Involvement of the Ureter

CT has proved very useful in the study of ureter obstruction caused by metastatic involvement, since this technique is able to visualize the retroperitoneum and the periureteral tissues very clearly (PUECH et al. 1987).

Several mechanisms can lead to ureter obstruction in metastatic disease from primaries such as cancer of the prostate, bladder, cervix, rectum and ileal carcinoid:

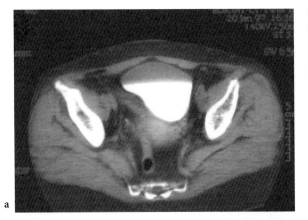

a

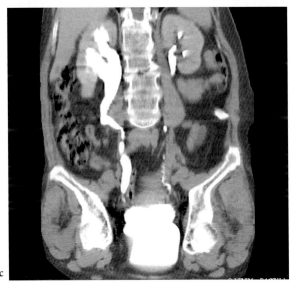

c

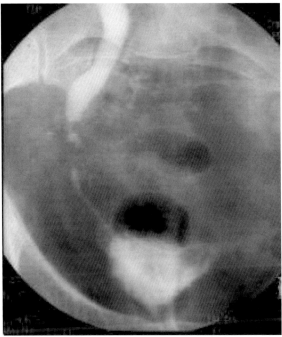

b

Fig. 27.44a–c. Periureteral extension of a bladder cancer. **a** Axial spiral CT at the excretory phase: retraction and thickening of the lateral bladder wall; periureteral circumferential soft-tissue mass. **b**. Excretory urography: stenosis and irregularities of the right ureter 3 cm above the ureterovesical junction. **c** MPR along the axis of the right ureter demonstrates the continuity between periureteral infiltration and bladder carcinoma. Spiral CT allows differentiation between this situation and a second tumor location in the ureter

- Metastatic retroperitoneal infiltration can elicit a reactive fibrosis (malignant retroperitoneal fibrosis).
- Bulky retroperitoneal lymph node metastases and secondary periureteral soft-tissue infiltration can compress the ureter (retroperitoneal lymph node metastases).
- The ureter wall can be the site of hematogenous metastases (ureteral metastases).

Spiral CT. The CT features differ according to the mechanism leading to the ureter obstruction:
- Retroperitoneal fibrosis: extensive periaortic and paracaval soft-tissue infiltration,
- Malignant obstruction by lymph node metastases: irregular retroperitoneal mass and infiltration,
- Ureteral metastases: thickening of the ureter wall

with no change in the adjacent retroperitoneal fat tissue.

27.3.3
Urolithiasis

Place of Spiral CT Among Imaging Techniques. Plain radiography is the most commonly used imaging modality for the detection of urinary tract stones. Calcifications outside the urinary tract, such as gallstones, costochondral calcifications, phleboliths, and calcified mesenteric lymph nodes often make the diagnosis difficult, so that excretory urography is needed. US is useful in determining the character of a radiolucent intraluminal filling defect at excretory urography. It helps to pinpoint the location of small stones close to the pyeloureteral junction or the ureterovesical junction. However, because it provides only incomplete coverage of the entire ureter, more sophisticated imaging techniques, such as spiral CT, are frequently indicated for the detection of stones and even the follow-up after treatment (REMER et al. 1997).

Native spiral CT has proved to be an accurate technique for the diagnosis of renal colic (LEVINE et al. 1997; OLCOTT et al. 1997; PREMINGER et al. 1998; YILMAZ et al. 1998). It is also useful in determining the character of a radiolucent intraluminal defect. CT detects most urinary stones, regardless of their calcium content. 3D display of the CT data set allows optimal visualization of stones, especially staghorn stones or multiple calculi, and monitoring of percutaneous access for minimally invasive treatment (LIBERMAN et al. 1997).

Technical Procedure. The most useful CT reconstruction algorithm is curved multiplanar reconstruction of the ureters to determine whether a ureteral stone is present. Spiral CT performed during a single breath-hold has no interslice gap. We perform native dual-slice CT (Elscint, Haifa, Israel), with neither intravenous nor oral contrast medium. The abdomen and pelvis are scanned from the midportion of the T-12 vertebral body to the midportion of the symphysis pubis with 5.5-mm slice thickness and a pitch of 1.5. The data acquisition time lies between 20 and 25 s and is achieved during a single breath-hold. Following patient scanning and primary image reconstruction at 2.5-mm intervals, data are transferred to a workstation, where a radiologist performs secondary image reconstruction using 2D and 3D algorithms (SOMMER et al. 1995).

Findings on Spiral CT. The findings on spiral CT are shown in Figs. 27.46–27.50. Hydronephrosis, hydroureter, perinephric fluid, and ureteral stones are considered as positive findings establishing the diagnosis of renal colic. The most important problem relates to the demonstration of whether a suspected calcification along the expected course of the ureter really lies within the latter.

Several features of native CT are helpful in this context. In phleboliths, CT findings include a central region of low attenuation (on magnified images with adequate bone window settings, i.e. level, 300 HU, width, 1,500 HU), a bifid peak on the histogram and a comet sign (adjacent eccentric, tapering soft-tissue mass corresponding to the noncalcified portion of the pelvic vein containing the phlebolith). Conversely, a mean attenuation value greater than 300

HU and a soft-tissue rim sign indicate a ureteral stone (BELL et al. 1998). However, attenuation values of calculi and phleboliths overlap, and caution is therefore required.

"Stranding" or a "tissue rim" around the stone are important secondary signs. Stranding represents inflammatory changes in the periureteral fat (Fig. 27.47). The soft-tissue rim is believed to represent edema within the ureter wall.

Dilatation of the collecting system and ureter may be present without detectable intraureteral stone, when the latter has already passed into the bladder or has even been eliminated without being noticed by the patient.

Work-up of Ureteral Stone Disease. CT urography may be useful in atypical presentation of renal colic or in the preoperative work-up. In an experimental in vitro study, the chemical composition of urinary tract stones was determined by CT. This was performed using the absolute CT value at 120 kV as well as the subtraction between the CT values at the energy levels of 80 and 120 kV, respectively. Uric acid calculi were the only stones that could be distinguished from other stones by using the absolute CT value, but dual-energy CT allowed a distinction between struvite, cystine, calcium oxalate monohydrate or dihydrate, and brushite calculi (MOSTAFAVI et al. 1998).

The accurate measurement of stone size is very important for treatment selection. Lithotripsy is used for calculi smaller than 25 mm, whereas complications occur with larger calculi.

Volumetric information and size of renal calculi has been determined with a mean of error of only 4.8%, so that spiral CT is considered the best technique to determine stone volume (OLCOTT et al. 1997).

27.3.4
Inflammatory Conditions of the Ureter

27.3.4.1
Urinary Tract Infection

Ureteritis. Either discrete thickening of the ureter wall or no change is seen on CT.

Tuberculosis. Excretory urography is the best imaging method to analyze the retraction, scarring and strictures of the collecting system and ureters. Spiral

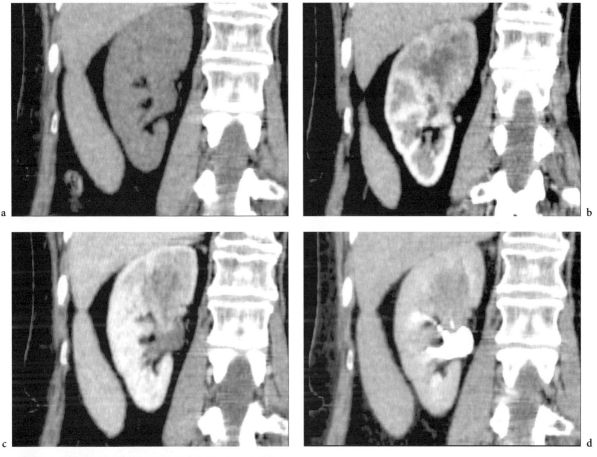

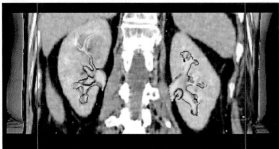

Fig. 27.45a–e. Transitional cell carcinoma of the kidney in a 72-year-old woman with hematuria. **a** Native spiral CT: obliteration of the renal sinus fat at the level of the superior calix. **b** Spiral CT at the cortical phase: weak enhancement of the cortex at the upper pole. **c** Spiral CT at the tubular phase: homogeneous nephrogram at the lower pole but persistence of the cortical phase at the upper pole due to the focal obstruction. **d** Spiral CT at the excretory phase: infiltration of the upper part of the renal sinus. **e** Volume rendering demonstrating the entire pelvicaliceal system

CT is indicated particularly in nonfunctioning kidneys or when contrast medium concentration is insufficient at excretory urography. The association of renal lesions with ureteral and bladder involvement is highly suggestive of tuberculosis. Renal cavities with thick walls, thickening of the ureter and bladder wall are the characteristic features in spiral CT. Retraction and scarring are more difficult to assess on CT than on excretory urography.

Fungal Disease. Fungus balls in the collecting system present as noncalcified lucent filling defects, non-visible on native CT images but clearly depicted on delayed CT images.

Corynebacterium infection. Calcification and diffuse thickening of the ureter wall are suggestive of this rare condition.

27.3.4.2
Ureteral and Periureteral Inflammation

Extensive ureteral and periureteral inflammatory reaction can be observed in patients with postoperative ureter and after renal transplantation.

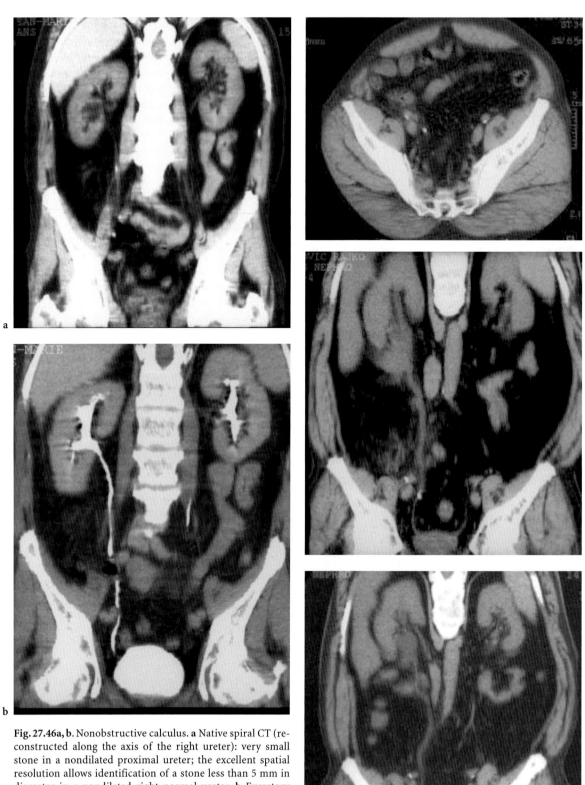

Fig. 27.46a, b. Nonobstructive calculus. **a** Native spiral CT (reconstructed along the axis of the right ureter): very small stone in a nondilated proximal ureter; the excellent spatial resolution allows identification of a stone less than 5 mm in diameter in a nondilated right normal ureter. **b** Excretory phase (reconstructed along the axis of the right ureter)

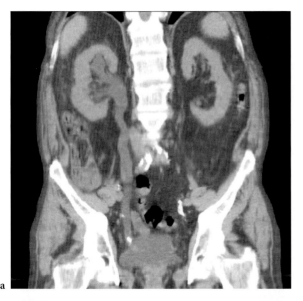

a

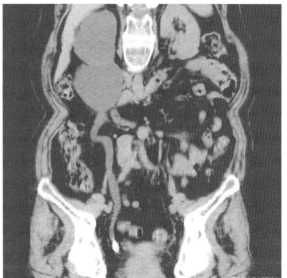

b

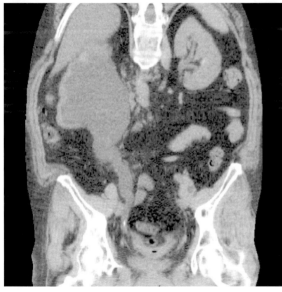

b

Fig. 27.48a–c. Urolithiasis: value of MPRs along the axis of the ureter in different patients. **a** MPR of native spiral CT clearly demonstrates both stone and dilatation of collecting system and ureter. **b** MPR of native spiral CT clearly demonstrates both stone in the distal part of the right ureter and massive dilatation of right collecting system; renal parenchyma is so severely atrophic that it can no longer be identified. **c** MPR of native spiral CT clearly demonstrates both stone in the distal part of the right ureter and massive dilatation of right collecting system: the small stone is impacted above the site of radiation fibrosis; severe loss of renal function with thinning of parenchyma

◁ ——————————————————————

Fig. 27.47a–c. Investigations in a patient with acute right lumbar pain: normal plain film and US; hyperthermia 48 h after initial symptoms. **a** Native spiral CT: 5-mm stone with periureteral fat infiltration. **b** Native spiral CT (reconstructed along the axis of the right ureter): mild dilatation of the collecting system and ureter with periureteral infiltration. **c** Native spiral CT (reconstructed along the axis of the right ureter): 1 week later, the small stone has progressed to the distal ureter

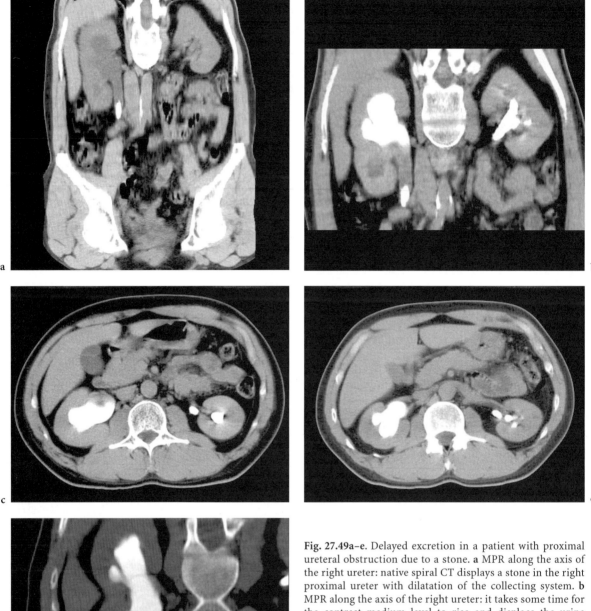

Fig. 27.49a–e. Delayed excretion in a patient with proximal ureteral obstruction due to a stone. **a** MPR along the axis of the right ureter: native spiral CT displays a stone in the right proximal ureter with dilatation of the collecting system. **b** MPR along the axis of the right ureter: it takes some time for the contrast medium level to rise and displace the urine above; the contrast medium tends to accumulate in the most dependent part of the renal collecting system with lack of opacification of inferior calix and proximal ureter. **c** Axial spiral CT: round pseudomass at the anterior part of the right pelvis due to delayed contrast medium excretion. **d** Late axial spiral CT at the same level as in **c**: homogeneous opacification of the pelvis. **e** Reconstructed spiral CT at the late excretory phase displays stone and complete opacification of the collecting system

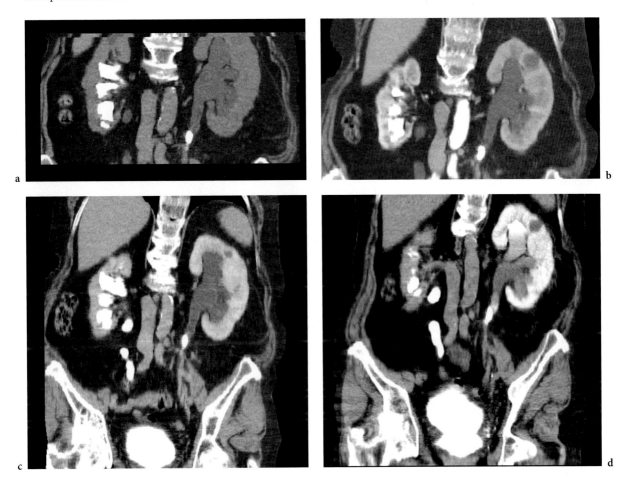

Fig. 27.50a–d. Acute obstruction: classic findings on CT urography performed in the work-up of renal colic: mild left flank pain and urinary infection. **a** Native spiral CT: stone in the upper lumbar ureter with dilatation of the collecting system. **b** Spiral CT at the cortical phase: faint enhancement of the cortex. **c** Spiral CT at the early excretory phase (5 min): no opacification of left collecting system. **d** Spiral CT at the excretory phase 2 h later: delayed excretion with faintly opacified collecting system and increasingly denser nephrogram

27.3.4.3
Fistulas

CT provides several unique criteria for diagnosing ureteral injuries. It is often capable of differentiating liquefying hematomas from lymphatic or urine collections. Postcontrast images with a delay of up to 3 h are required to detect leakage of contrast medium-containing urine and to find the precise site of the fistula.

27.3.5
Endometriosis

Pathology. The incidence of ureteral involvement by endometriosis is 1.2%. Usually, the utero-sacral liga-

ments are also involved. Distinction has been made between the so-called intrinsic and extrinsic forms. The latter includes encasement or displacement of the ureter by endometriosis of the surrounding structures; the ureteral wall and mucosa remain intact. Invasion of the ureter, possibly with penetration of the mucosa, is considered the intrinsic form. In both forms, dense fibrosis is found histologically. This is the result of a desmoplastic reaction (SHOOK and NYBERG 1988; STILLWELL et al. 1986).

Radiological Appearance of Ureteral Endometriosis. The appearance is relatively specific: it consists of a 0.5- to 2-cm stricture located within the last 2–5 cm of the ureter. This stricture usually begins 3 cm distal to the inferior aspect of the sacroiliac joint at the level of the utero-sacral ligaments (PATEL et al.

1992). A typical feature is medial attraction of the ureter with a J-shaped course at the level of utero-sacral ligaments. Hydronephrosis and hydroureter can widely vary from severely nonfunctioning kidney to only moderate ureter obstruction. Excretory urography is the main imaging procedure for demonstrating endometriosis of the ureter. On MRI, diagnosis of endometrial cyst can be strongly suggested, since hemorrhagic fluid has a characteristic behavior. Small foci of endometriosis are not readily apparent by any imaging technique.

Findings at Spiral CT. Delayed CT images demonstrate the site and extent of the ureter obstruction: close proximity to the uterus, medial attractions of the ureter and adnexal cysts are regarded as features very suggestive of endometriosis (Fig. 27.51).

Place of Spiral CT Among Imaging Techniques. MRI is clearly superior to CT for the diagnosis of endometriosis. The unique T1 and T2 relaxation times of the hemorrhagic fluid make it possible to determine the age of the hemorrhagic components. MR urography is a useful tool to indicate the precise location and extent of the stricture.

27.3.6
Postradiation and Postoperative Ureteritis

27.3.6.1
Postradiation Ureteritis

Pathology. The ureters are relatively resistant to radiation. However, radiation-induced changes do occur, most often in the form of strictures. Ureteral strictures have been reported in 1–3% (or even less) of patients treated with brachytherapy or external-beam radiation therapy for pelvic malignancies. Chronic radiation-induced ureteral injuries typically occur approximately 6 months after treatment but may be seen as late as 10 years or longer thereafter. Strictures are the most common manifestation of chronic post-radiation ureteral injury and typically involve the distal ureter at or just above the ureterovesical junction. The strictures can be up to 8 cm long and usually have smooth margins.

Findings on Spiral CT. Diffuse and circumferential thickening of the ureter wall is the main feature (Fig. 27.52). Strong enhancement is clearly identified at early phase CT after contrast medium injection (CAPPS et al. 1997). Rarely, iliac artery aneurysms

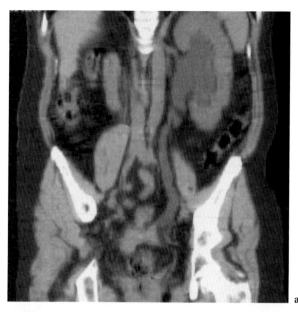

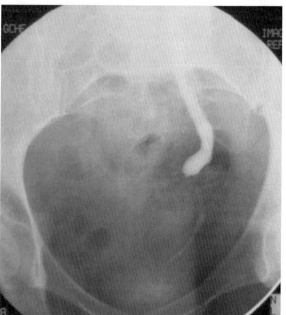

Fig. 27.51a, b. Endometriosis: nonfunctioning kidney and medial attraction of the left ureter close to a pelvic fibrous soft-tissue mass. **a** Spiral CT clearly depicts the site of obstruction. **b** Antegrade pyelography gives similar information on the site of obstruction

are observed after ureteral stent and radiation therapy (MARINO et al. 1987) (Fig. 27.52).

27.3.6.2
Postoperative Ureter

Spiral CT is a good complement to US in the radiological work-up of complications after urinary di-

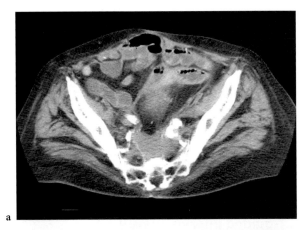

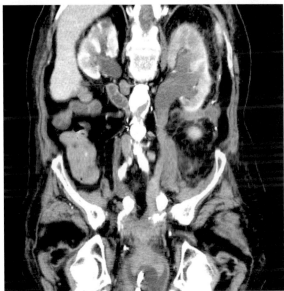

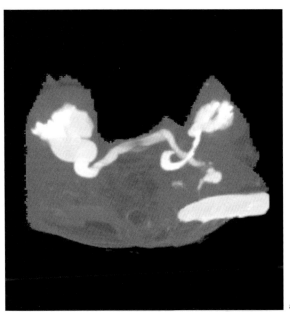

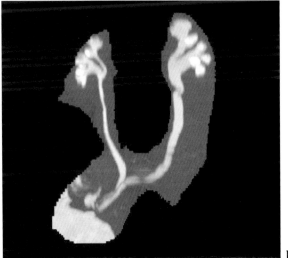

Fig. 27.52a, b. A 70-year-old man was hospitalized with gross hematuria. Radiation-induced ureteral stricture after administration of 45 Gy to the pelvis for rectal carcinoma was treated by retrograde stent. Persistent gross hematuria after retrieval of the stent. Spiral CT study (20-s acquisition time, 5.5-mm slice thickness, pitch 1.5). **a** Axial spiral CT at the early phase of contrast medium injection: increased antero-posterior diameter (>1 cm) of the presacral space. Aneurysm of left internal iliac artery. **b** MPR along the axis of the left ureter: increased attenuation of the lumbar part of the left internal iliac artery suggests presence of blood – dilatation of the initial portion of the artery. Embolization of the internal iliac artery immediately stops the hematuria

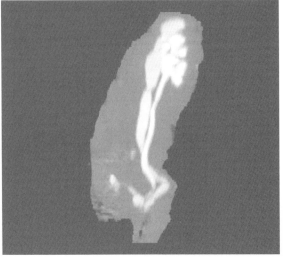

Fig. 27.53a–c. MIP representation of ileal loop diversion (Bricker loop): bilateral obstruction due the configuration of the loop, which is too narrow and tubular. **a** Axial MIP. **b** Coronal MIP. **c** Sagittal MIP. Note the external collecting bag placed over a stoma

version (Fig. 27.53) or renal transplantation (Figs. 27.54–27.57). Ureter obstruction, fistulas, lymphoceles and pseudoaneurysms of renal artery are well depicted.

27.3.7
Congenital Anomalies of the Ureter

Spiral CT has not often been performed in the workup of patients with congenital anomalies of the ureters, because sufficient information is usually provided by US and excretory urography. However, the capabilities of spiral CT to depict the collecting system are sometimes useful (BRAVERMAN and LEBOWITZ 1991) (Fig. 27.58). Delayed enhanced spiral CT is particularly appropriate when the renal function is poor, either because of obstruction of the

collecting system or because the renal parenchyma is severely atrophic. In the following situations, spiral CT is of great help (CRONAN et al. 1986):

- Ectopic ureter arising from the upper-pole system: CT shows intra- or extravesical implantation (Fig. 27.59).
- Dysplasic ectopic kidney with ectopic implantation in the seminal vas (SCHWARTZ et al. 1988).
- Retrocaval ureter (LAUTIN et al. 1988) (Fig. 27.60).

27.4
CT-guided Interventions

Because of respiratory misregistration, precise visualization of the needle tip during retroperitoneal biopsy or placement of a catheter drainage system is

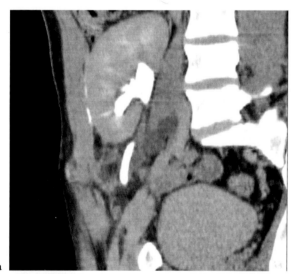

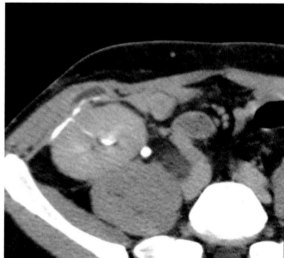

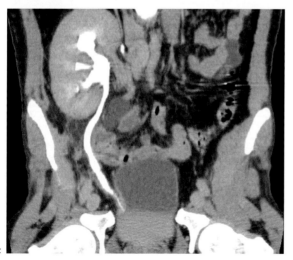

Fig. 27.54a–c. Renal transplantation: obstruction at the ureterovesical anastomosis was treated by percutaneous drainage; follow-up spiral CT after retrieval of drainage catheter (20-s acquisition time, 2.7-mm slice thickness, pitch 1.5). **a** Coronal reconstruction through the transplant kidney: urine leak along the transplant. **b** Axial reconstruction: extravasated urine surrounds the lateral border of the transplant kidney. **c** MPR along the axis of the ureter: mild obstruction at the ureterovesical anastomosis

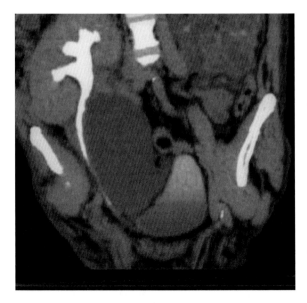

Fig. 27.55. Renal transplantation with postoperative obstruction: lymphocele. Reconstructed spiral CT at the excretory phase: displacement and compression of the ureter through a huge lymph collection

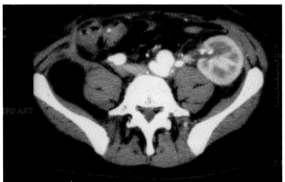

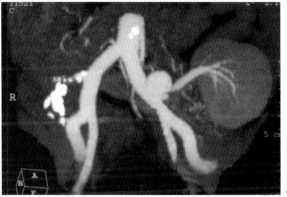

Fig. 27.57a, b. Renal transplant and mycotic aneurysm of the iliac artery: acute hypogastric pain and perineal hematoma in a renal transplant patient. No renal failure. a Axial plane at the early arterial phase demonstrates the iliac aneurysm. b MIP confirms the anastomotic aneurysm

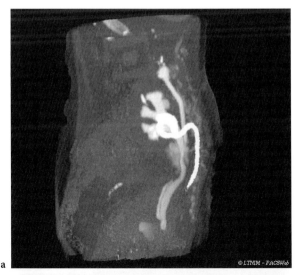

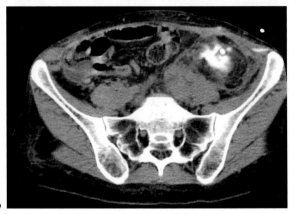

Fig. 27.56a, b. Renal transplant, complete duplication of collecting system: obstructive renal failure, fistula from lower-pole ureter, pyelostomy of the inferior collecting system. a MIP at the excretory phase: double ureter with dilatation of the inferior collecting system and extravasation of contrast just below the pyeloureteral junction. b Axial plane at the excretory phase demonstrates the extravasation around the ureter. Fistula related to ischemic necrosis of the ureter

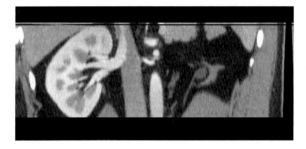

Fig. 27.58. Hypoplasia of the left kidney. MPR displays the pyelon and the initial segment of the left ureter of a severely hypoplastic left kidney

often time-consuming with conventional CT. Furthermore, following puncture, placement of the catheter drain requires considerable time during the different steps of the procedures (dilatation of the needle path, placement of the catheter and verification of its optimal position).

In our experience, real-time CT fluoroscopy combined with laser guidance reduces the duration of the image-guided percutaneous procedures significantly (LEMAITRE et al. 1998).

A third-generation spiral CT scanner (CT Twin *flash*, Elscint, Haifa, Israel) equipped with a slip-ring and two 526-channel solid-state detector arrays was upgraded by adding a high-speed array processor (real-time reconstruction unit) to increase the image reconstruction speed. This technique makes it possible to reconstruct CT data acquired with a continuous exposure and display them in real time. To achieve a higher response speed and lower sensitivity to needle partial-volume artifacts, the two raw data files are used together to reconstruct one single fused image. The reconstruction matrix is 256×256, which is interpolated to 512×512 for display purposes.

As a result, a display rate of six images/s with a delay time of 0.7 s is achieved. The gantry aperture diameter is 700 mm and, thanks to its flared shape, interventions with large angulation of the gantry are possible. Both couch sliding and gantry tilting up to 30° are feasible during CT-fluoroscopic procedures.

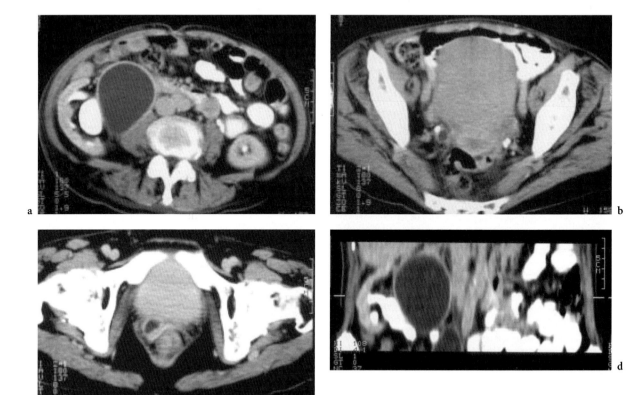

Fig. 27.59a–d. Complete duplication of right collecting system with ectopic orifice into the vagina. a Obstruction of the medially located upper kidney. b Severe dilatation and absence of opacification of the medially located upper-pole ureter. c The upper-pole ureter is recognized close to the vagina. d MPR

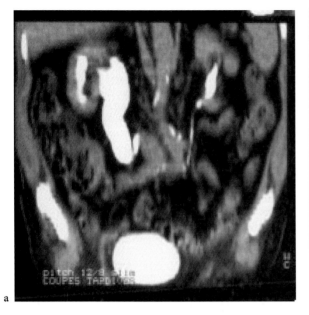
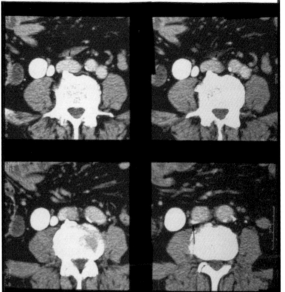

a   b

Fig. 27.60a,b. Retrocaval ureter. a MPR along the axis of the ureter: ureter is seen looping medially. b Four successive axial images at the excretory phase: the ureter goes around the inferior vena cava with dilatation of the upper collecting system

In the early phase of our experience, we used the following parameters: 120 kV and 25 mA, resulting in an exposure of 12 mAs per image, 5-mm slice collimation.

Use of a special laser-guidance system (Laser-Guide, Elscint) installed on the gantry directs an external laser-beam marker towards the lesion. The position and the angulation of the laser beam relative to the patient and the depth of needle penetration are simulated on previously acquired axial images. After positioning and angulation of the laser beam on a cutaneous marker, a puncture is made while the laser beam is directed onto the external extremity of the needle and the angulation is maintained during the course of the puncture. Verification of the needle tip localization is obtained during CT fluoroscopy, and the path can be maintained with or without a needle holder: cranial or caudal couch-sliding allows the progression of the guide and then of the catheter to be followed into the pelvicaliceal system.

CT fluoroscopy allows routine, efficient and safe percutaneous nephrostomy placement, especially when access to the pelvicaliceal system proves difficult. In our experience, the mean time necessary for the procedure was 26 min, not including patient setting-up and postprocedure control. The average duration of CT fluoroscopy per nephrostomy placement was 49 s (LEMAITRE et al. 1998).

In our study, using needle holder or intermittent fluoroscopy made it possible to minimize or avoid irradiation of the operator's hand. The radiation dose to the operator's hand with or without the use of a needle holder was estimated by using scattered radiation information supplied by the manufacturer. The irradiation of the patient and of the operator was kept low by the use of the high-attenuation bow-tie filter, short exposure times and the lowest possible scanning parameters (tube voltage of 80 kV and tube current 30 mAs).

The advantage of CT-guided procedures is that they provide the best access site for percutaneous lithotripsy and for transpapillary puncture in order to reach the cup of the selected calyx.

The advent of spiral CT has brought new applications for interventional procedures and will further greatly increase the central role of CT in patient management.

27.5
Conclusion

Spiral CT improves imaging of the retroperitoneum through the elimination of respiratory misregistration and the reduction of partial volume averaging. The high data acquisition speed makes it possible to cover the entire abdomen and pelvis in less than 25 s with 5-mm effective slice thickness during a single breath-hold. Exploration of the urinary tract can include CT angiography and CT urography.

The advent of multiple arcs of detectors in the very near future will improve the quality of the information yielded by CT even further.

References

Baron RL, McClennan BL, Lee JKT et al (1982) Computed tomography of transitional-cell carcinoma of the renal pelvis and ureter. Radiology 144:125–130

Bell TV, Fenlon HM, Davison BD et al (1998) Unenhanced helical CT criteria to differentiate distal ureteral calculi from pelvic phleboliths Radiology 207:363–367

Bosniak MA, Megibow AJ, Ambos MA et al (1982) Computed tomography of ureteral obstruction. AJR Am J Roentgenol 138:1107–1113

Braverman RM, Lebowitz (1991) Occult ectopic ureter in girls with urinary incontinence: diagnosis by using CT. AJR Am J Roentgenol 156:365–366

Capps GW, Fulcher AS, Szucs RA et al (1997) Imaging features of radiation-induced changes in the abdomen. Radiographics 17:1455–1473

Chambers TP, Baron RL, Lush RM (1994) Hepatic CT enhancement. II. Alterations in contrast material volume and rate of injection within the same patients. Radiology 193:518–522

Chen HH, Panella JS, Rochester D et al (1988) Non-Hodgkin lymphoma of ureteral wall: CT findings. J Comput Assist Tomogr 12:157–15

Cronan JJ, Amis ES, Zeman RK et al (1986) Obstruction of the upper-pole moiety in renal duplication in adults: CT evaluation. Radiology 161:17–21

Cullenward MJ, Scanlan KA, Pozniak MA et al (1986) Inflammatory aortic aneurysm (periaortic fibrosis): radiologic imaging. Radiology 159:75–82

Degesys GE, Dunnick NR, Silverman PM et al (1986) Retroperitoneal fibrosis: use of CT in distinguishing among possible causes. AJR Am J Roentgenol 146:57–60

Ditonno P, Smith RB, Koyle MA et al (1992) Extrarenal angiomyolipomas of the perinephric space. J Urol 147:447–450

Dorfman RE, Alpern MB, Groos BH et al (1991) Upper abdominal lymph nodes: criteria for normal size determined with CT. Radiology 180:319–322

Frank R, Stenzl A, Frede T et al (1998) Three-dimensional computed tomography of the reconstructed lower urinary tract: technique and findings. Eur Radiol 8:657–663

Fukuya T, Honda H, Hayashi T et al (1995) Lymph-node metastases: efficacy of detection with helical CT in patients with gastric cancer. Radiology 197:705–711

Glanz I, Grünebaum M (1976) Ureteral changes in polyarteritis nodosa as seen during excretory urography. J Urol 116:731–733

Kenney PJ, Stanley RJ (1987) Computed tomography of ureteral tumors. J Comput Assist Tomogr 11:102–107

Kottra JJ, Dunnick NR (1996) Retroperitoneal fibrosis. Radiol Clin North Am 34:1259–1275

Lautin EM, Haramati N, Frager D et al (1988) CT diagnosis of circumcaval ureter. AJR Am J Roentgenol 150:591–594

Lemaitre L, Ernst O, Dubrulle F et al (1998) Percutaneous nephrostomy: placement under laser guidance and real time CT fluoroscopy. 6th European symposium on uroradiology, 12–16 Sept 1998, Strasbourg

Levine JA, Neitlich J, Verga M et al (1997) Ureteral calculi in patients with flank pain: correlation of plain film radiography with unenhanced helical CT. Radiology 204:27–31

Liang Y, Kruger RA (1996) Dual-slice spiral versus single-slice spiral scanning: comparison of the physical performance of two computed tomography scanners. Am Assoc Phys Med 23:205–216

Liberman SN, Halpern EJ, Sullivan K et al (1997) Spiral computed tomography for staghorn calculi. Urology 50:519–524

Marino R, Mooppan UMM, Zein TA et al (1987) Urological manifestations of isolated iliac artery aneurysms. J Urol 137:232–234

McNicholas MMJ, Raptopoulos VD, Schwartz RK et al (1998) Excretory phase CT urography for opacification of the urinary collection system. AJR Am J Roentgenol 170:1261–1267

Mostafavi MR, Ernst RD, Saltzman B (1998) Accurate determination of chemical composition of urinary calculi by spiral computerized tomography. J Urol 159:673–675

Munechika H, Honda M, Kushihashi T et al (1987) Computed tomography of retroperitoneal cystic lymphangiomas. J Comput Assist Tomogr 11:116–119

Naegeli CH, Cordasco EM, Meden G et al (1990) Lymphangiomyomatosis-newer concepts in pathogenesis and management-case reports. Angiology 41:957–960

Olcott EW, Sommer FG, Napel S (1997) Accuracy of detection and measurement of renal calculi: in vitro comparison of three-dimensional spiral CT, radiography and nephrotomography. Radiology 204:19–25

Patel A, Thorpe P, Ramsay JWA et al (1992) Endometriosis of the ureter. Br J Urol 69:495–498

Perlman ES, Rosenfield AT, Wexler JS et al (1996) CT urography in the evaluation of urinary tract disease. J Comput Assist Tomogr 20:620–626

Pode D, Caine M (1992) Spontaneous retroperitoneal hemorrhage. J Urol 147:311–318

Preminger GM, Vieweg J, Leder RA et al (1998) Urolithiasis: detection and management with unenhanced spiral CT – a urologic perspective. Radiology 207:308–309

Puech JL, Song MY, Joffre F et al (1987) Ureteral metastases-computed tomographic findings. Eur J Radiol 7:103–106

Randazzo RF, Neustein P, Koyle MA (1987) Spontaneous perinephric hemorrhage from extrarenal angiomyolipoma. Urology 29:428–431

Remer EM, Herts BR, Streem SB et al (1997) Spiral noncontrast CT versus combined plain film radiography and renal US after extracorporeal shock wave lithotripsy: cost-identification analysis. Radiology 204:33–37

Rubin GD, Silverman SG (1995) Helical spiral CT of the retroperitoneum. Radiol Clin North Am 33:903–932

Schwartz LM, Kenney PJ, Bueschen AJ (1988) Computed tomographic diagnosis of ectopic ureter with seminal vesicle cyst. Urology 31:55–56

Shook TE, Nyberg LM (1988) Endometriosis of the urinary tract. Urology 31:1–6

Smith PA, Marshall FF, Fishman EK (1998) Spiral computed tomography evaluation of the kidneys: state of the art. Urology 51:3–11

Som P (1992) Detection of metastasis in cervical lymph nodes: CT and MR criteria and differential diagnosis. AJR Am J Roentgenol 158:961–969

Sommer FG, Jeffrey RB, Rubin GD et al (1995) Detection of ureteral calculi in patients with suspected renal colic: value of reformatted noncontrast helical CT. AJR Am J Roentgenol 165:509–513

Steinkamp HJ, Hosten N, Richter C et al (1994) Enlarged cervical lymph nodes at helical CT. Radiology 191:795–798

Stillwell TJ, Kramer SA, Lee RA (1986) Endometriosis of ureter. Urology 28:81–85

Vassallo P, Wernecke K, Roos N et al (1992) Differentiation of benign from malignant superficial lymphadenopathy: the role of high-resolution US. Radiology 183:215–220

Waldron JA, Newcomer LN, Katz ME et al (1983) Sclerosing variants of follicular center cell lymphomas presenting in the retroperitoneum. Cancer 52:712–720

Whalen RK, Althausen AF, Daniels GH (1992) Extra-adrenal pheochromocytoma. J Urol 147:1–10

Wilms G, Oyen R, Waer M et al (1986) CT demonstration of aneurysms in polyarteritis nodosa. J Comput Assist Tomogr 10:513–515

Wong-You-Cheong JJ, Wagner BJ, Davis CJ (1998) Transitional cell carcinoma of the urinary tract: radiologic-pathologic correlation. Radiographics 18:123–142

Yilmaz S, Sindel T, Arslan G et al (1998) Renal colic: comparison of spiral CT, US and IVU in the detection of ureteral calculi. Eur Radiol 8:212–217

Zeman RK, Zeiberg A, Hayes WS et al (1996) Helical CT of renal masses: the value of delayed scans. AJR Am J Roentgenol 167:771–776

28 Adrenals

H.-M. HOOGEWOUD

CONTENTS

28.1   Anatomy *319*
28.1.1 Cortex *319*
28.1.2 Medulla *320*
28.1.3 Anatomic Variants: Ectopic Locations *320*
28.2   Imaging the Adrenal Glands with Spiral CT *320*
28.2.1 Intravenous Contrast Material *320*
28.2.2 Attenuation Values of Adrenals *320*
28.3   Endocrinological Aspects
        of Adrenocortical Disease *321*
28.3.1 Hypercorticism *321*
28.3.2 Hyperaldosteronism *322*
28.3.3 Virilization *322*
28.3.4 Feminization *322*
28.3.5 Mixed Endocrine Syndromes *323*
28.3.6 Cortical Hypofunction *323*
28.4   Adrenal Cortical Tumours
        and Tumour-like Conditions *323*
28.4.1 Hyperplasia *323*
28.4.2 Multinodular Adrenal with Hypercortisolism *324*
28.4.3 Multinodular Adrenals *325*
28.4.4 Adrenal Cortical Adenoma *325*
28.4.5 Incidentalomas *325*
28.4.6 Adrenal Cortical Carcinoma *326*
28.4.7 Nonneoplastic Adrenal Enlargement *329*
28.5   Adrenal Medullary Tumours *330*
28.5.1 Phaeochromocytomas *330*
28.5.2 Neuroblastomas *332*
28.5.3 Ganglioneuroblastomas *333*
28.5.4 Ganglioneuromas *333*
        References *333*

28.1
Anatomy

The two adrenal glands are located at the medial and superior aspects of the kidneys and are generally completely surrounded by perirenal fat. Occasionally fusion with the liver or with the renal capsule is encountered. The right adrenal lies posterior to the inferior vena cava, between the right liver lobe and the crus of the diaphragm. The left adrenal lies on the same level as the right, but anteromedial to the left kidney. It is located lateral to the aorta and the left crus of the diaphragm, cranial to the left renal vein.

The combined weight of both adrenals tends to be about 8 g in the case of sudden death and 12 g after prolonged illness. There is no difference between the sexes in adrenal weight.

The adrenals have an abundant arterial supply, with arteries arising from the renal artery, the aorta and the phrenic artery. Additional arterial branches from the spermatic or ovarian artery can be found on the left side, and branches from the intercostal branches on the right side. The right adrenal vein drains directly into the inferior vena cava, whereas the left adrenal vein drains mostly either into the left renal vein or into the inferior vena cava.

28.1.1
Cortex

Classically the cortex is divided into three histological layers, the zona glomerulosa, the zona fasciculata and the zona reticularis. The zona glomerulosa is the outermost layer. It is not clearly demarcated from the inner zone, and its identification is sometimes difficult, as the zona fasciculata may reach the capsule. The zona fasciculata is the thickest of all three histological layers, presenting as long columns of cells oriented radially around the adrenal vein. Generally, in unstressed subjects, the cells are clear, with a large amount of cytoplasm containing lipids. In stress, or after administration of ACTH, the cells lose their lipids and resemble the cells of the zona reticularis. The zona reticularis, the innermost zone, is well separated from the zona fasciculata in unstressed patients. The eosinophilic cells are embedded in a thick reticulin framework. The histological zones of the adrenals are not closed compartments with different hormone types specifically attributed

H.-M. HOOGEWOUD, MD; Département de Radiologie, Hôpital Cantonal, CH-1708 Fribourg, Switzerland

to each zone. It appears that most of the cell division occurs in the outermost zones and that most of the cells die in the zona reticularis.

28.1.2
Medulla

About 8–10% of the volume of the gland is occupied by medulla. Medullary tissue is not evenly distributed through the glands and is mostly concentrated in their medial aspects. There is generally a clear delineation between the cells of the medulla and those of the zona reticularis. The chromaffin medullary cells are grouped as small nests of cells surrounded by a rich capillary network. The cells, which have a granular basophilic cytoplasm, are round or polyhedric.

28.1.3
Anatomic Variants: Ectopic Locations

Accessory adrenal tissue contains mostly cells of the cortical type. Ectopic adrenal tissue can be found in the retroperitoneum around the coeliac plexus, in and around the kidney, and in the genitalia, the broad ligaments, the spermatic cord and the epididymis.

28.2
Imaging the Adrenal Glands
with Spiral CT

Speed is not an issue in CT scan examinations of the adrenals. The main advantage of helical scanning is the reduction of misregistration due to patient movement or intestinal peristalsis.

Adrenal glands are generally small, thin structures and require high-quality imaging with good resolution. Generally, routine precontrast scans of the upper abdomen are performed with 7–10 mm slice thickness before contrast injection. They give a clue to the pathology to be expected. Because of the importance of precontrast and postcontrast attenuation densitometry and of the necessity to minimize partial volume effects, we use a helical protocol with 3-mm slice thickness, a pitch of 1.4–2.0 at 120 kV, 190–240 mA, 0.8 s per rotation and a reduced field of view. Images are reconstructed every 3 mm. This protocol can be adapted, and 5-mm slices are used in

the presence of larger adrenal masses. Unenhanced normal adrenal glands have an attenuation of about 25 HU. Differentiation of cortex and medulla is not possible. Adrenal glands generally resemble an inverted "Y", "V" or "L" and are mostly readily recognized in their typical location. Although with state-of-the-art CT scanners both adrenals are generally easily recognized, parts of adrenal gland limbs may be truncated or be confused with veins or soft tissue strands in the perirenal fat. Recognition of the adrenals may sometimes be difficult in slim patients with low body fat.

28.2.1
Intravenous Contrast Material

Contrast material (1.5–2 ml/kg body weight with an iodine content of 300 g/l) is injected into the antecubital vein of patients with normal renal function. Imaging starts about 25–35 s after the beginning of the injection. Contrast material helps to delineate vascular structures, especially adjacent veins, from the adrenals and to avoid confusing them with adrenal limbs, which can happen in patients with few body fat.

Intravenous Contrast Material and Phaeochromocytoma. In the presence of known secreting phaeochromocytoma it is prudent to administer alpha and beta adrenergic blockade prior to contrast material injection, as an adrenergic hypertensive crisis can occur. The response of plasma epinephrine levels to intravenous injections of contrast material is unpredictable. Recently, however, it has been shown that specific blockade may not be required before contrast medium-enhanced scanning with iohexol (MUKHERJEE et al. 1997).

28.2.2
Attenuation Values of Adrenals

28.2.2.1
Nonenhanced Scans

In the recent literature, considerable attention has been given to attenuation values of adrenal tissue on unenhanced scans. In general, adenomas have relatively low attenuation values on unenhanced CT scans, due to their lipid content. The low attenuation values may help to differentiate adenomas from nonadenomas, as on average, adenomas have attenuation values of about 2.2 – 8.6 HU and non-adenomas, about 30–40 HU (LEE et al. 1991; SINGER et al. 1994; KOROBKIN et al. 1996). Overlaps are rare. For characterizing benign adrenal masses a threshold CT attenuation value of 0 HU has a sensitivity/specificity ratio of 33–47%/100%, whereas a threshold attenuation of 10 HU has a ratio of 73–79%/96%. A diagnosis based solely on unenhanced attenuation values can be misleading, as cystic phaeochromocytoma, for example, may show values between 5 and 15 HU (MUNDEN et al. 1993).

28.2.2.2
Enhancement of Adrenal Lesions After Contrast Material

In distinguishing benign from malignant adrenal disease, it is generally agreed that early contrast enhancement does not contribute anything, except for delineation from the kidney or from adjacent vessels. Both benign and malignant lesions, adenomas and nonadenomas, show enhancement after bolus injection of contrast material. The mean attenuation of nonadenomas is significantly greater than that of adenomas on scans acquired 60–90 s after injection of contrast material. There is, however, a greater overlap in attenuation values of the adenomas and nonadenomas than on unenhanced images. Imaging in the early contrast enhancement phase is helpful in distinguishing the adrenals from adjacent structures such as kidney or vessels.

Delayed scanning after contrast material injection (Table 28.1) is helpful to distinguish adenoma from nonadenoma, malignant from benign adrenal

tumours. Proposed scanning delays range between 15 min and 60 min after injection. KOROBKIN studied the washout curves of adrenal adenomas and nonadenomas. There was no significant difference between the two groups in peak enhancement. With over 5 min of delay the attenuation measured was significantly lower in the adenoma group than in the nonadenoma group. With 150 ml of 300 mg iodine/ml contrast medium injected at a rate of 2–3 ml/s and a threshold of 37 HU, the specificity/sensitivity ratio for the diagnosis of adenoma on the 15 min delayed scan was 96%/96% (KOROBKIN et al. 1998).

28.3
Endocrinological Aspects of Adrenocortical Disease

28.3.1
Hypercorticism

Adrenal hyperproduction of the principal glucocorticoid, cortisol, characterizes Cushing's syndrome. Hypercorticism can have different causes, such as iatrogenic steroid medication, pituitary overproduction of ACTH and consequently adrenal hyperplasia (Cushing's disease), ectopic ACTH production and autonomous production of cortisol by neoplasms of the adrenal cortex. Clinically, the syndrome is characterized by a combination of following symptoms: glucose intolerance, hypertension, truncal obesity, muscle weakness and fatiguability, abdominal striae, oedema and osteoporosis. Cushing's syndrome is

Table 28.1. Summary of information needed for delayed scanning

Delay	Attenuation at delayed scans of adenomas	Attenuation at delayed scans of nonadenomas	Proposed threshold	Specificity / sensitivity	Reference
60 min	11±13 HU	49±8.3 HU	30 HU	100%/95%	KOROBKIN et al. 1996
30 min	<37 HU	>41 HU	<37 HU	100%/100%	SZOLAR and KAMMERHUBER 1997
14 min	–	–	24 HU	96%/98%	BOLAND et al. 1997
0	–2±13 HU	30±8 HU			
40–80 s	64±29 HU	63±16 HU			
5 min	21±12 HU	61±16 HU			
10 min	16±12 HU	59±13 HU			KOROBKIN et al. 1998
15 min	15±14 HU	64±23 HU	37 HU	96%/96%	
30 min	16±14 HU	52±14 HU			
45 min	13±13 HU	49±11 HU			

confirmed by increased production of cortisol in the absence of stress and low ACTH. In normal individuals there is a diurnal variation of cortisol and ACTH production, the highest blood cortisol level being measured in the morning. In patients with Cushing's syndrome the levels in the evening may be as high as those earlier in the day. After administration of dexamethasone, a synthetic glucocorticoid, a decrease in production of cortisol is noted in patients with pituitary-dependent Cushing's syndrome (Cushing's disease). Tumours producing ACTH ectopically do not respond to dexamethasone, and neither do tumours that secrete cortisol autonomously, such as adrenal cortical neoplasms.

About 80% of cases of endogenous hypercorticism are related to pituitary overproduction of ACTH: 10–15% have ACTH production by non-pituitary tumours, most often small cell carcinomas of the lung. Hypercorticism due to cortical adrenal neoplasms is rare, being caused by adrenal carcinoma in about 4% of cases and by adrenal adenomas in 5–10%. The differential diagnosis is dealt with in Table 28.2.

male sex ratio is about 3:1, and the mean age range between 30–50 years. Over 90% of patients with adenoma have a solitary nodule. Most of the others have a second nodule on the same side. Bilateral disease is rare. In this patient group the mean age is older and the sex ratio is nearly even. An important but rare cause of primary hyperaldosteronism is a dominantly inherited enzyme disease that can be relieved by dexamethasone (SUTHERLAND et al. 1966).

28.3.3
Virilization

Virilization is the appearance of male characteristics in females of any age or in prepubertal males. Virilization of adrenal origin is associated either with congenital adrenal hyperplasia (an enzymatic disorder) or with adrenal neoplasms producing androgens or androgen precursors. In adults the majority of neoplasms are malignant. Dexamethasone does not suppress secretion of plasma androgens or uri-

Table 28.2. Differential diagnosis of adrenal adenoma

Differential diagnosis	Criteria
Adrenal nodule (incidentaloma)	On CT can mimic adenoma but may be multiple. There is no atrophy or hyperplasia of adjacent adrenal tissue. Lesions larger than 5 cm are suggestive of malignancy.
Adrenal cortical carcinoma	Small carcinoma may mimic adenoma (see discussion below).
Multinodular hyperplasia	Multiple nodules within a hyperplastic adrenal. Often associated with hypercorticism.
Phaeochromocytoma (see below)	Rather homogeneous aspect. May have foci of necrosis or haemorrhage. All sizes, can be bilateral or ectopic.
Multiple endocrine neoplasia	Often bilateral.
Metastatic carcinoma	Often bilateral.

28.3.2
Hyperaldosteronism

Hyperaldosteronism is a condition defined by inappropriate secretion of aldosterone, independently of the renin-angiotensin system. Clinically, the signs of hyperaldosteronism are hypertension, potassium depletion and suppression of plasma renin activity. Normokalaemic forms of the disease exist and may mimic essential hypertension. In over 80% of cases, primary hyperaldosteronism is caused by a unilateral, predominantly solitary, cortical adenoma (Conn's syndrome; CONN et al. 1964). The female/

nary 17-ketosteroids in patients with adrenal virilizing tumours.

28.3.4
Feminization

Feminization of adrenal origin, characterized by feminizing hair changes, testicular atrophy, gynaecomastia and loss of libido, is rarely seen in adult males and is mostly due to a malignant adrenal neoplasm. In children feminization of adrenal origin is generally caused by an adrenal adenoma. When feminization is caused by an adrenal neoplasm 17-ketosteroids are elevated, the highest levels being attained in the presence of carcinoma.

28.3.5
Mixed Endocrine Syndromes

Mixed endocrine syndromes are rare. They can be seen in association with carcinomas of the adrenal cortex.

28.3.6
Cortical Hypofunction

Adrenal cortical insufficiency (Addison's disease) characterized by low cortisol and elevated ACTH can be divided into chronic (more than 2 years), sub-acute (less than 2 years) and acute insufficiency. Autoimmune-based atrophy is the most common cause of chronic adrenal cortical hypofunction. On CT, atrophy of the adrenals without calcifications is found (Fig. 28.1). Bilateral small adrenals are suggestive for autoimmune atrophy. Granulomatous infection of the adrenals is also a common cause of adrenal hypofunction. In late stages of the disease, the adrenals become atrophic and present with coarse dense calcifications. The most frequent cause of granulomatous infection of the adrenals is tuberculosis, although in the southern parts of the USA histoplasmosis may be more frequent. Calcifications secondary to granulomatous infections are indistinguishable from idiopathic calcifications. Adrenal cortical hypofunction may be seen in patients with haemochromatosis. The adrenals are hypotrophic and may be hyperdense as a result of iron deposition in the parenchyma. Bilateral metastasis to the adrenals induces adrenal cortical hypofunction only in about 20% of patients; generally adrenal function is well preserved.

The most frequent cause of subacute adrenal cortical insufficiency is the active inflammatory stage of granulomatous adrenalitis. Both adrenals are generally enlarged with hypodense zones interspersed representing areas of necrosis. Subacute Addison's disease due to cytomegalovirus, *Mycobacterium avium* and *Mycobacterium intracellulare* adrenalitis has also been described in AIDS patients. CT should be performed in all cases of subacute adrenal cortical insufficiency. The presence of enlarged adrenals bilaterally is indicative of granulomatous infection. A fine needle aspiration biopsy is helpful to detect

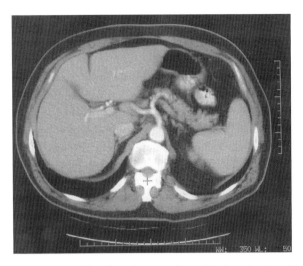

Fig. 28.1. Atrophic adrenals in a patient with chronic adrenal cortical hypofunction. The right adrenal gland is very thin, and the left can hardly be distinguished from adjacent vessels

the pathogen and establish the diagnosis.

Missing the diagnosis of acute adrenal cortical insufficiency may be fatal. Clinical symptoms such as nausea, vomiting, diarrhoea, hypotension and weakness are quite unspecific. The most frequent cause is adrenal haemorrhage seen after severe hypotension, shock and septicaemia. On CT the adrenals are enlarged and hyperdense owing to the presence of blood.

28.4
Adrenal Cortical Tumours and Tumour-like Conditions

28.4.1
Hyperplasia

Hyperplasia is defined as an increased number of cells in an organ and is thus generally associated with increased function. A large number of patients lack evidence of hypersecretion from the adrenals, however, despite the presence of enlarged nodular adrenal glands. The term "nodule" is reserved for such cases of focally increased adrenal cells without proven alteration of secretory function.

28.4.1.1
Congenital Adrenal Hyperplasia

There are various forms of congenital adrenal hyperplasia. They are the result of congenital errors in the various steps of biosynthesis of cortisol, androgens and/or aldosterone. These metabolic errors are due to reduced effectiveness or absence of different enzymes necessary for the biosynthesis of cortisol. Compensatory hypersecretion of precursor metabolites is the result of reduced production of cortisol common to all these situations and causes hyperplasia of the adrenals. As various cortisol precursors have mineralocorticoid and androgenic activity, hypertension and virilization are common in both males and females. At autopsy the glands have a cerebriform appearance with extensive infolding of cortex and predominance of compacta cells extending to the periphery. As most patients are treated the glands have a normal appearance on CT.

28.4.1.2
Hyperplasia and Hypercorticism Due to Pituitary ACTH Hypersecretion

In Cushing's disease, ACTH-dependent hypercorticism, ACTH produced in excess overstimulates the adrenals, which in turn become symmetrically enlarged and hypersecrete cortisol. Most patients are aged between 30 and 40 years, and the sex ratio shows a female predominance of 3:1. The adrenals are not massively enlarged, seldom exceeding the doubling of the organ volume. Normally the combined weight of the adrenals is 8 g. In Cushing's disease the combined weight ranges between 12 and 16 g, just occasionally reaching 24 g. On CT enlargement of the organs can be recognized, sometimes with a slight degree of nodularity.

28.4.1.3
Hyperplasia and Hypercorticolism Due to Ectopic ACTH

The appearance of the adrenals hyperstimulated by ectopically produced ACTH (often a small cell cancer of the lungs) is quite similar to that seen in Cushing's disease. The combined weight of the glands ranges between 24 and 30 g. The thickness of the cortex often exceeds 4 mm.

28.4.1.4
Hyperplasia and Hyperaldosteronism

Inappropriate release of excess amounts of aldosterone is generally due to an adrenal cortical adenoma. Diffuse hyperplasia of both glands can be found in the absence of adenoma, but is rare. However, hyperplasia and adenomas often coexist in hyperaldosteronism.

28.4.2
Multinodular Adrenal with Hypercortisolism

In a few patients with bilateral adrenal disease and Cushing's syndrome nodules can be found. In these patients there is an overlap between adenoma and hyperplasia.

28.4.2.1
Multinodular Hyperplasia with Hypercorticism

Both adrenals are grossly enlarged in the presence of this combination, because of irregularly distributed nodules. Anatomically, the cortex can hardly be recognized because of the large numbers of nodules. The dexamethasone test is not effective. The patients suffering from this condition do usually respond to ACTH and metyrapone, however. It is classified as hyperplasia, as the cortex between the nodules is active and hyperplastic. The size of the nodules may range from a few millimetres up to 30 mm. The combined gland weight generally ranges between 60 and 100 g. A combined weight of 167 g has been reported. CT demonstrated bilaterally enlarged adrenal glands distorted by multiple bumps (TERZOLO et al. 1997).

28.4.2.2
Microadenomatous Adrenal with Hypercorticism

In this condition, the adrenals have an almost normal weight. The morphology of the glands is characterized by many evenly dispersed nodules with a diameter of 1–5 mm, combined with apparently inactive internodular cells. These patients with low plasmatic ACTH suffer from hypercorticism, which does not respond to any hormonal manipulation. The hormonal situation is similar to that in adrenal neoplasm. Different terms have been coined for this condition, such as "familial pigmented nodular hyperplasia" and "micronodular cortical adenomatosis". The appearance on CT is that of normal adrenals, as the size of the nodules does not allow their recognition and the weight of the gland is normal. As in this condition the adrenals act in an autonomic way, bilateral adrenalectomy has been advocated as the treatment of choice.

28.4.2.3
Relations Between Hyperplasia and Neoplasia

Except in congenital types of hyperplasia, there is little evidence that hyperplasia progresses to neoplasia. Adrenal hyperplasia may present in the form of nodules, which may even be encapsulated and mimic adenomas. The histological distinction between adenoma and hyperplasia can be difficult in these situations. Only functional autonomy or the presence of metastases can prove the existence of a neoplasm. Imaging techniques are not helpful.

28.4.3
Multinodular Adrenals

Nodules are frequently encountered in the adrenals. Their size varies between less than 1 mm and 3–4 cm. Nodules are frequently multiple and bilateral, few reaching a larger size. There is often side-to-side asymmetry in the size of the nodules. Histologically, distinction from adenomas may sometimes be difficult. The incidence of nodularity of the adrenal glands increases with age, as does the number and the size of the nodules. No evidence of adrenal dysfunction is found. These nodules, formerly only discovered at autopsy, account for the vast majority of the so-called incidentalomas seen during CT examinations of the upper abdomen. On native CT scans the nodules have a low attenuation (Fig. 28.2), and on delayed scans their attenuation is also low, making distinction from true adenomas impossible.

28.4.4
Adrenal Cortical Adenoma

An adrenal adenoma is a benign neoplasm with cells resembling those of normal adrenal tissue and presenting functional autonomy. True adenomas are very rare. Syndromes associated with adenomas are, in decreasing frequency: hyperaldosteronism, hypercorticism, virilization and feminization. Cushing's disease is most frequently associated with bilateral adrenal hyperplasia, and seldom with an adrenal adenoma. In contrast, Conn's syndrome is most frequently associated with an adenoma, and rarely with adrenal hyperplasia. CT shows the presence of an adenoma, but only clinical and biological methods permit diagnosis of the type of adenoma. Adenomas in Conn's disease tend to be small and unilateral. In a series of 29 patients with hyperaldosteronism, the sensitivity of detection of the adenomas was 82% (DUNNICK et al. 1993). With CT, adrenal adenoma in Cushing's disease are easier to detect because of their larger size. Adenomas in nontreated congenital adrenal hyperplasia are even

larger, and their separation from carcinoma, which is more frequent in this entity, can be difficult.

Differential Diagnosis. Table 28.2 is devoted to the differential diagnosis of adrenal cortical adenoma, which is difficult and involves such different entities as incidentalomas, carcinomas and metastases. No single criterion permits separation of these entities in every case. Biological, histological and clinical criteria are often needed in addition to imaging techniques to obtain a definite diagnosis.

28.4.5
Incidentalomas

Incidentalomas are nodules of the adrenals with no endocrine activity, found incidentally during abdominal imaging. A multicentre retrospective study conducted in Northern Italy analysed the medical records of patients with adrenal incidentalomas over a 5-year period; 210 medical records were analysed. Adrenal cortical carcinoma was found in 13% and phaeochromocytoma in 10% of the patients operated on. The tumour diameter was highly correlated with the risk of cancer. The cut-off size of 5 cm had a sensitivity of 93% and a specificity of 64% in the discrimination between malignant and benign adrenal cortical lesions (TERZOLO et al. 1997). Cut-off sizes raise the question of whether the histological size of the adrenal tumour corresponds to the size estimated at the preoperative CT. A Greek

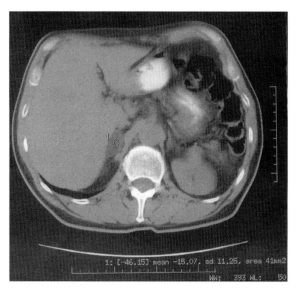

Fig. 28.2. Incidentaloma of the right adrenal gland. On the native scan the mean absorption value is –15 HU

Table 28.3. Differential diagnosis of adrenal cortical carcinoma

Differential diagnosis	Criteria
Renal adenocarcinoma	Renal adenocarcinoma distorts renal calices whereas adrenal cortical carcinoma tends to displace the normal kidney
Islet cell carcinoma	Islet cell carcinoma may be confused with ectopic adrenal cortical carcinoma, but the endocrine situation is different. Distinction is possible with biochemical tests and biopsy
Hepatocellular carcinoma	Ectopic adrenal cortical carcinoma may arise from liver and be confused with a hepatocellular carcinoma. Huge bulging hepatocellular carcinoma may be confused with adrenal cortical carcinoma on the right side. The renal capsule may, however, be recognized with helical CT (especially using multiplanar reconstruction), US, or MR. CT, or US-guided biopsy is helpful
Metastatic carcinoma	Metastases to the adrenal can be confused with adrenal cortical carcinomas. Bilateral involvement of the adrenal is more frequently seen in metastatic disease than in adrenal carcinomas. CT- or US-guided biopsy is helpful
Phaeochromocytoma and paraganglioma	Phaeochromocytoma and adrenal cortical carcinoma may be confused in CT

study addressed this problem and found in 76 tumours that CT had underestimated the histological size by over 23%. Moreover, the authors found 3 carcinomas smaller than 2.9 cm, that is to say smaller than often proposed cut-off sizes (Linos and Stylopoulos 1997).

Fine needle aspiration biopsy can be helpful in selection of patients who need operations (Gaboardi et al. 1991).

28.4.6
Adrenal Cortical Carcinoma

Carcinoma of the adrenal cortex is a very rare tumour, accounting for less than 0.1% of all malignant neoplasms (Hutter and Kayhoe 1966). Carcinomas are rarely bilateral and of ectopic origin (see below). There are two age peaks: in childhood, generally before the age of 5 years, and between 40 and 50 years.

About 20–40% of adrenal cortical carcinomas do not produce an endocrine syndrome. These can thus attain a large size before clinical detection. Most carcinomas give rise to various endocrine abnormalities, such as Cushing's syndrome, virilization and metabolic disturbances due to excretion of various steroids and their precursors.

The distinction between benign and malignant adrenal cortical neoplasm is virtually impossible when the tumour is small. Large size of the tumour is a sign of malignancy, but it should be borne in mind that there is considerable overlap, especially in sex

hormone-secreting tumours. In children carcinoma may be confused with adrenal congenital hyperplasia.

Necrosis and intratumour haemorrhage are indirect signs of malignancy. Carcinomas of the adrenal cortex may mimic renal cell carcinoma, and it is sometimes impossible to distinguish between the two either with CT or with other imaging modalities. The behaviour of adrenal cortical carcinomas after contrast medium is similar to that of renal cell carcinoma. Some tumours have cystic parts and show nearly no enhancement, while others demonstrate a strong early arterial enhancement with fast-filling draining veins. The pattern of metastatic spread is similar to that of renal cell carcinoma with nodal or haematogenous metastases. Predilection sites for metastases are liver (50%), lung (52%), local spread (50%), local lymph nodes (17%), peritoneum (15%), distant lymph nodes (14%), bone (11%), kidney (7%) and brain (4%) (Page et al. 1986). Vascular invasion, especially in the inferior vena cava, has been described. The prognosis is poor, and patients die from uncontrollable endocrine disorders or from their metastases. The differential diagnosis of adrenal cortical carcinoma is presented in Table 28.3.

28.4.6.1
Ectopic Adrenal Cortical Carcinoma

Carcinomas can also arise from ectopic adrenal cortical tissue. Ectopic tumours have been described within the kidney, the liver, the pancreas, the paraaortic region and the gonads. These tumours behave like their normotopic counterparts and may or may not produce endocrine syndromes. Only in the presence of such a syndrome is the adrenal nature of these tumours easy to ascertain. Any mass effect is dependent on the site of the tumour.

28.4.6.2
Metastases to the Adrenals

Metastases to the adrenals are frequent and often clinically silent. Metastases are the most frequent cause of malignant lesions in the adrenals. Per gram of tissue, the adrenals are the most common site for metastases of many malignant tumours. After lung, liver and bone, the adrenals are the most common site for metastatic disease from all neoplasms. Although metastatic involvement is often bilateral (Fig. 28.3a, b), adrenal insufficiency is rare, as residual cortical tissue is nearly always present. The tumours that most frequently present with adrenal metastases are listed in Table 28.4.

Table 28.4. Incidence of adrenal metastases found at autopsy depending on the type of the primary tumour

Primary tumour	Incidence	Reference
All neoplasms	27%	ABRAMS et al. 1950
Breast cancer	36%	CHO and CHOI 1980
Lung cancer	34%	AUERBACH et al. 1975
Malignant melanoma	50%	DASGUPTA and BRASFIELD 1964
Renal cell carcinoma	7–19%	CAMPBELL et al. 1983
Gastrointestinal	10–16%	CEDERMARK et al. 1977

In CT, the presentation pattern of metastases to the adrenals varies widely. On native CT they present with soft tissue density. Lesions with water-like density due to intensive necrosis and cystic transformation are often seen. Contrast enhancement pattern is also varied and depends on the type of the primary cancer (Figs. 28.4a, b, 28.5).

28.4.6.3
Unusual Tumours of the Adrenal Cortex

MYELOLIPOMA

Myelolipoma is a benign tumour or tumour-like lesion composed of matured fat cells and bone marrow cells. The cells of the haematopoietic line, as in active bone marrow, are at different stages of maturation. The incidence at autopsy ranges between 0.08% and 0.2%. The size of the lesion varies between some millimetres and 30 cm, 5 cm being the average (NOBEL et al. 1982). There are no specific symptoms associated with myelolipoma. When present, symptoms are mostly related to the mass effect (SHARMA et al. 1997). Retroperitoneal and intralesional haemorrhage has been described (CATALANO 1996). The lesion is usually found incidentally during upper abdomen CT and presents as a nonenhancing mass with fat density. Attenuation values depend on the proportion of fat and bone marrow cells. A pseudocapsule may be present. Some lesions present with considerable amounts of calcification. Detection of fat within the lesion generally establishes the diagnosis (Fig. 28.6). In lesions where fat is largely predominant, myelolipoma

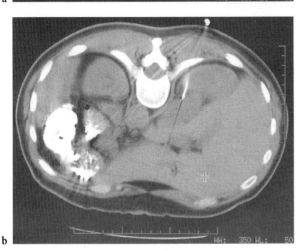

Fig. 28.3. a Bilateral necrotic metastases to the adrenal glands from a bronchial carcinoma. b Fine needle aspiration biopsy of the right adrenal gland of the same patient

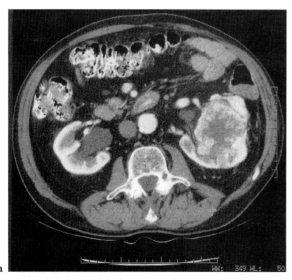

a

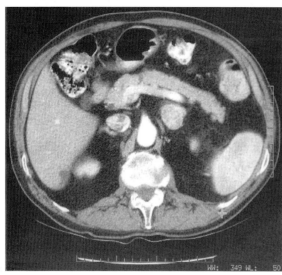

b

Fig. 28.4. a Hypernephroma in left kidney. **b** Same patient: metastasis of hypernephroma to homolateral adrenal gland

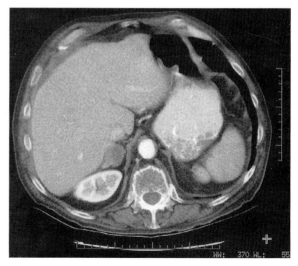

Fig. 28.5. Metastasis to right adrenal gland of a bronchial carcinoma

tween 2 cm and 15 cm (diameter). Symptoms are associated with the size and the mass effect and with intralesional haemorrhage. On native CT the smoothly marginated lesion has heterogeneous attenuation values ranging between 15–20 HU. Calcifications are either phleboliths or associated with previous episodes of intralesional haemorrhage. On contrast-enhanced CT the lesion shows a mixed picture of enhancing and nonenhancing zones. Peripheral rim enhancement on the postcontrast scan has been described (Marotti et al. 1997). In cavernous haemangioma a progressive enhancement from the periphery to the centre of the tumour, similar to the contrast enhancement of the liver, can be noticed (Rieber and Brambs 1995).

Other Rare Tumours of the Adrenal Stroma. Various rare and unusual tumours can grow within the adrenal glands. Leiomyoma and leiomyosarcoma presumably originate from the musculature of the adrenal vasculature (Choi and Liu 1981). Other neoplasms, such as teratoma, fibroma, fibrosarcoma, and neurofibroma have also been described.

Lymphoma. Primary adrenal lymphoma is extremely rare, only 16 cases having been reported in the last 40 years (Truong et al. 1997). Secondary involvement of the adrenals is more frequent, being seen at autopsy in about 25% of patients with lymphoma. The most common type of lymphoma to involve the adrenals is non-Hodgkin lymphoma. Involvement is bilateral in about 46% of patients (Feldberg et al. 1986). On native CT, attenuation

sometimes cannot be distinguished from liposarcoma. Confusion with a renal upper pole angiomyolipoma occurs sometimes. Fine needle aspiration biopsy helps to establish the diagnosis in cases where haematopoietic cells can be detected.

Diverse Connective Tissue Tumours
Angioma. Very occasionally, connective tissue neoplasms may originate in the adrenal cortex. They comprise capillary or cavernous haemangiomas and lymphangiomas. Phleboliths are characteristic for the lesion, which is generally found incidentally during upper abdomen CT. The lesion size varies be-

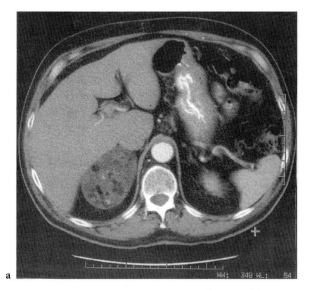

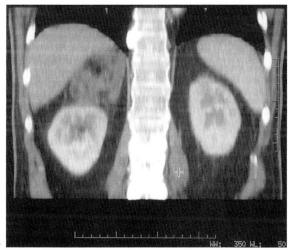

Fig. 28.6a, b. Fat-containing myelolipoma of right adrenal gland. (Courtesy of Dr F. Sadry)

values range between 40 and 60 HU, and there is little enhancement after intravenous contrast material administration. As in lymphomatous manifestations in other parts of the body, necrosis can be seen in rapidly growing lesions.

28.4.7
Nonneoplastic Adrenal Enlargement

28.4.7.1
Adrenal Cystic Lesions

Cysts of the adrenal glands are rare (1:1400 at autopsy), mostly non-functional and found inciden-

tally. About 45% of the cysts are of the endothelial type. They are predominantly small, asymptomatic, lymphangiomatous cysts. Nearly 40% of adrenal cysts are pseudocysts that lack an endothelial lining and can be considered the end-stage of a remote haemorrhage. Some adrenal cysts are true epithelial cysts and comprise retention cysts and cystic transformation of embryonic remnants. Parasites such as *Echinococcus* may also manifest as cystic adrenal lesions. Adrenal cysts can also be found as a manifestation of hepatorenal polycystic disease (BASTIDE et al. 1997). Although most adrenal cysts are small, some can be quite large and symptomatic. On unenhanced CT scans it may be difficult to distinguish between a benign cyst (Fig. 28.7) and a low-attenuation adenoma. About half of the benign cysts, and most pseudocysts or parasitic cysts, show mural, septal or even central calcifications. Wall thickness seldom exceeds 3 mm. A mural enhancement, but no intralesional enhancement, is found in about one third of cysts. The majority of cysts are unilocular and have reached a size of about 5–6 cm at detection (ROZENBLIT et al. 1996).

Cystic adrenal lesions can, however, also have other, rare, origins: cystic adenomas, cystic adrenal carcinoma, cystic metastases, cystic phaeochromocytoma, cystic neurogenic choristoma (SHERAZI and DICKS MIREAUX 1997).

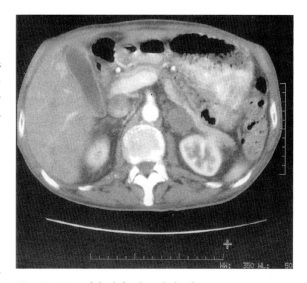

Fig. 28.7. Cyst of the left adrenal gland

28.4.7.2
Haemorrhage and Necrosis

Haemorrhage is the commonest cause of adrenal mass in neonates. The occurrence is relatively uncommon. It is said to be associated with neonatal bradycardia and asphyxia. Symptoms may be either absent or dramatic. In the presence of a massive haemorrhage, shock and hypotension may occur. If bacteraemia occurs an abscess may develop, usually about 4–6 weeks after birth (ATKINSON et al. 1985).

In adults, haemorrhage in the adrenals is rare, but it is seen after severe hypoperfusion, hypotension, shock, burns and trauma and is frequently associated with centrolobular necrosis in the liver and renal tubular necrosis. Extensive haemorrhage is seen in association with septicaemia in Waterhouse-Friderichsen syndrome. In anticoagulant-associated adrenal haemorrhage, the bleeding is apparently not due to excessive anticoagulation. It generally occurs in the first 3 weeks of treatment and is probably due to stress-induced increased production of ACTH.

Traumatic adrenal haemorrhage occurs unilaterally in about 80% and mostly on the right side. Bilateral haemorrhage may induce adrenal insufficiency (IKEKPEAZZU et al. 1996).

Adrenal haemorrhage often culminates in adrenal pseudocysts. On CT, the adrenals appear round or oval, being similar to adenomas and metastases in size and shape (Fig. 28.8). The attenuation value depends on the time gap between the CT scan and the time of the bleeding. High values of attenuation are found soon after the bleeding episode. With time, attenuation values decrease, as in other organs.

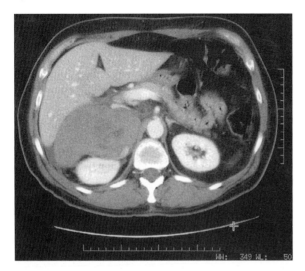

Fig. 28.8. Haemorrhage in right adrenal gland. (Courtesy of Dr F. Sadry)

28.4.7.3
Granulomatous Infection

Adrenals involved in infections producing granulomatous reaction are generally enlarged during the active inflammatory stage. Areas of necrosis are often present and can be seen as hypodense zones within the adrenals. The most common infections are tuberculosis and histoplasmosis. In the end-stages of the diseases extensive calcifications may be found in CT. Granulomatous disease is an important cause of adrenal insufficiency (see 28.3.6).

28.5
Adrenal Medullary Tumours

Adrenal medullary tumours are divided into the phaeochromocytoma type and the neuroblastoma type. Primitive cells (sympathogonia) deriving from the neural crest may differentiate either into sympathoblasts and later sympathetic ganglion cells or into phaeochromoblasts and later into phaeochromocytes. Neoplasms deriving from the most primitive cells are the most malignant and are generally seen in infancy (i.e. neuroblastoma).

28.5.1
Phaeochromocytomas

Phaeochromocytoma is a neoplasm that produces, contains and secretes catecholamines. Of neuroectodermal origin, it arises from chromaffin cells that are found in the adrenal medulla and in a large number of sympathetic ganglia in the body. In autopsy series the incidence of phaeochromocytoma is about 0.1%. About 0.1% of patients with hypertension are found to have a phaeochromocytoma. It is probable that the presence of a certain number of these tumours remains unsuspected because of low or absent endocrine activity. Most phaeochromocytomas remain clinically undetected, as shown in a series of 54 phaeochromocytomas confirmed at autopsy. Their presence had been clinically unsuspected in 41 of these patients although 22 had hypertension (ST. JOHN SUTTON et al. 1981). As a mnemonic, the rule of 10% may be helpful: 10% are bilateral, 10% are ectopic, 10% are malignant and about 10% are inherited. There is a strong association with von Recklinghausen neurofibromatosis, with von Hippel-Lindau haemangioblastomatosis and with

Sturge-Weber syndrome. These diseases have an autosomal dominant mode of transmission.

Bilateral phaeochromocytoma is frequently associated with MEN, a familial syndrome manifesting as <u>m</u>ultiple <u>e</u>ndocrine <u>n</u>eoplasms of various glands, especially MEN types IIa and IIb (Fig. 28.9). In MEN II, phaeochromocytomas are usually bilateral, be multicentric and can associated with medullary hyperplasia. CT is a precise and sensitive method of detecting phaeochromocytomas. It has sensitivity and specificity of about 90%. These figures are based on older series using 18-s or 5-s scanners. Helical CT, with its inherently better resolution and its decreased sensitivity for patients' movements, should logically perform much better. There is, however, no

larger study to corroborate this hypothesis. When the results of the most recent studies were combined, it was found that CT had been able to localize phaeochromocytomas correctly in more than 90% of the cases (Martin Marquina Aspiunza et al. 1997; Goretzki et al. 1997; Neumann and Langer 1997).

Phaeochromocytomas present either as small masses emerging from a limb of an adrenal or as a mass replacing the entire adrenal (Fig. 28.9). Phaeochromocytomas may become large and displace adjacent organs. Generally, phaeochromocytomas have a homogeneous aspect, although some may present with hypodense foci, caused by earlier episodes of haemorrhage, as necrosis, or even as cys-

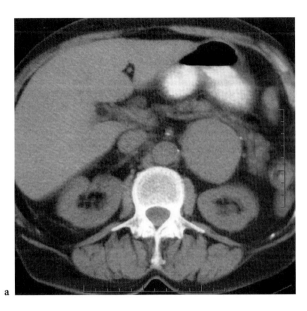

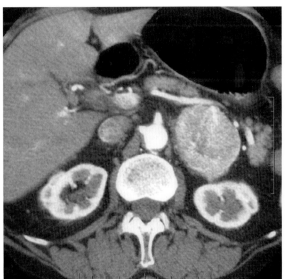

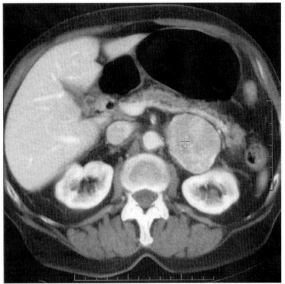

Fig. 28.9. a Phaeochromocytoma in left adrenal, native scan. **b** Arterial phase. **c** Parenchymal phase

tic tumours. The amount of degeneration is in proportion to the size of the tumour, small tumours tending to be solid whereas larger tumours tend to be partly or highly cystic. In a series of 84 phaeochromocytomas, 46% were solid, 44% were cystic and 19% were highly cystic. It appeared also that the pattern of excretion of vasoactive substances and the pattern of hypertension varied with the amount of degeneration (Ito et al. 1996).

Intravenous contrast material may be useful to delineate the inferior vena cava or the renal upper pole in patients with low body fat. It is, however, prudent to avoid its use (see 28.2.1). Oral contrast media should be given in sufficient quantity to opacify all bowel loops, as extra-adrenal phaeochromocytomas may be misdiagnosed as insufficiently opacified bowel loops. Extraadrenal phaeochromocytomas may also "hide" in the bowel wall or in the pericardial cavity. Thoracic lesions are easily recognized. With a sensitivity of about 90% and a specificity of about 95%, iodine-131 metaiodobenzylguanidine (MIBG) scintigraphy is a excellent imaging method for localization of phaeochromocytomas (Nielsen et al. 1996), especially when they are metastatic or multicentric (Quint et al. 1987).

28.5.1.1
Recurrent and Malignant Phaeochromocytomas

Most patients treated surgically for phaeochromocytomas will be cured. Any postoperative increase of catecholamines should arouse the suspicion of either recurrence or distant metastases. The recurrence rate is about 10%. Recurrences appear 5–6 years after tumour resection. It is not possible to predict whether or not there will be a recurrence on the basis of the histology of the primary tumour (Remine et al. 1974). Larger tumours more frequently tend to be malignant. The growth rate of malignant phaeochromocytomas is relatively low. They metastasize to liver, lymph nodes and bones.

28.5.1.2
Phaeochromocytomas in Childhood

Phaeochromocytomas must be suspected in children with sustained hypertension. The tumour is rare in children and is more frequently bilateral (20%) and extraadrenal (31%) than in adults. The vast majority of tumours are small (1.3 – 2.0 cm) and do not differ histologically from the tumours seen in adults (Stackpole et al. 1963). Some of the phaeochromocytomas seen in childhood are related to MEN II, to von Hippel-Lindau disease or to neurofibromatosis. MIBG scintigraphy, CT and ultrasound are the accurate methods of diagnosis and localization.

28.5.2
Neuroblastomas

Neuroblastomas are malignant neoplasms that arise from the adrenal medulla and from the sympathetic ganglia. They account for most of the solid tumours found in the abdomen in childhood. Between 25% and 30% of the tumours are found within the first year of life, and 25% between the ages of 1 and 2 years. The remainder are found at all ages. The tumours present as abdominal masses in half the patients, and with fever and pain in about a third. The tumours may be quite highly differentiated and contain ganglion cells (ganglioneuroblastoma) or be undifferentiated and infiltrate the bone marrow in such a way as to be confused with leukaemia.

Extension of neuroblastoma is generally classified according to the staging system proposed by Evans' group (Evans 1980; Evans et al. 1971):

Stage I: tumour confined to organ of origin

Stage II: tumour extending in continuity beyond the organ or structure of origin but not crossing the midline, with or without ipsilateral lymph node involvement

Stage III: tumours extending in continuity beyond the midline, with or without bilateral lymph node involvement

Stage IV: remote disease involving skeleton, viscera, soft tissue, or distant lymph node groups

Stage IVS: disease that would otherwise be stage I or stage II, except that there is remote disease confined to one or more of the following sites: liver, skin or bone marrow (without radiographic evidence of bone involvement)

Neuroblastoma is a rather special tumour. The prognosis has improved in the last 20 years, even with disseminated disease (in about two thirds of the cases at time of the diagnosis), and especially in children less than 1 year old. It has the propensity occasionally to undergo spontaneous regression and spontaneous or induced differentiation to a benign ganglioneuroma (De Grazia et al. 1997).

On native CT, attenuation of neuroblastoma is equal to or less than that of liver. The tissue is generally heterogeneous, with areas of necrosis and haemorrhage. Calcifications are found in 85% of the tumours (BOUSVAROS et al. 1986); they are finely stippled and linear or ring-shaped. Enhancement after intravenous contrast material is moderate (BOECHAT et al. 1985). CT is the imaging modality of choice. It helps to display the full extent of the tumour, to monitor the response of therapy and to detect recurrences after treatment.

28.5.3
Ganglioneuroblastomas

Ganglioneuroblastoma is a complex tumour containing both mature ganglion cells such as are found in ganglioneuromas and primitive neuroblastic cell lines, together with cells of intermediate differentiation. Ganglioneuroblastomas are seen in children less than 10 years old. The tumour is generally located in the retroperitoneum (65%), and otherwise in the mediastinum, neck and adrenals (STOWENS 1957). Some authors consider them as neuroblastomas with maturation and ganglionic differentiation (ASHLEY 1978).

28.5.4
Ganglioneuromas

The mature ganglioneuroma is a benign neoplasm. It is composed of sympathetic ganglion cells with sheathed neurites with or without myelin. It may contain Schwann cells and collagen. It generally arises from sympathetic chains extending from the base of the skull, along the neck, the posterior mediastinum, the retroperitoneum and the adrenal glands. Ganglioneuromas can also be found in other organs, such as uterus, ovary, skin or gastrointestinal tract. Adrenal ganglioneuromas occur predominantly between the third and fifth decades. They are mostly asymptomatic and frequently calcify. Urinary catecholamines and their metabolites may be increased. On CT, ganglioneuromas appear as solid masses, which can simulate primary adrenal carcinoma, but with no signs of local or vascular extension. The specific diagnosis can only be made after biopsy or surgical removal (JOHNSON et al. 1997).

References

Abrams HL, Spiro R, Goldstein N (1950) Metastases in carcinoma: analysis of 1000 autopsied cases. Cancer 3:74–85
Ashley DJB (1978) Histological appearance of tumours. Churchill Livingstone, Edinburgh
Atkinson GO Jr, Kodroff MB, Gay BB Jr, Ricketts RR (1985) Adrenal abscess in the neonate. Radiology 155:101
Auerbach O, Garfinkel L, Parks VR (1975) Histologic type of lung cancer in relation to smoking habits, year of diagnosis and sites of metastases. Chest 67:382–387
Bastide C, Boyer L, Djellouli N, Baguet JC, Viallet JF (1997) Kystes surrénaliens bilateraux et polykystose hepatorenale. Presse Med 26(15):711–712
Boechat MI, Ortega J, Hoffman AD et al (1985) Computed tomography in Stage III neuroblastoma. AJR Am J Roentgenol 145:1283
Boland GW, Hahn PF, Pena C, Mueller PR (1997) Adrenal masses: characterization with delayed contrast-enhanced CT. Radiology 202(3):693–696
Bousvaros A, Kirks DR, Grossman H (1986) Imaging of neuroblastoma: an overview. Pediatr Radiol 16:89
Campbell CM, Middleton RG Rigby OF (1983) Adrenal metastasis in renal cell carcinoma. Urology 21:403–405
Catalano O (1996) Retroperitoneal hemorrhage due to a ruptured adrenal myelolipoma. A case report. Acta Radiol 37(5):688–690
Cedermark BJ, Blumenson LE, Pikren JW, Elias EG (1977) The significance of metastases to the adrenal gland from carcinoma of the stomach and esophagus. Surg Gynecol Obstet 145:41–48
Cho SY, Choi HY (1980) Causes of death and metastatic patterns in patients with mammary cancer. Am J Clin Pathol 73:232–234
Choi SM, Liu K (1981) Leiomyosarcoma of the adrenal gland and its angiographic features. A case report. J Surg Oncol 16:145–148
Conn JW, Knopf RF, Nesbit RM (1964) Clinical characteristics of primary aldosteronism from an analysis of 145 cases. Am J Surg 107:159–172
DasGupta T, Brasfield R (1964) Metastatic melanoma. Cancer 17:1323–1339
De Grazia-E, Cimador-M, De-Bernardi-B (1997) Recenti acquisizioni sul neuroblastoma retro-peritoneale. [Recent advances on retroperitoneal neuroblastoma.] Arch Ital Urol Androl 69(4):233–240
Dunnick NR, Leight GS Jr, Roubidoux MA, Leder RA, Paulson E, Kurylo L (1993) CT in the diagnosis of primary aldosteronism: sensitivity in 29 patients. AJR Am J Roentgenol 160(2):321–324
Evans AE, D'Angio GJ, Randolf J (1971) A proposed staging for children with neuroblastoma. Cancer 17:374–378
Evans AE (1980) Staging and treatment of neuroblastoma. Cancer 45:1799–1802
Feldberg MAM, Hendriks MJ, Klinkhamer AC (1986) Massive bilateral non-Hodgkin's lymphomas of the adrenals. Urol Radiol 8:85–88
Gaboardi F, Carbone M, Bozzola A, Galli L (1991) Adrenal incidentalomas: what is the role of fine needle biopsy? Int Urol Nephrol 13:197–207
Goretzki PE, Simon D, Roher HD (1997) Operatives Konzept beim sporadischen und familiären Phaochromozytom.

334 H.-M. Hoogewoud

[Surgical concept in sporadic and familial pheochromocytoma.] Zentralbl Chir 122(6):467–472

Hutter AM Jr, Kayhoe DE (1966) Adrenal cortical carcinoma. Am J Med 41:572–580

Ikekpeazzu N, Bonadies JA, Sreenivas VI (1996) Acute bilateral adrenal hemorrhage secondary to rough truck ride. J Emerg Med 14(1):15–18

Ito Y, Obara T, Yamashita-T, Kanbe-M, Iihara (1996) M Pheochromocytomas: tendency to degenerate and cause paroxysmal hypertension. World J Surg 20(7):923–926, discussion 927

Johnson GL, Hruban-RH, Marshall-FF, Fishman-EK (1997) Primary adrenal ganglioneuroma: CT findings in four patients. AJR Am J Roentgenol 169(1):169–171

Korobkin M, Brodeur F, Francis IR, Quint LE, Dunnick NR, Londy F (1998) CT-time attenuation washout curves of adrenal adenomas and nonadenomas. AJR Am J Roentgenol 170:747–752

Korobkin M, Brodeur FJ, Francis IR, Quint LE, Dunnick NR, Goodsitt M (1996) Delayed enhanced CT for differentiation of benign from malignant adrenal masses. Radiology 200(3):737–742

Korobkin M, Brodcur FJ, Yutzy GG, Francis IR, Quint LE, Dunnick NR, Kazerooni EA (1996) Differentiation of adrenal adenomas from nonadenomas using CT attenuation values. AJR Am J Roentgenol 166(3):531–536

Lee MJ, Hahn PF, Papanicolaou N, Egglin TK, Saini S, Mueller PR, Simeone JF (1991) Benign and malignant adrenal masses: CT distinction with attenuation coefficients, size, and observer analysis. Radiology 179(2):415–418

Linos DA, Stylopoulos N (1997) How accurate is computed tomography in predicting the real size of adrenal tumors? A retrospective study. Arch Surg 132(7):740–743

Marotti M, Sucic Z, Krolo I, Dimanovski J, Klaric R, Ferencic Z, Karapanda N, Babic N, Pavlekovic K (1997) Adrenal cavernous hemangioma: MRI, CT, and US appearance. Eur Radiol 7(5):691–694

Martin Marquina Aspiunza A, Sanz Perez G, Diez Caballero Alonso F, Robles Garcia JE, Zudaire Berjera JJ, Rodriguez Rubio Cortadellas FI, Abad Vivas Perez JI, Rosell Costa D, Berian Polo JM (1997) Pheochromocytoma. Actas Urol Esp 21(7):715–718

Mukherjee JJ, Peppercorn PD, Reznek RH, Patel V, Kaltsas G, Besser M, Grossman AB (1997) Pheochromocytoma: effect of nonionic contrast medium in CT on circulating catecholamine levels. Radiology 202:1, 227–231

Munden R, Adams DB, Curry NS (1993) Pheochromocytoma: radiologic diagnosis. South Med J 86(11):1302–1305

Neumann K, Langer R (1997) Bildgebende Verfahren zur Diagnostik des Phaochromozytoms. [Imaging methods in diagnosis of pheochromocytoma.] Zentralbl Chir 122(6):438–442

Nielsen JT, Nielsen-BV, Rehling (1996) Location of adrenal medullary pheochromocytoma by I-123 metaiodobenzylguanidine SPECT. M Clin Nucl Med 21(9):695–699

Nobel MJ, Montague DK, Levin HS (1982) Myelolipoma: an unusual surgical lesion of the adrenal gland. Cancer 49:952–958

Page DL, DeLellis RA, Hough A (1986) Tumors of the adrenal. Atlas of tumor pathology. AFIP, Washington DC, p 136

Quint LE, Glazer GM, Francis IR, Shapiro B, Chenevert TL (1987) Pheochromocytoma and paraganglioma: comparison of MR imaging with CT and I-131 MIBG scintigraphy. Radiology 165(1):89–93

Remine WH, Chong GC, van Heeren JA, Sheps SG, Harrison EG Jr (1974) Current management of pheochromocytoma. Ann Surg 179:740–748

Rieber A, Brambs HJ (1995) CT and MR imaging of adrenal hemangioma. A case report. Acta Radiol 36(6):659–661

Rozenblit A, Morehouse HT, Amis ES Jr (1996) Cystic adrenal lesions: CT features. Radiology 201(2):541–548

Sharma MC, Kashyap S, Sharma R, Chumber S, Sood R, Chahal R (1997) Symptomatic adrenal myelolipoma. Clinicopathological analysis of 7 cases and brief review of the literature. Urol Int 59(2):119–124

Sherazi ZA, Dicks Mireaux C (1997) Suprarenal cystic masses: unusual causes. Clin Radiol 52(12):953–955

Singer AA, Obuchowski NA, Einstein DM, Paushter DM (1994) Metastasis or adenoma? Computed tomographic evaluation of the adrenal mass. Cleve Clin J Med 61(3):200–205

St John Sutton M, Sheps S, Lie J (1981) Prevalence of clinically unsuspected pheochromocytoma. Review of a 50-year autopsy series. Mayo Clin Proc 56:354

Stackpole RH, Melikow MM, Uson AC (1963) Phaeochromocytoma in children. J Pediatr 63:315–330

Stowens D (1957) Neuroblastoma and related tumours. Arch Pathol 63:451–459

Sutherland DJA, Ruse JL, Laidlaw JC (1966) Hypertension, increases aldosterone secretion and low plasma renin activity relieved by dexamethasone. Can Med Assoc J 95:1109–1119

Szolar DH, Kammerhuber F (1997) Quantitative CT evaluation of adrenal gland masses: a step forward in the differentiation between adenomas and nonadenomas. Radiology 202(2):517–521

Terzolo M, Ali A, Osella G, Mazza E (1997) Prevalence of adrenal carcinoma among incidentally discovered adrenal masses. A retrospective study from 1989 to 1994. Gruppo Piemontese Incidentalomi Surrenalici. Arch Surg 132(8):914–919

Terzolo M, Boccuzzi A, Ali A, Bollito E, De Risi C, Paccotti P, Angeli A (1997) Cushing's syndrome due to ACTH-independent bilateral adrenocortical macronodular hyperplasia. J Endocrinol Invest 20(5):270–275

Truong B, Jolles PR, Mullaney JM (1997) Primary adrenal lymphoma: gallium scintigraphy and correlative imaging. J Nucl Med 38(11):1770–1771

29 Detection and Staging of Renal Neoplasms

H.Trillaud, J. Palussiere, N.Grenier

CONTENTS

29.1   Introduction   *335*
29.2   Advantages of Helical CT   *335*
29.3   Limitations of Helical CT   *338*
29.4   Renal Cell Carcinomas   *339*
29.5   Cystic Renal Neoplasms   *339*
29.6   Other Renal Tumors   *342*
29.6.1 Transitional Cell Carcinoma   *342*
29.6.2 Angiomyolipoma   *343*
29.6.3 Lymphoma   *343*
       References   *344*

29.1
Introduction

CT is widely used in the detection and staging of renal neoplasms (Smith et al. 1989; Stuart Wolf 1998). In comparison with conventional CT, helical CT has further improved the evaluation of renal masses, and particularly the detection and characterization of small renal neoplasms (Bosniak and Rofsky 1996; Curry 1995; Davidson et al. 1997; Szolar et al. 1997; Urban 1997). Thanks to optimal visualization of the renal lesions and their associated vascular component, helical CT provides the necessary information for surgical management, considering the increasing use of nephron-sparing procedures (Smith et al. 1997). However, in order to take full advantage of helical CT, a dedicated renal protocol must be used. Such care is also important to avoid the potential pitfalls of this method (Bosniak 1997).

H. Trillaud, MD, PhD; Service de Radiologie, Groupe Hospitalier Pellegrin, Place Amélie Raba-Léon, F-33076 Bordeaux Cédex, France
Jean Palussiere, MD; Service de Radiologie, Institut Bergonié, F-33076 Bordeaux Cédex, France
N. Grenier, MD; Service de Radiologie, Groupe Hospitalier Pellegrin, Place Amélie Raba-Léon, F-33076 Bordeaux Cédex, France

29.2
Advantages of Helical CT

Helical CT acquires a volumetric data set during a single breath-hold. The elimination of respiratory misregistration ensures that the entire volume of interest is examined, avoiding the omission of areas of the kidney lying between consecutive slices from the imaging, which can happen with conventional CT. In addition, lesion detection is potentially improved, because of the reduction of partial volume averaging obtained with the use of overlapping reconstruction intervals (Figs. 29.1–29.3). The chance of identifying small lesions (Szolar et al. 1997) or subtle, but diagnostically important, features, such as slight wall or septal nodularity (Bosniak 1997), is maximized.

The faster scanning obtained with helical CT also allows multiphasic renal imaging. Thus, images obtained at the same anatomical level can be compared before and in several phases after intravenous administration of contrast medium (Fig. 29.4). In particular, images can be acquired during peak levels of contrast material enhancement. Older CT equipment is inconsistent in the demonstration of the short-lived cortical phase of the nephrogram, because of insufficient temporal resolution. In contrast, helical CT makes it possible to distinguish the two distinct phases of renal parenchymal enhancement (Cohan et al. 1995). During the earlier phase (usually 40–70 s after contrast medium injection), the renal cortex can be differentiated from the medulla because of its earlier and stronger enhancement. Vessels are also optimally visualized. The later phase, i.e., nephrographic phase shows an homogeneous nephrogram (100–200 s after contrast medium injection, Fig. 29.4).

Whereas earlier investigators have emphasized the utility of images obtained during the corticomedullary phase (Kauczor et al. 1994), recent studies have shown the nephrogenic phase to be superior to the corticomedullary phase for the detection of renal masses (Cohan et al. 1995; Birnbaum and

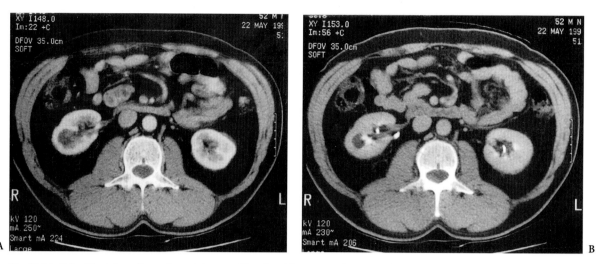

Fig. 29.1A, B. Incidental small renal cyst. 52-year-old male with a 15 mm lesion in the right kidney. **A** In the corticomedullary phase, 40 s after bolus injection the cyst is less well characterized than in **B** in the later phase, at 380 s after contrast agent injection

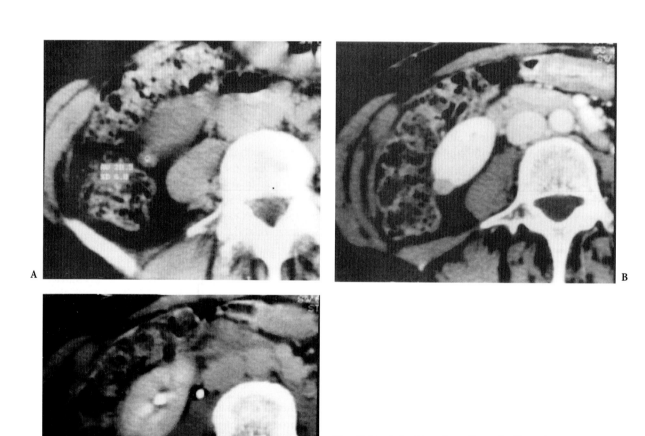

Fig. 29.2A–C. Incidental small renal cell carcinoma in a 62-year-old woman with a 1-cm tumor in the right kidney. The lesion has a density of 20 HU on the unenhanced scan (**A**), 104 HU in the nephrographic phase (**B**) and 84 HU in the excretory phase (**C**) after contrast media injection. Thin collimation and lack of breathing artifact with helical CT allows accurate measurement and characterization of this small tumor

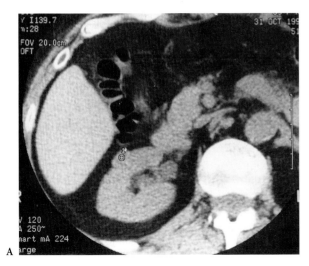
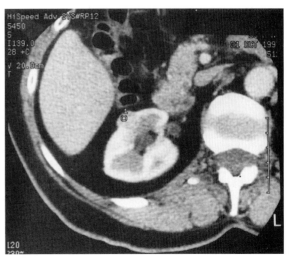

Fig. 29.3A, B. Incidental small mass in a 50-year-old woman: **A** before and **B** after contrast medium administration. The mass was hyperechoic on ultrasonography. **A** No fat was detected on unenhanced helical CT. **B** In the corticomedullary phase a 12-mm tumor is seen in the right kidney and shows a strong enhancement. The mass was subsequently removed and was found to be an angiomyolipoma

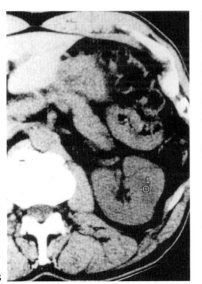
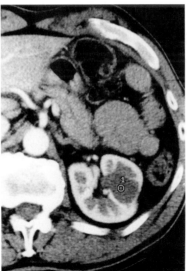
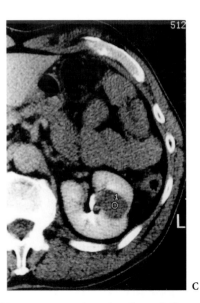

Fig 29.4. A Hypovascular renal cell carcinoma in a 60-year-old man, with an area of low attenuation (8 HU) in the medulla on unenhanced image. **B** After contrast medium administration note the low attenuation (25 HU) adjacent to a cortical scar suggesting a renal mass on the corticomedullary image. **C** The solid renal mass can be easily detected on the nephrographic image obtained at the same level (35 HU)

JACOBS 1996; KOPKA et al. 1997; SZOLAR et al. 1997; ZEMAN et al. 1996) (Fig. 29.5). However, the corticomedullary phase should not be eliminated from a dedicated renal imaging protocol, because it can be useful in differentiating normal variants, such as prominent columns of Bertin or dromedary humps, from renal masses. Asymmetric cortical enhancement attributable to renal artery stenosis or ob-

struction is often better visualized in the corticomedullary phase (URBAN 1997).

Helical CT image acquisition also allows three-dimensional surface rendering of renal tumors, the surrounding structures and the vascular supply to the kidney (SMITH et al. 1997; Fig. 29.6). Such information can be of help in planning a partial nephrectomy.

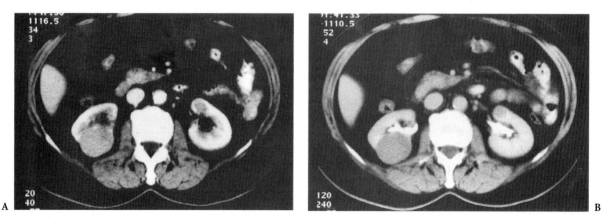

Fig. 29.5. Bilateral tumors in a 53-year-old woman whose corticomedullary phase (**A**) shows a 4-cm tumor in the right kidney. The 15-mm left tumor was better seen on the delayed phase (**B**). This tumor was missed on a previous examination without delayed phase. The right tumor was proven at surgery to be an oncocytoma, and the left tumor was a renal cell carcinoma

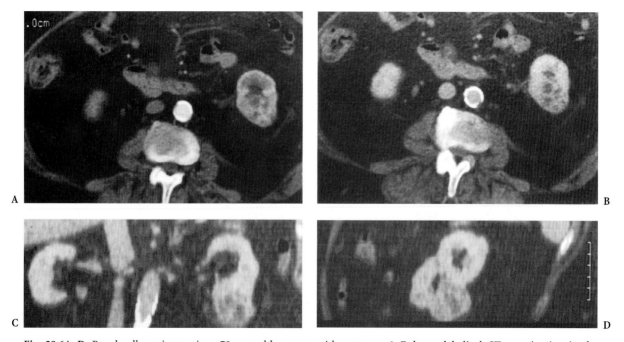

Fig. 29.6A–D. Renal cell carcinoma in a 78-year-old woman with a tumor. **A** Enhanced helical CT examination in the corticomedullary phase suggests a mass. **B** Delayed nephrographic phase and multiplanar imaging with **C** coronal and **D** sagittal reconstruction improves lesion detection

29.3
Limitations of Helical CT

Lesion enhancement after the administration of a contrast medium allows the distinction between a cyst and a neoplasm. Enhancement of a renal mass, indicating neovascularity, is the hallmark of a renal tumor. The lower dose of radiation used with helical

CT decreases the signal-to-noise ratio and diminishes the accuracy of attenuation measurements in regions of interest (BIRBAUM and JACOBS 1966; BOSNIAK and ROFSKY 1996; BRINK et al. 1992; JAMIS-Dow et al. 1996). Another factor might also affect the reliability of attenuation measurements: partial volume effects are increased in a particular slice with helical CT through flattening and broadening of the section sensitivity profile. However, this adverse effect can be offset by more consistent imaging of the center of the lesion. For these reasons, many authors have stressed the usefulness of axial cluster imaging (fast step-by-step slice imaging) during the nephrographic phase, with a high tube current to improve image quality and attenuation measurements (BOSNIAK and ROFSKY 1996).

29.4
Renal Cell Carcinoma

A major advantage of helical CT over conventional CT is the increased sensitivity for the detection of small renal cell carcinomas (<3 cm) (SZOLAR et al. 1997; Figs. 29.2, 29.5). This leads to a more favorable prognosis for these small tumors than for large symptomatic renal tumors. On helical CT, the most common appearance of a small renal cell carcinoma is a noncalcified lesion with an attenuation value of 20 HU or higher and enhancement by more than 10 HU after intravenous injection of contrast medium (SILVERMAN et al. 1994). Previous investigations have shown nephrographic-phase and excretory-phase renal imaging to be superior to corticomedullary-phase imaging for the detection of a renal mass. COHAN et al. (1995) demonstrated that small (<2 cm) medullary lesions may be missed on images obtained during the corticomedullary phase and that disparate enhancement of the renal medulla compared with that of the adjacent cortex can give rise to medullary pseudolesions during that phase, mimicking a tumor, for example. In some cases of hypovascular tumor the enhancement after injection of contrast medium can be missed if imaging is performed only in the corticomedullary phase, because hypovascular lesions require a sufficient time period before a significant amount of contrast medium concentrates in the tumor and alters its attenuation value (BOSNIAK and ROFSKY 1996). BIRNBAUM and JACOBS (1996) reported that only 69% of neoplasms showed enhancement by more than 10 HU during the corticomedullary phase, whereas all neoplasms demonstrate a definite enhancement during the nephrographic phase (Fig. 29.4). Furthermore, small hypervascular cortical tumors can be missed on the early phase because they are interpreted as a prominent column of Bertin. For renal masses greater than 3 cm, helical CT increases specificity in the diagnosis of a neoplastic lesion. The pseudolesions mimicking a pathologic process on ultrasound or conventional CT are dismissed as a normal variant by using overlapping slices and thin collimation at the peak contrast enhancement of the normal parenchyma.

Another advantage of helical CT is to improve depiction of tumor extension into the renal vein and inferior vena cava by optimal vascular opacification during peak contrast enhancement (WELCH and LEROY 1997; Figs. 29.7–29.9). A thrombus is better recognized in the renal vein during the corticomedullary phase, when the renal vein is at peak contrast enhancement by capillary-venous shunting in the renal tumor. The later phase allows detection of vena cava thrombosis. In addition, helical CT enables distinction between tumor thrombus and blood clot by the detection of enhancing tumor vessels in the tumor thrombus (REZNEK 1966; ZAGORIA et al. 1995; WYATT et al. 1995; Fig. 29.10). In some cases, the inflow of nonopacified blood in the renal vein or in the inferior vena cava can cause diagnostic difficulties on helical CT. Indeed, a false-positive diagnosis of a flow defect can result from the mixture of slow-flowing, not yet opacified blood from a capsular vein merging into the already opacified blood flow of the renal vein. The flow defect in the inferior vena cava is related to the mixture of unopacified blood originating from below the renal veins with contrast-enhanced blood coming from the renal veins (Fig. 29.11). For that reason, delayed scans, i.e. systematic second helical acquisition after the corticomedullary phase, are required.

29.5
Cystic Renal Neoplasms

Cystic renal cell cancers are better differentiated from complicated benign cysts using helical CT. For small lesions between 1 cm and 3 cm, the advantage of overlapping intervals and thin collimation in a single breath-hold is evident. In some cases, a cyst protrudes from the surface of the kidney and can be encircled by an effaced wedge of renal parenchyma. It is possible to distinguish this aspect from the thick wall of a cystic neoplasm using 3D reconstructions. The difficulty of determining tissue enhancement in some cases of small renal cyst has already been mentioned above. Septa, the wall of the cyst and areas of nodularity are better visualized with thin slices at peak contrast enhancement (BOSNIAK 1997; DAVIDSON et al. 1997; Fig. 29.12).

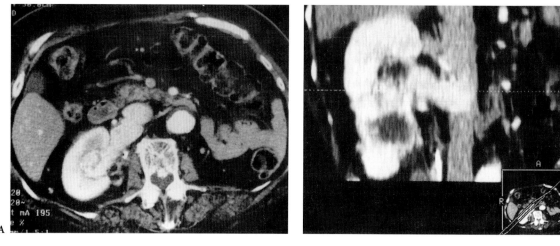

Fig. 29.7. A Renal cell carcinoma with vascular invasion in a 74-year-old woman with a renal tumor that has invaded the right renal vein and the inferior vena cava at the level of the renal vein. **B** Coronal reconstruction helps to visualize the vascular invasion

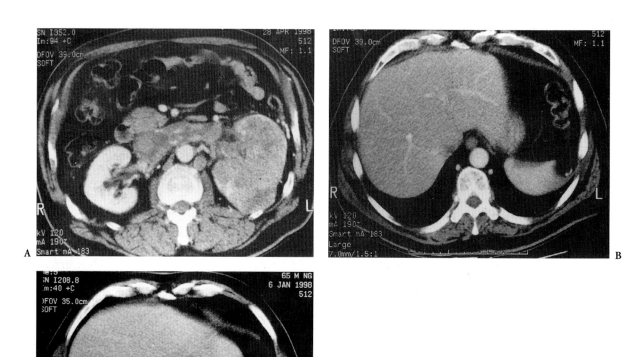

Fig. 29 8. A Renal cell carcinoma with vascular invasion in a 65-year-old man with a large cancer that has invaded the left renal vein. **B** The thrombus extension is not seen early after bolus injection. **C** Scan at the peak contrast enhancement provides optimal vena cava opacification and reveals the thrombus

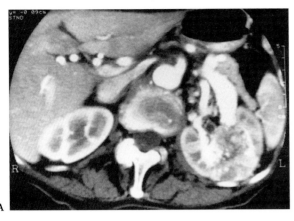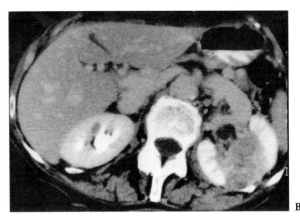

Fig. 29.9A,B. Renal cell carcinoma in an 80-year-old woman examined by helical CT during the corticomedullary phase, showing the hypervascular component of the tumor on the left kidney. Note the peak contrast enhancement on the large left renal vein without thrombus in **A** compared with **B**

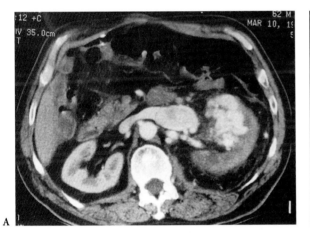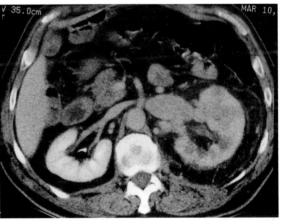

Fig. 29.10. **A** Renal cell carcinoma in a 62-year-old man whose helical CT during corticomedullary phase shows dense enhancement suggestive of capillarovenous shunting in the tumor. In addition, the tumor thrombus in the renal vein is better visualized during the corticomedullary phase than on the delayed image (**B**). Note the tumor thrombus enhancement (**A**)

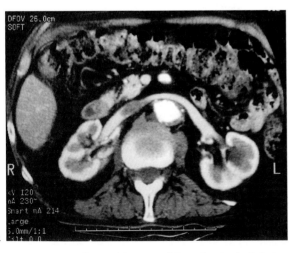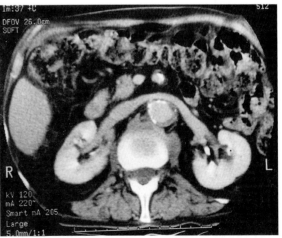

Fig. 29.11A, B. False-positive case of thrombus in the inferior vena cava with helical CT. **A** Flow defect in the inferior vena cava during the corticomedullary phase in this 85-year-old man. **B** The false image disappears in the later phase

29.6
Other Renal Tumors

29.6.1
Transitional Cell Carcinoma

Transitional cell carcinoma depicted with CT can be revealed as a sessile mass, a ureteral wall thickening, or an infiltrating mass (URBAN et al. 1997b; WYATT et al. 1995). These three patterns are better visualized on delayed scans for collecting system opacification and with a small field of view centered on the lesion when detected by intravenous urography (Fig. 29.13). A dedicated protocol for patients with hematuria or the suggestion of an intraluminal filling defect on intravenous urography must also include excretory-phase CT. In some cases the infiltrative mass is better visualized with a 3D model (SMITH et al. 1997; Fig. 29.14).

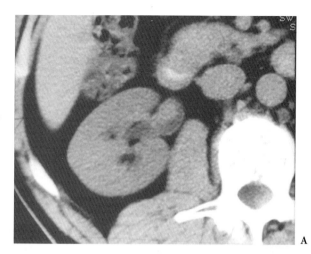

A

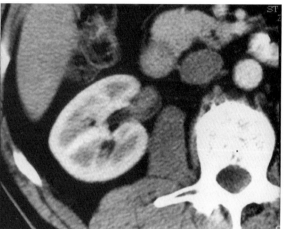

B

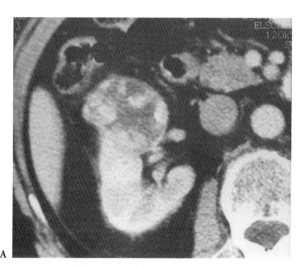

A

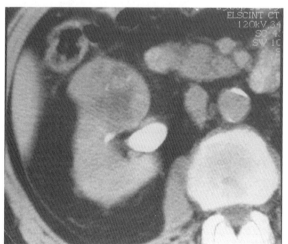

B

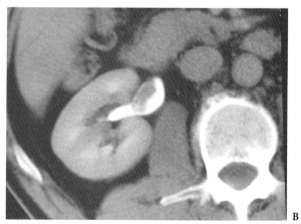

B

Fig. 29.13A–C. Transitional cell carcinoma in a 51-year-old man in whom helical CT **A** before and **B** soon after contrast administration suggest a subtle mass in the right renal pelvis. **C** Delayed scan shows the tumor more reliably

Fig. 29.12A, B. Cystic renal cell carcinoma in a 71-year-old man manifesting a cystic right renal mass. Note that the enhancing nodularity, which is suggestive of malignancy, is better seen during the corticomedullary phase (**A**) than during the delayed phase (**B**)

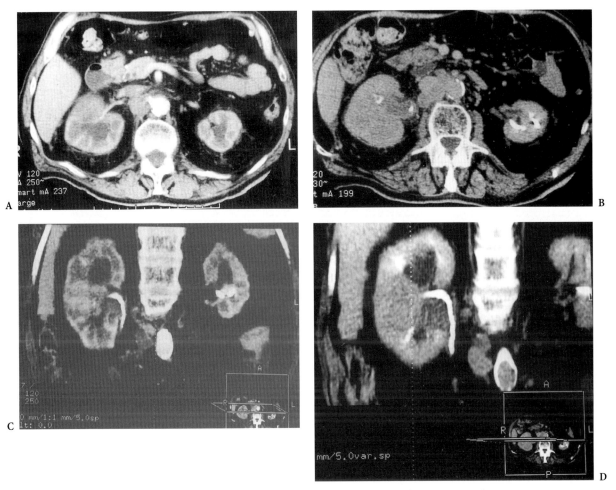

Fig. 29.14A–D. Transitional cell carcinoma in an 83-year-old man with renal pelvis probe for hydronephrosis. **A** After bolus injection helical CT reveals a mass in the right kidney. Appearance is indistinguishable from primary renal cell carcinoma. **B** Delayed scan suggests a filling defect in the renal pelvis. Coronal reconstructions (**C**) after bolus injection and (**D**) in the delayed phase improve lesion evaluation

29.6.2
Angiomyolipoma

Renal angiomyolipomas are benign neoplasms with macroscopic aggregates of fat in 95% of cases (LEMAITRE et al. 1995; WILLS 1995). When a small hyperechoic lesion is noted on ultrasonography examination, this lesion must be evaluated with unenhanced CT to look for the presence of fat, which indicates a benign angiomyolipoma (Fig. 29.15). When no fat is detected by CT, the lesion can be another solid neoplasm; obviously, there are important implications for the patient's treatment. Helical CT with thin collimation in a single breath-hold may improve the detection of subtle foci of fat within a renal mass. Furthermore, the optimal vascular opacification early after contrast media injection improves evaluation of the vascularity of this tumor.

29.6.3
Lymphoma

CT features of focal renal lymphoma are similar to those of renal cell carcinoma. As for conventional CT, helical CT should indicate renal lymphoma when an involvement of abdominal lymph nodes and a perirenal mass are noted (DIMOPOULOS et al. 1995).

344

H. Trillaud et al.

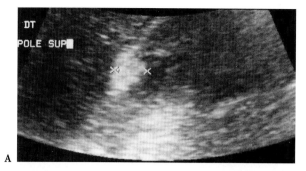

A

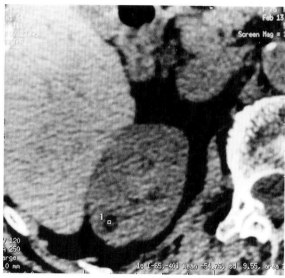

B

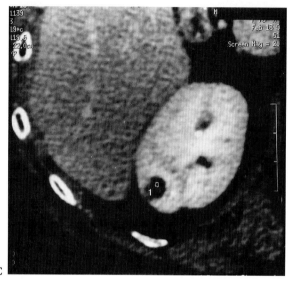

C

Fig. 29.15A–C. Small angiomyolipoma in a 75-year-old woman with an 11-mm tumor demonstrated in the superior pole of the right kidney. A This lesion was detected by ultra sonography as an hyperechoic tumor. B Unenhanced helical CT with thin collimation allows accurate densitometry of the lesion and demonstrates small foci of fatty tissue. C Optimal enhancement highlights borders of the tumors and shows the vascular component

References

Birnbaum BA, Jacobs JE (1996) Multiphasic renal CT: comparison of renal mass enhancement during the corticomedullary and nephrographic phases. Radiology 200:753–758

Bosniak MA (1997) Diagnosis and management of patients with complicated cystic lesions of the kidney. AJR Am J Roentgenol 169:819–821

Bosniak MA, Rofsky NM (1996) Problems in the detection and characterization of small renal masses. Radiology 198:638–641

Brink JA, Heiken JP, Balfe DM et al (1992) Spiral CT: decreased spatial resolution in vivo due to broadening of section sensitivity profile. Radiology 185:469–474

Cohan RH, Sherman LS, Korobkin M, Bass JC, Francis IR (1995) Renal masses: assessment of corticomedullary-phase and nephrographic-phase CT scans. Radiology 196:445–451

Curry NS (1995) Small renal masses (lesions smaller than 3 cm): imaging evaluation and management. AJR Am J Roentgenol 164:355–362

Davidson AJ, Hartman DS, Choyke PL, Wagner BJ (1997) Radiologic assessment of renal masses: implications for patient care. Radiology 202:297–305

Dimopoulos MA, Moulopoulos LA, Costantidinides C, Deliveliotis C, Pantazopoulos D, Dimopoulos C (1996) Primary renal lymphoma: a clinical and radiological study. J Urol 155:1865–1867

Jamis-Dow CA, Choyke PL, Jennings, SB, Marston Linehan W, Thakore KN, Walther MM (1996) Small (≤3 cm) renal masses: detection with CT versus US and pathologic correlation. Radiology 198:785–788

Kauczor HU, Schwickert HC, Schweden F, Schild HH, Thelen M (1994) Bolus-enhanced renal spiral CT: technique, diagnostic value and drawbacks. Eur J Radiol 18:153–157

Kopka L, Fischer U, Zoeller G, Schmidt C, Ringert RH, Grabbe E (1997) Dual-phase helical CT of the kidney: value of the corticomedullary and nephrographic phase for evaluation of renal lesions and preoperative staging of renal cell carcinoma. AJR Am J Roentgenol 169:1573–1578

Lemaitre L, Robert Y, Dubrulle F, Claudon M, Duhamel A, Danjou P, Mazeman E (1995) Renal angiomyolipoma: growth followed up with CT and/or US. Radiology 1997:598–602

Reznek RH (1996) Imaging in the staging of renal cell carcinoma. Eur Radiol 6:120–128

Silverman SG, Lee BY, Seltzer SE, Corless CL, Adams DF (1994) Small (_3 cm) renal masses: correlation of spiral CT features and pathologic findings. AJR Am J Roentgenol 163:597–605

Smith SJ, Bosniak MA, Megibow AJ, Hulnick DH, Horii SC,

Nagesh Raghavendra B (1989) Renal cell carcinoma: earlier discovery and increased detection. Radiology 170:699–703

Smith SJ, Marshall FF, Urban BA, Heath DG, Fishman EK (1997) Three-dimensional CT stereoscopic vizualization of renal masses: impact on diagnosis and patient treatment. AJR Am J Roentgenol 169:1331–1334

Stuart Wolf J (1998) Evaluation and management of solid and cystic renal masses. J Urol 159:1120–1133

Szolar DH, Kammerhuber F, Altziebler S, Tillich M, Breini E, Fotter R, Schreyer HH (1997) Multiphasic helical CT of the kidney: increased conspicuity for detection and characterization of samll (<3 cm) renal masses. Radiology 202:211–217

Urban BA (1997) The small renal mass: what is the role of multiphasic helical scanning? Radiology 202:22–23

Urban BA, Buckley J, Soyer P, Scherrer A, Fishman EK (1997a) CT appearance of transitional cell carcinoma of the renal pelvis. 1. Early-stage disease. AJR Am J Roentgenol 169:157–161

Urban BA, Buckley J, Soyer P, Scherrer A, Fishman EK (1997b) CT apperance of transitional cell carcinoma of the renal pelvis. 2. Advanced-stage disease. AJR Am J Roentgenol 169:163–168

Welch TJ, Leroy AJ (1997) Helical and electron beam CT scanning in the evaluation of renal vein involvement in ptients with renal cell carcinoma. JCAT 21:467–471

Wills JS (1995) Management of small renal neoplasms and angio-myolipoma: a growing problem. Radiology 197: 583–586

Wyatt SH, Urban BA, Fishman EK (1995) Spiral CT of the kidneys: role in characterization of renal disease, part II: neoplastic disease. Crit Rev Diagn Imaging 36:39–72

Zagoria RJ, Bechtold RE, Dyer RB (1995) Staging of renal adeno-carcinoma: role of various imaging procedures. AJR Am J Roentgenol 164:363–370

Zeman RK, Zeiberg A, Hayes WS, SilvermanPM, Cooper C, Garra BS (1996) Helical CT of renal masses: the value of delayed scans. AJR Am J Roentgenol 167:771–776

Renal Tumors:
The Role of Spiral CT and Controversies

30 The Case for Ultrasonography

J.-Y. MEUWLY

CONTENTS

30.1   Introduction   *349*
30.2   Cystic Masses   *349*
30.3   Solid Masses   *352*
30.4   Pseudomasses   *355*
30.5   Infectious Processes   *356*
30.6   Conclusion   *357*
       References   *357*

30.1
Introduction

Over the course of the last few years, the number of incidentally detected renal cancers has increased markedly, thanks to new imaging techniques. Tumours discovered in this way are smaller and still at an earlier stage than those suspected clinically (UEDA et al. 1991).

According to SMITH et al. (1989) and REUSS (1994), the use of ultrasonography (US) and computerized tomography (CT) has resulted in the diagnosis of five times as many small cancers (<3 cm) as previously. This improvement in diagnostic performance has directly affected patient survival (KESSLER et al. 1994).

If one compares the two imaging techniques, US is as sensitive as CT in the detection of renal masses with diameters of 25–30 mm (JAMIS-DOWN et al. 1996), but less sensitive than CT for smaller tumours. In the series reported by SMITH et al. (1989), 30% of small tumours were detected by US, while in that of UEDA et al. (1991), the proportion was 69%.

Thanks to its low cost and high availability and performance, US occupies an important position among the imaging techniques. The number of US explorations greatly exceeds the number of investigations performed with CT and magnetic resonance

J.-Y. MEUWLY, MD; Department of Radiology, University Hospital, CHUV Lausanne, Switzerland

imaging (MRT) combined (SCHAPPERT 1997). Considering the impact of the incidental discovery of asymptomatic renal masses on patient survival, it is essential that the ultrasonographer be familiar with the semiology of renal masses. It is the only way to be able to recognize a suggestive image, even if it is unrelated to the clinical context of the US examination.

The purpose of this chapter is to describe and illustrate the echographic characteristics of renal masses in such a way that the reader will be able to recognize them and to take suitable diagnostic and therapeutic actions. The main role of US is to characterize renal masses as liquid or solid and to determine which require more detailed investigation.

30.2
Cystic Masses

Simple cysts are the most frequently diagnosed renal masses, and their incidence increases with age. They are found in 25–33% of patients over the age of 50 years (TADA et al.1983). Usually asymptomatic and discovered incidentally, simple cysts can become symptomatic when they compress the kidneys, become infected or bleed (BOSNIAK 1986; HAYDEN and SWISCHUK 1991).

To be characterized as a simple cyst, the mass should be perfectly anechogenic with posterior enhancement, have clearly defined thin walls and be round or oval in shape. A massive caliceal dilatation, a haematoma or an aneurysm, or even a false aneurysm, may mimic the appearance of a simple cyst. Simple cysts can be localized intraparenchymatously (cortical cysts) or sinusally, in which case they are known as parapyelic cysts if they are cortical cysts with an intrasinusal projection or peripyelic cysts if they originate in the sinus (AMIS and CRONAN 1988); the latter correspond to lymphatic dilatations.

If internal echoes (other than artefacts), septations, nodularities, thick walls or calcifications are present, the diagnosis of a simple cyst cannot be made and another pathology must be suspected. These different types of cysts have been well described by BOSNIAK (1986) on the basis of CT criteria, and this classification is widely used in the US literature (Table 30.1).

Type 1 lesions are simple cysts, which require no further evaluation, as they are entirely benign (Fig. 30.1). Type 2 lesions (minimally complicated cysts) should be monitored radiologically, as some turn out to be cancers (Fig. 30.2). Type 3 lesions (complicated cysts) should be explored surgically, since 50% turn out to be cancers (Fig. 30.3). Type 4 lesions are considered malignant until proved otherwise (Fig. 30.4). Several assessments of this classification have been published, confirming its value despite certain limitations (BELLMAN et al. 1995; WILSON et al. 1996), and it remains the best noninvasive method for assessing cystic kidney lesions.

Simple cysts can also be multiple and bilateral; whether single or multiple, they are harmless and do not require treatment unless they become symptomatic. The treatment of simple cysts is dealt with later in this chapter. Other multiple cysts must be recognized, because they are associated with either renal tumours or other diseases. The first group includes acquired renal cysts in patients undergoing chronic dialysis (acquired cystic kidney disease; ACKD) and those associated with Von Hippel-Lindau's disease and tuberous sclerosis. Polycystic kidney disease, nephronophthisis, medullary sponge kidney, the

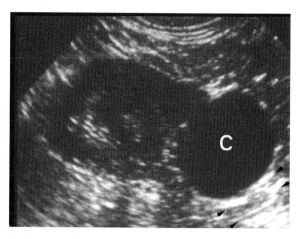

Fig. 30.1. Sagittal sonogram of the right kidney shows an anechoic mass of the lower pole (*C*), with regular margins, thin wall and posterior acoustic enhancement (*arrowheads*):

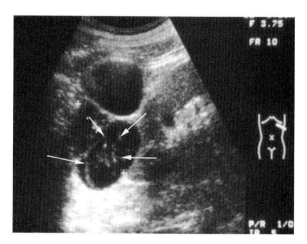

Fig. 30.2. Transverse sonogram of the left kidney shows four cysts on the upper pole. One cyst contains multiple thin septations (*arrows*): minimally complicated cyst

Table 30.1. Bosniak classification of cystic renal masses, modified for ultrasound

Category	Criteria
Type 1 Simple cysts	Cysts with echo-free contents, clear-cut margins, thin wall and posterior enhancement
Type 2 Minimally complicated cysts	Minimally calcified wall, septated cysts, echogenic cysts
Type 3 More complicated cysts	Cysts with thickening of the wall, nodularities, coarse calcifications, Doppler signal within the wall
Type 4 Cystic carcinoma	Irregularity of the margins, large solid areas and irregular thickening of the wall

glomerulocystic diseases and multicystic dysplasias belong in the second group. All these cysts have the same US characteristics as a simple cyst, and it is only their number and distribution and the age at which they are discovered that direct the diagnosis (Fig. 30.5).

With few exceptions, all these multiple cysts are bilateral and cannot be confused with renal tumours; nevertheless, it is necessary to know how to distinguish one disease from the other, as their prognoses differ. It is especially important to pay particular attention to the US exploration of cystic diseases linked to an increased incidence of renal tumours.

ACKD is seen in patients with chronic renal failure. The prevalence is 50% after 5 years of dialysis

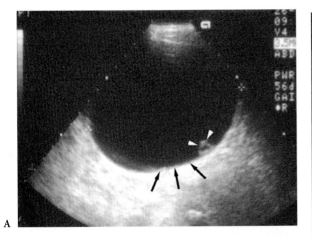

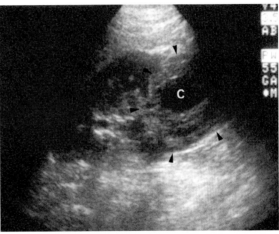

Fig. 30.4. Sagittal sonogram of the right kidney shows a cystic mass at the upper pole. There is a thick irregular margin (*arrowheads*) and a small hypoechoic central component (*c*): cystic carcinoma

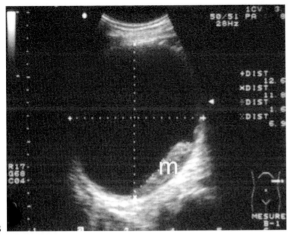

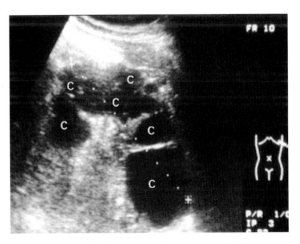

Fig. 30.3. **A** Transverse sonogram of the left kidney shows a large cystic mass with minimal thickening of the wall (*arrows*) and a small bud (*arrowhead*): complicated cyst. **B** The patient refused any treatment, and 2 years later, the cyst was becoming larger and there was a frank echoic mass within

Fig. 30.5. The left kidney is no longer recognizable on this transverse sonogram. Multiple cystic masses (*c*) with a thin wall are deforming the normal architecture of the kidney. There is a massive enlargement of the kidney: autosomal dominant polycystic kidney disease (ADPKD)

and 90% after 5–10 years (MATSON and COHEN 1990). ACKD is diagnosed as bilateral involvement, with at least three cysts on each side. The incidence of metastatic or invasive renal carcinomas (RCC) in patients with ACKD is up to 6 times as high as in the general population (LEVINE et al. 1991). Although large tumours can be recognized sonographically by their solid appearance, small tumours are easily confused with haemorrhagic cysts, which appear in about 50% of ACKD carriers; the differential diagnosis can be made by CT. The development of US contrast agents will perhaps allow this distinction to be made by US in the future.

In tuberous sclerosis, renal involvement (cysts and/or angiomyolipomas) is seen in 50% of cases.

The angiomyolipomas are hyperechogenic, and their lipid content can be characterized by CT (BERNSTEIN 1993). The presence of an echogenic cyst in cases of tuberous sclerosis, Von Hippel-Lindau disease or ACKD should suggest a malignant tumour, as should the absence of lipid in a solid mass.

The incidence of renal carcinoma is not increased in other cystic kidney diseases. This question has been raised several times with reference to autosomal dominant polycystic kidney disease (ADPKD; BERNSTEIN et al. 1987). In fact, the incidence of renal tumours is no higher in patients with ADPKD than in the general population (CABALLERO et al. 1997), but the expression of the tumours is unusual, with an earlier age at presentation, fever, night sweats and weight loss (KEITH et al. 1994). Since fever is much more common as the first symptom of a renal tumour in patients with ADPKD (32%) than in the general population (7%), caution is necessary when faced with an echogenic cyst in this clinical context. In such cases, US-guided fine needle puncture can help in determining whether the nodule is infectious or haemorrhagic. Calcifications, frequently seen in ADPKD, never have the same significance as for simple cysts.

Complicated cysts (Bosniak types 2, 3 and 4) can be haemorrhagic cysts, haematoma (Fig. 30.6), superinfected cysts, hydatid cysts, multilocular cystic nephromas, Wilms' cysts or cystic kidney carcinomas. In this group, only hydatid cysts can be recognized with certainty by US criteria; CT or surgery are generally required for the diagnosis of the other types.

The US semiology of hydatid cysts has been well described by GHARBI et al. (1981). Hydatid cysts can be anechogenic (type I) and indistinguishable from simple cysts, but a parasitic nature should be suspected if they are found in an area of endemic echinococcal infection. Type II hydatid cysts have a germinal membrane that becomes detached (water lily sign). Type III cysts have an alveolar appearance and must not be confused with polycystic disease. Type IV cysts are heterogeneous, and type V cysts have a calcified wall. ÖDEV has shown that these different appearances are seen with renal hydatid cysts (ÖDEV et al. 1996), although these are rare, with echinococcosis of the kidney representing only 2–3% of involvement, compared with 65% for the liver and 25% for the lungs.

Ultrasonography can help determine the choice for percutaneous treatment of patients in whom the diagnosis can be made with certainty (GOEL et al. 1995). This therapeutic objective is the best indication for fine needle puncture (WOLF 1998). In the case of hydatid cysts, as for simple cysts, this treatment consists in aspiration of the cyst contents and injection of a sclerosing agent, normally 95% ethanol (PFISTER et al. 1996). Various alcohol treatment procedures, variations on that initially described by BEAN (1981), have been suggested. For both simple cysts and hydatid cysts, the authors recommend fine needle puncture followed by insertion of a large-calibre drain by the method of Seldinger. The timing of drainage is variable. HANNA recommends a sec-

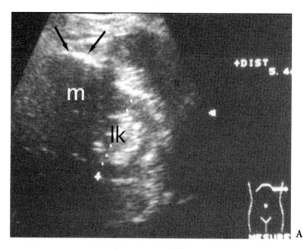

A

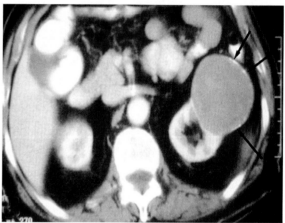

B

Fig. 30.6. A Transverse sonogram of the left kidney (*lk*) shows an homogenous echoic mass (*m*) with a thin hyperechoic rim (*arrows*). **B** There is no enhancement on CT scanning. A calcified wall is clearly visible (*arrows*). The history of the patient revealed an episode of trauma many years ago: calcified renal haematoma

ond alcohol treatment session via the drain before it is removed (HANNA and DAHNIYA 1996), which eliminates all recurrence of simple cysts.

30.3
Solid Masses

Any solid renal mass should, a priori, be considered malignant. However, certain solid renal masses (adenomas, oncocytomas and angiomyolipomas) are benign. None of these tumours can be distinguished with certainty from a malignant tumour by US, but some US signs make it possible to orient the diagnosis and to encourage a conservative surgical approach.

Sonographically, oncocytomas appear as homogeneous hypoechogenic masses within which radial scarring can be defined (GOINEY et al. 1984). Doppler does not give a definitive diagnosis (DENYS et al. 1991). US contrast agents will perhaps allow better characterization, but may have the same limitations as angiography (AMBOS et al. 1978). Needle biopsy is not sufficient, since a well-differentiated renal adenocarcinoma may contain areas of tissue with an oncocytic appearance, and often only the analysis of the whole excised fragment can lead to a definitive diagnosis.

Angiomyolipoma (AML) is the only benign renal tumour that can be diagnosed radiologically. This tumour is normally single, but can also be multiple and bilateral in tuberous sclerosis. It is usually asymptomatic, but may reveal itself as painful haematuria secondary to intratumour haemorrhage. Using US, angiomyolipoma appears as a homogeneous hyperechogenic nodule without a peripheral border (Fig. 30.7), producing, when large, a posterior acoustic shadow. However, this appearance is not specific and AML cannot be distinguished from renal carcinoma by US criteria (SIEGEL et al. 1996). The differential diagnosis is made by CT, which demonstrates either the lipid component of the tumour (SILVERMANN et al. 1996) or its characteristic homogeneity (JINZAKI et al. 1997). Paradoxically, it seems that this way to come to a definitive diagnosis is rarely attempted (IKEDA et al. 1995).

Adenocarcinoma is the most frequently encountered primary tumour in adults (80–85% of cases) and generally manifests as pain in the side, haematuria and a palpable mass in the elderly patient. The US appearance of a renal carcinoma is that of a well-delineated, heterogeneous solid mass, more or less echogenic than the adjacent parenchyma, that deforms the outline of the kidney (Fig. 30.8). In 10% of cases, the tumour contains calcifications that are usually central and punctiform, but may sometimes

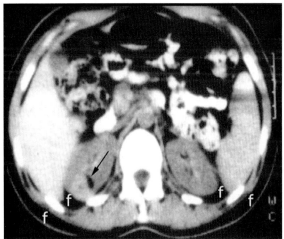

Fig. 30.7. A Sagittal sonogram of the right kidney shows a hyperechoic mass 1 cm in size of the lower pole (*arrowheads*). **B** CT scan demonstrates that this mass (*arrow*) is of the same density as the surrounding and subcutaneous fat (*f*): angiomyolipoma

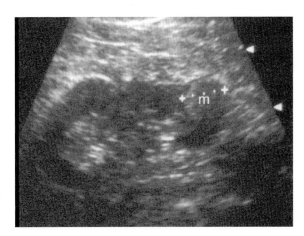

Fig. 30.8. A small hyperechoic mass (*m*) is depicted on this sagittal sonogram of the left kidney. No definite characterization can be done on this ultrasonographic image. Surgery revealed a small renal cell carcinoma (RCC)

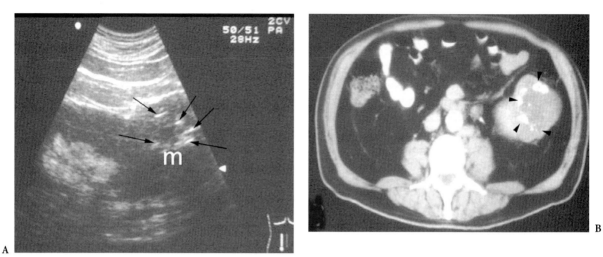

Fig. 30.9. A Sagittal sonogram shows an heterogeneous mass (*m*) at the lower pole of the left kidney. Coarse calcifications within the mass (*arrows*) depict the malignant nature of the tumour. **B**. The calcifications (*arrowheads*) are clearly visible on the CT scan

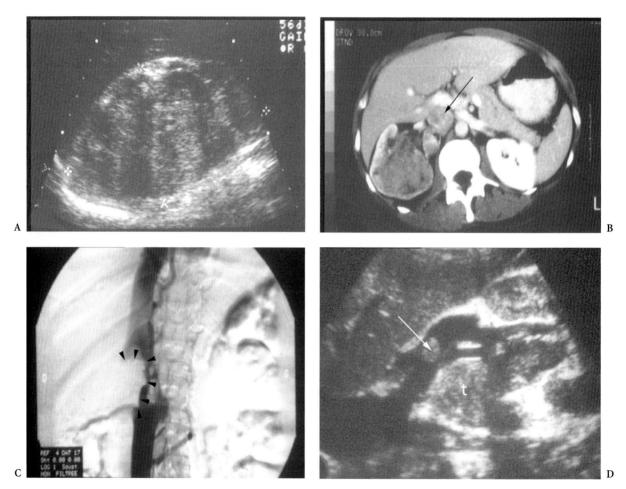

Fig. 30.10. A Sagittal sonogram of the right kidney shows complete replacement of the normal renal architecture by an heterogeneous process. **B** The mass is clearly visible on the CT scan. The inferior vena cava is enlarged (*arrow*) and its lumen is filled with some heterogeneous material. **C** Digital subtracted venography shows the filling defect (*arrowheads*). **D** Sagittal sonogram of the inferior vena cava shows tumour tissue beside the vein (*t*) and inside (*arrow*)

be linear and peripheral (Fig. 30.9). Diagnosis can be made by US in the case of large tumours, but not of small tumours. Several Doppler criteria [displacement of the 2.5 kHz frequency peak (KIER et al. 1990; KUIJPERS et al. 1994), or even the 4 kHz peak (KUIJPERS and JASPERS 1989)], can help to characterize a malignant tumour. Colour Doppler US and US contrast agents often make it possible to distinguish the intratumoral vessels accurately. Whether in spectral mode, colour or power mode, Doppler improves the performance of B-mode US, but has the same limitations as angiography in characterizing renal masses (DENYS et al. 1991).

Careful screening must be performed for tumour extension to the vena cava (5–10% of cases) and for a contralateral localization (4–5 % of cases) (MADAYAG et al. 1979). US is less useful than CT or MRI in the staging of renal tumours (REZNEK 1996), but its role in screening for tumour extension to the IVC should be emphasized (Fig. 30.10) (HABBOUB et al. 1997). The introduction of US contrast agents should give US pride of place in the initial screening for renal tumours (ROBBIN 1997). With the exception of the characterization of a stage T4 tumour in a patient having a high surgical risk, percutaneous biopsy is not indicated in the case of suspected RCC.

Wilms' tumour and sarcoma (Fig. 30.11) are more rare and cannot be distinguished sonographically from renal carcinoma.

Renal lymphoma is also rare. Lymphomatous infiltration of the kidney can be primary or secondary to the extension of retroperitoneal adenopathy. In the case of a primary pathology, the most common appearance is that of multiple hypoechogenic masses distributed throughout the parenchyma (Fig. 30.12; EISENBERG et al. 1994). The mass can be solitary or show a diffuse infiltration with a large hypoechogenic kidney. The presence of retroperitoneal adenopathy should suggest the diagnosis. When faced with a suspicion of renal lymphoma, a percutaneous needle biopsy could be performed under US guidance.

Intrarenal metastases, often multiple and bilateral, are frequent. They usually originate in the lungs, breast or contralateral kidney and are most often discovered on autopsy. When visible on US, they appear as more or less homogeneous iso-, hyper-, or hypoechogenic nodules. Given a history of primary tumour, the diagnosis is simple. The metastases can sometimes be voluminous and solitary.

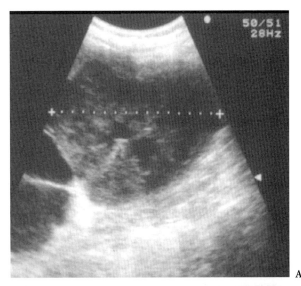
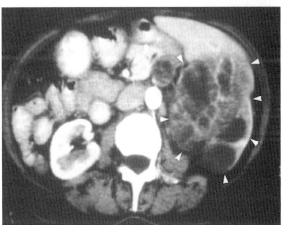

Fig. 30.11. A Sagittal sonogram of the left kidney shows a large heterogeneous mass of the lower pole. B On the contrast-enhanced CT scan, the left kidney is replaced by an heterogeneous mass, indistinguishable from RCC (*arrowheads*). Surgery revealed a sarcoma

30.4 Pseudomasses

Images of pseudomasses should be distinguished from those of true tumour masses. Hypertrophy of the column of Bertin (Fig. 30.13), a cortical scar or fetal lobulation can be difficult to recognize by US. Colour Doppler can help to identify them by demonstrating the absence of disorganization of vascular architecture. Occasionally, they can only be recognized by CT or MRI. Infectious processes can also produce images of mass effect. The diagnosis must therefore be oriented by the clinical context and confirmed by percutaneous biopsy.

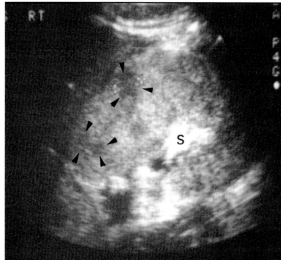

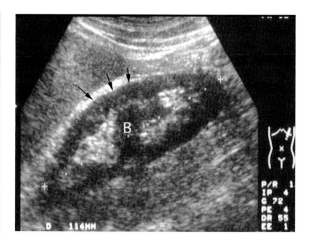

Fig. 30.13. A column of Bertin (*B*) occupies the renal sinus on this sagittal sonogram of the left kidney. Note the lack of deformity of the renal contour (*arrows*)

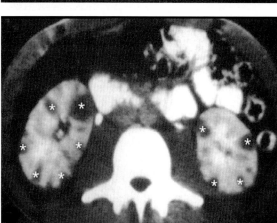

Fig. 30.12. A Sagittal sonogram of the right kidney shows a massively enlarged kidney with obliterated sinus (*s*). Multiple lymphomatous masses appear as hypoechoic nodules (*arrowheads*). **B** The lymphomatous masses are hypodense (*∗*) on this contrast-enhanced CT scan

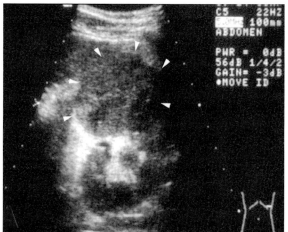

30.5
Infectious Processes

Several kinds of alterations of the renal parenchyma (normal kidney, acute stage oedematous large kidney and scarring stage atrophic small kidney with increased or decreased cortico-medullary differentiation, focal hypoechogenicity and renal mass) may occur during infectious processes. Decreased mobility of the kidney within the renal compartment is a good indication of an inflammatory process (GOLDMAN and FISHMAN 1991).

In focal nephritis, a segment of the renal parenchyma becomes oedematous, giving an image of a

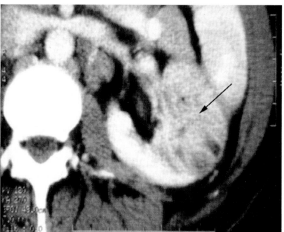

Fig. 30.14. A Transverse sonogram of the left kidney shows an ill-defined enlargement of the upper pole of the kidney (*arrowheads*), related to pyelonephritis. **B** The contrast-enhanced CT scan clearly depicts the focal nephritis (*arrow*)

poorly delimited hypo- or isoechogenic mass (Fig. 30.14). In the event of haemorrhage in the infectious focus, the mass can appear hyperechogenic and a differential diagnosis must be made against a complicated cyst, a carcinoma or a lymphoma.

Renal abscess can develop from a focus of focal nephritis or during the course of severe pyelonephritis with diffuse involvement of the renal parenchyma. It can be solitary or multiple and intra- or perirenal. Ultrasonography may disclose a mass with a more or less thick wall and more or less echogenic contents. The presence of hyperechogenic punctuations with reflection echoes indicates the presence of gas, which is characteristic of an infectious process, in the absence of history of any recent interventional procedure.

Other, rarer, infectious processes (tuberculosis, malacoplakia and xanthogranulomatous pyelonephritis) can mimic tumours.

Renal tuberculosis can appear in the form of a complicated cyst or a mass. With renal tuberculosis, a loss of differentiation between parenchyma and sinusal fat, an abscess or pyelonephrosis may also be seen (BECKER 1988). Needle aspiration can confirm the diagnosis in patients with negative urine cultures (DAS et al. 1992).

Malacoplakia is seen in immunosuppressed patients, diabetics and chronic alcoholics and results from a poor immune response to the infectious agent, with inclusion in the histiocytes of incompletely destroyed bacteria. Rounded hypoechogenic parenchymatous masses appear in the kidneys and deform them. Central necrosis with calcifications may be seen (HARTMAN et al. 1980; OTTAVIOLI et al. 1990).

Xanthogranulomatous pyelonephritis is caused by chronic infection of a blocked kidney, often due to a staghorn calculus. The renal parenchyma is progressively replaced by a granulomatous material rich in lipid-filled macrophages. On US, the kidney appears dedifferentiated and the dilated cavities are often filled with echogenic material. The calculus is usually clearly visible (COUSINS et al. 1994; VANKIRK et al. 1980).

30.6
Conclusion

Ultrasonography has a place in the diagnosis of renal masses. It allows the detection of a large number of such masses before any clinical manifestation. US

is of limited use in the characterization of solid masses and tumour staging, but it is essential in distinguishing between benign simple cysts and and lesions suggested to be a mass requiring additional investigations. US can also be used to guide needle aspiration or biopsy when indicated. In the future, US contrast agents will perhaps allow a more precise characterization of renal tumours, making it possible to avoid the use of more onerous techniques, such as CT or MRI.

References

Ambos MA, Bosniak MA, Valensi QJ et al (1978) Angiographic patterns in renal oncocytomas. Radiology 129:614–622

Amis ES, Cronan JJ (1988) The renal sinus: an imaging review and proposed nomenclature for sinus cysts. J Urol 139:1151–1159

Bean WJ (1981) Renal cysts: treatment with alcohol. Radiology 138:329–331

Becker JA (1988) Renal tuberculosis. Urol Radiol 10:25–30

Bellman GC, Yamaguchi R, Kaswick J (1995) Laparoscopic evaluation of indeterminate renal cysts. Urology 45:1066–1070

Bernstein J (1993) Renal cystic disease in the tuberous sclerosis complex. Pediatr Nephrol 7:490–495

Bernstein J, Evan AP, Gardner KD Jr (1987) Epithelial hyperplasia in human polycystic kidney disease. Am J Pathol 129:92–101

Bosniak MA (1986) The current radiological approach to renal cysts. Radiology 158:1–10

Caballero AJ, Gonzalez HC, Padilla LM, Marchal EC (1997) Renal-cell carcinoma and polycystic disease in an adult. Actas Urol Esp 21:410–414

Cousins C, Somers J, Broderick N et al (1994) Xanthogranulomatous pyelonephritis in childhood: ultrasound and CT diagnosis. Pediatr Radiol 24:210–212

Das KM, Vaidyanathan S, Rajwanshi A, Indudhara R (1992) Renal tuberculosis: diagnosis with sonographically guided aspiration cytology. AJR Am J Roentgenol 158:571–573

Denys A, Helenon O, Souissi M et al (1991) Doppler pulsé et couleur des masses rénales: corrélation angiographique et anatomo-pathologique. J Radiol 72:599–608

Eisenberg PJ, Papanicolaou N, Lee MJ, Yoder IC (1994) Diagnostic imaging in the evaluation of renal lymphoma. Leuk Lymphoma 16:37–50

Gharbi HA, Hassine W, Brauner MW, Dupuch K (1981) Ultrasound examination of the hydatic liver. Radiology 139:459–463

Goel MC, Agarwal MR, Misra A (1995) Percutaneous drainage of renal hydatid cyst: early results and follow-up. Br J Urol 75:724–728

Goldman SM, Fishman EK (1991) Upper urinary tract infection: the current role of CT, ultrasound and MRI. Semin Ultrasound CT MR 12:335–360

Goiney RC, Goldberg L, Cooperberg PL et al (1984) Renal

oncocytomas, sonographic analysis of 14 cases. AJR Am J Roentgenol 143:1001

Habboub HK, Abu-Yousef MM, Williams RD et al (1997) Accuracy of color Doppler sonography in assessing venous thrombus extension in renal cell carcinoma. AJR Am J Roentgenol 168:267–271

Hanna RM, Dahniya MH (1996) Aspiration and sclerotherapy of symptomatic simple renal cysts: value of two injections of a sclerosing agent. AJR Am J Roentgenol 167:781–783

Hartman DS, Davis CJ, Lichtenstein JE, Goldman SM (1980) Renal parenchymal malakoplakia. Radiology 136:33–42

Hayden CK, Swischuk LE (1991) Renal cystic disease. Semin Ultrasound CT MR 12:361–373

Ikeda AK, Korobkin M, Platt JF et al (1995) Small echogenic renal masses: how often is computed tomography used to confirm the sonographic suspicion of angiomyolipoma? Urology 46:311–315

Jamis-Down CA, Choyke PL, Jennings SB et al (1996) Small (<or = 3 cm) renal masses: detection with CT versus US and pathologic correlation. Radiology 198:785–788

Jinzaki M, Tanimoto A, Narimatsu Y et al (1997) Angiomyolipoma: imaging findings in lesions with minimal fat. Radiology 205:497–502

Keith DS, Torres VE, Kling BF et al (1994) Renal cell carcinoma in autosomal dominant kidney disease. J Am Soc Nephrol 4:1661–1669

Kessler O, Mukamel E, Gillon G et al (1994) Effect of improved diagnosis of renal cell carcinoma on the course of the disease. J Surg Oncol 57:201–204

Kier R, Taylor KJ, Feyock AL, Ramos IM (1990) Remal masses: characterization with Doppler US. Radiology 176:703–707

Kuijpers D, Jaspers R (1989) Renal masses: differential diagnosis with pulsed Doppler US. Radiology 170:59–60

Kuijpers D, Kruyt RH, Oudkerk M (1994) Renal masses: value of duplex Doppler ultrasound in the differential diagnosis. J Urol 151:326–328

Levine E, Slusher SL, Grantham JJ et al (1991) Natural history of acquired renal cystic disease in dialysis patients: a prospective longitudinal CT study. AJR Am J Roentgenol 156:501–506

Madayag MA, Ambos MA, Lefleur RS, Bosniak MA (1979) Involvement of the inferior vena cava in patients with renal carcinoma. Radiology 133:321–326

Matson MA, Cohen EP (1990) Acquired cystic kidney disease: occurrence, prevalence, and renal cancers. Medicine 69:217–226

Ödev K, Kilinc M, Arslan A et al (1996) Renal hydatid cysts and the evaluation of their radiologic images. Eur Urol 30:40–49

Ottavioli JN, Cart P, Fauchart JP et al (1990) Renal parenchymal malakoplakia: a case report. J Urol 96:393–396

Pfister C, Sibert L, Thoumas D et al (1996) Place de la sclérothérapie alcoolique par ponction percutanée dans le traitement des kystes rénaux symptomatiques. Prog Urol 6:543–547

Reuss J (1994) Der Nierentumor als sonographischer Zufallsbefund. Ultraschall Med 15:163–167

Reznek RH (1996) Imaging in the staging of renal cell carcinoma. Eur Radiol 6:120–128

Robbin ML (1997) The promise of sonographic contrast agents in the kidney. In: Nanda NC, Schlief R, Goldberg BB (eds) Advances in echo imaging using contrast enhancement. Kluwer Academic, Dordrecht, pp 525–541

Schappert SM (1997) Ambulatory care visits to physician offices, hospital outpatient departments, and emergency departments: United States, 1995. Data from the National Health Care Survey, no 129. National Center for Health Statistics, Hyattsville

Siegel CL, Middleton WD, Teefey SA, McClennan BL (1996) Angiomyolipoma and renal cell carcinoma: US differentiation. Radiology 198:789–793

Silvermann SG, Pearson GD, Seltzer SE et al (1996) Small (<or = 3 cm) hyperechoic renal masses: comparison of helical and conventional CT for diagnosing angiomyolipoma. AJR Am J Roentgenol 167:877–881

Smith SJ, Bosniak MA, Megibow AJ et al (1989) Renal carcinoma: earlier discovery and increased detection. Radiology 170:699–703

Tada S, Yamagishi J, Kobayashi H et al (1983) The incidence of simple renal cyst by computed tomography. Clin Radiol 34:437–439

Ueda T, Yasumasu T, Uozumi J, Naito S (1991) Comparison of clinical and pathological characteristics in incidentally detected and suspected renal carcinoma. Br J Urol 68:470–472

VanKirk OC, Go RT, Wedel VJ (1980) Sonographic feature of xanthogranulomatous pyelonephritis. AJR Am J Roentgenol 134:1035–1039

Wilson TE, Doelle EA, Cohan RH et al (1996) Cystic renal masses: a reevaluation of the usefulness of the Bosniak classification system. Acad Radiol 3:564–570

Wolf JS (1998) Evaluation and management of solid and cystic renal masses. J Urol 159:1120–1133

31 The Case for Spiral CT

H. Trillaud, J. Palussière, N Grenier

Helical CT is widely accepted as the state-of-the-art technique for the detection and staging of renal neoplasms. CT examinations are accessible, fast and noninvasive. Like ultrasonography, this technique has made it possible to detect renal carcinomas at an early stage, while the tumor is still small . This facilitates the treatment and improves the prognosis (Davidson et al. 1997; Szolar et al. 1997).

More accurate renal imaging thanks to helical CT has led to a re-evaluation of the traditional surgical approach to renal neoplasms (Smith et al. 1989; Stuart Wolf 1998). In the past, the only treatment was total nephrectomy in potentially curable patients. Currently, partial nephrectomy can be performed in small tumors, when they appear well marginated and circumscribed on helical CT. No worsening of the prognosis was observed after this parenchyma- preserving surgical management. In patients with renal cell carcinoma in a solitary kidney or who have decreased renal function, helical CT helps to define the resection border for partial nephrectomy.

Helical CT have also modified the evaluation of cystic renal masses. In 1986 Bosniak proposed a classification of cystic renal masses into four categories based on CT findings (Bosniak 1986). Currently, helical CT is used after ultrasonography to define the cystic lesions better and help clinicians to decide which lesions are benign (category I and II), potentially malignant (category III), or clearly malignant (category IV). This information has obvious implications for patient management.

Helical CT with a dedicated renal imaging protocol, including preliminary native scans followed by scans obtained after a bolus injection of contrast medium, with the same parameters as the native ones and thin (5-mm) slices, improves accuracy in determination of the category of a cystic mass according to the Bosniak classification (Bosniak 1997).

Siegel et al. (1997) confirmed in a recent study that the Bosniak classification was useful for evaluating cystic renal masses. However, these authors noted important interobserver disagreement in the categorization of cystic masses, particularly concerning categories II and III. In this study, it was suggested that high-quality examination and experienced reviewers are required to improve the utility of this classification.

Although helical CT with thin slices allows characterization of small renal tumors between 1.5 cm and 3 cm in diameter, it also frequently shows incidental masses that are too small (<1–1.5 cm) to be characterized. In most cases, these are benign cysts. However, if in a given case the mass cannot be characterized by ultrasonography, the management of such a small lesion is difficult and controversial. In a young patient, most authors perform a follow-up CT examination after 1 year to monitor interval growth (Bosniak and Rofsky 1996). In other patients, except the very old and those with severe underlying disease, there are no widely accepted rules concerning the most appropriate management.

The major controversy appears to be an economic one. The current trend towards increased use of ultrasonography and CT in patients with nonrenal complaints has resulted in the more frequent incidental detection of asymptomatic renal tumors. The accurate characterization of these tumors, i.e. the differentiation between renal neoplasms, minimally complicated cysts, and simple cysts, has become an increasingly frequent indication for dedicated renal CT exams. This strategy, of course, has economic consequences, which still need to be evaluated.

H. Trillaud, MD, PhD; Service de Radiologie, Centre Hospitalier Universitaire de Bordeaux, Groupe Hospitalier Pellegrin, Place Amélie-Raba-Léon, F-33076 Bordeaux Cédex, France
J. Palussière, MD; Service De Radiologie, Institut Bergonié, F-33076 Bordeaux Cédex, France
N Grenier, MD; Service de Radiologie, Centre Hospitalier Universitaire de Bordeaux, Groupe Hospitalier Pellegrin, Place Amélie-Raba-Léon, F-33076 Bordeaux Cédex, France

References

Bosniak MA (1986) The current radiological approach to renal cysts. Radiology 158:1

Bosniak MA (1997) Diagnosis and management of patients with complicated cystic lesions of the kidney. AJR Am J Roentgenol 169:819–821

Bosniak MA, Rofsky NM (1996) Problems in the detection and characterization of small renal masses. Radiology 198:638–641

Davidson AJ, Hartman DS, Choyke PL, Wagner BJ (1997) Radiologic Assessment of renal masses : implications for patient care. Radiology 202:297–305

Siegel CL, McFarland EG, Bring JA et al (1997) CT of cystic renal mass: analysis of diagnostic performance and interobserver variation. AJR Am J Roentgenol 169:813–818

Smith SJ, Bosniak MA, Megibow AJ, Hulnick DH, Horii SC, Nagesh Raghavendra B (1989) Renal cell carcinoma: earlier discovery and increased detection. Radiology 170:699–703

Stuart Wolf J (1998) Evaluation and management of solid and cystic renal masses. J Urol 159:1120–1133

Szolar DH, Kammerhuber F, Altziebler S, Tillich M, Breini E, Fotter R, Schreyer HH (1997) Multiphasic helical CT of the kidney: increased conspicuity for detection and characterization of small (<3 cm) renal masses. Radiology 202:211–217

32 The Case for MRI

W. Okuno, H. Hricak

CONTENTS

32.1   Introduction *361*
32.2   Advances in MRI Technology *361*
32.3   Tumor Detection *361*
32.4   Tumor Characterization *361*
32.5   Renal Cell Carcinoma Staging *362*
32.6   Advantages of MRI over CT *363*
32.7   MRI: Still a Problem-Solving Modality *364*
32.8   Conclusion *364*
        References *364*

32.1
Introduction

Since the introduction of magnetic resonance imaging (MRI) into clinical use, much attention has been given to renal imaging. A number of papers have demonstrated the ability of MRI to show normal renal parenchyma and to detect and stage renal tumors. During the past decade, advances in MRI technology have further improved the efficiency of renal MRI.

32.2
Advances in MRI Technology

Fast, single-breath-hold MRI techniques, such as half-Fourier acquisition single-shot turbo spin-echo (HASTE) and fast multiplanar spoiled gradient-recalled acquisition in the steady state (FMPSPGR), have improved image quality, interpretability, and reproducibility. In addition, these rapid MRI sequences allow increased patient throughput and thus have the potential to reduce the cost of renal MRI.

W. Okuno, MD; Department of Radiology, Box 0628, L-308, 505 Parnassus Avenue, San Francisco, CA 94143-0628, USA
H. Hricak, MD, PhD; Department of Radiology, Box 0628, L-308, 505 Parnassus Avenue, San Francisco, CA 94143-0628, USA

Another development in MRI technology is in-phase and opposed-phase gradient echo imaging. This technique is more sensitive for fat detection than computed tomography (CT) or fat-suppressed MRI, and it may play a future role in renal tumor characterization. Another gradient echo technique, gradient-recalled acquisition in the steady state (GRASS), can detect blood flow without intravenous contrast medium. This GRASS sequence is the most reliable, noninvasive method to detect vascular invasion by renal cell carcinomas (Goldfarb et al. 1990).

32.3
Tumor Detection

The ability of MRI and CT to detect renal masses is nearly equivalent, and both are superior to US for this purpose (Jamis-Dow et al. 1996; Semelka et al. 1993). Both CT and MRI can detect approximately 90% of renal tumors over 1 cm in diameter. The use of gadolinium chelates with fast MRI sequences has further improved the ability of MRI to detect and characterize small (<3 cm) renal lesions (Yamashita et al. 1995). In some cases, it is difficult to determine the origin of a renal fossa mass on CT even after reformations into multiple planes. In these cases, the superior tissue contrast of MRI and its direct multiplanar imaging capabilities may be helpful in determining the organ of origin and thus aid in tumor characterization (Fig. 32.1).

32.4
Tumor Characterization

For renal tumor characterization, MRI is most useful in situations where iodinated contrast agents are contraindicated or when CT is inconclusive. Since CT requires bolus injection of intravenous contrast medium medi for accurate renal tumor character-

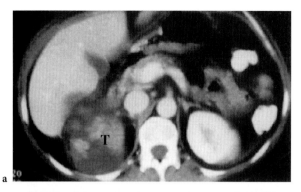

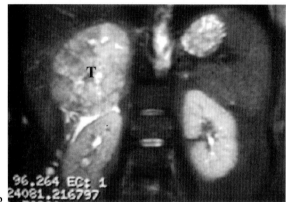

Fig. 32.1a, b. Value of multiplanar MRI in determination of lesion origin. **a** CT scan shows a right upper quadrant mass (*T*) contiguous with the upper pole of the right kidney and posterior segment of the right lobe of the liver. Renal cell carcinoma was a clinical concern. **b** Coronal SSFSE T2-weighted MR image shows that the mass (*T*) is separate from the right kidney and arises from the liver. Hepatocellular carcinoma was proven on pathology

ization, MRI with gadolinium chelate is the preferred study for characterizing solid or complex cystic renal tumors in patients with a history of contrast reactions, renal insufficiency, or poor IV access.

The role of MRI in the diagnosis of renal angiomyolipoma (AML) is uncertain at this time. Angiomyolipoma is the only common renal neoplasm that contains macroscopic fat, so that the identification of fat in a renal lesion by CT or fat-suppressed MRI is diagnostic of a benign lesion. In-phase and opposed-phase MRI can detect microscopic amounts of intralesional fat. Although this increases its sensitivity for detecting AMLs, it also reduces its specificity. The problem is that some renal cell carcinomas contain microscopic fat but none contain macroscopic fat. Thus, in contrast to the detection of macroscopic fat in a renal lesion, the detection of microscopic intralesional fat is not diagnostic of AML (OUTWATER et al. 1997).

32.5
Renal Cell Carcinoma Staging

For renal tumor staging, MRI is the best study, but whether the incremental benefit of MRI over CT is worth the added cost is uncertain. To our knowledge, no cost analysis comparing CT and MRI for renal tumor staging has been performed. MRI and CT have comparable accuracies for determining perinephric extension, with sensitivities about 50% and specificities about 95% (JOHNSON et al. 1987; HRICAK et al. 1988). Since both MRI and CT rely on lymph node size to detect lymphatic metastases, these tests have similar accuracy (about 90%) for determining lymph node metastases . The two studies are comparable in their ability to detect intra-abdominal metastases, but clearly CT is better for detecting thorax metastases.

The major advantage of MRI over CT in renal cell carcinoma staging is the ability of MRI to detect vascular invasion without the need for contrast medium. Incomplete mixing of blood with contrast in the inferior vena cava (IVC) or renal vein may mimic the appearance of thrombus, leading to overstaging by contrast-enhanced CT or gadolinium-enhanced MRI (Fig. 32.1). In addition, studies requiring contrast medium to enhance vessels cannot reliably distinguish bland thrombus from tumor thrombus, because incomplete mixing of contrast with blood may simulate thrombus enhancement and erroneously suggest tumor thrombus. Furthermore, a dilated IVC is a nonspecific finding that can be caused by many conditions, such as right ventricular failure, increased blood flow secondary to renal cell carcinoma hypervascularity, venous thrombus, and tumor thrombus.

Since MRI using GRASS sequences show bright vessels without intravenous contrast medium, many of the problems of vascular imaging by CT are eliminated. Studies have shown that MRI using this sequence is superior to contrast-enhanced MRI or CT for the detection of vascular invasion (GOLDFARB et al. 1990; ROUBIDOUX et al. 1992; KALLMANN et al. 1992; MYNENI et al. 1991). More importantly, MRI is more accurate than CT for determining the cephalad extent of tumor thrombus. Involvement of the distal renal veins or IVC by tumor and the cephalad extension of tumor within the IVC are important determinants of the surgical approach to renal cell carcinoma. MRI is 94–100% accurate at predicting the extent of IVC thrombus, whereas CT is only 33–73% accurate (GOLDFARB et al. 1990; MYNENI et al. 1991). In addition, GRASS sequences can distinguish bland

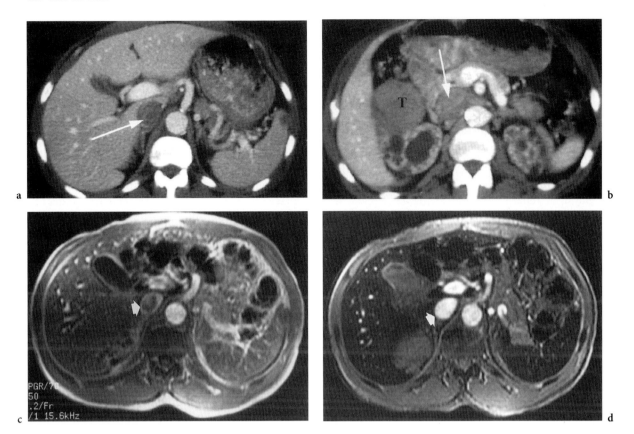

Fig. 32.2a–d. Value of gradient echo imaging in the evaluation of vascular patency. **a, b** CT scans performed during the portal venous phase of enhancement (70 s delay) at the level of the **a** splenic vein and **b** the origin of the superior mesenteric artery (SMA). There is a solid renal mass (*T*) arising from the anterior aspect of the right kidney. There is right hydronephrosis and innumerable bilateral renal cysts in this patient with acquired cystic renal disease secondary to hemodialysis. The inferior vena cava (*arrow*) is enlarged and has an apparent filling defect suggesting thrombus. The small lesion in the anterior aspect of the spleen is a cyst. **c.** Delayed (2 min) gadolinium-enhanced FMPSPGR T1-weighted MR image at the same level as in **b** (SMA origin) shows an apparent filling defect in the IVC suggesting thrombus (*arrow*). **d.** Axial GRASS image at the same level shows flow in the IVC (*arrow*). The apparent filling defect on the contrast-enhanced CT and MRI represents pseudothrombus due to incomplete mixing of blood and contrast

thrombus from tumor thrombus. Tumor thrombus has an intermediate signal intensity on GRASS sequences, similar to the signal of the primary tumor. In contrast, bland thrombus has very low signal on GRASS sequences.

32.6
Advantages of MRI Over CT

There are two important advantages of MRI over CT that define the current niche of MRI for renal tumor imaging. First, CT requires the intravenous bolus administration of relatively large volumes (>80 ml) of iodinated contrast agents for accurate renal imag-

ing. These contrast agents are potentially nephrotoxic and are associated with adverse reactions in up to 5% of patients. In contrast, MRI contrast agents are gadolinium chelates, which are not nephrotoxic and are associated with less adverse reactions. Gadolinium contrast agents may be safely used in patients allergic to iodinated contrast and in patients with renal insufficiency. The volume of gadolinium required for renal MRI (about 10 ml) is substantially less than the volume of iodinated contrast required for renal CT. Thus, patients unable to tolerate a large volume load, such as those with severe right heart failure, may be safely imaged with MRI. Furthermore, adequate contrast-enhanced MRI studies of the kidneys can be performed without the bolus injection of contrast medium, so that MRI may be useful in patients with poor intravenous access. Finally, MRI can reliably image blood vessels and flow without intravenous contrast medium.

The second advantage of MRI is its direct multiplanar imaging capabilities. This capability improves the ability of MRI to detect small renal neoplasms located at the kidney pole and to assess invasion of adjacent structures. Although spiral CT with reformations can show these polar tumors and adjacent organ invasion, the need for these reformations are not known a priori. Consequently, the routine reading of renal CT images in the axial plane will miss a few of these small polar tumors and subtle adjacent organ invasion that MRI would detect.

32.7
MRI: Still a Problem-Solving Modality

Based on literature review, MRI is the most accurate imaging modality for the detection, characterization, and staging of renal tumors. However, despite these technological advances and evidence-based data, MRI remains a problem-solving tool for renal tumor imaging.

Several factors have kept CT the imaging modality of choice for renal tumor imaging. Parallel improvements in CT technology, particularly helical CT, have dramatically improved the ability of CT to image renal neoplasms. In addition, MRI examination generates more images than CT, and this increases the time needed to read renal MRI studies. Furthermore, since CT is more widely used for abdominal imaging than MRI, most radiologists are more comfortable reading abdominal CT than MRI. This greater confidence in the results of CT may be conveyed to the referring physician in both the written report and verbal consultation. Whether the benefits of MRI over CT for renal tumor imaging justify the additional costs remains to be shown.

32.8
Conclusion

Despite dramatic improvements in MRI technology over the past decade, this modality remains a problem-solving tool for renal tumor imaging. At present, MRI is mostly used to stage patients with renal cell carcinoma when contrast-enhanced CT is contraindicated or inconclusive. But as the cost of MRI declines and physicians become more comfortable interpreting the studies, MRI may eventually replace CT for the staging of patients with renal cell carcinoma.

References

Goldfarb DA, Novick AC, Lorig R et al (1990) Magnetic resonance imaging for assessment of vena caval tumor thrombi: a comparative study with venacavography and computerized tomography scanning. J Urol 144:110–113

Hricak H, Thoeni RF, Carroll PR et al (1988) Detection and staging of renal neoplasms: a reassessment of MR imaging. Radiology 166:643–649

Jamis-Dow CA, Choyke PL, Jennings SB et al (1996) Small<or 3-cm renal masses: detection with CT versus US and pathologic correlation. Radiology 198:785–788

Johnson CD, Dunnick NR, Cohan RH et al (1987) Renal adenocarcinoma: CT staging of 100 tumors. AJR 148:59–63

Kallman DA, King BF, Hattery RR et al (1992) Renal vein and inferior vena cava tumor thrombus in renal cell carcinoma: CT, US, MRI and venacavography. J Comput Assist Tomogr 16:240–247

Myneni L, Hricak H, Carroll PR (1991) Magnetic resonance imaging of renal cell carcinoma with extension into the vena cava: staging accuracy and recent advances. Br J Urol 68:571–578

Outwater EK, Manoj B, Siegelman ES et al (1997) Lipid in renal clear cell carcinoma: detection on opposed-phase gradient-echo MR images. Radiology 205:103–107

Roubidoux MA, Dunnick NR, Sostman HD et al (1992) Renal carcinoma: detection of venous extension with gradient-echo MR imaging. Radiology 182:269–272

Semelka RC, Shoenut JP, Magro CM et al (1993) Renal cancer staging: comparison of contrast-enhanced CT and gadolinium-enhanced fat-suppressed spin-echo and gradient-echo MR imaging. J Magn Reson Imaging 3:597–602

Yamashita Y, Miyazaki T, Hatanaka Y et al (1995) Dynamic MRI of small renal cell carcinoma. J Comput Assist Tomogr 19:759–765

33 Synthesis

F. TERRIER

To define the respective roles of the different imaging modalities in the work-up of patients with renal tumors, it is useful to recapitulate some relevant facts on their histological types and biological behavior (WALSH et al. (1992).

Adenocarcinomas are by far the most frequent malignant renal tumors (>90%). They originate from the renal parenchyma and are usually slow-growing tumors. Since the advent of US and CT, renal adenocarcinomas are now mostly found incidentally in patients who are undergoing imaging studies of the abdomen for unrelated clinical symptoms (NAKANO et al. 1992; OEZEN et al. 1993).

Transitional cell carcinomas, which develop from the excretory system, are second in frequency, but represent less than 10% of all malignant renal tumors.

According to autopsy findings, the incidence of renal metastases is higher than usually suspected. With the exception of involvement by lymphomas, they nearly always occur in the terminal stages of disease, mostly in melanoma or in bronchus and breast cancer.

Solid benign renal tumors are rare, the most frequent being angiomyolipomas, which contain fatty tissue.

Percutaneous biopsy of a renal mass is indicated only in a few specific situations: in an advanced neoplastic stage, when the tumor has obviously grown beyond the stage where surgical treatment is still a realistic option (i.e., tumor is already grossly infiltrating adjacent structures or there are proven distant metastases already) and when histological confirmation is needed before irradiation or chemotherapy. It may also be indicated when the clinical context or concomitant radiological findings strongly suggest that a renal mass is a lymphoma or

a renal metastasis and histology is needed before the appropriate therapy can be decided upon. Taking all this into account, the roles of the different imaging techniques, namely US, CT and IRM, are described below.

US is an excellent technique for the detection of solid renal tumors. When a renal adenocarcinoma is suspected on the grounds of a clinical examination it can be confidently confirmed or excluded by US (for example in patients with symptoms such as hematuria and back pain or in those with bone or lung metastases of unknown origin). US allows accurate differentiation of a solid renal tumor from a benign renal cyst. In the case of a noncomplicated cyst (classes 1 and 2 according to the Bosniak classification) no further investigation is needed (BOSNIAK 1986). If, on the other hand, US shows that the mass is solid, the study then has to focus on the renal vein and the inferior vena cava, taking advantage of color and power Doppler, in order to look for a tumor thrombus. If such a thrombus is demonstrated (which is a very strong indication that a renal adenocarcinoma is present), its extent should be very precisely determined. It is especially important to demonstrate whether it reaches the inferior vena cava and, if so, the precise position of its end relative to the openings of the hepatic veins. This information is needed for the planning of surgery. US-guided percutaneous biopsy for histological diagnosis is not indicated; rather, it is necessary to proceed to CT for the purpose of staging. This latter technique will also show intratumoral fat in the case of an angiomyelolipoma.

Spiral CT is a very sensitive technique for demonstrating renal tumors. Even lesions under 1 cm in diameter can be accurately detected. However, characterization, which means mainly the differential diagnosis between solid tumor and cyst, may be fraught with difficulties if an adequate imaging protocol has not been followed. Both the cortical and nephrographic phases are needed, and density measurements comparing pre- and postcontrast values, should be performed.

F. TERRIER, MD; Department of Radiology, Division de Radiodiagnostie et Radiologie Interventionnelle, Hôpital Cantonal, Rue Micheli-du-Crest 24, CH-1211 Genève 14, Switzerland

Because CT is an all-round technique, it is the procedure of choice for staging of renal tumors, allowing the detection of enlarged retroperitoneal lymph nodes (caused by metastatic involvement or reactive hyperplasia) and also of distant metastases in lung, liver, adrenals or bones. If flow artifacts hamper confident determination of whether a tumor thrombus is present in the renal vein and inferior vena cava, and if so its exact extent, Doppler US can be a very adequate complement to the CT examination.

Thus, US and CT perform extremely well when used in tandem in the evaluation of patients with suspected or proven solid renal tumors. Most of the time, the next step will be surgery, without histological confirmation, if the most probable diagnosis suggested by the imaging data is renal adenocarcinoma. Because it is a slow-growing tumor, a "wait and see" strategy is sometimes preferred in very old patients.

Is there a role for MRI? Definitely, when the use of intravenous iodinated contrast agents is contraindicated, for example in the case of renal failure or when a patient has a history of a severe contrast medium reaction. But otherwise? MRI can be useful in the case of a very large tumor, because of its high soft-tissue contrast and its flexibility regarding the imaging plane, to determine the organ of origin, e.g. the kidney, the adrenal or the liver, and to define its extent, in particular whether the psoas muscle or the liver is infiltrated. It allows superb depiction of a thrombus in the renal vein reaching into the inferior vena cava, but color and power Doppler can do the same. Thus, in the vast majority of cases, combined US and CT provide adequate information for proper patient management and MRI is not required.

In one particular situation, the great potential of MRI for tissue characterization is doubtless of value: to differentiate a complicated renal cyst (class 3 and 4 according to the Bosniak classification) from a cystic or necrotic carcinoma. This differential diagnosis can be very difficult with the other imaging techniques, especially when the cystic mass is calcified. On MRI, enhancing nodules in the wall of the cystic mass, which are regarded as a sign of malignancy, are detected with high sensitivity, even in the presence of calcification; on CT, calcification would considerably hinder the analysis of the soft-tissue component of the mass.

For the diagnosis of transitional cell carcinoma of the kidney, intravenous urography (IVU) remains the most appropriate technique, because of its high spatial resolution and its exquisite demonstration of the excretory system. If properly performed, spiral CT in the urographic phase is also a sensitive technique for demonstrating a neoplastic mass in the pyelocaliceal system. In addition, in the nephrographic phase it allows demonstration of the extraluminal infiltration of the tumor, which obviously is not possible with IVU alone. At present, MRI does not have much to offer in the case of transitional cell carcinoma, even when used in the technique of MR urography, because of insufficient spatial resolution. Only in a nonfunctioning kidney, caused for example by hydronephrosis as a consequence of tumor growth, does MRI have any advantage over CT and allow better demonstration of the cause of obstruction and the extent of the tumor.

References

Bosniak MA (1986) The current radiological approach to renal cysts. Radiology 158:1–10

Nakano E, Iwasaki A, Seguchi T, Kokado Y, Yoshioka T, Sugaop H, Koide T (1992) Incidentally diagnosed renal cell carcinoma. Eur Urol 21:294–298

Oezen H, Colowick A, Freiha FS (1993) Incidentally discovered solid renal masses: what are they? Br J Urol 72:274–276

Walsh PC, Retik AB, Stamey TA, Vaughan ED Jr (1992) Campbell's urology, 6th edn. Saunders, Philadelphia

Gastro-intestinal Tract

34 CT Enteroclysis

G.A. Rollandi, E. Biscaldi

CONTENTS

34.1   General Introduction   369
34.1.1 Why Use CT to Study the Digestive System?   369
34.1.2 Why CT Enteroclysis?   369
34.2   Basic Principles   370
34.2.1 CT Versus Conventional Radiology in the Study
        of the Small Intestine   370
34.2.2 The Choice of Endoluminal Contrast Medium   371
34.3   Examination Technique   371
34.3.1 Preparation of the Intestine   371
34.3.2 Administration Route of the Contrast
        Medium   372
34.3.3 Infusion of the Contrast Medium   373
34.3.4 Endoluminal Contrast Medium   373
34.3.5 CT Technique   373
34.3.6 Post-processing   374
34.4   Crohn's Disease   374
34.4.1 Introduction   374
34.4.2 CT Semeiotics   375
34.5   Tumours   377
34.5.1 Introduction   377
34.5.2 Benign Tumours   378
34.5.3 Malignant Tumours   380
34.5.4 Lymphomas   381
        References   382

34.1
General Introduction

34.1.1
Why Use CT to Study the Digestive System?

The use of computerized tomography to study the digestive system is still controversial and not widespread, even though the technical and cultural conditions that once seriously limited its application have changed substantially in recent years.

The most significant technical change is without doubt the advent of spiral technology. The speed of acquisition and the large number of images obtain-able in the unit of volume explored have definitively eliminated any possibility of artefacts due to intestinal peristalsis, have achieved ideal enhancement, and have paved the way to multiplanar vision of the intestinal loops, which has sometimes proved indispensable in the evaluation of intestinal pathology. Moreover, the evolution of detectors, in terms of efficiency and accuracy of measurement, has brought the spatial resolution of CT images within a range that is useful for the assessment of diseases of the digestive system.

Some cultural aspects have also played an important part. In the past, CT was mainly carried out by "technical specialists", who built up the CT semeiotics of organs that were otherwise difficult to explore (liver, pancreas, kidneys, etc.). In the 1970s and 1980s, the training ground of these "technical specialists" was decidedly separate from that of the "organ specialists", who studied the digestive system by means of traditional techniques that are "poorer" but require particularly long and dedicated training. In the 1990s, the development of endoscopy, and the consequent marked reduction in the number of conventional radiological examinations of the digestive tract, diverted many specialists who were already experts on the digestive system towards CT, which had meanwhile advanced in terms of technical quality and clinical importance.

The substantial technical improvement in computerized tomography and the availability of doctors specialized in CT who are culturally "sensitive" to digestive tract pathology are therefore comparatively recent phenomena. Thus, international centres have been created in which specific techniques and semeiotics for the CT study of the digestive system have been developed.

34.1.2
Why CT Enteroclysis?

The segment of the digestive tract that is of the most radiological interest is the one running from the

G.A. Rollandi, MD; Second Service of Radiology, S. Martino Hospital, Largo R. Benzi 10, I-16132 Genoa, Italy
E. Biscaldi, MD; Department of Radiology, Giannina Gaslini Children's Hospital, Largo Gaslini 5, I-16148 Genoa Italy

lower bend of the duodenum to the transverse colon, because it is the segment in which endoscopy encounters the greatest technical difficulties. In performing CT examinations of the small intestine, there are some basic rules to be obeyed. These have been amply discussed and recognized in conventional radiology, and are aimed at avoiding errors and endowing the techniques adopted with the maximum diagnostic potential. In particular, the question of how to administer the contrast medium – orally or by means of oro-jejunal intubation – has to be tackled in CT too.

Published reports on large series of patients examined by means of enteroclysis techniques date back to the 1950s. However, the development of new materials and innovative forms of naso-jejunal probes, from the early experiments to the more recent trials by HERLINGER (1978), MAGLINTE (1984) and NOLAN (1984), has largely overcome the main obstacles to jejunal intubation, namely the discomfort caused to the patient by insertion of the nasal catheter and the difficulty of reaching the jejunum on account of the poor manoeuvrability of the probe inside the stomach.

Now that these two obstacles have been overcome, artificial distension of the intestinal lumen offers a few undeniable advantages:

1. It is possible to overcome any rate of gastric emptying (natural or drug-induced) by infusing the endoluminal contrast medium at the desired speed and avoid its being degraded by the digestive enzymes.
2. Forced distension of the intestinal lumen highlights reduced distensibility of the wall due to ulcers or tumours.
3. Visualization of all the intestinal loops in the distended state enables us to detect distortions or kinks in their outline due to adherences.
4. Loops that have collapsed as a result of peristaltic waves are not mistaken for tumorous stenoses.

These advantages are also common to CT enteroclysis techniques. In addition, any pathological thickening of the intestinal wall can be unmistakably detected.

In our view, therefore, whatever contrast medium is utilized to distend the intestinal lumen (see below), this should preferably be administered through a naso-jejunal probe whenever CT examination of the small intestine is to be carried out.

34.2
Basic Principles

34.2.1
CT Versus Conventional Radiology in the Study of the Small Intestine

In the study of the digestive system, there are a few fundamental differences between CT and conventional radiology; these stem essentially from the intrinsic features of the systems that form the images (Table 34.1).

In the study of the digestive tract, CT offers a whole series of advantages. These range from the view of the intestinal wall below the mucous layer, to the direct observation of the contiguous organs, and to the absence of overlapping of the ileal loops, which continues to constitute one of the main difficulties in conventional examination of the small intestine. Nevertheless, the chief obstacle to the acceptance of CT as a tool for directly examining the small intestine stems from its poor spatial resolution in comparison with that of conventional radiology. Indeed, this insufficient spatial resolution may actually render small protruding (polyps) or excavating (ulcers) lesions of the intestinal mucosa *invisible*.

However, CT is endowed with high contrast resolution, which may be further improved by the refined contrast enhancement made possible by spiral technology. Enhancement of the intestinal wall may therefore be used to investigate alterations in the local micro-circulation, which nearly always extends to a much larger area than the ulcers or polyps. We may consider how perilesional wall enhancement is

Table 34.1. Some differential properties of the two techniques for small bowel study (*DC* double contrast)

Computed tomography	X-Ray
Low spatial resolution	High spatial resolution
High contrast resolution	Low contrast resolution
No overlapping of loops (tomographic technique)	Overlapping of loops even with DC technique
Poor overall view of intestinal loops	Very good overall view
Good overall view of organs surrounding digestive tract	Extra-intestinal organs not directly visible
Direct view of intestinal wall	Indirect view of intestinal wall

used as an indicator for the radiological detection of a lesion, in much the same way as the endoscopy specialist is guided by the reddening of the mucosa around the lesion due to simple inflammatory mechanisms. The application of this concept enables diagnostic sensitivity to be improved significantly, which more than offsets the shortcoming in spatial resolution, as has been shown by preliminary studies on clinical application, both in the case of inflammatory pathology and in the case of neoplastic disease (ROLLANDI et al. 1995, 1996; SCHOBER et al. 1996) (Figs. 34.1, 34.2).

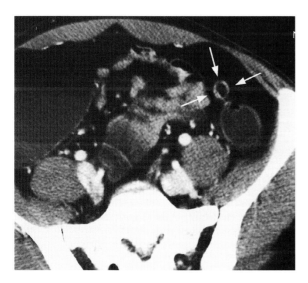

Fig. 34.1. Focal enhancement of the wall of a diverticulum (*arrows*) of the left colon: the increased enhancement is correlated with an inflammatory hyperaemia

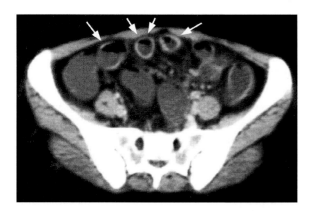

Fig. 34.2. Diffuse enhancement of the small bowel wall (*arrows*): the increased enhancement is correlated with an inflammatory hyperaemia due to salmonellosis infection

34.2.2
Choice of Endoluminal Contrast Medium

The function of the endoluminal contrast medium is to distend the intestinal loops in order to improve the view of stenoses and to eliminate false positives or negatives due to peristalsis. Moreover, following the logic of the easier detection of lesions by means of the greater perilesional enhancement provided by the i.v. injection of an iodine contrast medium, it is easy to see that the choice of contrast medium is necessarily restricted to those with a CT attenuation value similar to or less than 0 HU.

Although water has an attenuation value that meets these needs, it is absorbable by the intestinal mucosa, and thus engenders a serious risk of altering the blood volume. The most widely used contrast media are therefore aqueous solutions of nonreabsorbable salts or aqueous suspensions of low-density long-chain molecules, such as cellulose (Figs. 34.3, 34.4) (ROLLANDI et al. 1995; SCHOBER et al. 1996). A few experiments with contrast media based on fatty acids (EZ-FAT) have had no practical follow-up (RAPTOPOULOS et al. 1987).

The use of air as a transparent contrast medium is not indicated, both on account of the difficulty and discomfort encountered by the patient during administration and elimination from the intestine, and because its attenuation value is too low and too different from that of the intestinal mucosa, and too wide an observation window would therefore be required (ANGELELLI and MACARINI 1988).

34.3
Examination Technique

34.3.1
Preparation of the Intestine

This question is controversial. Some authors (HERLINGER and MAGLINTE 1989) maintain that a fast of at least 10 h is sufficient to prepare the small intestine for examination. Other authors, including ourselves, are convinced that the small intestine and colon must be cleansed before any examination of the small intestine is performed (GARVEY, 1985). Indeed, a clean colon facilitates the flow of the contrast medium through the small intestine, and ensures greater comfort for the patient, who does not feel strong stimuli to evacuate during distension of the small intestine. Moreover, it avoids pollution due to

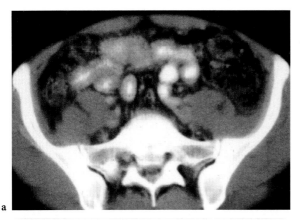

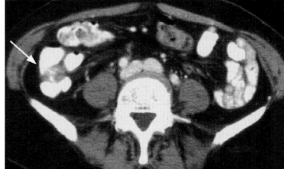

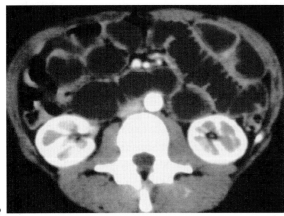

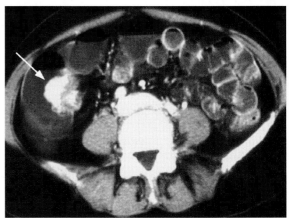

Fig. 34.3a, b. Comparison between **a** a standard CT examination of the small bowel, with oral administration of dense intraluminal contrast medium and **b** a dedicated examination with distension of loops with cellulose, administered by naso-jejunal catheter.

Fig. 34.4 a, b. Same patient as in Fig. 34.3, examined **a** with conventional spiral technique and **b** with transparent enteroclysis CT, with a carcinoid tumour (*arrow*) of the ileocolic valve. Detectability of the tumour increases with transparent endoluminal contrast medium

faecal reflux from the colon to the last ileal loop, which may aggravate diagnostic difficulties in this delicate intestinal segment. Finally, it should be pointed out that precise diagnostic information is very often necessary with regard to the ascending colon as well as the small intestine during the same examination session, and that therefore this segment should also be properly prepared.

Nevertheless, we recognize that cleansing of the colon need not be so rigorous as for radiological examination of the colon itself. Consequently, we use a nonabsorbable iso-osmolar solution-based preparation 6–7 h before the examination. As well as being well tolerated by the patient, this preparation has no irritant effect on the mucosa of the small intestine and the colon, which could give rise to confusion or diagnostic difficulty.

Intestinal preparation is not performed in patients with intestinal obstruction, who are examined only in basal conditions without any enteroclysis.

34.3.2
Administration Route of the Endoluminal Contrast Medium

CT examination of the small intestine is performed with a single volume acquisition. When scanning takes place, all the loops must be uniformly and adequately distended. For this reason, the contrast medium cannot be administered orally, since the insufficient speed of administration and the discontinuity of gastric emptying would have a negative influence on the quality of the examination. In our view, therefore, the use of a transgastric catheter is clearly essential.

Indispensable features of this catheter are:

– Sufficient length to allow the tip of the catheter to be positioned at least at the level of Treitz's arch, after a passage through the stomach that may necessarily be tortuous;

- Great flexibility, in order to negotiate the often acute flexures at the level of the duodenal apex;
- Small outer calibre, in order to minimize damage and discomfort during insertion or when in position;
- Large inner calibre, so as to ensure an adequate flow of the contrast medium;
- Sliveness of guidewire, to allow its modulated insertion into the catheter also when the catheter follows several curves. Modulated insertion can change the flexibility of the catheter's tip to across difficulties of the blind insertion in the jejunum. The torsional control of the precurved tip of the guidewire allows to orient the tip of the couple catheter-guidewire easily rotating by fingers the side outside the mouth of the patient;
- An inflatable balloon at the tip of the catheter with a calibre large enough to prevent reflux of the contrast medium into the duodenum and stomach (causing nausea and vomiting) in the distension phase of the intestinal loops.

A large number of catheters have been specially designed for examination of the small intestine, and these have evolved over time as a result of improvements in manufacturing techniques, the availability of new materials, and the experience of various authors. Indeed, numerous users who are keenly involved in this issue have proposed new models of catheters with slight personalized technical modifications; we ourselves are no exception (Rollandi et al. 1999). However, the choice of catheter, as of any other invasive device, remains a personal matter. The objective is to perform the intubation manoeuvre as efficiently as possible and with the least possible discomfort to the patient. As the success of this operation does not depend solely on technical factors, we may claim that, within certain limits, the "best" catheter does not exist.

The insertion route of the catheter is, however, well codified. It has been scientifically demonstrated (MAGLINTE 1984) and corroborated by precise personal experience that nasal insertion of the catheter is tolerated by the patient much better than oral insertion. The oral route will then only be used if it is really necessary.

34.3.3
Infusion of the Intraluminal Contrast Medium

The endoluminal contrast medium must be infused at a temperature of 37°C and at a constant flow rate

of 60–100 cc per minute. The constant flow rate is easily ensured by using peristaltic-type automatic injectors similar to those used in haemodialysis.

The quantity of contrast medium needed to distend the small intestine properly is 1700–2300 cc (ROLLANDI et al. 1995, 1996a, b, 1999; SCHOBER et al. 1996), especially if they are injected as hypotonic agents (see section 34.3.5). Since the progress of the transparent contrast medium cannot be observed by means of fluoroscopy, in the early stages of regulating our technique we used echographic monitoring to avoid dangerous overdistension of prestenotic intestinal loops. Subsequent experience, however, has revealed that this precaution is unnecessary: every time a serious problem of passage is encountered, the discomfort of the patient becomes evident well before any observable echographic sign.

34.3.4
Endoluminal Contrast Medium

The reasons for choosing a "negative" contrast medium have already been illustrated above. From among these "negative" contrast media, we have chosen a type of cellulose (hydroxypropyl methylcellulose Methocel E-Z-EM, Westbury N.Y., USA) at a concentration of 0.5% in water, which is already well known and widely used in the double contrast enema for investigation of the small intestine in conventional radiology. It is, therefore, a contrast medium that meets the density needs of CT enteroclysis, is well tolerated, and has an acceptable degree of water absorption.

34.3.5
CT Technique

The CT acquisition phase is preceded by drug-induced hypotonicity of the small intestine by means of i.v. injection of 10 mg of hyoscine methylbromide (Buscopan). This is done to eliminate intestinal peristalsis and consequent segmentation of the loops. Unlike what happens during small intestine enema in conventional radiology, during which the operator can choose when to acquire the images by fluoroscopically monitoring the pattern of peristalsis, volumetric acquisition in CT is single, as is observation of the loops. One of the easiest false-positive errors to make is confusing segmentation due to peristalsis with organic stenosis. Inducing hypotonicity greatly reduces, though it does not eliminate, this kind of pitfall.

A further advantage of induced hypotonicity is that it shows up the difference between the calibre of normal loops and that of segments rendered less distensible by inflammatory, scarring or infiltrating pathologies.

When contrast enhancement is performed, the ratio between the amount of iodine injected and the patient's body weight must be rigorously observed: about 3.5 g of iodine per kilogram of body weight is injected, which is equivalent to about 1.5 cc of contrast medium per kilogram at a concentration of 370 g of I/100 cc. The contrast medium is injected at a temperature of 37°C, at a flow rate of 3 cc/s, with delay times that allow imaging in the portal phase (50 s delay time). The delay time may be prolonged to 60 s, and the flow rate reduced to 2.5 cc/s, in elderly patients.

The volumetric acquisition parameters depend on the equipment used, and in particular on the thermal capacity of the X-ray tube, and on the quality and efficiency of the detectors. While these parameters may vary, volumetric acquisition must be carried out with a layer thickness of 7 mm, pitch of 2 and a reconstruction interval of 3 mm, while the patient holds a single breath. If the area to be examined is limited (follow-up examination of known disease or suspicion of inflammatory ileal pathology etc.), the layer thickness may be reduced to 5 mm, or the pitch to 1.5 mm, thus improving the quality of the images without obliging the patient to hold his or her breath too long.

With the new multislice detector bars, better performance in terms of global scan time and of thickness of slices will be possible.

34.3.6
Post-processing

The large number of images produced by the volumetric acquisition technique is aimed at yielding high-quality multiplanar volumetric reconstruction (MPVR). Multiplanar images and the analysis of axial images enable us to follow the complex task of unravelling the tangle of jejunal and ileal loops step

by step and may reveal themselves to be essential to our understanding of the normal and pathological morphology of post-surgical anastomoses (Fig. 34.5a, b).

34.4
Crohn's Disease

34.4.1
Introduction

Crohn's disease is an inflammatory disease that can involve any part of the gastrointestinal tract, but which shows a clear preference for the terminal ileum (CROHN, 1932).

From the histological point of view, the most characteristic sign of the disease is the presence of noncaseating granulomas of the submucosa, though these are found in only 60% of cases (HAMILTON and MORSON 1985).

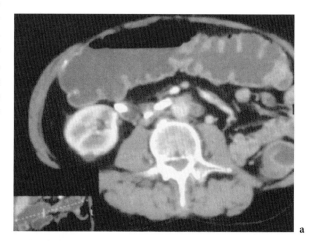

a

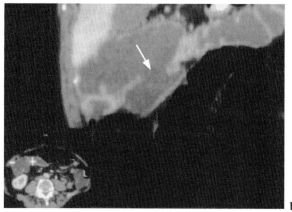

b

Fig. 34.5a, b. The good quality of the multiplanar reconstruction allows accurate analysis of the anastomosis of right hemicolectomy (a). Passage from small to large bowel (*arrow*) is better seen on reconstruction on coronal plane (b)

The earliest and most significant macroscopic sign is the presence of aphthoid ulcers. However, in the early stages, the tissue surrounding the ulcer, while of normal appearance on radiological and endoscopic examination, already shows histological signs of marked inflammatory infiltration (HAMILTON and MORSON 1985). This is of great importance in understanding the natural history of the disease, and explains why CT is able to detect these small invisible ulcers early, by means of enhancement of the surrounding areas.

In the early stages of the disease, the inflammatory process is confined to the submucosal layer. It subsequently tends to extend to all the layers of the intestinal wall, from the mucosa to the outer surface of the serosa. The ulcers broaden, coalesce, deepen and intersect, taking on a cobblestone appearance. Further progression of the disease is characterized by marked oedema of the submucosal layer and by the proliferation of nerve tissue (neuromatosis) in the submucosa, lymphocyte infiltrate and non-caseating granulomas. Stenoses then form as a result both of intrinsic fibrosis at the intestinal wall and of compression due to inflammatory proliferation of the loose cellular tissue of the mesenterium (creeping), which tends to isolate the inflamed loops from one another.

Sometimes, in the phase of acute inflammation emerging to the serous layer, the fibrin deposited on the outer surface of the loops causes the loops to adhere to one another, thus giving rise to passage difficulty, on account of the resulting sharp bends, and paving the way to the formation of entero-enteric fistulas.

34.4.2
CT Semeiotics

34.4.2.1
Early Lesions

Although the diagnostic role of CT in the early stages of Crohn's disease is controversial, the experience of some groups suggests that the diagnostic sensitivity of specialized CT techniques (ROLLANDI et al. 1995; SCHOBER et al. 1996) is greater than that obtainable by means of traditional radiological methods. This high degree of sensitivity, even in the early stages, can be explained by the natural history of the disease; it has been shown (ADMANS et al.1980 STEINHARDT et al.

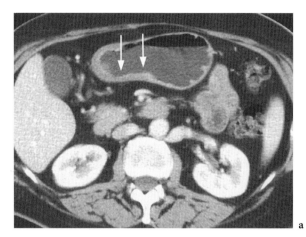

a

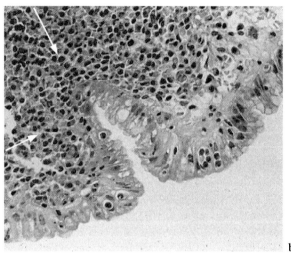

b

Fig. 34.6a, b. Spiral CT of a case of gastric localization of Crohn's disease. On CT images (**a**) the wall of the antrum (*arrows*) seems multilayered, with intense enhancement of mucosal side, increased thickness of submucosal layer and global thickening of the wall. The endoscopic examination (**b**) was negative, and only examination of a deep biopsy revealed a lymphocytic infiltration (*arrow*) of the submucosal space characteristic of Crohn's disease, with a normal mucosal layer. This case reminds us that Crohn's disease starts as a submucosal disease, and reduces the importance of detection of the mucosal aphthoid ulcers as sign of early stage of the disease

1985) that patients come in for radiological examination not earlier than 2–4 years after the onset of symptoms, which are often subtle and atypical. It is therefore almost impossible that wall involvement might be restricted to the single and poorly detectable aphthoid ulcers. In this phase, CT examination is able to detect changes in wall thickness and vascularization, even when the endoscopic appearance is normal (Fig. 34.6a, b). However, the initial lesions are often completely nonspecific and are manifested only by an increase in the enhancement of

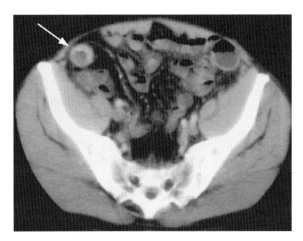

Fig. 34.7. Partial thickening of the wall of the last loop, with increased enhancement, in a case of early stage of Crohn's disease

the mucosa and a scarcely perceptible thickening of the wall (Fig. 34.7).

34.4.2.2
Intermediate Lesions

The second stage of the disease (ENGELHOM et al. 1989) is characterized by accentuation of the early CT signs, in particular by the increase in the thickness of the intestinal wall, which shows evident stratification. CT reveals a thin layer on the mucosa side, which is characterized by intense enhancement (at least 100 HU), a hypodense underlying layer, which may be 2 or 3 times as thick as the former, and an outer layer of intermediate density and thickness (ROLLANDI et al. 1999). Histological examination of surgical specimens reveals that the layer with the greatest enhancement is made up of mucosa, and that the hypodense intermediate layer is due to the lymphocytic infiltration, oedema and neuromatosis of the submucosa (Fig. 34.8a, b).

In this phase, as in all the others, the mucous ulcers are not directly visible, although alteration of the wall is evident.

A characteristic feature of the disease is seen in the alternation of pathological segments and apparently healthy segments Figs. 34.9, 34.10).

34.4.2.3
Advanced Lesions

In the advanced stage, involution phenomena of the intestinal wall are accentuated (Figs. 34.11, 34.12). Tight stenoses may be present, with prestenotic dilatation of the intestinal loop. Fibro-fatty proliferation

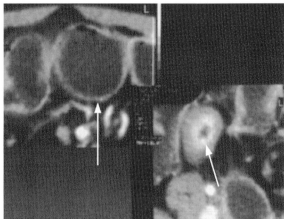

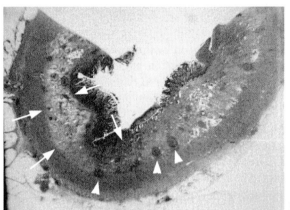

Fig. 34.8a, b. Intermediate lesion of Crohn's disease. Compare the aspect of a normal wall (*arrow*) (a *left*) with the thickening of the pathological wall (*arrow*) (a *right*). The specimen of the same case (**b**) reveals significant thickening of the submucosal layer by neuromatosis (*arrows*) and granulomatosis (*arrowheads*) and allows interpretation of the radiological sign of layering

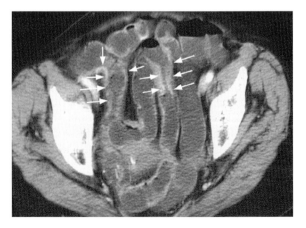

Fig. 34.9. Skip lesions: thickened, enhanced and layered segments (*arrows*) alternate with other, normal alternate ones

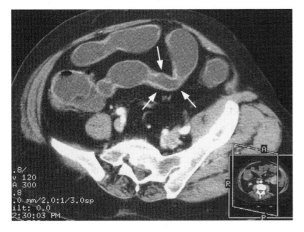

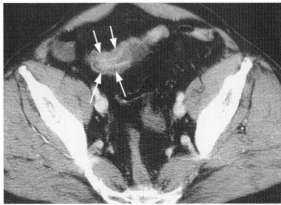

Fig. 34.10. Skip lesions: alternation of thickened, enhanced and layered segments (*arrows*), with mild dilatation of the loops before the narrowed points. Note the fibro-fatty proliferation of the mesenteric tissue

Fig. 34.12. Narrowed segment (*arrows*) of small bowel affected by advanced Crohn's disease: the inflammatory condition arises on the surface of serosal side, which has lost its smooth shape. Important mesenteric fatty proliferation

(creeping) of the local loose mesenteric tissue is particularly frequent. This is probably due to a reaction to the chronic inflammatory stimulus (Maccioni et al. 1997), caused by the breakthrough of inflammation to the serosa of the diseased segments. A frequent finding is that of enlarged lymph nodes within the thickened mesenterium.

Fistulas and abscesses frequently appear in the advanced stage of Crohn's disease. The fistulous tract may be difficult to detect in the case of enteroenteric fistulas; communication is established between two intestinal loops rendered contiguous by "sticking" of the inflamed, fibrin-covered serosal surfaces. The tract is therefore very short. Brief fistulous tracts are difficult to pick out on CT examination, especially if a hypodense endoluminal contrast

medium is used. Longer fistulas are easier to detect. These appear in the form of dense streaks within the mesenteric tissue of adipose density, which creates good natural contrast even when a dense contrast medium is not used (Fig. 34.13a, b).

34.4.2.4
Activity of the Disease

Crohn's disease is characterized by the alternation of phases of intense inflammatory activity with phases of relative remission. Several systems have been drawn up on the basis of scores correlated with clinical and haematological parameters, but with no real success. From the radiological standpoint, attempts have also been made to correlate imaging with disease activity (Rollandi et al. 1997), but no significant results have been achieved. Some hope is offered by the measurement of the resistance indexes of the superior mesenteric artery at Doppler US and by magnetic resonance imaging (Maccioni et al. 1997).

34.5
Tumours

34.5.1
Introduction

Primary tumours of the small bowel are considered rare, especially in view of the large surface area of the intestinal mucosa. The reported incidence of

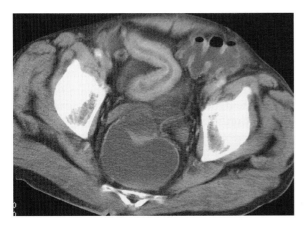

Fig. 34.11. Intense enhancement of the mucosa of a long tract of ileal loop affected by Crohn's disease

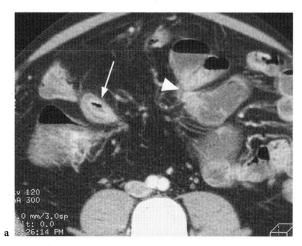

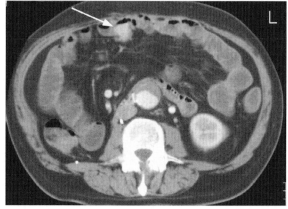

Fig. 34.14. Small enhancing mass (*arrow*) in the small bowel: metastases from lung cancer

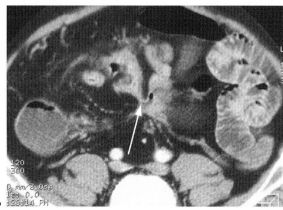

Fig. 34.13a, b. Advanced case of Crohn's disease: thickening of the bowel wall (**a** *arrow*), adhesions and angled shape of the loops (**a** *arrowhead*), fatty proliferation of the mesenteric tissue, and entero-enteric fistula (**b** *arrow*)

these tumours ranges from 2% to 6% of all tumours of the digestive tract. To date, this low incidence has not been explained (CALMAN 1974).

The subtle and often nonspecific symptoms of these tumours, together with their rarity and the complexity of the techniques capable of reaching the small bowel, make their diagnosis difficult.

Secondary tumours of the small bowel have also been thought to be very rare. Some autopsy statistics, however, have shown that this is not so (McNEILL et al. 1987; ASH and WIEDEL 1964). In our experience too, secondary lesions from melanomas, bronchogenic or breast cancers are not as rare as one might expect (ROLLANDI et al. 1997). It could well be that the availability of more sophisticated investigative techniques, together with the increasingly painstaking follow-up of the various primary neoplasms, has

led to more accurate detection of secondary lesions located in the small bowel wall, and that no real increase in their incidence has occurred (Fig. 34.14).

34.5.2
Benign Tumours

There are numerous histological types of benign bowel tumours, the most important in terms of incidence and frequency of malignant transformation being leiomyomas and adenomas (OLMSTED et al. 1987). Lipomas and hamartomas are less frequent.

The most indicative symptoms are bleeding, invagination and occlusion. In the majority of cases, these tumours are diagnosed at the time of surgical intervention for occlusion.

Differential diagnosis among these types of tumour is practically impossible on the basis of morphology alone. Better results are achieved when morphological data are supplemented by other data, such as the site of the tumour, the modality of growth and, for what concerns lipomas with a high lipid content, the degree of attenuation seen on CT examination.

34.5.2.1
Leiomyomas (Gastrointestinal Stromal Tumours GIST, Smooth-muscle Type, Benign)

These originate in the muscular coat of the bowel wall, and tend to grow by separating the muscle fi-

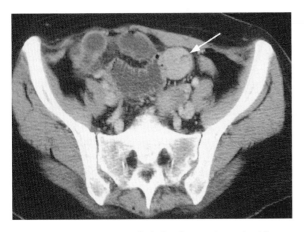

Fig. 34.15. Leiomyomas: well-defined mass (*arrow*) with medium enhancement. Mild dilatation of the loops proximal to the tumour

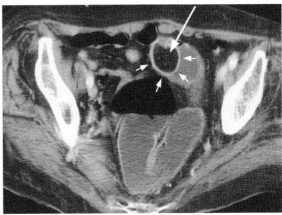

Fig. 34.16. Typical lipoma: round and regular mass, with fatty density (*arrow*), surrounded by normal mucosal layer (*small arrow*)

bres without infiltrating them. They may grow towards the intestinal lumen, be contained within the muscle wall, or they may develop mainly outside the bowel in the peritoneal cavity, while still being contained by the serous coat.

In the first case, symptoms appear when the calibre of the lumen is reduced by more than one third, or when bleeding occurs from the frequent small dystrophic ulcers of the mucosa that surrounds them. In the second case, symptoms appear late, usually in the form of a mass which becomes palpable when it reaches 10 cm or more in size. When the mass exceeds 5 cm in size or there are signs of involvement of contiguous structures, a malignant form must be taken into consideration.

On CT examination, the tumour appears as a well-defined mass with medium-high enhancement (Fig 34.15).

Differential diagnosis is against carcinoid tumours, leiomyosarcomas and metastases. In the first case, the differential diagnosis can be made on CT examination only in the presence of desmoplastic streaks, which are pathognomonic of carcinoid tumours. In the other two cases, the differential diagnosis cannot be made on the basis of morphology alone.

34.5.2.2
Lipomas

These arise from the adipose tissue of the submucosa, and tend to grow very slowly and, being of submucosal origin, bulge towards the intestinal lumen, giving rise to subocclusive or painful symptoms due to transitory invagination.

If the lipid component predominates, the negative attenuation value on CT examination is pathognomonic and enables the definitive diagnosis to be made (Fig. 34.16). If, however, the tumour presents a marked fibrous component that brings the degree of attenuation back to positive values, the differential diagnosis may be difficult.

Intestinal liposarcomas are exceedingly rare. Abdominal liposarcomas, though rare, develop almost exclusively at the expense of the adipose tissue of the mesentery. However, the appearance of streaks of density and increased enhancement on CT examination (described as signs of malignancy in adipose neoplasms of the mesentery) cannot, at least in principle, be distinguished from the fibrous component frequently found in benign intestinal lipomas.

34.5.2.3
Hamartomas

These are dismorphic polyps in which the glands are supported by broad bands of smooth muscle fibres. Frequently found in the jejunum, they are often associated with polyposis (Peutz-Jeghers syndrome, juvenile hamartomatosis). They appear as small masses inside the intestinal lumen, sometimes with very intense enhancement due to their angiomatous component. Small calcifications are occasionally detected, which facilitates and supports the diagnosis.

34.5.2.4
Adenomas

These are classified as tubular or villous according
to their histological pattern. On account of their
glandular origin and considerable surface area (especially in the villous variety), they are regarded as
benign tumours with a high risk of malignant transformation. They are usually located in the duodenum and the first segment of the jejunum. Their
usually small size (about 2 cm) makes them difficult
to detect in segments other than the duodenum.

On CT examination, these tumours appear as a luminal filling defect with moderate enhancement and
regular borders. The absence of any further typical
characteristics hinders differential diagnosis against
the tumours described previously.

34.5.2.5
Neurogenic Tumours

Arising from the submucosal and myenteric nerve
plexuses, these neoplasms are most frequently neurofibromas which appear in multiples during the
course of Recklinghausen's disease or other systemic
neurofibromatoses (DUDIAK et al. 1989).

The radiological appearance does not differ from
that of leiomyomas, making radiological differential
diagnosis virtually impossible.

34.5.3
Malignant Tumours

These are the most disastrous tumours of the digestive system. Symptoms are subtle and nonspecific, and obstruction is manifested late (the small
bowel propels liquid, so that the lumen is not obstructed until the tumour is advanced). Moreover,
the rich vasculature of the mesentery facilitates
liver metastases. As a result, the diagnosis is often
made late. The rate of mortality 5 years after diagnosis is high.

34.5.3.1
Adenocarcinomas

These are the most common malignant tumours of
the small bowel. They tend to narrow the lumen, almost always causing subocclusive symptoms. When
the tumour is first diagnosed, secondary adeno-
megaly, liver metastases or direct infiltration of the
surrounding structures are often found (Fig. 34.17).

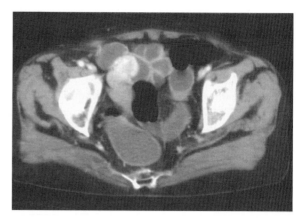

Fig. 34.17. Adenocarcinoma of an ileal loop. Note the intense
and irregular enhancement. At the time of examination the
patient had already liver metastases

34.5.3.2
Leiomyosarcomas (Gastrointestinal Stromal Tumours, GIST Smooth-muscle Type, Malignant)

These are relatively rare intestinal tumours. The lesion is usually single and grows slowly. It grows
mainly outside the lumen and symptoms are manifested late in relation to the size that it can attain
(more than 50% of these tumours are palpable at the
time of diagnosis) (GOURTSOYIANNIS 1997).

On CT examination, considerably heterogeneous
enhancement is often observed, with areas of necrosis and bleeding, partly due to the size of the lesion
and partly due to its malignant transformation. In
spite of these characteristics, differential diagnosis
against leiomyomas is particularly difficult.

34.5.3.3
Carcinoid Tumours

These arise from the chromaffin cells found at the
base of Lieberkühn's crypts.

Generally small, such tumours mainly occur in
the appendix, in the distal ileum or inside a Meckel's
diverticulum. The likelihood of malignant transformation is related to the size of the lesion. Although
nonsecreting carcinoid tumours are sometimes encountered, as a rule these tumours secrete serotonin,
kallikrein or other amines. However, the quantity of
amines secreted is rarely sufficient to determine evident systemic symptoms.

At the site of the lesion, the serotonin that comes
into contact with the fibres of the muscular coat of
the bowel wall induces chronic stimulation of fibro-

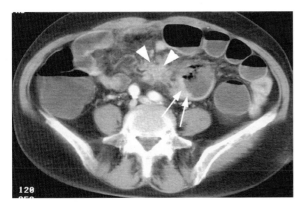

Fig. 34.18. Stenosis with irregular, nonlayered thickening of the ileal wall (*arrows*). Note the desmoplastic streaks (*arrowheads*) in the mesentery, a typical sign of carcinoid tumour

cyte production, which is characteristic of these tumours. The desmoplastic streaks radiate from the lesion along the wall or in the mesentery, taking on the appearance of rays of sunlight. On CT examination, these streaks are pathognomonic of carcinoid tumours (Fig. 34.18). A thorough search must be carried out for loco-regional lymphadenomegaly (a frequent finding), secondary hepatic lesions (especially if systemic symptoms are present), and other intestinal localizations.

34.5.4
Lymphomas

Lymphomas account for about 22% of primary malignant tumours of the ileum. Lymphomas can be classed as *primary* (intestinal localisation, no involvement of lymph-nodes, blood or parenchymal organs) and *secondary* (intestinal localization contemporary with or subsequent to other disease localizations).

Primary lymphomas of the small bowel most commonly affect the middle-aged (sixth decade) and children. The most frequent localization is the distal segment of the ileum, on account of the presence of abundant lymphatic tissue.

The most common histotype is non-Hodgkin (NHD). A distinct type of primary lymphoma is *Mediterranean* lymphoma or "alpha-chain disease" (plasmacytoid), which affects Arab or Jewish populations of Middle Eastern or North African origin. Showing a predilection for young subjects, this lymphoma determines a malabsorption syndrome (steatorrhoea) and the production of monoclonal heavy chains of IgA.

All lymphomatous neoplasms arise from the lymphatic tissue of the submucosa, subsequently infiltrating the wall and forming mucous ulcers. At the level of the ileum, lymphomas present various radiological pictures (DODD 1990):

1. Pseudo-aneurysmal form: this is the most frequent form and involves neoplastic spread within the submucous and muscular coats. As a result, the wall is weakened and tends progressively to bulge outwards. Thickening of the wall is caused by infiltration of the full thickness, from the submucosa to the serosa (Fig. 34.19).

2. Polypoid form: the expansive growth of the lymphoid tissue of the submucosa tends to give rise to a mass which protrudes into the intestinal lumen. This mass takes on a polypoid shape, but is lined with almost normal mucosa. The lymphomatous polyp may cause narrowing of the ileal lumen.

3. Constrictive form: this rare form is generally observable in histiocytic lymphomas and in forms associated with malabsorption. It occurs more commonly in the jejunum and may be found in coeliac disease evolving towards lymphoma. In this variety, considerable amounts of fibrotic tissue are present, probably due to the chronic inflammatory stimulus exerted by the coeliac disease. This tissue causes stenosis, which is atypical in other forms of lymphomatous diseases.

4. Mesenteric form: the lymphoid tissue grows mainly towards the serous coat. The neoplastic tissue, which is sometimes very abundant, fills the spaces between the intestinal loops and tends to involve the mesentery (Fig. 34.20).

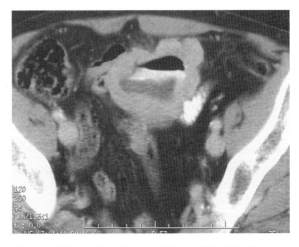

Fig. 34.19. Primary lymphoma of the small bowel, with weakening of the wall and pseudo-aneurysmal form

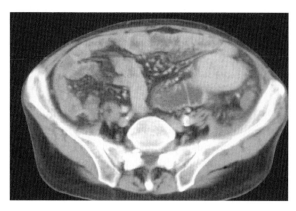

Fig. 34.20. Primary lymphoma of the small bowel. Mesenteric form: the lymphoid tissue grows mainly towards the serous coat

lymphoadenitis and carcinoid tumours. In this latter case, perilesional desmoplastic proliferation, which is pathognomonic of carcinoid tumours, must be sought.

The CT appearance of lymphoma is characterized by a single (rarely diffuse) transparietal thickening of an ileal loop. Contrast enhancement is relatively homogeneous and is not stratified as in Crohn's disease. Pseudo-aneurysms and the absence of dilatation of the bowel segments proximal to the location of the disease can easily be identified on CT examination, too.

The nonstenotic ileal lumen is an important factor in the differential diagnosis against adenocarcinomas, Crohn's disease and intestinal tuberculosis, all of which generally cause stenosis of the lumen.

The detection and staging of forms which develop outwards from the wall is very easy. Their appearance is pathognomonic of lymphoma. The neoformation exhibits scant and irregular enhancement; the intestinal loops are dislocated and the wall is infiltrated, but there are no direct or indirect signs of stenosis.

Lymphomatous forms which determine a tight stenosis of the intestinal lumen are not distinguishable from adenocarcinomas, especially if there is no voluminous mesenteric or retroperitoneal lymphadenopathy suggestive of lymphoma. The presence of an eccentric stenosis of polypoid morphology may point to carcinoma.

Polypoid forms are only visible when they exceed 1.5–2 cm in size. Ulcerations of the mucosa are not directly visible on CT examination; sometimes, however, enhancement of the periulcerative wall may be indirectly observed, though this sign is aspecific and difficult to detect.

The differential diagnosis of lymphoma will also include specific and nonspecific inflammatory

References

Admans H, Whorwell PS, Wright HO, et al (1980) Diagnosis of Crohn's disease. Dig Dis Sci 25:911–915
Angelelli G, Macarini L (1988) CT of the bowel: use of water to enhance depiction. Radiology 169:848–849
Ash MJ, Wiedel PD (1964) Gastrointestinal metastases from carcinoma of the breast: autopsy study and 18 cases requiring operative intervention. Arch Surg 159:477–480
Calman KC (1974) Why are small bowel tumours rare? An experimental model. Gut 15:552–554
Crohn DB, Ginzburg L, Oppenheimer GD (1932) Regional ileitis: a pathological and clinic activity. JAMA 99:1323–1329
Dodd GD (1990) Lymphoma of the hollow abdominal viscera. Radiol Clin North Am 28:771–778
Dudiak KM, Johnson CD, Stephens DH (1989) Primary tumours of the small intestine: CT evaluation . AJR Am J Roentgenol 152:995–998
Engelhom L, De Toeuf J, Herlinger H, Maglinte DDT (1989) Crohn's disease of the small bowel. In: Herlinger H, Maglinte D (eds) Clinical radiology of the small intestine. Saunders, Philadelphia
Garvey CS, De Lacey G, Wilkins RA (1985) Preliminary colon cleansing for small bowel examinations: results and implications of a prospective survey. Clin Radiol 36:503–506
Gourtsoyiannis NC (1997) Primary malignant neoplasms. In Gourtsoyiannis NC, Nolan DJ (eds) Imaging of small intestinal neoplasms. Elsevier, Amsterdam, pp 105–189
Hamilton SR, Morson BC (1985) Crohn's disease pathology. In: Bokus gastroenterology, 4th edn. Saunders, Philadelphia
Herlinger H (1978) A modified technique for the double contrast small bowel enema. Gastrointest Radiol 3:201–207
Herlinger H, Maglinte D (eds) Clinical radiology of the small intestine. Saunders, Philadelphia
Maccioni F, Broglia L, Bezzi M, Viscido A, Caprilli R, Rossi P (1997) Accuracy of MR imaging in the evaluation of the clinical activity of Crohn's disease. Radiology 205:(p)286
Maglinte DDT (1984) Balloon enteroclysis catheter. AJR Am J Roentgenol 143:761–762
McNeill PM, Wagmann LD, Neifeld JP (1987) Small bowel metastases from primary carcinoma of the lung. Cancer 59:1486–1489
Nolan DJ (1984) Radiological atlas of gastrointestinal disease. Wiley, New York
Olmsted WW, Ros PR, Hjermstad BM, McCarthy MJ (1987) Tumours of the small intestine with little or no malignant predisposition: a review of the literature and report of 56 cases. Gastrointest Radiol 12:231–239
Raptopoulos V, Davi MA, Davidoff A, Karellas A, Hays D, D'Orsi CJ, Smith EH (1987) Fat density oral contrast agent for abdominal CT. Radiology 164:653–656
Rollandi GA, Curone PF, Bertolotto M, Talenti A, Derchi LE (1995) Crohn disease: evaluation with spiral CT and transparent bowel enema. Radiology 197:(p)314

Rollandi GA, Curone PF, Biscaldi E, Bonifacino E, Nardi F. Derchi LE (1996) Malignant tumors of small bowel. Evaluation with spiral CT and transparent enema study. Radiology 201:(p)322

Rollandi GA, Curone PF, Crespi G; Biscaldi E, Bonifacino E, Gandolfo N (1996) Spiral CT and transparent small bowel enema: correlation between imaging and CDAI (Crohn Activity Index) Radiology 201(p):381

Rollandi GA, Biscaldi E, Curone PF, Gandolfo N, Bonifacino E, Nardi F, Ferrando R (1997) Malignant tumours of small bowel: evaluation with spiral CT and transparent enema. Eur Radiol [Suppl] 7:119

Rollandi GA, Curone PF, Biscaldi E, Nardi F, Bonifacino E, Conzi R, Derchi LE (1999) Spiral CT of the abdomen after distension of small bowel loops with transparent enema in patients with Crohn disease. Abdom Imaging 1999, 24:6, (in press)

Schober E, Turetschek K, Oberhuber G, Vogelsang H, Moeschl P, Mostbeck GH (1996) Enteroclysis spiral CT: diagnostic yield in the preoperative assessment of Crohn disease. Radiology 201:(p)380

Steinhardt JH, Loetschke K, Kasper et al (1985) European Cooperative Crohn's Disease Study: clinical features and natural history. Digestion 31:97–108

35 Virtual Colonoscopy

H.-J. BRAMBS

CONTENTS

35.1 Introduction *385*
35.2 Virtual Reality Imaging *385*
35.2.1 Patient Preparation *386*
35.2.2 Data Acquisition *386*
35.2.3 Rendering *387*
35.2.4 Interpretation *388*
35.2.5 Clinical Assessment *389*
35.2.6 Perspectives *392*
      References *392*

35.1
Introduction

Recent refinements in spiral CT technology and parallel improvements in computer graphics hardware and software tools stimulated interest in nonconventional means of data visualization. One of the most revolutionary technologies of modern imaging is virtual endoscopy (VE). The first report on the technical feasibility of colon imaging with helical CT and virtual reality was published by VINING et al. (1994). This method uses high-resolution spiral CT scanning and sophisticated computerized rendering techniques to construct a three-dimensional model of different structures and organs that can be examined in various fashions, including flying through and around normal and pathologic anatomy. VE provides a realistic 3D surface view of the inner walls of hollow structures, simulating conventional endoscopy.

A variety of novel CT approaches to the large bowel have recently been described, with new and somewhat confusing terminology:
- CT pneumocolon is a significant refinement of the previously performed conventional dynamic CT of the large bowel for the staging of colorectal cancer. These studies were of only limited value owing to retained feces and collapsed bowel,

which made accurate staging difficult (FREENY et al. 1986; BALTHAZAR et al. 1998). The crucial prerequisites of the new type of study are bowel cleansing, i.v. administration of a smooth muscle relaxant, and rectal air insufflation (AMIN et al. 1996; HARVEY et al. 1998). Compared with barium enema CT pneumocolon is technically easier and less invasive, is quick and has a lower radiation dose, and it seems to be a useful method particularly for the staging of colonic carcinomas (AMIN et al. 1996). CT data are displayed and interpreted in the conventional fashion without additional postprocessing. Because the data gathered by this procedure are truly volumetric, without information gaps or slice-to-slice misregistrations, they can be used as a source of image manipulation, multiplanar reformatting, and three-dimensional reconstruction.
- CT colonography is the next step in the refinement of the technique, using volumetric CT data combined with advanced imaging software to create 2D and 3D reconstructions of the bowel (Fig. 35.1). The rationale behind such developments is the desire to compress the vast amount of data into a more manageable form of imaging. Both 2D and 3D CT colonography have been shown to be feasible techniques for detection of colorectal polyps and tumors (Fig. 35.2). Therefore, this technique is currently being widely investigated as a potential method for colonic cancer screening.

35.2
Virtual Reality Imaging

Virtual reality imaging (virtual colonoscopy) is the most recent development in volumetric analysis of spiral CT data combined with novel computer graphics; it provides a form of interactive approach simulating fiberoptic viewing (Fig. 35.3). Virtual reality imaging does not add any new information to

H.-J. BRAMBS; Abteilung Röntgendiagnostik, Radiologische Klinik und Poliklinik, Universitätsklinikum Ulm, Steinhövelstrasse 9, D-89075 Ulm, Germany

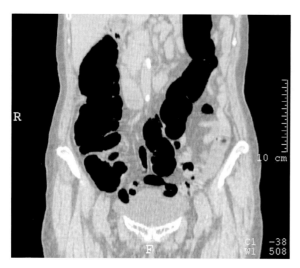

Fig. 35.1. Two-dimensional coronal reconstruction (CT colonography) shows typical appearance of a normal air-insufflated and distended colon

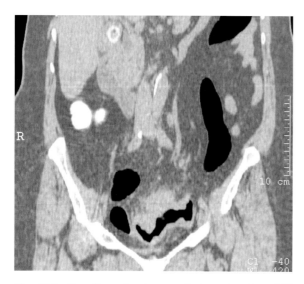

Fig. 35.2. Two-dimensional coronal reconstruction (CT colonography) showing a marked concentric thickening of the bowel wall of the sigmoid colon with a irregular stenosis of the lumen

that supplied by axial source images. Like other 3D reconstructions, its main role is in permitting optimal visualization of complex anatomic structures.

35.2.1
Patient Preparation

CT colonography requires a meticulously cleansed and dry bowel for optimal results, because retained fecal matter or fluid can lead to diagnostic error. Usually a standard barium enema preparation is

recommended, whereas standard cathartic agents for colonoscopy (for example GoLytely) have the disadvantage that excessive intraluminal fluid can remain and can cause significant perceptual problems.

Adequate colonic distension is crucial for high-quality virtual colonography. Prior to CT scanning an enema tip is inserted into the rectum and air is instilled to near maximum patient tolerance in the moments just before initiation of scanning. The degree of distension can be assessed on the CT pilot view. If large amounts of fluid or collapsed loops are encountered on reviewing the axial images, the colon can be reinflated and the patient can be placed in the prone position and re-imaged. Some authors recommend routinely imaging with patients in both the supine and the prone position to get adequate bowel distension and to increase the sensitivity for polyp detection (CHEN et al. 1999; DACHMAN et al. 1998; FENLON and FERRUCCI 1997). This technique helps to differentiate mobile fecal material from polyps and provides a second look at suspected abnormalities identified on one of the two examinations.

The use of spasmolytic agents is essential for adequate and lasting colonic distension. Hyoscine-*n*-butyl bromide (Buscopan, at a dose of 20–40 mg i.v.) is preferred in Europe, whereas in the US glucagon (at a dose of 1.0 mg i.v.) is widely used to suppress intestinal motility.

35.2.2
Data Acquisition

Proper data acquisition is integral to the creation of 3D spiral CT images. The acquisition of an uninter-

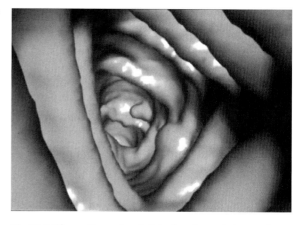

Fig. 35.3. Three-dimensional virtual endoscopic image shows the characteristic triangular appearance of a normal transverse colon

rupted volume of data without respiratory and peristaltic motion is required. In the abdomen the performance of spiral acquisition during a single breath-hold has significantly improved the results. Scanners with new technology are capable of subsecond rotations and have multidetector arrays, which facilitate longer coverage in the longitudinal axis.

The "optimal" technique is a balance between ideal image quality on the one hand, and radiation dose and large data sets on the other. Using thin sections and thin reconstruction intervals (Fig. 35.4) will improve image quality (Table 35.1).

Reported patient scanning protocols have typically utilized 5 mm collimation with variable pitch settings ranging between 1 and 1.5 (Table 35.2). Narrow collimation, in the order of 2.5–5 mm, is essential to create displays with sufficient resolution (in depicting small polyps and demonstrating tumor stenoses). Increased reconstruction intervals and table speeds degrade both 2D and 3D image quality,

Table 35.2. Variations in data acquisition depending on techniques of examination and technical equipment

Examination	Collimation (mm)	Pitch	Reconstruction interval (mm)
Spiral CT pneumocolon (Harvey et al. 1998)	5	1.5	2.5
CT colonography + VE (Hara et al. 1996)	5	1.5	2.5
CT colonography + VE (Dachman et al. 1998)	5	1	1
Virtual colonoscopy (Fenlon et al. 1998)	5	1.25	2
VE using multidetector CT (Ulm 1999)[a]	2.5	0.8	1.6

[a]Corresponding preliminary experience with a multidetector CT (MX 8000, Picker)

and the degradation becomes most marked when 2D images are reformatted along oblique planes.

Overlapping reconstruction intervals improve multiplanar and 3D images by decreasing volume-averaging artifacts and yielding smooth 3D images, which have been shown to facilitate detection of small lesions. A minimal overlap of 50% is required to minimize partial-volume effects. With standard spiral CT equipment using a collimation of 5 mm at a pitch of 1.25, coverage of an average adult large bowel requires a single breath-hold of approximately 50 s (!), which obviously is not practical for most patients. Alternative strategies involve acquiring data during 2–4 breath-holds or increasing the pitch.

Radiation dose is an important issue if the method is eventually aimed at cancer screening. A major disadvantage of CT colonography is that, for routine use, a narrow collimation data set would result in an unacceptable radiation dose. Tube current is a parameter that can affect image quality and examination efficiency. However, the high contrast between the air-filled bowel and the colon wall permits a significant reduction of radiation dose. Images obtained at a low dose setting (70 mA) have an only slightly degraded image quality and decrease radiation to a level comparable with that incurred by a standard barium enema (HARA et al. 1997; JOHNSON et al. 1997).

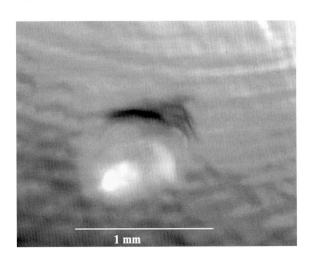

Fig. 35.4. With adequate acquisition parameters even very small polyps (diameter 1 mm) can be depicted with thin collimation (in vitro preparation of a pig bowel)

Table 35.1. Scanning parameters for CT colonography. (After DACHMAN et al. 1998; FENLON and FERRUCCI 1997; HARA et al. 1997)

Parameter	Spiral CT	
	One detector	Multiple detectors
Slice thickness	5 mm	2.5 mm
Reconstruction interval	2–3 mm	1.6 mm
Pitch	1.25–1.5	1–0.8
mA	70–120	85–120
kVp	120	120

35.2.3
Rendering

Data rendering to create the 3D endoluminal images can be performed using either surface rendering or volume rendering techniques (DACHMAN et al. 1998). With surface rendering, contiguous CT images are manipulated using a marching cubes algorithm to create a wire frame model of the surface of the bowel wall, as shown in Fig. 35.5. Depending on the threshold value selected, tissues of different density can be either included or removed from the final 3D image. This technique has one major advantage over volume rendering: since any extraneous data are discarded before the model is created, it uses only about 10% of the available data, so decreasing the computer burden.

Volume rendering uses the entire data set, preserving the original dynamic range of acquired data and therefore providing a more reliable representation of anatomy and pathology. A 50- to 100-fold increase in processing speed is required for perspective volume rendering to become an interactive technique (RUBIN et al. 1996). With both techniques perspective rendering is possible, which approximates the human visual system. However, manual planning of flight paths is a tedious and time-consuming task.

A novel variant of volume rendering is tissue transition projection (TTP). Images obtained with this technique resemble those obtained in conventional fluoroscopic double-contrast studies with a translucent bowel wall (ROGALLA et al. 1999).

35.2.4
Interpretation

Differences among investigators' methods of interpretation may be important. Radiologists have the choice of viewing solely the nonreformatted axial CT images, only the 2D reformatted views, only the 3D reformatted views, or a combination of these aspects. The initial interpretation can be made from the axial images and endoluminal views can be used only when necessary to help distinguish normal folds from polyps (Dachman et al. 1998). An alternative method is simultaneous viewing of axial and standard multiplanar reconstructions. Further, multiplanar reconstructions can be viewed simultaneously with the endoluminal view.

Two-dimensional images seem to be particularly useful for lesion characterization and for detecting lesions behind haustral folds. Three-dimensional images are helpful in differentiating colonic folds from polyps and may be more sensitive than 2D CT colonography for detecting small lesions (JOHNSON et al. 1997). Probably a combined 2D and 3D image display provides the most robust method of polyp

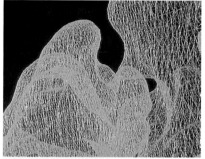
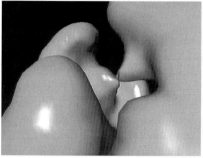

a

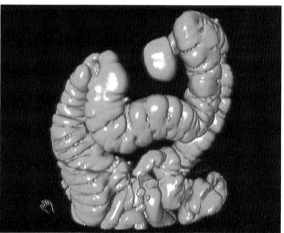

b

Fig. 35.5a,b. a The surface of the bowel wall consists of multiple tiny polygons that, when summed together, form the three-dimensional topography of the issue. Tumor stenosis at the right colonic flexure. **b** 3D surface rendering of the entire colon and the terminal ileal loops

detection and diagnosis of colorectal cancer (JOHNSON et al. 1997; ROYSTER et al 1997). Virtual colonoscopy examines the internal surface of the colonic lumen, whereas 2D CT colonography clearly provides a more accurate assessment of colonic wall thickness.

However, because experience with VE is limited and most radiologists are not familiar with the endoscopic view, interpretative criteria have to be developed. Polyps are identified as well-defined intraluminal projections, which are best seen in profile. Tumors are characterized as large intraluminal masses that vary widely. Review of both axial CT images and virtual colonoscopy images is necessary to improve identification of subtle colorectal lesions.

Poorly distended bowel loops may simulate stenoses, and residual intraluminal fluid and retained fecal material can both disguise and mimic abnormalities of the bowel wall. Additional artifacts on virtual colonoscopy may be caused by the use of inappropriate scan parameters, or as a function of the reconstruction algorithms used (FENLON et al. 1998). A frequently observed phenomenon is stair-step artifact, which produces a series of concentric rings that are most prominent where a rapid change in bowel contour occurs.

Diagnostic interpretation time remains long with the present technologies, and novel methods of colonic display will be required to improve the efficiency of interpretation.

35.2.5
Clinical Assessment

The clinical potential of VE in the evaluation of the colon is enormous, and it is hoped that the information derived from a spiral CT scan of the air-distended colon will be able to reproduce the findings of conventional endoscopy adequately. To be a clinically valuable means of evaluating the colon for polyps and tumors, it must be feasible to obtain, display, and interpret the images in a cost-effective and time-effective fashion using readily available hardware and software.

35.2.5.1
Tumor Diagnosis and Staging

The accuracy of CT colonoscopy in diagnosing colorectal cancer (Fig. 35.6 and 35.7) has not yet been sufficiently assessed. Reports in small series of patients indicate that tumors can be detected with a high sensitivity (HARVEY et al. 1998). ROYSTER et al. (1997) compared the diagnostic accuracy of axial 2D CT, virtual colonoscopy, and conventional colonoscopy in 20 patients with colorectal cancer. With the 2D axial CT images of the air-distended colon, all tumors (size range, 2.5–6.0 cm) were identified, but it is uncertain whether improved tumor staging will be possible using this method.

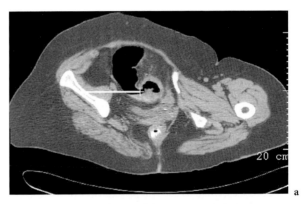

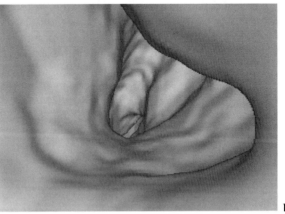

Fig. 35.6a,b. Axial scan and virtual colonoscopy at the edge of a tumor with severe stenosis at the "endoscopic" view

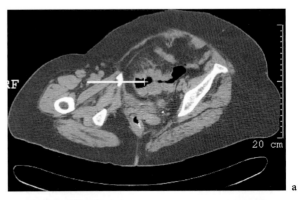

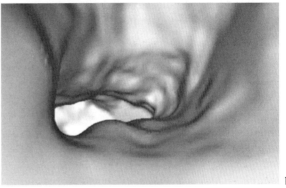

Fig. 35.7a,b. Axial scan and virtual colonoscopy of a significant tumor stenosis with slightly irregular contours at the "endoscopic" view

Virtual colonoscopy could be a safe and accurate method of evaluating the large bowel proximal to occlusive tumors which occur predominantly in the distal colon. Several studies have shown that in occlusive colon cancers the entire colon is visualized on colonoscopy in only about 50% of patients. A small percentage of patients with colorectal carcinoma have a second synchronous bowel tumor, and about one third have multiple coexistent adenomatous polyps. A preoperative examination of the entire colon is obviously essential to prevent local recurrences, to decrease the probability of the development of distant metastases, and to achieve longer survival times. With barium enema a preoperative total colon examination in occlusive carcinoma is technically difficult and associated with some risk. The majority of patients do not undergo adequate total colon evaluation prior to surgery. By detecting synchronous polyps and cancers, virtual colonoscopy could direct appropriate surgical management (FENLON et al. 1999b).

35.2.5.2
Screening

Colonic cancer is a major public health concern, and the need for screening is well documented. It is increasingly recognized that screening asymptomatic persons for colorectal cancer results in a 25–50% reduction in cancer mortality. The aim of screening is to detect and remove precancerous polyps and so prevent the development of invasive tumor growth. However, widespread colorectal screening is hampered by several practical impediments, including limited resources, methodological inadequacies, poor patient acceptance and compliance.

Virtual colonoscopy has conceptual appeal for polyp detection (Fig. 35.8–35.10), and several studies have shown promising results (Table 35.3). If it can be shown that the accuracy of CT colonography can approach that of colonoscopy for detection of polyps, this method could potentially replace the currently used and recommended techniques for screening.

Johnson and Hara's group evaluated the sensitivity and specificity of virtual colonoscopy in 70 patients with 35 known polyps and compared their results with those of colonoscopy, which served as the gold standard (JOHNSON et al. 1997). The sensitivity and specificity of virtual colonoscopy for patients with lesions of 10 mm or more in diameter were found to be 75% and 90%, respectively. Another study by HARA et al. (1996) evaluated 30 endoscopi-

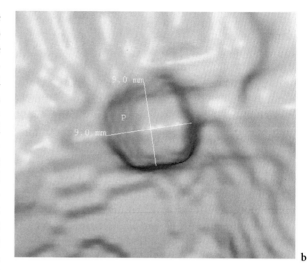

b

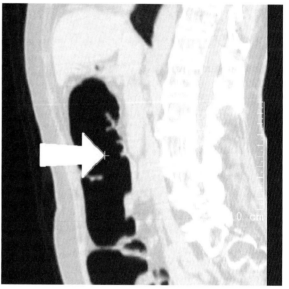

b

Fig. 35.8a,b. Small colonic polyp at the colonoscopic view. The small polyp is only faintly depicted at the two-dimensional reconstruction which does not permit unequivocal differentiation between a simple fold and a polyp

cally proven polyps in ten patients and detected 100% of all polyps that were greater than 1 cm in diameter, 71% of polyps that were between 5 and 9 mm, and 28% of polyps that were less than 5 mm. ROYSTER et al. (1997) found comparably good results in the detection of polyps smaller than 1 cm using axial CT images and virtual colonoscopic images, but in their study there was a substantially higher rate of false-positive diagnoses of polyps with use of only the axial CT examination.

Preliminary results of virtual colonoscopy for polyp detection are better than those of barium enema investigation and can rival those yielded by

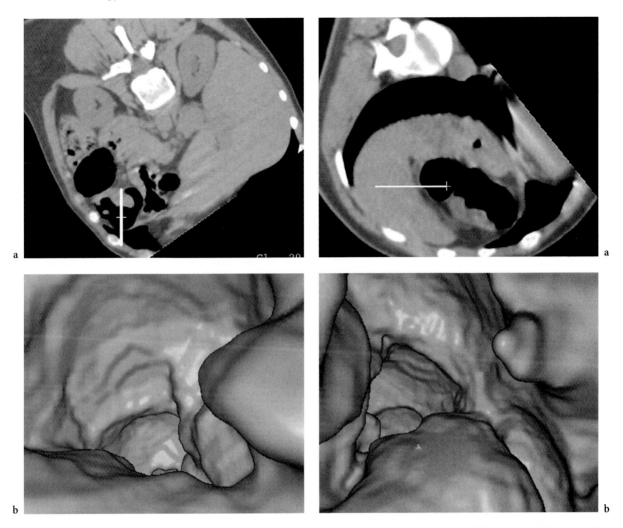

Fig. 35.9a,b. Large colonic polyp at the left flexure in axial image and virtual colonoscopy

Fig. 35.10a,b. Tumor-like polypoid lesions in axial view and virtual depiction

Table 35.3. Sensitivity and specificity in detecting colorectal polyps and masses

Authors	Number of patients	Sensitivity	Specificity	Polyp size
Hara et al. 1996	10	100%	–	>10 mm
Johnson et al. 1997	70	75%	90%	>10 mm
Royster et al. 1997	20	100%	–	>20 mm
		91%	–	<20 mm
Dachman et al. 1998	44	83%	100%	> 8 mm
Fenlon et al. 1998	35	100%	–	> 6 mm

conventional colonoscopy (Fenlon et al. 1999a; Johnson et al. 1997). However, polyps smaller than a few millimeters in diameter and subtle wall thickening are difficult to portray accurately, because of current imaging resolutions and partial-volume effects. Flat lesions will continue to be a challenge. Polypoid lesions must be elevated at least 2 mm above the normal surface to be identified (Johnson et al. 1997).

False-positive results are most frequently caused by misinterpretation of retained stool, respiratory artifacts, or normal colonic folds (misinterpreted as polyps.

35.2.6
Perspectives

Virtual reality imaging is an emerging technology that promises to revolutionize medical imaging. So far, however, its clinical usefulness is limited by lengthy image processing times and data storage requirements. The eventual solution of this problem will be the use of faster, more expensive computers to increase efficiency. Another approach is to refine scanning protocols and software capabilities.

It is theoretically possible that labeling fecal material with a specific contrast agent might permit the subsequent subtraction of fecal matter from the CT images and thus obviate the need for any type of bowel cleansing. Such a development would perhaps be the greatest advantage of using VE as a screening procedure, as it is widely believed that the reason for the current poor uptake for colorectal cancer screening amongst the general population is the reluctance to ingest bowel cleansing agents.

Further reduction in interpretation time may be supported by the development of computer-aided diagnostic techniques (VINING et al. 1997). For example, novel techniques for rapid and automatic computation of flight paths for guiding VE exploration of the 3D medical images have to be developed.

For the future, MR colonography appears to have considerable potential with regard to screening for colonic polyps. As in the case of CT colonography, improvements in diagnostic accuracy are likely with the routine addition of virtual colonoscopic viewing (LUBOLDT et al. 1998). Preliminary results suggest that MR colonography could become an alternative to CT colonography.

References

Amin Z, Boulos PB, Lees WR (1996) Technical report: spiral CT pneumocolon for suspected colonic neoplasms. Clin Radiol 51:56–61

Balthazar EJ, Megibow AJ, Hulnick D, Naidich DP (1988) Carcinoma of the colon: detection and preoperative staging by CT. AJR Am J Roentgenol 150:301–306

Chen SC, Lu DSK, Hecht JR, Kadell BM (1999) CT colonography: value of scanning in both the supine and prone positions. AJR Am J Roentgenol 172:595–599

Dachman AH, Kuniyoshi JK, Boyle CM, Samara Y, Hoffmann KR, Rubin DT, Hanan I (1998) CT colonography with three-dimensional problem solving for detection of colonic polyps. AJR Am J Roentgenol 171:989–995

Fenlon HM, Ferrucci JT (1997) Virtual colonoscopy: what will the issues be? AJR (Am J Roentgenol) 169:453–458

Fenlon HM, Clarke PD, Ferrucci JT (1998) Virtual colonoscopy: imaging features with colonoscopic correlation. AJR Am J Roentgenol 170:1303–1309

Fenlon HM, Barish MA, Blake MA, Ferrucci JT (1999a) Colorectal poyp detection: prospective comparison of virtual and conventional colonoscopy. Eur Radiol 9 [Suppl 1]:144–145

Fenlon HM, McAneny DB, Nunes DP, Clarke PD, Ferrucci JT (1999b) Occlusive colon carcinoma: virtual colonoscopy in the preoperative evaluation of the proximal colon. Radiology 210:423–428

Freeny PC,. Marks WM, Ryan JA, Bolen JW (1986) Colorectal carcinoma evaluation with CT: preoperative staging and detection of postoperative recurrence. Radiology 158:347–353

Hara AK, Johnson CD, Reed JD, Ahlquist DA, Nelson H, Ehman RL, McCollough CH, Ilstrup DM (1996) Detection of colorectal polyps by computed tomographic colography: feasibility of a novel technique. Gastroenterology 110:284–290

Hara AK, Johnson CD, Reed JE, Ahlquist DA, Nelson H, Ehman RL, Harmsen WS (1997) Reducing data size and radiation dose for colonography. AJR Am J Roentgenol 168:1181–1184

Harvey CJ, Amin Z, Hare CMB, Gillams AR, Novelli MR, Boulos PB, Lees WR (1998) Helical CT pneumocolon to assess colonic tumors: Radiologic-pathologic correlation. AJR Am J Roentgenol 170:1439–1443

Johnson CD, Hara AK, Reed JE (1997) Computed tomographic colonography (virtual colonoscopy): a new method for detecting colorectal neoplasms. Endoscopy 29:454–461

Luboldt W, Steiner P, Bauerfeind P, Pelkonen P, Debatin JF (1998) Detection of mass lesions with MR colonography: preliminary report. Radiology 207:59–65

Rogalla P, Beneder A, Schmidt E, Hamm B (1999) Comparison of virtual colonoscopy and tissue transition projection (TTP) in colorectal cancer. Eur Radiol 9 [Suppl 1]:S144

Royster AP, Fenlon HM, Clarke PD, Nunes DP, Ferrucci JT (1997) CT colonoscopy of colorectal neoplasms: two-dimensional and three-dimensional virtual-reality techniques with colonoscopic correlation. AJR Am J Roentgenol 169:1237–1243

Rubin GD, Beaulieu CF, Argiro V, Ringl H, Norbash AM, Feller JF,. Dake MD, Brooke Jeffrey R, Napel S (1996) Perspective volume rendering of CT and MR images: applications for endoscopic imaging. Radiology 199:321–330

Vining DJ, D.W. Gelfand RE, Bechthold, et al (1994) Technical feasibility of colon imaging with helical CT and virtual reality (abstract). AJR Am J Roentgenol 162:104

Vining DJ, Hunt GW, Ahn KD, Stelts BS, Hemler PF (1997) Computer-assisted detection of colon polyps and masses. Radiology 205(P):705–706

36 Mesenteric Ischemia

P. Taourel, B. Gallix, J.M. Bruel

CONTENTS

36.1 Introduction 393
36.2 Pathophysiology of Mesenteric Ischemia 393
36.2.1 Macroscopic Circulation 393
36.2.2 Microscopic Circulation 394
36.2.3 Response to Drop in Blood Pressure 394
36.2.4 Radiologically Detectable Effects of Ischemia 394
36.3 Etiology of Mesenteric Ischemia 394
36.4 Acute Mesenteric Ischemia 395
36.4.1 Caused by Arterial Occlusion 395
36.4.2 Nonocclusive 398
36.4.3 Caused by Venous Occlusion 399
36.4.4 Caused by Strangulating Obstruction 401
36.5 Subacute Mesenteric Ischemia 402
36.5.1 Ischemic Colitis 402
36.5.2 Ischemic Enteritis 403
36.6 Chronic Mesenteric Ischemia 404
36.7 Conclusion 404
References 404

36.1
Introduction

In 1926, the view was expressed that occlusion of the mesenteric vessels had to be regarded as one of those conditions in which the diagnosis is impossible, the prognosis hopeless, and treatment almost useless (COKKINIS 1926). This pessimism is still shared by many physicians more than 70 years later. Such an attitude results partly from the fact that the diagnosis of mesenteric ischemia is fraught with difficulty. Indeed, patients with mesenteric ischemia exhibit a wide spectrum of clinical symptoms, ranging from a relatively innocuous episode of mild abdominal pain to a full-blown abdominal catastrophe, depending on the duration, severity and location of the bowel ischemia. Therefore, there is a need

P. TAOUREL, MD; Imagérie Médicale, Hôpital Saint-Eloi, CHU de Montpellier,F-34295 Montpellier, France
B. GALLIX, MD; Imagérie Médicale, Hôpital Saint-Eloi, CHU de Montpellier,F-34295 Montpellier, France
J.M. BRUEL, MD; Imagérie Médicale, Hôpital Saint-Eloi, CHU de Montpellier,F-34295 Montpellier, France

for imaging techniques that will make the diagnosis of mesenteric ischemia more accurate. As a consequence of the increased availability and use of high-resolution spiral CT in patients with acute abdomen, data are now available about the technique of spiral CT and the results obtained with it, and on the indications for spiral CT in the diagnosis of mesenteric ischemia. After a short review of the physiopathology and the causes of mesenteric ischemia, this chapter will focus on the CT semiology of mesenteric ischemia, on the value and limitations of spiral CT in the diagnosis, and on the current role of CT, as opposed to other examination techniques, in the evaluation of patients with suspected mesenteric ischemia.

36.2
Pathophysiology of Mesenteric Ischemia

36.2.1
Macroscopic Circulation

The sources of collateral flow between the celiac and mesenteric vessels and between the splanchnic vessels and the systemic circulation are numerous and constitute one of the major protectors against ischemic injury to the gut. The primary potential pathway of collateral flow between the celiac axis and superior mesenteric artery (SMA) is through the gastroduodenal and pancreaticoduodenal arteries. The major anatomic pathways between the SMA and inferior mesenteric artery (IMA) are the marginal artery of Drummond, which runs parallel to the mesenteric border of the colon, and the arc of Riolan joining the middle and left colic arteries, which also lies within the mesentery but is more centrally located. At the splenic flexure there are fewer arcades linking the superior with the inferior mesenteric distribution, which explains why one of the common sites for ischemic colitis is the splenic flexure. Moreover, in the ileo-cecal region the vasa recta, which are end-arteries arising from the marginal artery of Drummond, are fewer in number and are located farther from the bowel wall, explaining why this region is vulnerable to nonocclusive ischemia associated with systemic shock (LUDWIG 1995).

36.2.2
Microscopic Circulation

There is an extensive network of vessels within the bowel wall, arising from the vasa recta on the mesenteric border of the bowel and passing through the muscularis propria to form a rich submucosal plexus. A central arteriole originates from the submucosal plexus, loses its muscularis coat, and arborizes into a capillary network that supplies the mucosal villi. This system is conspicuously redundant, to the extent that only about 20% of the mucosal capillaries are actually in use at any particular instant (PATEL 1992).

36.2.3
Response to Drop in Blood Pressure

Collateral pathways open in territories adjacent to the occluded vessel in response to the fall in arterial pressure distal to the obstruction; the precapillary sphincters dilate, reducing peripheral resistance and maintaining flow despite reduction of a pressure head. At the same time, every available capillary opens so that oxygen extraction can be maximized. In general, the intramural blood flow in regional ischemia redistributes to favor the mucosa. The prolonged perfusion time explains the increased staining of the mucosa (shock bowel) on CT after intravenous injection of contrast medium (MIRVIS 1994).

Autoregulation of flow can be maintained for only a brief period. During this time, the blood flow in the bowel wall is almost always sufficient for intestinal viability. However if the low-flow state is prolonged active vasoconstriction occurs, which may persist even after correction of the primary cause of the decreased flow.

36.2.4
Radiologically Detectable Effects of Ischemia

Regardless of the cause of acute ischemia, the earliest response of any portion of the bowel is a spasm of the muscularis propria. This persistent spasm produces initial cramping pain and may cause rapid transit with diarrhea and an abdomen free of gas on abdominal plain film (SCHOLZ 1993).

Later in the ischemic period, the ischemic segment of bowel loses its ability to contract and swallowed air will remain in the now atonic dilated segment. This produces a clinical and radiographic picture of paralytic ileus or even of small bowel obstruction. During the same period, there is a generalized increase in capillary permeability. The extravasated blood may come from the ischemic but nonoccluded vessels or from collateral vessels. This produces submucosal edema and hemorrhage and is responsible for the pattern of bowel wall thickening and thumbprinting seen on imaging studies.

If the ischemia persists, the mucosal blisters rupture, leading to an ulcerated mucosa. Later, the blisters will coalesce, dissecting the mucosa from the serosa and resulting in infarction of the mucosa. Finally, with persistent ischemia, transmural infarction of the wall may occur, in which case the bowel perforates, causing free intraperitoneal air.

36.3
Etiology of Mesenteric Ischemia

Bowel ischemia may be caused by arterial or venous occlusive disease.

Arterial occlusive disease is the most frequent cause of mesenteric ischemia. It can be due to narrowing, thrombosis or embolism involving the arterial tree that supplies the bowel. SMA embolism accounts for nearly 50% of episodes of acute mesenteric ischemia (KALEYA 1992). Emboli may arise from aortic plaques or result from the migration of an intracardial mural thrombus. As shown by angiographic studies (BAKAL 1992), emboli to the SMA tend to lodge at points of normal anatomic narrowing, usually immediately distal to the origin of a major branch. Emboli located in the SMA proximal to the origin of the ileocolic artery are considered major, whereas emboli located in the SMA distal to this point or in branches of the SMA are considered minor. Minor emboli account for only about 15% of the emboli responsible for acute mesenteric ischemia. Proximal narrowing or occlusion of main visceral arteries are usually caused by arteriosclerotic plaques, but can also be caused by other vascular conditions, such as an aortic dissection or a complication of surgery for aortic aneurysm. Occasionally, mesenteric tumors, vasculitis, and thromboangiitis obliterans after radiation therapy may occlude the smallest peripheral visceral vessels (Scholz 1993).

Nonocclusive arterial disease responsible for mesenteric ischemia is due to low-flow states. Their cause is usually decreased cardiac output of any etiology, including primary cardiac disease, infarction, arrhythmia and hypovolemia. In addition, secondary mesenteric vasoconstriction may worsen ischemia. This vasoconstriction may be a consequence of cardiotonic medications such as digitalis, vasopressin or other pressor agents. Exceptionally, peripheral mesenteric flow may be diminished by mesenteric arterial-to-arterial steal or arterial-to-venous shunting despite normal or even high cardiac output.

Mesenteric venous occlusion is the cause of bowel ischemia in 5–15% of patients. The main conditions associated with mesenteric venous thrombosis are previous abdominal surgery and hypercoagulable state (Rhee 1994). Other causes include abdominal trauma, pancreatitis, regional infectious processes, tumors that compress or invade the mesenteric vein, and cirrhosis.

Intestinal ischemia also occurs in strangulation as a complication of mechanical obstruction. It occurs in about 10% of patients with small bowel obstruction and is associated with closed-loop obstruction caused by adhesions, internal or external hernias, or idiopathic small-bowel volvulus. In these patients venous drainage is impaired and draining mesenteric veins are then occluded, leading to severe congestive changes affecting the wall of the bowel and the mesentery. Increased venous and capillary pressure leads to edema, rupture of small vessels, and intramural and mesenteric hemorrhage. Arterial insufficiency usually follows, aggravating the anoxia and contributing further to the rapid development of ischemia, infarction, and perforation (Balthazar 1994).

36.4
Acute Mesenteric Ischemia

36.4.1
Caused by Arterial Occlusion

36.4.1.1
Clinical Findings

Abdominal pain, which may initially be crampy, is usually the first clinical sign. Bloody diarrhea may also be present. Fever and signs of peritonitis occur as the ischemia persists, and finally bowel wall infarction develops. Arterial occlusion by an embolus tends to be sudden, severe, and extensive, but rarely produces prodromal syndromes. Conversely, patients with severe arterial occlusion from arteriosclerosis tend to have a history of chronic low-grade nonspecific abdominal symptoms that culminate in a severe ischemic episode. In the case of very far distal arterial occlusions, as seen in scleroderma or in radiation enteritis, it may be that bowel motor function alone is affected, causing diarrhea or small bowel obstruction.

36.4.1.2
Semiology of CT

It is more than 10 years since several papers reported the CT findings in bowel ischemia and infarction (Alpern 1988; Clark 1987; Federle 1984; Perez 1989; Smerud 1990) and established their relative frequency.

Dilatation of the bowel lumen is a common CT finding, reflecting the interruption of peristaltic activity in ischemic segments. The dilated bowel may be gas-filled or fluid-filled with minimal intraluminal gas, because blood and fluid exudate into the lumen of the ischemic bowel. However, dilatation of the bowel lumen is not specific to ischemia. Ascites and infiltration of the mesentery fat are other nonspecific findings often seen in ischemia.

Abnormalities of the bowel wall are more informative findings of ischemia. Bowel wall thickening is the most frequently described abnormality. In ischemia resulting from arterial occlusion it is an early finding, and it reflects the combination of intramural edema and acute submucosal hemorrhage (Bartnicke 1994). However, bowel wall thickening is not specific, being present in inflammatory, infectious and neoplastic conditions. Like others (Klein et al 1995), we have shown (Taourel 1996) that the focal lack of enhancement of the bowel wall after contrast medium injection is a more specific finding in ischemia with an arterial origin (Fig. 36.1). This pattern is probably caused by the lack of perfusion (Klein 1995). It is associated with a very thin wall, which is not seen on CT when the loop is fluid-filled ("virtual wall"). Contiguous to the ischemic bowel there is an infiltration of the mesenteric fat. Intramural gas is a later finding in mesenteric ischemia. Its frequency varies between 5% and 50% in the literature, according to the severity of the condition in patients included in the studies. The intramural gas,

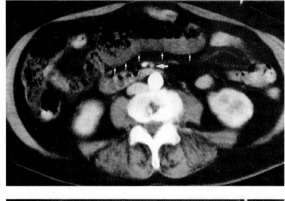

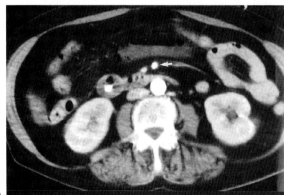

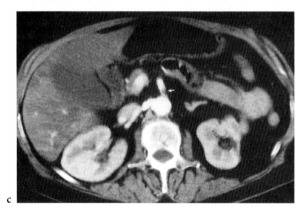

Fig. 36.1a–c. Nonenhancing bowel wall owing to embolus of the SMA. **a** CT scan demonstrates that the wall of a dilated bowel loop is not enhanced (*thin arrows*). Note also the absence of opacification of the SMA (*arrow*). **b** CT scan at an upper level shows patency of the superior mesenteric artery (*arrow*), indicating that the embolus is relatively distal. **c** CT scan at the level of the liver detects thrombus at the ostium of the SMA (*thin arrow*), suggesting that the embolus has migrated from an arteriosclerotic thrombus

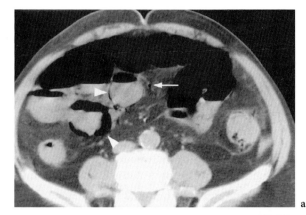

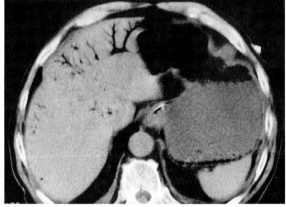

Fig. 36.2a, b. Intramural and intraportal gas. **a** CT scan of the pelvis shows pneumatosis involving the ileum as a linear air collection (*arrowheads*) between fluid-filled ileum and mesenteric fat. Note also bubbles of gas in the mesentery (*thin arrow*) owing to air in peripheral mesenteric veins. **b** CT scan of the liver shows intraportal gas

or pneumatosis intestinalis, is caused by diffusion of luminal gas into the bowel wall across the compromised mucosa. The detection of intramural gas on CT is improved by using a large window setting. On CT, pneumatosis intestinalis appears as cystic, linear, or curvilinear intramural gas collections in a cir-cumferential distribution around the bowel lumen (Fig. 36.2). Intramural gas is not pathognomonic of ischemia, since it can be seen in other conditions, including pulmonary disease, intestinal obstruction, peptic ulcer, collagen vascular disease, and steroid administration (CONNOR 1984). Mesenteric or portal venous gas may be associated with pneumatosis intestinalis. It represents the propagation of intramural gas into the mesenteric venous system (Fig. 36.2). Although mesenteric gas is often due to bowel infarction, it can also be seen in any condition in which there is mucosal disruption, such as abdominal abscesses, gastric ulcers, and ulcerative colitis (BARTNICKE 1994).

Occlusion of the main trunk of the SMA is easily demonstrated by contrast-enhanced CT scans; consequently, CT is accurate in diagnosis of thrombosis and proximal embolus of the SMA (Fig. 36.3). Conversely, the accuracy of CT in diagnosing more distal embolus is debatable. In our personal series (TAOUREL 1996), we diagnosed only 7 of the 19 arterial occlusions shown by surgery (Fig 36.1). KLEIN et al. (1995), in contrast, found a good sensitivity of CT in diagnosing peripheral emboli. The helical technique improves the detection of emboli in the mesenteric arterial branches, because scanning is performed soon after the initiation of contrast medium injection (25–40 s), i.e. during the arterial phase. However, because mesenteric veins are not enhanced during the arterial phase, dual-phase helical CT of the abdomen is necessary for detection of occlusion of both mesenteric arteries and veins (BRUEL 1998).

36.4.1.3
Accuracy of CT

Most of the published studies were retrospectively conducted in patients with known bowel ischemia or infarction; thus, they do not allow determination of the sensitivity and specificity of CT in the prospective evaluation of intestinal ischemia. Moreover, although these studies may demonstrate the relative frequency of various CT findings in intestinal ischemia, data may be biased by the study design. Initial reports suggesting that CT was accurate in the diagnosis of acute mesenteric ischemia included only patients with CT findings suggestive of bowel necrosis for the most part, therefore excluding false-negative studies from the analysis. Furthermore, because the study groups described in the published reports comprised only patients with known intestinal ischemia, it is impossible to determine the speci-

ficity of the various findings present in intestinal ischemia. For all these reasons, we have performed a study including both a group of patients with acute mesenteric ischemia and a group of patients without acute mesenteric ischemia but with a clinical condition consistent with this entity. We have shown that a thrombus or embolus in the SMA, intramural gas, intraportal gas, lack of enhancement of the bowel wall, and findings of ischemia in solid organs such as spleen, liver, or kidney had a specificity in excess of 95% in the diagnosis of acute mesenteric ischemia (TAOUREL 1995). Even if each of these findings has an individual sensitivity inferior to 30%, when the presence of any of these findings is used as a criterion for the diagnosis of acute mesenteric ischemia, the sensitivity of CT rises to 64%, while the specificity remains equal to 92%. Although encouraging, these results should be validated in a prospective clinical trial.

36.4.1.4
Comparison with Other Examination Techniques

Angiography remains the gold standard in the evaluation of the arterial splanchnic circulation. The value of angiography relative to CT in patients with suspected acute mesenteric ischemia is diagnostic and therapeutic: angiography can show peripheral arterial occlusion not diagnosed by CT; it allows selective thrombolysis when needed. Therefore, the role of angiography is central in the diagnosis and management of acute mesenteric ischemia. Thus, in patients with a strong clinical suspicion of acute mesenteric ischemia, emergency angiography is recommended (BAKAL 1992). However, in clinical practice, patients are often seen with nonspecific signs of an acute abdomen: mesenteric ischemia is then only one of several possible diagnoses. In this clinical setting, CT can show findings of acute mesenteric ischemia and rule out alternative diagnoses.

36.4.1.5
Impact of CT

Improved outcome of acute mesenteric ischemia can be achieved only if surgery is performed before irreversible ischemic changes of the bowel wall have occurred (LEVY 1990). Early diagnosis remains the cornerstone of successful treatment and is achieved by early aggressive use of angiography in patients with high suspicion and by extensive use of CT in patients with lower suspicion of acute mesenteric ischemia.

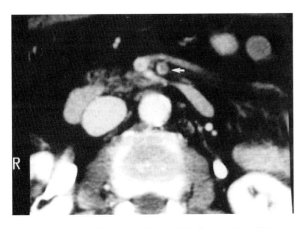

Fig. 36.3. Direct depiction of arterial obstruction. CT scan demonstrates the absence of opacification of the SMA (*arrow*) despite obvious enhancement of the aorta. The position of the defect, distal to the origin of the superior mesenteric artery, suggests an embolus as the cause of the obstruction

36.4.2
Nonocclusive

36.4.2.1
Clinical Findings

As in the case of mesenteric ischemia caused by arterial obstruction, abdominal pain out of proportion to the physical findings is a cardinal symptom in patients with nonocclusive acute mesenteric ischemia (BASSIOUNY 1997). Unexplained abdominal distension, fever, diarrhea, nausea, vomiting, or diminished bowel sounds are other common but nonspecific manifestations. Because clinical findings are nonspecific, the clinical diagnosis of nonocclusive acute mesenteric ischemia requires a high index of suspicion in the case of elderly patients with any of the following risk factors: acute myocardial infarction with shock, congestive heart failure, dysrhythmia, hypovolemia resulting from burns, sepsis, pancreatitis, hemorrhagic shock, and medication with splanchnic vasoconstrictors such as adrenergic agents or digitalis (BASSIOUNY 1997).

36.4.2.2
Semiology of CT

The CT findings in nonocclusive acute mesenteric ischemia have been reported mainly in adults or children with posttraumatic shock (SIVIT 1992; MIRVIS 1994). Lesions involve the small bowel or the right colon, considered by some authors (LANDRENEAU 1990; LUDWIG 1995) as a target organ of nonocclusive mesenteric ischemia. In such patients, the small bowel has been described as diffusely dilated, fluid-filled, with thickened walls and mucosal folds and overall abnormally intense contrast enhancement of the bowel wall (Fig. 36.4). Other reported CT manifestations of hypoperfusion include diminished caliber and increased enhancement of the inferior vena cava (JEFFREY 1988) and aorta (Fig. 36.4), and intense contrast enhancement of the kidneys and mesentery. The CT appearance of the small bowel is consistent with the increased permeability demonstrated by BULKLEY (1985) in a canine model of hypoperfusion. Increased permeability leads to wall thickening, increased enhancement after intravenous injection of contrast medium (owing to both slowed perfusion and increased interstitial leak of contrast material), and accumulation of intraluminal fluid (probably resulting from reduced resorption capacity). At this stage, both in the study of SIVIT (1992) and in that of MIRVIS (1994), when

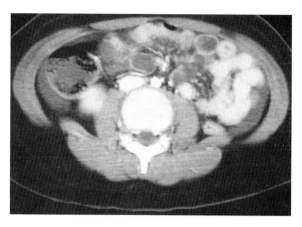

Fig. 36.4. Shock bowel in a 13-year-old girl involved in a motor vehicle collision. CT scan shows intense contrast enhancement of the small bowel wall and of the vena cava. Note also the diminished caliber of the aorta and the presence of peritoneal fluid

surgery was performed the bowel recovered a normal appearance. The recovery of a normal morphologic appearance and of an apparently normal function indicates the ability of the small bowel to tolerate prolonged periods of hypoperfusion resulting from hypovolemic shock. In a later phase, the bowel wall may be thickened with reduced enhancement (KLEIN 1995) or thin and nonenhanced (Fig. 36.5), as in ischemia caused by arterial occlusion.

36.4.2.3
Accuracy of CT

The accuracy of CT in the evaluation of nonocclusive mesenteric ischemia is subject to some limitations, mainly because of the lack of surgical correlations, since nonocclusive mesenteric ischemia is usually not seen as an indication for surgery and because the changes observed in shock bowel on CT may not be evident on visual inspection at laparotomy. Consequently, no data are available on the accuracy of CT in nonocclusive mesenteric ischemia. However, we can assume that the accuracy of CT is lower in nonocclusive than in occlusive ischemia, because the direct vascular changes (e.g. embolus) observed in occlusive ischemia are very helpful in the diagnosis of acute mesenteric ischemia.

36.4.2.4
Comparison with Other Examination Techniques

Definitive diagnosis of nonocclusive acute mesenteric ischemia requires expeditious arteriographic

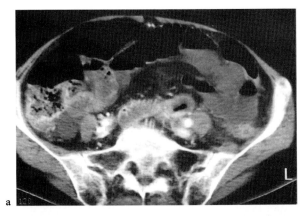

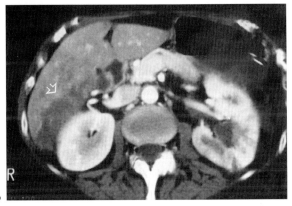

Fig. 36.5a, b. Nonocclusive acute mesenteric ischemia in a patient with myocardial infarction. **a** CT scan shows the nonenhancement of the wall of most of the small bowel loops. By comparison the wall of the colon and of some posterior loops is normally enhanced. **b** CT scan at the level of the liver also demonstrates ischemia of the liver (*open arrow*)

study of the aorta and mesenteric vessels. The advantages of angiography are that it allows diagnosis and treatment of vasospasm. SIEGELMAN et al. (1974) have described four reliable arteriographic criteria for the diagnosis of mesenteric vasospasm: narrowing of the origin of the SMA branches, alternate dilatation and narrowing of these branches, spasm of the mesenteric arcades, and impaired filling of the intramural vessels. The treatment of nonocclusive acute mesenteric ischemia is essentially pharmacological and is readily achieved by selective infusion of papaverine into the SMA. Thus, because of these two advantages, arteriography is clearly superior to CT in the diagnosis and management of nonocclusive acute mesenteric ischemia.

36.4.2.5
Impact of CT

From these data, we can assume that the impact of CT in the diagnosis and management of non-occlusive acute mesenteric ischemia is relatively weak, for the following reasons: the finding of an abnormally enhanced bowel wall in a patient with shock is not helpful as an argument for surgery versus conservative treatment; CT is inferior to angiography for the diagnosis of mesenteric vasospasm; and, last but not least, in contrast to angiography, CT does not allow treatment of nonocclusive acute mesenteric ischemia.

36.4.3
Caused by Venous Occlusion

36.4.3.1
Clinical Findings

Patients with acute mesenteric venous thrombosis may present with typical signs and symptoms of acute bowel ischemia, characterized by pain out of proportion to the physical findings, nausea, vomiting and bloody diarrhea. However, the symptoms are often less severe, and patients typically present with diffuse intermittent pain lasting several days (RHEE 1994).

36.3.3.2
Semiology of CT

The trunk and the larger branches of the superior mesenteric vein are well identified on CT scans performed during the portal phase. Lack of enhancement of these vessels indicates thrombosis. The thrombosis can be complete (Fig. 36.6) or partial (Fig. 36.7), with a nonopacifying filling defect in the lumen of the vein. The walls of the veins opacify around the nonopacifying thrombus (VOGELZANG 1988). In addition to defining the presence of any portal and mesenteric thrombi, CT may suggest the age of a thrombus. In the first days after its formation, a fresh thrombus shows high attenuation values on native CT, because of the recent incorporation of blood into it (HADDAD 1992). Extravascular abnormalities associated with mesenteric venous thrombosis include bowel wall thickening with abnormally high enhancement and infiltration of the mesenteric fat. These features correlate well with published pathological reports, which have shown that in venous thrombosis the bowel wall becomes edema-

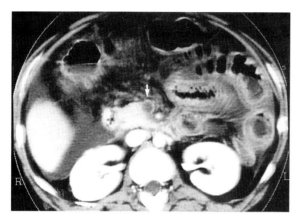

Fig. 36.6. Mesenteric venous thrombosis. CT scan demonstrates the absence of opacification of the superior mesenteric vein, which is enlarged (*arrow*). Note also thickening of the wall of the small bowel loops and strandings in the mesenteric fat

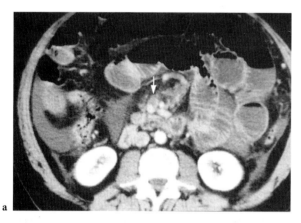

a

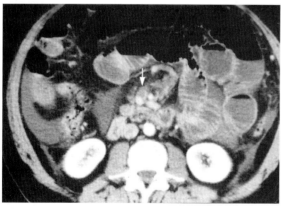

b

Fig. 36.7a, b. Mesenteric venous thrombosis. CT scans (a, b) demonstrate partial venous thrombosis located at the anterior part of the superior mesenteric vein (*thin arrow*). Note also the presence of dilated fluid-filled bowel loops and strandings in the mesenteric fat. By comparison with the dilated bowel in Fig. 36.5, the wall of the loops are normally enhanced

tous, cyanotic and thickened with intramural hemorrhage (BOLEY 1992), while necrosis of the bowel wall is a more prominent feature of arterial occlusion (MITSUDO 1992).

36.4.3.3
Accuracy of CT

The accuracy of CT in the diagnosis of acute venous thrombosis is very high. The published sensitivity varies between 90% and 100% in studies including 10–20 patients (HARWARD 1989; VOGELZANG 1988; RHEE 1994). Some false-negative results may be due to rare cases of thrombosis limited to the peripheral branches of the superior mesenteric vein. The specificity is also very high, since although superior mesenteric occlusion may occur in patients without leading to bowel wall ischemia, the presence of this finding in association with bowel wall thickening is diagnostic for venous mesenteric ischemia in the proper clinical setting (BARTNICKE 1994).

36.4.3.4
Comparison with Other Examination Techniques

CT is the diagnostic test of choice in acute mesenteric venous thrombosis. Although ultrasonography with color duplex may be used as the first-line test with very good accuracy for the diagnosis of portal thrombosis, its ability to diagnose mesenteric venous thrombosis is inferior. Mesenteric arteriography with venous phase was once central to the diagnosis of venous thrombosis. However, arteriography is less sensitive than CT and is actually no longer often used (RHEE 1994).

36.4.3.5
Impact of CT

Mesenteric venous thrombosis is recognized more frequently now because of the widespread availability of high-resolution CT and its frequent use in patients with nonspecific symptoms. Accurate diagnosis allows the use of anticoagulation, which is particularly effective in the case of a fresh thrombus, since it has been shown that the only factor that alters early survival is anticoagulation (RHEE 1994). Prompt diagnosis of mesenteric venous thrombosis, institution of anticoagulant therapy, follow-up imaging to assess recanalization, and the search for causes that may be correctable have led to decreased mortality and morbidity of mesenteric ischemia (MATOS 1986, RHAMOUNI 1992).

36.4.4
Caused by Strangulating Obstruction

36.3.4.1
Clinical Findings

Ischemia complicating small bowel obstruction is a crucial event since, as noted by MUCHA (1987), in almost every reported series of small intestinal obstruction the most critical factor affecting outcome is whether the obstruction has progressed to the point of strangulation. Classic signs of strangulation are intense abdominal pain, fever, tachycardia, and hyperleukocytosis. However, fever, tachycardia and hyperleukocytosis are lacking in more than half the patients. Furthermore, these findings may be present without strangulation.

36.4.4.2
Semiology of CT

CT signs indicative of strangulation pertain to abnormalities involving the wall of the incarcerated bowel and to characteristic changes occurring in the small bowel mesentery (Fig. 36.8). The wall of the bowel may be slightly and circumferentially thickened, it may show increased attenuation, it may exhibit concentric rings of slightly different densities (target or halo sign), or in advanced cases lack of enhancement or pneumatosis intestinalis may develop. Congestive changes of the mesentery vary in severity from increased haziness with blurring of the mesenteric vessels to total obliteration of the fatty mesentery and its vessels caused by the mesenteric hemorrhage (BALTHAZAR 1994).

36.4.4.3
Accuracy of CT

The accuracy of CT in detecting bowel ischemia caused by strangulating obstruction remains a controversial topic, with wide variations in the few reported series. The sensitivity of CT has been reported to range from 63% to 100% (BALTHAZAR 1992; TAOUREL 1995; FRAGER 1996; BALTHAZAR 1997). Subtle CT signs can be differently interpreted, explaining these variations. A rigid interpretation of less specific and questionable changes increase sensitivity to the detriment of specificity. The 100% sensitivity in the study of FRAGER (1996) was associated with a specificity of only 61%. Any discrepancy between CT and pathological data may be explained by the time interval between CT and surgery, and also

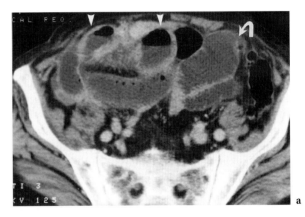

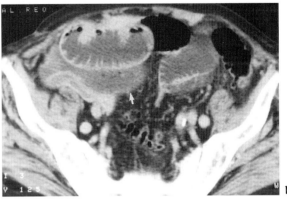

Fig. 38.8a, b. Strangulated small bowel. CT scans show distended fluid-filled intestinal loops in midpelvis with bowel thickening (*arrowheads*) and localized mesenteric effusion (*arrow*). Dilatation of fluid-filled proximal loops is also present with normal bowel wall thickness (*arrow*)

by limitations of surgical visual evaluation, since the appearance of the bowel can be normal in cases of early, nontransmural necrosis, as demonstrated by pathological studies (MITSUDO 1992).

36.4.4.4
Comparison with Other Examination Techniques

Despite these limitations, CT is actually largely superior to other examinations in the diagnosis of strangulation, even to color Doppler, although the latter is currently under evaluation for assessment of the bowel wall vascularization, particularly for intussusception in children.

36.4.4.5
Impact of CT

The impact of CT in the diagnosis of strangulation has been well emphasized by BALTHAZAR (1997). In all patients in whom CT signs of ischemia are detected, emergency exploratory laparotomy should be performed, even though about one-fifth of the patients in this group will have only simple mechanical small bowel obstruction without strangulation. In patients without CT findings of ischemia, the initial approach might be one aimed at conservation, depending on the cause of the obstruction. However, in these cases, exploratory laparotomy should not be unduly postponed if the patient's condition deteriorates, even in the absence of CT signs of ischemia.

36.5
Subacute Mesenteric Ischemia

36.5.1
Ischemic Colitis

36.5.1.1
Clinical Findings

Usually, ischemic colitis presents clinically in an insidious fashion, with abdominal pain, distension and diarrhea, which is typically bloody. Abdominal pain may be missing and distension the only symptom. Patients are often elderly males afflicted with cardiovascular conditions, diabetes mellitus, and/or renal failure. In the majority of patients with ischemic colitis, symptoms resolve with conservative treatment (TOURSARKISSIAN 1997). In some severe forms of ischemic colitis there is transmural gangrenous necrosis of a colonic segment, which rapidly leads to peritonitis necessitating surgical resection.

36.5.1.2
Semiology of CT

CT findings in ischemic colitis depend on the severity and duration of the process (BALFE 1997). In mild disease, CT demonstrates moderate segmental circumferential colonic wall thickening, and contrast enhancement is homogeneous or has the appearance of the target or halo sign (Figs. 36.9, 36.10). Thickening is associated with minimal inflammatory strandings in the surrounding fat. In more severe disease, submucosal hemorrhage appears as discrete high-attenuation masses, which are responsible for irregular and scalloped margins of the colon corresponding to the "thumbprinting" seen on barium studies. The infiltration of the pericolic fat

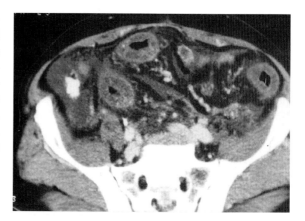

Fig. 36.9. Ischemic colitis involving the sigmoid colon. CT scan shows circumferential thickening of the sigmoid colon

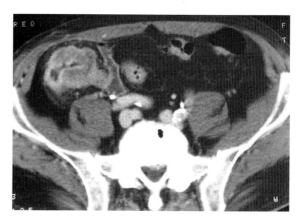

Fig. 36.10. Ischemic cecitis. CT scan shows circumferential thickening with target enhancement of the cecum

owing to the engorgement of the mesenteric veins is more obvious. In acutely ill patients, CT may show intramural gas or gas within the mesenteric venous tributaries suggestive of transmural infarction.

36.5.1.3
Accuracy of CT

The CT characteristics of the thickened colonic wall (its length, the severity of the thickening, the fact that the thickening is regular or irregular) generally allow differentiation of ischemic colitis from colic cancer and are particularly helpful in distinguishing tumorous from ischemic segments in patients with ischemic colitis proximal to colonic carcinoma (Fig. 36.11) (KO 1997). The main limitation of CT in ischemic colitis is the lack of specificity and the differential diagnosis with other forms of colitis, including mainly inflammatory and infectious colitis. The distribution of disease may give clues to the diagnosis. In ischemic colitis, wall thickening is not pancolic and is often limited to the left side of the colon, even though some studies have shown an increased incidence of right-sided disease (Fig. 36.10) (LANDRENEAU 1990).

36.5.1.4
Comparison with Other Examination Techniques

Although endoscopy and histological data obtained by biopsy are often not pathognomonic for ischemic colitis, the definitive diagnosis of ischemic colitis is frequently obtained by endoscopic examination (TOURSARKISSIAN 1997). Endoscopy can also be used to grade the severity of the disease. Barium enema may show thumbprinting caused by submucosal edema and hemorrhage, which is a classic finding in ischemic colitis. However, this examination is now rarely used in the evaluation of acute abdominal pain. Conversely, ultrasonography is more and more often used in the assessment of acute abdominal pain and allows the diagnosis of bowel disease. When the bowel wall is abnormally thickened in a symptomatic individual, Doppler sonography may be useful in determining whether the underlying process is inflammatory or ischemic in nature. TEEFEY et al. (1996) have shown that the thickened bowel wall exhibits no appreciable arterial signal in ischemia, whereas there is hypervascularity in inflammatory disease. However, as noted by BALFE (1997), this criterion is useful only during the early phase of ischemia, and not during the reperfusion phase, which is also characterized by hypervascularity. Angiography is sometimes per-

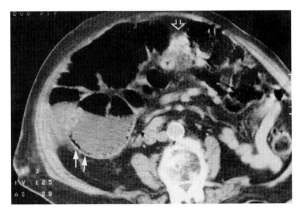

Fig. 36.11. Ischemic cecitis proximal to cancer of the transverse colon. CT scan shows air in the wall of the cecum (*thin arrows*). Ischemia is due to occlusion by a transverse colonic cancer demonstrated by a marked thickening of the wall of a short segment of the transverse colon (*open arrow*)

formed in the evaluation of ischemic colitis. It often reveals patent major visceral vessels, probably because most vascular lesions causing ischemic colitis are peripheral and therefore difficult to detect.

36.5.1.5
Impact of CT

Although CT findings are not specific, in clinical practice the pattern of a regular thickening of the left colon wall in the context of abdominal pain in a patient who is over 50 years old and has cardio-vascular risk factors is highly suggestive of ischemic colitis. Consequently, CT has a diagnostic impact and may indicate that coloscopy is needed for diagnostic confirmation and grading of a likely ischemic colitis.

36.5.2
Ischemic Enteritis

Subacute ischemic enteritis is characterized by preserved perfusion of the inner layers of the bowel wall. Clinical findings are less acute than in the aforementioned diseases and include abdominal pain, diarrhea or episodes of malabsorption that can resolve spontaneously. As we have seen, mesenteric venous thrombosis or nonocclusive ischemia may be responsible for such findings. However, in patients with recurrent symptoms, vasculitis affecting the small bowel may be evoked. Such patients may have any of a large group of diseases, such as polyarteritis nodosa, lupus erythematosus, rheumatoid vasculitis, Henoch-Schönlein purpura, Takayasu's disease, Buerger's disease and Behcet's disease (KRUPSKI 1997). Vasculitis can be distinguished by the associated extraintestinal pattern of involvement and by the type of mesenteric vessels affected. As examples, in Churg-Strauss vasculitis larger vessels are involved and patients give a history of allergy and have eosinophilia; in Henoch-Schönlein purpura postcapillary venulitis is the immediate cause of the intestinal changes and the clinical presentation is a triad of palpable purpura, arthritis, and abdominal pain; in Buerger's disease the affected vessels are peripheral arterial mesenteric branches and patients, who are typically young male smokers, have ischemia of the upper and lower extremities. Whatever the mechanism of ischemia, CT findings associate thickening of the small bowel wall and mesenteric fat strandings. These findings are not specific, and the diagnosis of vasculitis is made on the grounds of clinical and biological data associated with extra-abdominal imaging findings such as proximal obstruction of the branches of the aortic arch in Takayasu's disease or pleural and peritoneal fluid in lupus erythematosus.

36.6
Chronic Mesenteric Ischemia

Classic symptoms of chronic mesenteric ischemia include postprandial abdominal pain, weight loss, and diarrhea. Most patients have evidence of diffuse atherosclerotic disease. Compression by the arcuate ligament has also been described as a cause of abdominal angina, although celiac axis compression is a controversial entity because not all patients with occlusion of two or even three vessels are symptomatic (SCHOLZ 1993). Diagnosis of chronic mesenteric ischemia is based on duplex sonography and angiography. Few data are available on the CT findings and the role of this technique in patients with suspected chronic mesenteric ischemia. It has been shown that the diagnosis of celiac axis compression may be suggested by CT when narrowing or effacement of the celiac axis is produced by thickening of the crura anterior to the abdominal aorta and is associated with poststenotic dilatation of the celiac trunk and prominent peripancreatic collateral vessels (PATTEN 1991). In the same way, preliminary reports have shown that helical scan – with thin axial sections, reconstructions with overlap and 3D rendering techniques – is able to depict ostial stenosis of the celiac artery and SMA and, additionally, to demonstrate collateral pathways (RUBIN 1994). However, these promising results need further studies for confirmation and to determine the accuracy, the role and the impact of CT in the management of patients with suspected chronic mesenteric ischemia.

36.7
Conclusion

As yet, mesenteric ischemia obviously remains a potentially fatal disease, and an aggressive approach to its prompt diagnosis is warranted. In patients whose condition gives rise to a strong suspicion of acute mesenteric ischemia, emergency angiography is recommended. In other patients, who are more

numerous, since clinical findings are rarely very suggestive of ischemia, the role of CT appears to be that of a triage method. CT can document the presence of mesenteric vascular occlusion. We can already assume that helical CT allows the detection of more peripheral vascular occlusions because of the three basic advantages of helical CT over conventional CT for the study of abdominal organs: faster scanning time, smaller interscan intervals, and optimization of the use of contrast medium (ZEMAN 1998). CT can display the characteristic findings of abnormal perfusion of the bowel wall, despite being unable to allow assessment of bowel viability except in the most severe cases, where it shows bowel wall necrosis. Finally, CT is the most useful imaging procedure to detect a process mimicking ischemia, such as peritonitis, pancreatitis, diverticulitis or appendicitis.

References

Alpern MB, Glazer GM, Francis IR (1988) Ischemic or infarcted bowel : CT findings. Radiology 166:149

Bakal CW, Spayregen S, Wolf EL (1992) Radiology in intestinal ischemia. Surg Clin North Am 72:125–141

Balfe DM (1997) Acute ischemia of the bowel : radiologic diagnosis. Syllabus RSNA 1997

Balthazar EJ, Birnbaum BA, Megibow AJ, et al (1992) Closed-loop and strangulating intestinal obstruction : CT signs. Radiology 185:769–775

Balthazar EJ (1994) CT of small-bowel obstruction. AJR AM J Roentgenol 162:255–261

Balthazar EJ, Liebeskind ME, Macari M (1997) Intestinal ischemia in patients in whom small bowel obstruction is suspected : evaluation of accuracy, limitations, and clinical implications of CT in diagnosis. Radiology 205:519–522

Bartnicke BJ, Balfe DM (1994) CT appearance of intestinal ischemia and intramural hemorrhage. Radiol Clin North Am 32:845–860

Bassiouny HS (1997) Non occlusive mesenteric ischemia. Surg Clin North Am 77:319–326

Boley SJ, Kaleya RN, Brandt LJ (1992) Mesenteric venous thrombosis. Surg Clin North Am 72:183–202

Bulkley GB, Kvietys PR, Parks DA, Perry MA, Granger DN (1985) Relationship of blood flow and oxygen consumption to ischemic injury in the canine intestine. Gastroenterology 89:852–857

Bruel JM, Taourel P, Pradel JA (1998) CT of acute mesenteric ischemia. Abdom Imaging 23:334–336

Clark RA (1987) Computed tomography of bowel infarction. J Comput Assist Tomogr 11:757–762

Cokkinis AJ (1926) Mesenteric vascular occlusion. Bailliere, London, Tindall and Cox, pp 1–93

Connor R, Jones B, Fishman EK et al (1984) Pneumatosis intestinalis: Role of computed tomography in diagnosis and management. J Comput Assist Tomogr 8:269–275

Federle MP, Chun G, Jeffrey RB et al (1984) Computed tomography findings in bowel infarction. AJR Am J Roentgenol 142:91–95

Frager D, Baer JW, Medwid SW et al (1996) Detection of intestinal ischemia in patients with acute small-bowel obstruction due to adhesions or hernia : efficacy of CT. AJR Am J Roentgenol 166:67–71

Haddad MC, Clark DC, Sharif HS et al (1992) MR, CT, and ultrasonography of splanchnic venous thrombosis. Gastrointest Radiol 17:34–40

Harward TRS, Green D, Bergan JJ et al (1989) Mesenteric venous thrombosis. J Vasc Surg 9:328

Jeffrey RB, Federle MP (1988) The collapsed inferior vena cava : CT evidence of hypovolemia. AJR Am J Roentgenol 150:431–432

Kaleya RN, Sammartano RJ, Boley SJ (1992) Aggressive approach to acute mesenteric ischemia. Surg Clin North Am 72:43–64

Klein HS, Lensing R, Klosterhalfen B, Töns C, Günther RW (1995) Diagnosis imaging of mesenteric infarction. Radiology 197:79–82

Ko GH, Ha HK, Lee HJ, et al (1997) Usefulness of CT in patients with ischemic colitis proximal to colonic cancer. AJR Am J Roentgenol 168:951–956

Krupski WC, Selzman CH, Whitchill TA (1997) Unusual causes of mesenteric ischemia. Surg Clin North Am 77:471–502

Landreneau RJ, Fry WJ (1990) The right colon as a target organ of non occlusive mesenteric ischemia. Arch Surg 125:591–594

Levy PJ, Krausz MM, Manny J (1990) Acute mesenteric ischemia : improved results – a retrospective study analysis of ninety-two patients. Surgery 107:372–380

Ludwig KA, Quebbeman EJ, Bergstein JM, Wallace JR, Wittmann DH, Aprahamian C (1995) Shock-associated right colon ischemia and necrosis. J Trauma 39:1171–1174

Matos C, Van Gansbeke D, Zalcman M et al (1986) Mesenteric vein thrombosis : Early CT and US diagnosis and conservative management. Gastrointest Radiol 11:322–325

Mirvis SE, Shannuganathan K, Erb R (1994) Diffuse small-bowel ischemia in hypotensive adults after blunt trauma (shock bowel) : CT findings and clinical significance. AJR Am J Roentgenol 163:1375–1379

Mitsudo S, Brandt LJ (1992) Pathology of intestinal ischemia. Surg Clin North Am 72:43–64

Mucha P (1987) Small intestinal obstruction. Surg Clin North Am 67:597–620

Patel A, Kaleya RN, Sammartano RJ (1992) Pathophysiology of mesenteric ischemia. Surg Clin North Am 72:31–41

Patten RM, Coldwell DM, Ben-Menachem Y (1991) Ligamentous compression of the celiac axis : CT findings in five patients. AJR Am J Roentgenol 156:1101–1103

Perez C, Liauger J, Puig J, Palmer J (1989) Computed tomographic findings in bowel ischemia. Gastrointest Radiol 14:241–245

Philpotts LE, Heiken JP, Westcott MA, Gore RM (1994) Colitis : use of CT findings in differential diagnosis. Radiology 190:445–449

Rhamouni A, Mathieu D, Golli M et al (1992) Value of CT and sonography in the conservative management of acute splenorenal and superior mesenteric venous thrombosis. Gastrointest Radiol 17:135–140

Rhee RY, Gloviczki P, Mendonca CT et al (1994) Mesenteric venous thrombosis : still a lethal disease in the 1990 s. J Vasc Surg 20:688

Scholz FJ (1993) Ischemic bowel disease. Radiol Clin North Am 31:1197–1218

Siegelman SS, Sprayregen S, Boley SJ (1974) Angiographic diagnosis of mesenteric arterial vasoconstriction. Radiology 122:533–540

Sivit CJ, Taylor GA, Bulas DI, Kushner DC, Potter BM, Eichelberger MR (1992) Posttraumatic shock in children : CT findings associated with hemodynamic instability. Radiology 182:723–726

Smerud MJ, Johnson CD, Stephens DH (1989) Diagnosis of bowel infarction. AJR 154:99–103

Taourel PG, Fabre JM, Pradel JA et al (1995) Value of CT in the diagnosis and management of patients with suspected acute small-bowel obstruction. AJR Am J Roentgenol 165:1187–1192

Taourel PG, Deneuville M, Pradel JA, Regent D, Bruel JM (1996) Acute mesenteric ischemia : diagnosis with contrast-enhanced CT. Radiology 199:632–636

Toursarkissian B, Thompson RW (1997) Ischemic colitis. Surg Clin North Am 77:461–469

Zeman RK, Baron RL, Jeffrey RB, Klein J, Siegel MJ, Silverman PM (1998) Helical body CT : evolution of scanning protocols. AJR Am J Roentgenol 170:1427–1438

37 Synthesis: Impact of Spiral CT on Imaging of the GI Tract and Comparison with Other Imaging Modalities

D. Vanbeckevoort, L. Van Hoe, G. Verswijvel

CONTENTS

37.1   Introduction   407
37.2   Esophagus   407
37.3   Stomach   408
37.4   Small Bowel   410
37.5   Colon   412
37.6   Cost Effectiveness   413
37.7   Conclusion   414
        References   414

37.1
Introduction

Technological advances in CT have changed the practice of abdominal radiology. Traditionally, barium studies and fiberoptic endoscopy were the first examinations ordered in the evaluation of patients with suspected diseases of the bowel.

Today, with the introduction of spiral CT scanners, the work-up of these patients is being reconsidered. Although conventional barium studies and endoscopy remain superior to CT for evaluating intraluminal and mucosal disease, CT is far more accurate for evaluating the intramural and extraintestinal components, including the mesentery, peritoneal cavity, retroperitoneum, and solid organs (Balthazar 1991). Moreover, virtual endoscopy has emerged as a potential noninvasive alternative to both barium studies and endoscopy, at least for screening studies. In this chapter, the role of spiral CT in the investigation of the different parts of the GI tract is briefly reviewed.

D. Vanbeckevoort, MD; Department of Radiology, University Hospital Gasthuisberg, Herestraat 49, B-3000 Leuven, Belgium
L. Van Hoe, MD; Department of Radiology, University Hospital Gasthuisberg, Herestraat 49, B-3000 Leuven, Belgium
G. Verswijvel; Department of Radiology, University Hospital Gasthuisberg, Herestraat 49, B-3000 Leuven, Belgium

37.2
Esophagus

The value of conventional CT for staging of esophageal cancer remained controversial for a long time (Quint et al. 1985; Vilgrain et al. 1990). Some authorities have advocated CT as an effective decision-making tool, whereas others have rejected the ability of CT to stage esophageal cancer accurately (Halvorsen et al. 1987; Vilgrain et al. 1990).

Spiral CT outperforms conventional CT for several reasons: for example, the differentiation of vascular structures and lymph nodes is optimized, data gaps are avoided, and images can be calculated in an overlapping fashion. Thus, spiral CT leads to improved tumor staging and to earlier detection of tumor recurrence. It is especially valuable for demonstrating invasion of the trachea by tumor (Fig. 37.1). Multiplanar reconstructions give a better understanding of complex anatomical relationships (Fishman 1997).

Spiral CT also plays a fundamental part in selection of the most appropriate type of treatment (surgical versus nonsurgical, curative versus palliative) and in evaluation of the response to treatment (Van Hoe et al. 1997). In many medical centers a multimodal approach including chemotherapy and radiation therapy prior to surgery is used to treat esophageal carcinoma. In these cases, CT has a key role in assessment of the initial tumor bulk for radiation therapy planning and is useful in monitoring tumor response to cytoreductive therapy. However, CT does not always allow a distinction between a recurrent or residual neoplasm and changes resulting from radiation.

For optimal staging of esophageal carcinoma, endoscopic US is complementary to spiral CT. This technique depicts the different layers of the esophageal wall better and defines the degree of mural penetration by the tumor more precisely (Wojtowycz et al. 1995).

Another application of (spiral) CT is the evaluation of upper GI bleeding. Esophageal varices (Fig. 37.2) are usually easily detected and may be

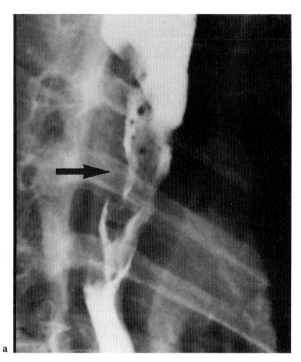

a

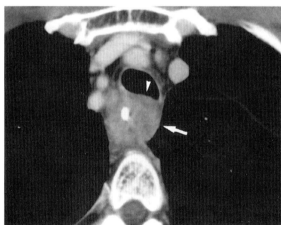

b

Fig. 37.1a, b. Primary squamous cell carcinoma of proximal esophagus with invasion of the trachea and mediastinum. **a** Esophagogram shows a large infiltrating tumor mass with severe narrowing of the esophageal lumen (*arrow*). **b** CT demonstrates marked circumferential but asymmetric esophageal wall thickening (*arrow*), indenting the posterior wall of the trachea inward (*arrowhead*). Fat planes surrounding the esophagus are obliterated

displayed by using the volume rendering technique (VRT) or maximum intensity projections (MIPs; Fishman 1997).

In the esophagus, CT allows localization and characterization of intramural and extramural esophageal lesions that appear submucosal on conven-

tional barium studies or endoscopy, such as esophageal leiomyomas. However, CT does not always allow differentiation between leiomyoma and leiomyosarcoma.

Currently, there is no clear evidence that CT plays any substantial part in the evaluation of esophagitis and disorders of the esophageal motility, such as achalasia and scleroderma. Esophagography and endoscopy remain the initial examinations in these conditions.

37.3
Stomach

The stomach is involved by a spectrum of pathologic processes ranging from inflammatory and infectious diseases to benign and malignant tumors.

Traditionally, CT has been used for better demonstration of a pathologic process shown up or suggested by conventional barium studies or endoscopy (Scatarige and DiSantis 1989; Kleinhaus and Militinau 1984; Fig. 37.3). CT not only clearly demonstrates the primary pathologic condition but also shows extension of the disease to adjacent or distant structures.

Nowadays, however, CT is being used routinely as the primary imaging technique in patients in whom abdominal pathology is suspected on the basis of clinical findings. In some of these cases, gastric dis-

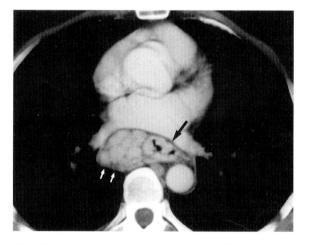

Fig. 37.2. Contrast-enhanced scan through the subcarinal space demonstrates enlarged, tortuous mediastinal varices (*small arrows*). The esophagus is partially distended by air and has a nodular appearance due to enlarged, submucosal, contrast-filled varices (*large black arrow*)

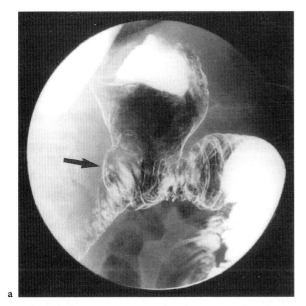

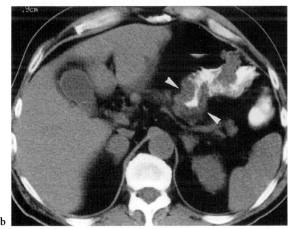

contrast material. Following the intravenous injection of contrast material, spiral CT provides a better assessment of the enhancement pattern of the gastric mucosa and the underlying gastric wall layers. As a result, tumors are commonly detected by CT even before conventional barium studies or endoscopy have been performed (ZEMAN et al. 1995).

Useful in detecting and staging gastric cancer, CT has also proved valuable in planning radiation fields and in assessing response to therapy (HUSBAND et al. 1996). NAKAJIMA et al. (1994) even used CT for the assessment of lymph node volume during chemotherapy in patients with inoperable advanced carcinoma.

CT has been shown to be valuable in the detection and differentiation of gastric conditions such as benign tumors, infections with *Helicobacter pylori* and other bacteria, various forms of gastritis (radiation, eosinophilic and emphysematous), ulcers, Ménétrier disease and varices (FISHMAN et al. 1996).

Following partial gastrectomy, CT plays an important role in the evaluation of early postoperative complications and in the detection of tumor recurrence (Fig. 37.5).

In the future, the respective role of endoscopic ultrasound and CT in evaluating the stomach will need to be further explored; however, CT is a cost-effective study and will remain an important imaging tool. Adequate gastric distention is essential for successful gastric CT.

Fig. 37.3 a, b. Metastatic carcinoma in a patient with a gastrojejunostomy for gastric ulcer. **a** Upper gastrointestinal tract examination demonstrates a tumor mass (*arrow*) at the gastrojejunal anastomosis. **b** CT scan shows an asymmetric circumferential thickening of the wall of the gastric stump near the anastomosis (*arrowheads*). Endoscopic biopsy revealed a metastatic large lung cell carcinoma

ease is first noted on the CT scan and may never have been considered in the clinical differential diagnosis before the CT examination (THOMAS et al. 1995). Recent advances in CT technology, such as spiral CT coupled with the use of water or a gas-producing agent to opacify the stomach with negative contrast, suggest that the value of CT in these applications will increase (Fig. 37.4).

Spiral CT performs better than conventional CT, owing to the optimized administration of iodinated

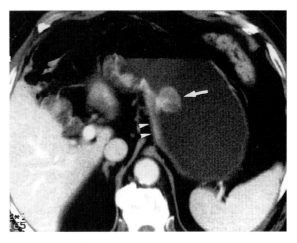

Fig. 37.4. Inflammatory pseudopolyp in a patient with a Billroth II gastrojejunostomy. CT scan using water as an oral contrast agent shows a pedunculated polyp (*arrow*) with adjacent thickening of the gastric wall (*arrowheads*)

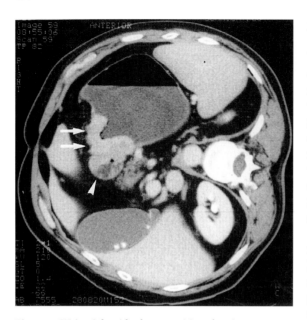

Fig. 37.5. CT in right-side-down position showing recurrent cancer following gastric resection (Billroth II) for carcinoma. The tumor encases the wall of the gastrojejunal anastomosis (*arrows*) and invades the adjacent duodenal loop (*arrowhead*)

37.4
Small Bowel

Radiologic imaging continues to play an important role in the diagnosis and management of diseases of the small bowel. The mesenteric small intestine remains the only gastrointestinal tract segment for which diagnostic study is not principally dependent on endoscopic viewing (LAPPAS 1992).

Barium contrast studies, particularly enteroclysis, remain the primary diagnostic methods in the small bowel for most clinical indications. CT often provides unique diagnostic information in patients with unusual or nonspecific complaints, unexplained bleeding, or clinical suspicion of disease undetected by barium studies.

Intestinal Obstruction. The diagnosis of small bowel obstruction is usually made on the basis of clinical signs and patient history. Plain abdominal films are used for confirmation (MUCHA 1987). If the latter are not diagnostic, or if the clinical picture is confusing, barium studies are usually performed.

CT has been shown to be useful in revealing the site, level, and cause of obstruction and has been increasingly used in patients with gastrointestinal obstruction (GAZELLE et al. 1994; FRAGER et al. 1994;

MAGLINTE et al. 1993; RUBESIN and HERLINGER 1991). In a series of 167 patients, the presence of bowel obstruction (based on findings of discrepant caliber between proximal and distal bowel) was correctly diagnosed in 60 patients using CT (94% sensitivity) and its absence, in 99 patients (96% specificity), yielding an overall accuracy of 95% (MEGIBOW et al. 1991). The cause of obstruction was predicted in most cases (73%). Evidence of a mass at the transition zone from dilated to nondilated bowel allowed an accurate diagnosis of a neoplastic etiology (Fig. 37.6), whereas the absence of specific focal findings suggested the presence of adhesions.

CT is a relatively expensive examination; therefore, guidelines for its rational use should be established. CT is most useful in patients with a history of abdominal malignancy and clinical symptoms suggestive of bowel obstruction (MEGIBOW et al. 1991). CT has a secondary role in postsurgical patients without cancer, who most probably have adhesive

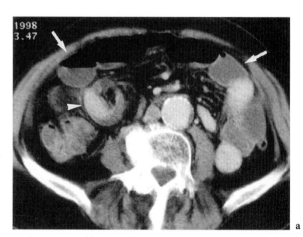

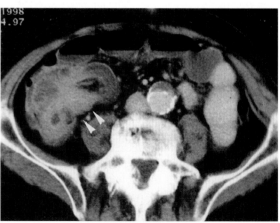

Fig. 37.6a, b. Obstruction caused by malignant tumor of terminal ileum with ileocolic intussusception. CT shows fluid-filled, distended small bowel loops (*arrows*) and a thick-walled, distal ileum invaginating into the colon (*arrowheads*)

obstruction. In addition, as noted by Rubesin and Herlinger, the relative advantages of CT and enteroclysis in the diagnosis of small bowel obstruction may well depend on the grade, duration, site, and cause of obstruction. CT is likely to be preferred to barium studies for evaluating long-lasting chronic obstruction associated with hypoperistalsis or high-grade obstruction, or in cases complicated by bowel infarction, in which prompt surgery is anticipated. In intermittent small bowel obstructions, enteroclysis is advocated because the luminal distension associated with this technique facilitates demonstration of low-grade obstructing lesions, especially adhesions (RUBESIN and HERLINGER 1991).

The role of CT in the diagnosis of bowel obstruction is evolving. Thanks to the volumic acquisition of data, spiral CT allows better imaging of the transition zone between dilated and nondilated intestinal segments, thereby helping to determine the cause of small bowel obstruction. Ciné display of data facilitates image analysis in these cases.

The impact of CT (versus barium enema studies) on the management of patients with obvious clinical symptoms of bowel obstruction remains to be defined.

Neoplasms. Neoplasms of the small intestine are uncommon and remain a difficult challenge for the clinician owing to their nonspecific clinical presentation. CT is an efficient and contributory tool in their diagnosis. In the past 10 years, the role of CT has expanded considerably. CT is much more accurate than conventional barium studies for evaluating the intramural and extraintestinal components of tumor. In known neoplastic disorders, CT provides additional information about tumor extension into the mesentery or adjacent organs and the presence of nodal or hepatic metastases (Fig. 37.7).

Conversely, conventional barium studies remains superior to CT for evaluating intraluminal and mucosal tumors. Barium examinations and CT should therefore be regarded as complementary techniques (COSCINA et al. 1986).

Sets of volumic data yielded by spiral CT allow for a detailed display of complex anatomical structures, which may enhance the ability to detect intestinal cancer. Similarly, optimizing vascular enhancement is important in defining the extent of tumor involvement, thus resulting in more accurate staging.

Inflammatory Disease. In adults, the clinical value of abdominal CT in the evaluation of inflammatory bowel disease is well established (LAPPAS 1992). CT,

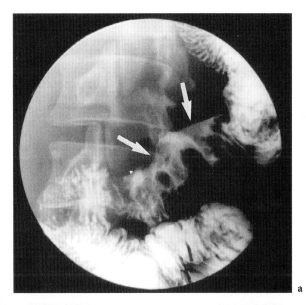

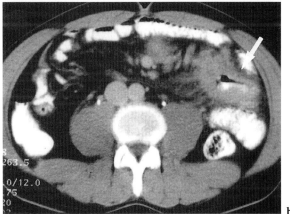

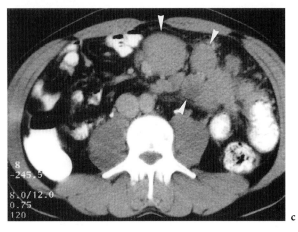

Fig. 37.7 a–c. Lymphoma in a patient with AIDS. **a** Small bowel series demonstrating the presence of a large ulcerated mass (*arrows*) in the jejunum without proximal obstruction. **b, c** Marked segmental wall thickening. Dilated lumen with wall ulceration (*arrow*), and several soft tissue masses (*arrowheads*) are seen in the adjacent mesentery on CT

by virtue of its superior contrast resolution and ability to directly image the bowel wall, lymph nodes, and surrounding mesentery, provides an important and often unique diagnostic perspective and therapeutic tool in the evaluation and management of these patients (BALTHAZAR 1986; FRAGER et al. 1983; GORE et al. 1985).

Conventional barium examinations remain superior to CT for evaluating intraluminal and mucosal disease. CT therefore should not be regarded as competing with, but as complementing, barium examinations of the gastrointestinal tract (BALTHAZAR 1991).

In a study of a large number of patients with clinically symptomatic Crohn's disease, CT demonstrated significant, previously unsuspected findings that led to a change of medical and surgical management in 28% of cases (FISHMAN et al. 1987). Additionally, CT proved reliable in confirming or excluding complications suggested clinically or by barium studies (FISHMAN et al. 1987; Fig. 37.8).

Following administration of intravenous contrast material, the enhancement pattern of the intestinal mucosa and underlying layers can be assessed with spiral CT. The clinical use of this technique is still under evaluation, but some authors have seen evidence of mucosal hyperemia owing to inflammatory bowel disease (ZEMAN et al. 1995).

The CT findings appear quite similar to those reported regarding bowel enhancement on MR imaging using paramagnetic contrast media (SEMELKA et al. 1991).

37.5
Colon

The role of CT in the evaluation of the colon is usually focused on neoplastic diseases. This technique provides useful information in the preoperative staging of patients with known colonic carcinoma. It has been shown that spiral CT increases the detection of metastatic disease (particularly in the liver), and improves the definition of tumor extent, thereby allowing more accurate staging of colon cancer. Optimization of contrast enhancement of vessels is useful in detecting small lymph node metastases, particularly in patients with primary tumors in the sigmoid and/or rectum, because these small nodules are more easily differentiated from the strongly enhanced vascular structures.

For the detection of colon carcinoma, barium enema and colonoscopy are still the primary techniques.

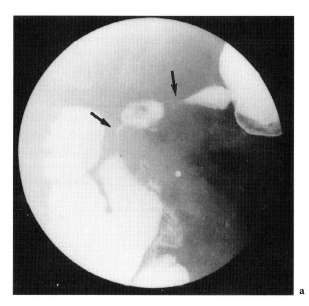

a

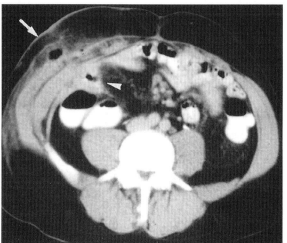

b

Fig. 37.8a, b. Recurrent Crohn's disease after partial right hemi-colectomy. a Small bowel follow-through study. Note marked luminal narrowing of the neo-terminal ileum with ulcerations typical of Crohn's disease (*black arrows*). b CT scan. The extent of the disease in the anterior abdominal wall (*arrow*) and the relationship of the abscess to the small bowel is better appreciated on CT (*arrowhead*)

Colon carcinomas almost invariably arise from pre-existing adenomatous polyps. There appears to be a lag time of 3–5 years between development of a colonic polyp and malignant degeneration of that polyp into colorectal cancer (CLARK et al. 1985). Removal of the polyp during this lag time eliminates the risk of malignant degeneration, and thus the risk of colon cancer (LIEBERMAN 1994).

A new technology called virtual colonoscopy shows great promise in detecting colon polyps and cancer, far less invasively than some current meth-

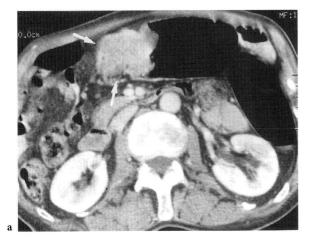

a

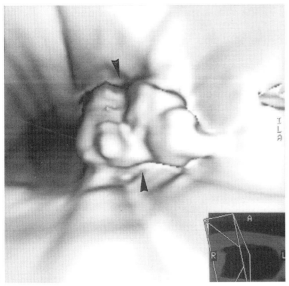

b

Fig. 37.9a, b. Nonstenotic adenocarcinoma of the transverse colon. **a** Axial scan shows a large tumor mass (*arrows*). **b** Virtual endoscopic image provides an intraluminal perspective and enables visualization of the surface of the polypoid tumor mass (*arrowheads*)

ods (Fig. 37.9). The procedure takes no more than a few minutes. The patient lies on the CT scan table. The colon is filled with air through a small tube placed into the rectum. The whole abdomen is imaged continuously and gapless using spiral technique. A computer program then reconstructs "endoscopic" images based on the CT data. This program enables the clinician to "fly" through the colon. In comparison with 'conventional' colonoscopy, virtual colonoscopy offers several advantages, which are mainly related to the noninvasive nature of this diagnostic tool.

However, virtual colonoscopy has not yet been tested against the current standard technique (colonoscopy) on a large scale. Such studies are necessary before virtual colonoscopy can be considered a valuable alternative for screening. MR colonoscopy is also a competing technique in this regard. Based upon the data of 23 patients, LUBOLDT et al. (1998) found a 100% sensitivity of MR colonoscopy in the detection of lesions larger than 10 mm, and 70% in lesions ranging between 5 and 10 mm.

After resection of rectal cancer (i.e. abdominal-perineal resection), spiral CT is ideal for follow-up and to plan radiotherapy in case of recurrence.

Finally, in the detection and evaluation of colitis, spiral CT can successfully define the degree of wall thickening and pericolic inflammation as well as the actual venous thrombosis in ischemic colitis (FISHMAN 1997). In patients with well-localized abscesses (Fig. 37.10), CT-guided percutaneous drainage helps to reduce morbidity associated with surgery.

37.6
Cost Effectiveness

Using current technology, spiral CT of the abdomen produces reproducible, high resolution images without motion artifacts in less than 10 min. CT can be cost effective if it can provide sufficient information to obviate more expensive diagnostic or surgical procedures. For example, TAOUREL et al. (1992) showed in France that the use of CT in the diagnosis of patients with an acute abdominal syndrome

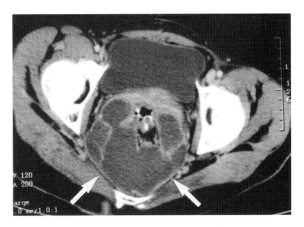

Fig. 37.10. Partial colectomy with colo-anal J-pouch. CT scan. Posterior and lateral to the pouch a low-density mass with an enhancing rim (*arrows*) represents a postsurgical abscess. Under CT guidance, the abscess was successfully drained percutaneously

modified the primary therapeutic strategy in 30% of cases and avoided a certain number of laparotomies. Appendiceal CT has also been shown, in a study performed in the United States, to be a cost-effective technique in the evaluation of patients with suspected acute appendicitis (Rao et al. 1998). It should be mentioned, however, that the results of these studies cannot be automatically extrapolated to other countries. In Europe, focused US will continue to be the primary diagnostic test in patients with acute right fossa pain.

CT can also be cost effective if it can replace a less expensive but less effective diagnostic test. For example, HULNICK et al. (1984) found that in patients with colonic diverticulitis, CT was preferable for demonstrating the extent of pericolic inflammation, which was underestimated with contrast enema in 41% of patients.

37.7
Conclusion

Although CT is established as one of the best-performing techniques for imaging of the gastrointestinal tract, it should be used selectively and in close cooperation between clinicians and radiologists. In many cases, CT may be complementary to more 'classic' studies such as barium examinations and endoscopy. The continuing development of techniques for image processing in virtual endoscopy will probably cause a dramatic change in the role of the different techniques: it is likely that cross-sectional modalities will be used not only for cancer staging but also for screening. Whether the technique of choice will be spiral CT or MRI remains an open question.

References

Balthazar EJ (1986) Colon. In: Megibow AL, Balthazar EJ (eds) Computed tomography of the gastrointestinal tract. Mosby, St. Louis, pp 279–386
Balthazar EJ (1991) CT of the gastrointestinal tract: principles and interpretation. AJR 156:23–32
Clark JC, Collan Y, Eide TJ, Esteve J, Ewen S, Gibbs NM, Jensen OM, Koskela E, Maclennan R, Simpson JG et al (1985) Prevalence of polyps in an autopsy series from areas with varying incidence of large-bowel cancer. Int J Cancer 36:179–186
Coscina WF, Arger PH, Levine MS et al (1986) Gastrointestinal tract focal mass lesions: role of CT and barium evaluations. Radiology 158:581–587
Fishman EK (1997) Spiral CT: clinical applications in the gastrointestinal tract. Clin Imaging 21(2):111–121
Fishman EK, Wolf EJ, Jones B et al (1987) CT evaluation of Crohn's disease: effect on patient management. AJR 148:537–549
Fishman EK, Urban BA, Hruban RH (1996) CT of the stomach: spectrum of disease. Radiographics 16:1035–1054
Frager DH, Goldman M, Beneventano TC (1983) Computed tomography in Crohn's disease. J Comput Assist Tomogr 7:819–824
Frager DH, Medwid SW, Baer JW, Mollinelli B, Friedman M (1994) CT of small-bowel obstruction: value in establishing the diagnosis and determining the degree and cause. AJR 162:37–41
Gazelle GS, Goldberg MA, Wittenberg J, Halpern EF, Pinkney L, Mueller PR (1994) Efficacy of CT in distinguishing small bowel obstruction from other causes of small-bowel dilatation. AJR 162:43–47
Gore RM, Cohen MI, Vogelzang RL, Neiman HL, Tsang TK (1985) The value of computed tomography in the detection of complications of Crohn's disease. Dig Dis Sci 30:701–709
Halvorsen RA Jr, Thompson WM (1987) Computed tomography staging of gastrointestinal tract malignancies. I. Esophagus and stomach. Invest Radiol 22:2–16
Hulnick DH, Megibow AJ, Balthazar EJ, Naidich DP, Bosniak MA (1984) Computed tomography in the evaluation of diverticulitis. Radiology 152:491–495
Husband JE, Nicolson VM, Minty I, Bamias A. (1996) CT evaluation of treatment response in advanced gastric cancer. Clin Radiol 51:215–220
Kleinhaus U, Militinau D (1984) Computed tomography in the preoperative evaluation of gastric carcinoma. Gastrointest Radiol 13:97–101
Lappas JC (1992) Small bowel imaging. Curr Opin Radiol 4(III):32–38
Lieberman D (1994) Screening /early detection model for colorectal cancer. Why screen? Cancer 74:2023–2027
Luboldt W, Steiner P, Bauerfeind P, Pelkonen P, Debatin JF (1998) Detection of mass lesions with MR-colonography: preliminary report. Radiology 207:59–65
Maglinte DD, Gage SN, Harmon BH, Kelvin FM, Hage JP, Chua GT, Ng AC, Graffis RF, Chernish SM (1993) Obstruction of the small intestine: accuracy and role of CT in diagnosis. Radiology 188:61–64
Megibow AJ, Balthazar EJ, Cho KC, Medwid SW, Birnbaum BA, Noz ME (1991) Bowel obstruction: evaluation with CT. Radiology 180:313–318
Mucha P (1987) Small intestinal obstruction. Surg Clin North Am 67:597–562
Nakajima T, Ishihara S, Motohashi H et al (1994) Neo-adjuvant chemotherapy for inoperable gastric cancer via local and general delivery routes (FLEP Therapy). In: Banzet P, Holland JF, Khayat D et al (eds) Cancer treatment: an update. Springer, Berlin Heidelberg New York, p 411
Quint L, Glazer G, Orringer M, Gross B (1985) Esophageal carcinoma: CT findings. Radiology 155:161–175
Rao PM, Rhea JT, Novelline RA, Mostafavi AA, McCabe CJ (1998) Effect of computed tomography of the appendix on treatment of patients and use of hospital resources. N Engl J Med 338(3):141–146
Rubesin SE, Herlinger (1991) CT evaluation of bowel obstruction: a landmark article: implications for the future. Radiology 180:307–308

Scatarige JC, DiSantis DJ (1989) CT of the stomach and duodenum. Radiol Clin North Am 27:687–706

Semelka RC, Shoenut JP, Silverman R et al (1991) Bowel disease: prospective comparison of CT and 1,5 T pre- and postcontrast MR imaging with T1-weighted fat-suppressed and breath-hold FLASH sequences. JMRI 1:625–632

Taourel P, Baron MP, Pradel J, Fabre JM, Seneterre E, Bruel JM (1992) Acute abdomen of unknown origin: impact of CT on diagnosis and management. Gastrointest Radiol 17:287–291

Thomas VIL, Cohen AJ, Wile AG (1995) CT detection of unsuspected gastric neoplasms. Appl Radiol 25:29–36

Van Hoe L, Van Cutsem E, Vergote I, Bellon E, Dupont P, Baert AL, Marchal G (1997) Size quantification of liver metastases in patients undergoing cancer treament: reproducibility of uni-, bi-, and three-dimensional measurements determined with spiral CT. Radiology 202:671–675

Vilgrain V, Mompoint D, Palazzo L et al (1990) Staging of esophageal carcinoma: comparison of results with endoscopic sonography and CT. AJR 155:277–281

Wojtowycz AR, Spirt BA, Kaplan DS, Roy AK (1995) Endoscopic US of the gastrointestinal tract with endoscopic, radiographic, and pathologic correlation. Radiographics 15:735–753

Zeman RK, Silverman PM, Cooper C, Weltman DI, Ascher SM, Patt RH (1995) Helical (spiral) computed tomography. Implications for imaging the abdomen. Gastroenterol Clin North Am 24):183–199

Abdominal Aorta and its Branches

38 Aorta and Visceral Arteries

M. Prokop

CONTENTS

38.1   Introduction   419
38.2   Examination Technique   420
38.3   Abdominal Aortic Aneurysms   420
38.3.1 Classification of AAA   421
38.3.2 Suspected Perforation of AAA   421
38.3.3 Inflammatory AAA   423
38.3.4 Planning of Surgery or Stent Grafting of AAA   424
38.3.5 Display Modes   425
38.4   Aortic Dissection   426
38.4.1 Abdominal Malperfusion   426
38.4.2 Display Modes   428
38.5   Occlusive and Inflammatory Diseases
        of the Aorta   429
38.5.1 Aortic Stenosis   429
38.5.2 Aortic Hypoplasia and Midaortic Syndrome   429
38.5.3 Leriche's Syndrome   429
38.5.4 Aortitis   430
38.6   Postoperative Findings   430
38.6.1 Endovascular Interventions   430
38.6.2 Abdominal Bypass Grafts   432
38.7   Pelvic Arteries   432
38.8   Visceral Arteries   432
38.8.1 Anatomic Variants   432
38.8.2 Tumor Involvement   433
38.8.3 Aneurysms   433
38.8.4 Celiac and Mesenteric Stenoses   434
38.8.5 Liver Transplantation   434
38.9   Renal Arteries   434
38.9.1 Renohypovascular Hypertension   434
38.9.2 Quantification of Stenoses   435
38.9.3 Display Modes   436
38.9.4 Living Renal Donors   437
38.9.5 Uretopelvic Junction Obstruction   437
38.10   Conclusion   437
        References   438

38.1 Introduction

Since the first applications of CT angiography (CTA) in the abdomen have been published (NAPEL et al. 1992a, b), CTA has become an established technique for minimally invasive imaging of the aorta and the renal and visceral arteries (Table 38.1). CTA can substitute for conventional angiography or intraarterial DSA for most diagnostic questions in the abdomen (BLUEMKE and CHAMBERS 1995). In many respects, it is in direct competition with Doppler ultrasound and MRA.

CTA is a highly reliable problem-solving tool for acutely ill patients with acute abdominal hemorrhage (UDEKWU et al. 1996), ruptured aortic aneurysms (HOLLAND et al. 1995), or abdominal side branch involvement in aortic dissection (PROKOP et al. 1993; KOEHLER et al. 1994; ZEMAN et al. 1995). It reliably detects acute or chronic aortic occlusion or postoperative complications of abdominal vascular surgery or radiologic interventions (BRINK 1997; RUBIN et al. 1994). CTA is an integral part of therapy planning in stent grafting of abdominal aneurysms (BALM et al. 1997; ARMON et al. 1998b; MARIN et al.

MATHIAS PROKOP, MD; Allgemeines Krankenhaus der Stadt Wien, Universitätsklinik für Radiodiagnostik, Abteilung Radiologie für konservative Fächer, A-1090 Wien, Austria

Table 38.1. Indications for CT angiography in the abdomen

Aortic aneurysm	Suspected rupture Planning of stent grafting / surgery Follow-up, suspected complications
Aortic dissection	Suspected abdominal malperfusion Planning of intervention / surgery Follow-up, suspected complications
Aortic stenosis / occlusion	Planning of intervention / surgery
Renal arteries	Suspected renovascular hypertension Planning of intervention / surgery Living renal donors: preoperative evaluation
Visceral arteries	Preoperative anatomy: hepatic arterial supply Staging of pancreatic cancer: vascular involvement Aneurysms, stenoses: planning of intervention / surgery Bypass grafts: suspected complications

1998), but may also be used to solve most preoperative questions in the abdominal vasculature (BROEDERS et al. 1998).

In patients with suspected renovascular hypertension, CTA may be used as a screening test and as a tool for optimizing subsequent intraarterial DSA and angioplasty of renal artery stenoses (KAATEE et al. 1996, 1997; POSTMA et al. 1997; PROKOP et al. 1997a). CTA can also be used as a minimally invasive single test for the preoperative evaluation of potential renal donors (RUBIN et al. 1995; COCHRAN et al. 1997; POZNIAK et al. 1998).

Using the data from the arterial phase of a biphasic liver CT, one is able, preoperatively, to determine the anatomy of the arterial supply of the liver and detect pathology of the celiac artery and the superior mesenteric artery (WINTER et al. 1995a, 1996; HOWLING et al. 1997; KOPECKY et al. 1997; SOUDACK et al. 1999). Similarly, the arterial phase of a biphasic pancreatic exam can be used to detect tumor encasement or invasion of the upper abdominal arteries (ZEMAN et al. 1994a; YOSHIMI et al. 1995).

The evaluation of peripheral vascular branches, in polyarteriitis nodosa for example, is not a proven indication for abdominal CTA. The same holds true for the detection of the anterior spinal artery prior to major thoraco-abdominal surgery. Here, the spatial resolution of CTA is not sufficient and arteriography remains the standard diagnostic imaging procedure.

38.2
Examination Technique

Evaluation of the aorta is technically simple and generally does not require elaborate scanning techniques. It can be done even with slow scanners that require 1.5 s or more for one revolution of the X-ray tube. The visceral and renal arteries require a more elaborate examination technique because the vessels of interest are small and often run parallel to the scan plane. However, good diagnostic results can also be obtained with slow scanners, even though the quality of 3D representations may not be prefect. Present advances, such as multirow detector systems with subsecond scanning, will lead to a dramatic improvement in image quality in all imaging planes and will allow for evaluation of vessels with less than 1 mm diameter.

CTA of the abdominal aorta should start above the celiac axis and should include the proximal iliac arteries, preferentially including the iliac bifurca-

tions. A low-dose pre-contrast scan is advisable to detect involvement of the thoraco-abdominal aorta and the iliac arteries and to adjust the scan range accordingly. The long scan range requires a high table speed and may thus lead to a reduced z-axis resolution. To overcome this limitation, a total scan time of 40–60 s should be used if available. Owing to this increased scan time, however, the intravascular contrast level close to the end of the examination may fall significantly. However, since the pelvic and femoral arteries run almost perpendicular to the scan plane in many patients, the diagnostic evaluation will almost never be hampered.

Even for a large effective slice thickness, identification of accessory renal arteries is reliably possible on transaxial images, given a reconstruction increment of ≤2 mm. Slice collimation should not exceed 5 mm and may even be reduced to 3 mm (PROKOP et al. 1997a) or below (VAN HOE et al. 1996). Larger collimations suppress fine detail and yield inferior results, especially for the assessment of renal or visceral artery stenoses. In CTA of the visceral arteries, detection of stenoses is the most critical imaging task and requires the smallest effective slice thickness possible. Therefore, some authors have suggested performing dual scans, with a high spatial resolution at the level of the abdominal side branches and a lower resolution below (ZEMAN et al. 1994b; VAN HOE et al. 1996; BROEDERS et al. 1998) if both the aortoiliac system and the visceral arteries have to be examined.

Table 38.2 gives an overview by scanner type of suggested scan parameters for the abdominal aorta, the renal and visceral arteries, and combined examination of the thoracoabdominal vasculature.

38.3
Abdominal Aortic Aneurysms

Abdominal aortic aneurysms (AAA) are a relatively common finding in the elderly population. In patients with marked arteriosclerotic disease, prevalence may range between 6% and 20%. Arteriosclerosis is also the most common cause of AAA. Other etiologies such as cystic media necrosis, mycotic origin or aortic dissection are much less frequent. Traumatic aneurysms are rare and usually due to direct trauma (shot gun or stab wounds). Most aneurysms are fusiform. Therapy is initiated if the size of an aneurysm exceeds 4–5 cm. The risk of rupture increases steadily with larger size of the aneurysms: if

Table 38.2. Suggested scanning techniques for CTA of the abdomen [*n* detector rows (*n*=2: split detector, *n*=4: multirow detector), *L* scan length, *TI* scan time, *SC* slice collimation / single detector width, *TF* table feed per rotation (TF / SC = pitch), *RI* reconstruction interval, *V* volume of contrast medium + saline flush, *F* flow rate; start delay is determined by test bolus or bolus triggering]

	n	L	TI	SC	TF	RI	V	F
Abdominal aorta								
1-s scanner	1	36 cm	60 s	3	6	2	150+75 ml	3 ml/s
1-s scanner	2	40 cm	50 s	2	8	2	150+75 ml	3.5 ml/s
0.5-s scanner	4	40 cm	33 s	1	6	1	120+60 ml	4 ml/s
Thoraco-abdominal aorta								
1-s scanner	1	60 cm	60 s	5	10	3	150+75 ml	3 ml/s
1-s scanner	2	60 cm	60 s	2.5	10	2	150+75 ml	3 ml/s
0.5-s scanner	4	60 cm	20 s	2.5	15	1.5	100+50 ml	5 ml/s
Renal / visceral arteries								
1-s scanner	1	12 cm	40 s	2	3	1	150+75 ml	4 ml/s
1-s scanner	2	15 cm	25 s	2	6	1	120+60 ml	4 ml/s
0.5-s scanner	4	20 cm	13 s	1	6	0.7	100+50 ml	5 ml/s

the aneurysm exceeds 10 cm, the risk approaches 60% (BLANKENSTEIJN et al. 1998). Saccular aneurysms often are of mycotic etiology and tend to grow faster. In the case of saccular aneurysms (cf. Fig. 38.10) surgery may be indicated earlier and is thus determined on an individual basis.

38.3.1
Classification of AAA

Aneurysms are classified according to their spatial relationship to the renal arteries (suprarenal, perirenal and infrarenal) since this determines whether an interventional radiological treatment is possible or a surgical approach is necessary (VAN HOE et al. 1996; BALM et al. 1997; WALTER et al. 1998). With involvement of renal or visceral arteries or with too short a distance of the AAA from the renal arteries a surgical treatment with re-implantation of the arteries in the graft becomes necessary. The involvement of the iliac arteries (ARMON et al. 1998a) determines whether a straight or Y-shaped graft will be implanted and whether a radiological intervention is feasible: in general, at least one internal iliac artery has to be preserved to ensure sufficient perfusion of the pelvic organs. For the purpose of radiological stent grafting, various classification schemes have been suggested (DORROS et al. 1997; SCHUMACHER et al. 1997).

38.3.2
Suspected Perforation of AAA

In acutely ill patients with AAA, the primary goal is to search for signs of perforation. A pre-contrast scan is mandatory for this indication.

Hemorrhage usually presents with streak-like densities in the para-aortic fat, which may extend into the paranephric space and the rest of the retroperitoneum, the root of the mesentery or even the peritoneal cavity. Cases of intraperitoneal hemorrhage may present with an isodense to hyperdense 'ascites' (i.e. fresh blood or hemorrhagic fluid). Various layers of density may form as (hemoglobin-rich and thus hyperdense) blood cells sediment posteriorly. A pure retroperitoneal hemorrhage is less life-threatening than a hemorrhage that has penetrated into the abdominal cavity (SATTA et al. 1997). Penetration into a bowel loop (usually the horizontal part of the duodenum) is rare and results in massive gastrointestinal hemorrhage. Penetration into the inferior vena cava is exceedingly rare and will lead to a massive shunt with rapid cardiac decompensation.

Hyperdense regions within a hematoma are relatively infrequent and occur mainly in subacute cases with repeated bleeding and enough time for blood clot formation. Fresh blood is usually isodense to the surrounding vessels since there is no separation between blood cells and serum (Fig. 38.1). Isodense hemorrhage can be considered a sign of hyperacute bleeding and requires rapid surgery in most cases.

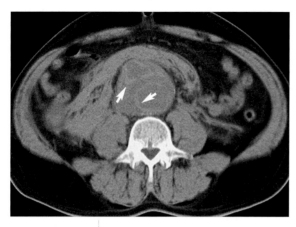

Fig. 38.1. Ruptured abdominal aortic aneurysm: the extravasated fresh blood on the pre-contrast scan is almost isodense to the soft tissues. This indicates a lack of clot formation and thus acute bleeding. The hyperdense lines within the aneurysm indicate fresh thrombus that marks the borders of the perfused lumen (*arrows*)

Since the indications for surgery depend upon the detection of an acute hemorrhage in the presence of an AAA, a contrast-enhanced CT angiogram is only indicated if the patient is hemodynamically stable and there is enough time to perform the examination. Usually less than 5 min is required to finish a contrast run in this situation. Since CTA may offer the surgeons important information, such as the presence of a retroaortic left renal vein (Fig. 38.2a) and the relation of the aneurysm to the renal and iliac arteries (Fig. 38.2b), we suggest performing a CTA whenever

the clinical situation of the patient allows it (BLUEMKE and CHAMBERS 1995; ERRINGTON et al. 1997; FITZGERALD and SPENCE 1996; HOLLAND et al. 1995; RUBIN et al. 1993). It is rare, however, to detect the site of rupture (Fig. 38.3) even if late scans are performed, and such an observation is often unreliable.

Direct trauma often causes saccular false aneurysms. Collateral damage to other abdominal organs and the vertebral column may occur (Fig. 38.4). Contrast-enhanced (late) scans are especially helpful for detecting contusions or lacerations in parenchymal organs.

Contained perforations are relatively frequent and may present as an incidental finding in the course of the work-up of an AAA. The typical sign is a soft-tissue dense or slightly hypodense, often rounded formation close to the aorta. This region corresponds to an old thrombus or partially resolved blood clot (Fig. 38.5).

Signs of impending rupture are minimum streak-like paraaortic densities (initial hematoma), a hyperdense rim in the periphery of the aneurysm (non-contrast-enhanced scans; c.f. Fig. 38.1), and perfused areas within the thrombosed peripheral portion of an aneurysm, which also are often found in perforated aneurysm (Fig. 38.6).

Most of the work-up for acute perforation of AAA does not depend on the use of CTA. However, the planning of surgery may be much improved if reliable information about the position of renal and visceral arteries relative to the aneurysm is available

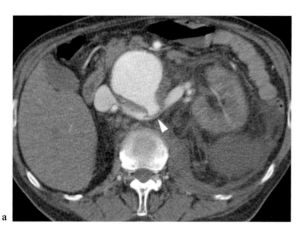

a

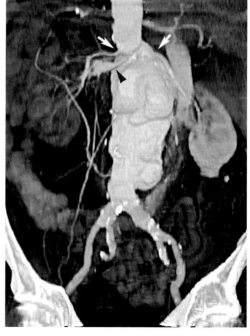

b

Fig. 38.2a, b. CT angiography in a patient with a ruptured aortic aneurysm provides important information for surgery: the axial sections (**a**) demonstrate a retroaortic renal vein (*arrowhead*) at the level of the aneurysm, while the volume-rendered image viewed from posterior (**b**) demonstrates involvement of the renal arteries (*arrows*), a hypoperfusion of the left kidney, and the highly obstructed retroaortic left renal vein (*arrowhead*)

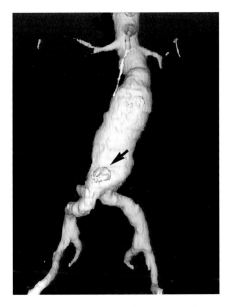

Fig. 38.3. CTA in a ruptured aortic aneurysm demonstrates the site of extravasation (*arrow*). Owing to hypoperfusion of the kidneys, the distal branches of the renal arteries and the kidney parenchyma do not exceed the chosen threshold level and are thus not displayed on the SSD of the aorta

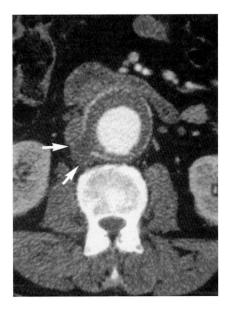

Fig. 38.5. In this patient with a known aortic aneurysm and abdominal pain, the axial image shows a blood clot next to the aorta (*arrows*), indicating a contained rupture. Note interruption of the aortic wall calcifications

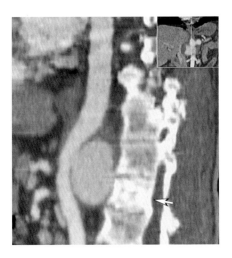

Fig. 38.4. Shotgun injury with traumatic saccular aortic aneurysm. Note the fracture of the adjacent vertebra (*arrow*)

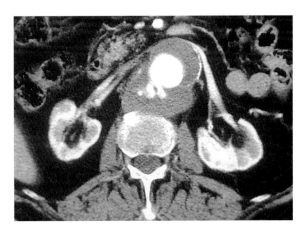

Fig. 38.6. In this contained rupture, signs that indicate an increased risk for perforation can be detected: there is an irregular and eccentric outpouching of the perfused lumen, an interruption of the calcifications of the aortic wall, and a large prevertebral thrombus

and the involvement of the aortic bifurcation and the iliac arteries is known. These questions can be easily and quickly answered using CTA.

38.3.3
Inflammatory AAA

Inflammatory aneurysms are characterized by a fibrous inflammatory reaction in the periaortic

tissues and may be related to retroperitoneal fibrosis.

They lead to a thickened aortic wall usually 0.5–1.5 cm wide. The thickening may be asymmetric or totally symmetric (Fig. 38.7). The aortic wall takes up contrast on a late scan phase. A single cut at a representative level is usually sufficient to confirm the late contrast enhancement. Often, however, the periaortic thickening may be readily appreciated on CTA scans even though no significant amount of contrast enhancement may yet be present in the arterial phase (Fig. 38.7). Calcifications of the aortic wall or wall-adherent thrombi within the AAA may be present. The inflammatory reaction may rarely involve adjacent bowel loops (increased risk of visceral hemorrhage) or may present similar findings to those in retroperitoneal fibrosis, including medialization and compression of the ureters (LACQUET et al. 1997).

With inflammatory AAA, it is important to determine the exact cranial to caudal extent of aortic involvement to facilitate preoperative planning. Surgical therapy often partially or completely resolves the inflammatory reaction. Radiologic stent grafting does not appear to be helpful. Steroid treatment may be effective to decrease inflammatory changes (STELLA et al. 1993).

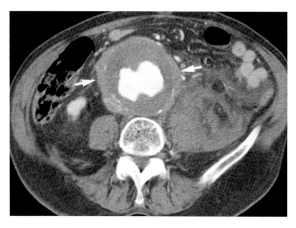

Fig. 38.7. Inflammatory aneurysms are characterized by a concentric or eccentric extraaortic rim of soft tissue (*arrows*) that becomes hyperdense after contrast administration. Note the wall calcifications internal to the soft tissue rim

38.3.4
Planning of Surgery or Stent Grafting of AAA

Again, the most important questions are the size, type and relationship of the aneurysm to the abdominal side branches (COSTELLO and GAA 1995; FITZGERALD and SPENCE 1996; MORITZ et al. 1996; MAY et al. 1996; ERRINGTON et al.1997; ARMON et al. 1998a).

Other important factors are the presence of accompanying stenoses of abdominal arteries (ERRINGTON et al 1997). Stenoses of the renal arteries require re-implantation or dilatation prior to surgery or radiological intervention. Stenoses of the superior mesenteric artery (Fig. 38.8) or the celiac artery may have serious effects if the origin of the inferior mesenteric artery is occluded during therapy: chronic ischemia with abdominal angina or even acute ischemic complications (left hemicolon, in 1.5%) may evolve if collateral pathways to the inferior mesenteric artery are cut off. Stenoses of the internal iliac arteries are only relevant if bilateral or if the other internal iliac artery has to be occluded during stent graft treatment.

For radiological interventions, the distance from the neck of the aneurysm to the renal arteries should (at present) exceed 1 cm (MARIN et al. 1998). Depending on the involvement of the aortic bifurcation or the iliac arteries either a straight stent graft or a bifurcated graft are implanted (FITZGERALD and SPENCE 1996; BALM et al. 1997; ARMON et al. 1998a, b). For exact planning of the size (diameter, length, noncovered proximal and distal portions) of the stent graft, measurements of a large number of distances has to be performed (BROEDERS et al. 1997; DORROS et al. 1997). New automated techniques that

a
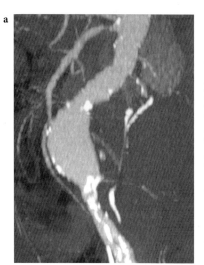
b
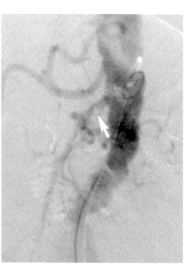

Fig. 38.8a, b. Stenosis of the superior mesenteric artery in a patient with AAA seen best on a lateral MIP (**a**): this finding was originally missed on preoperative angiography but subsequently proven by repeated DSA (*arrow*) (**b**)

measure the aortic diameter (both perfused and total lumen) and iliac diameter are presently being developed (RUBIN et al. 1998)

The measurements of diameters should be performed on multiplanar reformats perpendicular to
the aortic axis. Measurements of the length of the
graft may be difficult, especially in two scenarios:
kinking of the aorta (curved reformats may become
necessary) or very large aneurysms in which the
stent graft tends to move to the far side (usually anterior wall) of the aneurysm. Here, the necessary
length may be underestimated if the shortest distance from the neck to the distal end of the aneurysm is measured.

Maximum intensity projections (MIP) or shaded
surface displays (SSD) give a good overview of the
anatomic situation but are prone to projection effects that may lead to incorrect results. Distances between aneurysm and renal arteries may be underestimated, but never be overestimated on MIP or SSD
(DORFFNER et al. 1997).

38.3.5
Display Modes

Diagnosis of AAA and most related complications is
based on axial sections. Diameter and length measurements should be performed on (curved) reformats perpendicular or parallel to the aortic axis. All
two-dimensional cuts allow for a discrimination between perfused aortic lumen, thrombotic material,
wall calcifications or periaortic inflammatory reactions.

Three-dimensional displays such as MIP, SSD or
volume rendering techniques (VRT) are most helpful for presenting the findings to the referring physicians. 3D displays correlate well with intraoperative findings (GOMES et al. 1994; BROEDERS et al.
1998).

SSD require high intravascular contrast, thin sections and minimum noise for optimum results. They
have the advantage of an excellent anatomic orientation and generally do not require prior editing of the
skeleton (Fig. 38.9). They are especially helpful in
complex situations, such as in saccular aneurysms or
pronounced aortic kinking. Their disadvantage is
the strong dependence of the image on the chosen
threshold. This may lead to problems with aortic
side branches, such as renal and visceral arteries that
may seem stenosed or even occluded if too high a
threshold or too wide a section thickness have been
chosen.

MIP have an angiography-like appearance and
are excellent for detecting calcified plaques (Fig.
38.10). They are most helpful in simple fusiform
infrarenal aneurysms. They lack threshold-depen-

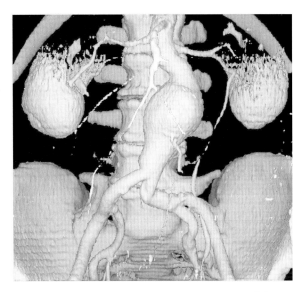

Fig. 38.9. Infrarenal AAA: excellent representation of the extent of the aneurysm and its relation to the branching vessels
(shaded surface display). The quality of the display depends
heavily on scan parameters, contrast enhancement and size
of branching vessels. Here, 3-mm slice collimation, 5-mm
table feed and 2-mm reconstruction increment were used

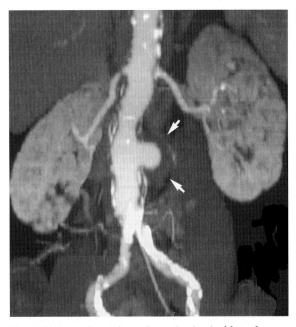

Fig. 38.10. A maximum intensity projection is able to demonstrate the calcified plaques as well as the perfused aortic lumen. If a narrow width of the displayed subvolume is used
even the thrombosed portion of the saccular aneurysm can
be seen (*arrows*). Also note the bilateral renal artery stenoses

dence and are able to display smaller vessels to better advantage. However, a host of other artifacts may occur (PROKOP et al. 1997b) that have to be kept in mind when interpreting those images. Also, removal of skeletal structures is necessary in order to obtain AP projections of the aorta and its side branches. This may require lengthy editing, depending on the available software. With modern algorithms, however, editing time can be cut down to 5 min or less.

VRT combines the advantages of both MIP and SSD (cf. Fig. 38.2): given correct opacity curves, a distinction between foreground and background is possible, calcifications may be visualized, and even small vessels can be accurately depicted (MARCUS et al. 1997). VRT, however, is a complex procedure that requires powerful computers and software for good results to be obtained within a reasonable amount of time.

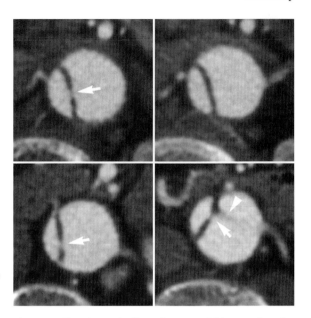

Fig. 38.11. Chronic aortic dissection: on axial images the relation of small branching vessels relative to the true and false channel can be determined. Note that there are holes in the membrane at or slightly below the level of arteries that arise from the false lumen (*arrows*). The reason for these holes is that the intimal flap has detached from the renal ostium. If there is incomplete detachment a web-like intimal flap may be detected in the false lumen (*arrowhead*)

38.4
Aortic Dissection

Aortic dissections are presently classified according to the Stanford criteria: involvement of the ascending aorta or aortic arch is classified as type A dissection, while dissections limited to the descending or abdominal aorta are type B dissections. Type A dissections require rapid surgical intervention, while a conservative approach is possible with type B disease.

For the imaging of abdominal aortic dissection, CTA is superior to angiography in most cases, because it allows for direct visualization of the intimal flap and thrombosed regions. Even small accessory renal arteries can be attributed to the true or false channel (Fig. 38.11). Owing to its higher spatial resolution and its insensitivity to flow artifacts, CTA is often superior to MRA with respect to small branching arteries and thrombus in the false lumen. CTA is ideal for monitoring of chronic dissection and for assessment before elective surgery (KOEHLER et al. 1994; PROKOP et al. 1993). In acute dissections, CTA is the fastest noninvasive imaging modality and has a high diagnostic yield (SOMMER et al. 1996; ZEMAN et al. 1995).

CTA reliably assesses the presence and course of one or even multiple intimal flaps with respect to branching arteries. Spatial resolution is often sufficient to detect the hole in the membrane at the site of a vessel that has detached from the intimal flap and now originates from the false channel (Fig. 38.11).

Aortic cobwebs are anatomic markers of the false lumen: they occur if fibrous bands within the aortic wall stay attached both to the intimal flap and to the outer portion of the wall (Figs. 38.11d, 38.13a). Their detection has become possible with spiral CTA. In iatrogenic dissection, CTA provides a noninvasive tool for assessing entry site and complications.

There is no general consensus as yet on whether an abdominal CTA should be performed routinely in every case of suspected acute dissection or whether a thoraco-abdominal examination is only necessary if there are abdominal symptoms, leg ischemia or laboratory signs of organ malperfusion.

38.4.1
Abdominal Malperfusion

The primary focus in acute dissection is the ascending aorta in order to rule out type A dissection. Abdominal involvement is relatively common in type A and type B disease but has rarely any therapeutic consequences. Organ malperfusion is the main reason for performing an abdominal examination in the acute setting. Malperfusion of the kidneys may lead to renal failure, and malperfusion of the celiac or mesenteric arteries may lead to bowel ischemia or liver damage if there is insufficient collateralization or two arterial territories are involved simultaneously. Organ malperfusion or leg ischemia requires rapid surgical or radiological intervention. Usually some type of aortic fenestration is performed, during which part of the dissection membrane is resected (HEINEMANN et al. 1994) or perforated and dilated via a transfemoral radiological approach (WILLIAMS et al. 1997).

Signs of organ malperfusion may develop in the subacute phase of an aortic dissection. CTA is indicated to prove this suspicion. It also serves as the most important technique to guide interventional treatment, since it is able to directly visualize the location and orientation of the dissecting membrane, the relative size of the two channels, the presence of thrombotic material, and often also preexistent holes in the dissecting membrane (Fig. 38.11) that may be dilated further instead of requiring needle perforation of an intact portion of the membrane.

Organ malperfusion can be suspected if the true or false channel is highly compressed or even thrombosed, or if the contrast enhancement of the dependent vascular territory is reduced (Fig. 38.12). Typically, the true channel is compressed anteriorly at the

origin of the celiac and superior mesenteric arteries (Figs. 38.12, 38.13). Bowel ischemia may present with decreased contrast medium uptake or with edematous swelling of the bowel wall or gas within the bowel wall (Fig. 38.13c). Splenic infarcts are rare. Liver perfusion may be decreased if both the mesenteric artery, and thus the portal venous flow, and the celiac artery, and thus the hepatic arterial flow, are obstructed. Clinical symptoms (rising lactate levels, abdominal pain) together with compression of the inflow have to be taken as serious indicators of malperfusion. Extension of the dissecting membrane into an abdominal side branch with formation of a blind sac in the false channel may also lead to arterial stenosis or even occlusion and is the most frequent cause of renal malperfusion or leg ischemia (usually at the level of the iliac arteries). In the renal arteries, intimal flaps that have not completely detached from the arterial orifice (Fig. 38.11) may lead to a (temporal) malperfusion of the artery.

Optimum assessment of the renal arteries, requires thin sections (of 3-mm collimation or less). With single-row spiral CT scanners this is only possible if just the abdominal aorta and not the entire thoraco-abdominal aorta has to be covered. In the latter cases, a wider collimation has to be used (Table 38.2) that may hamper direct evaluation of the side branches . However, the indirect signs, such as decreased contrast enhancement or difference in enhancement between right and left kidney, may help. With split detector scanners or newer, multirow detector scanners, 2.5 mm or even 1 mm collimation will become available for thoraco-abdominal CTA (Table 38.2).

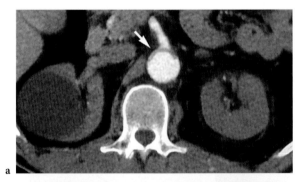
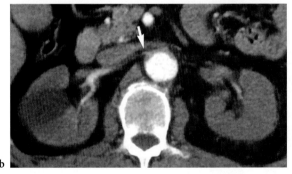

Fig. 38.12. Acute aortic dissection type B: the anteriorly located true channel is highly compressed (*arrows*). The renal arteries arise from this channel, which causes a severe malperfusion of both kidneys: virtually no contrast enhancement is present

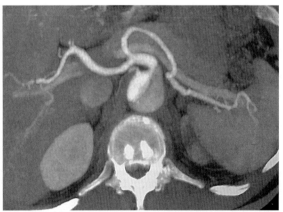

Fig. 38.14. Chronic aortic dissection type A: an axial MIP demonstrates differential opacification of both channels and the intimal flap, which is starting to extend into the orifice of the celiac artery

38.4.2
Display Modes

Transaxial sections are the primary display modality for assessment of vascular diameter, intimal flap, entry and re-entry sites, and perfusion of the true and false channels (Figs. 38.12, 38.13). MIP images are helpful to demonstrate the overall shape of the aorta and differential opacification of the channels (Fig. 38.14). MIP, however, only show the intimal flap if the viewing direction is parallel to the flap (Fig. 38.15a). SSD images may sometimes be advantageous for comprehensive display (Fig. 38.15b). Virtual angioscopy with perspective volume rendering may provide additional information in complex dissections with multiple entries and multiple membranes.

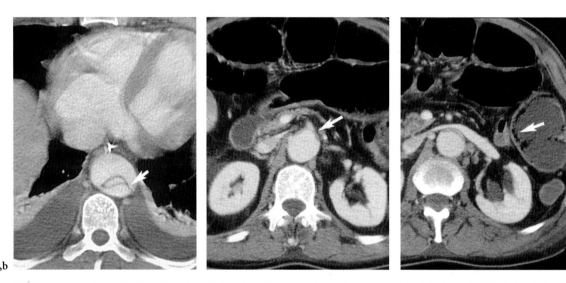

a,b   c

Fig. 38.13a–c. Acute aortic dissection type B: in this patient, there is an almost complete detachment of the intimal flap from the aortic wall at the level of the diaphragmatic hiatus. Note the web-like membrane (*arrow*) that attaches to both the true lumen and the aortic wall (**a**). Intraabdominally the true channel (*arrow*) is located anteriorly and is severely compressed at the level of the celiac artery and the superior mesenteric artery indicating the danger of abdominal malperfusion (**b**). Four days later, signs of gangrene with intramural gas (*arrow*) in small bowel loops developed (**c**)

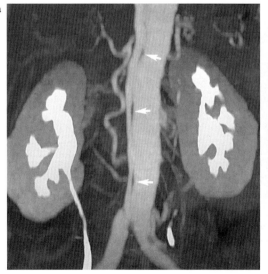

a

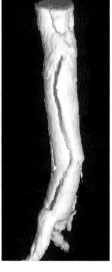

b

Fig. 38.15a, b. Chronic aortic dissection type B: MIPs are able to display the course of dissection only if the dissection membrane (*arrows*) runs perpendicular to the viewing plane (**a**). Shaded surface displays (**b**) may better demonstrate the dissection but high threshold values will have to be used in many cases. Thus, side branches often cannot be seen at all

38.5
Occlusive and Inflammatory Diseases of the Aorta

38.5.1
Aortic Stenosis

Aortic stenoses occur in the elderly as a consequence of severe arteriosclerosis, often accompanied by severe wall calcification (Fig. 38.16). Their typical location is in the infrarenal portion of the aorta. Soft and hard plaques are easily distinguished as the cause of an aortic stenosis. Thus, important information about the planning of radiological interventions is obtained (RUBIN et al. 1996b).

38.5.2
Aortic Hypoplasia and Midaortic Syndrome

Aortic hypoplasia is a congenital abnormality that usually involves both thoracic and abdominal portions of the aorta. Stenoses of more peripheral arteries or the pulmonary vasculature may be present.

In young patients aortic stenoses may also be due to the so-called midaortic syndrome, which has been attributed to fibromuscular changes of the aortic wall and main abdominal arteries (O'NEILL et al. 1995). Midaortic syndrome often involves the renal and visceral arteries. Inflammatory periaortic tissue such as is seen in inflammatory aneurysms or retroperitoneal fibrosis is not present.

For both indications, contrast-enhanced MRA should be preferred, since patients are young and radiation exposure is an issue.

38.5.3
Leriche's Syndrome

Leriche's syndrome is an acute occlusion of the aortic bifurcation, most often caused by an acute thrombosis on the basis of a severe arteriosclerotic aortic stenosis. An embolic etiology is less frequent. The diagnostic questions involve the location of the occlusion relative to the renal arteries, the presence of renal artery stenoses, and the demonstration of a suitable site for the distal anastomosis of a surgically implanted Y-graft.

A case of Leriche's syndrome is easily recognized, even on axial CT images. In acute Leriche's syndrome the occlusion is usually localized close to the aortic bifurcation. In the chronic state the aorta has often thrombosed right up to the orifices of the renal arteries (Fig. 38.17). Thrombotic and embolic occlu-

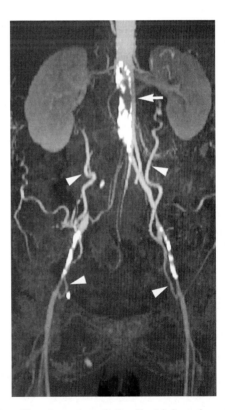

Fig. 38.17. Chronic aortic occlusion (Leriche's syndrome) with infrarenal thrombosis and calcification of the aorta. The MIP image shows extensive collaterals to the femoral circulation (*arrowheads*). Note the superimposing superior mesenteric artery (*arrow*)

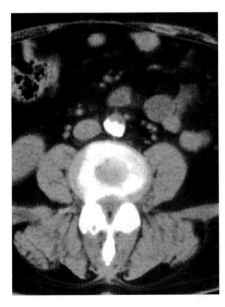

Fig. 38.16. Aortic stenosis (50%) due to massive calcified plaque seen on an axial pre-contrast image

sions can be distinguished if an intraluminal embolus is seen that usually presents as a partially occluding intraluminal lucency. In patients with acute emboli, the signs of aortic sclerosis are less pronounced. In chronic occlusion, there are extensive collaterals via the abdominal wall and the mesenteric arteries.

The simultaneous evaluation of the renal arteries and the proximal femoral arteries is not possible with older scanners. In this situation, DSA or contrast-enhanced MRA should be preferred. With subsecond scanners and multirow detector systems, CTA can answer all diagnostic questions with sufficient accuracy (Fig. 38.17). Multirow detectors will even allow for a simultaneous evaluation of the arterial system from the celiac artery down to the calves (100-cm scan length with 2.5-mm collimation in 33–53 s).

38.5.4
Aortitis

Takajashu's aortitis is a rare disease with a higher prevalence in the Asian population. It leads to a successive occlusion of thoracic, less frequently also of the abdominal arterial orifices. In clinically suggestive cases, CTA should be preferred even over arterial DSA, since involvement of the aortic wall can be detected earlier with CTA (PARK et al. 1997). Other causes of aortitis (e.g. giant cell arteritis) are possible but are indistinguishable from an imaging point of view.

Aortitis causes a concentric thickening of the aortic wall that has to be distinguished from circular thickening due to atheromatous plaques. This generally requires late scans in which contrast medium uptake in the aortic wall can be demonstrated. If Takayasu's disease is suspected, an additional CTA of the thoracic aorta and supraaortic branches should be scheduled at a later date.

38.6
Postoperative Findings

CTA is excellent for detecting any kind of postoperative complications (Figs. 38.18, 38.19), such as anastomotic aneurysms, perigraft perfusion, hemorrhage, graft occlusion or organ malperfusion (RUBIN et al. 1994b; BLUEMKE and CHAMBERS 1995; BRINK 1997). If a postoperative stenosis of an aortic side branch is suspected, however, the scan parameters have to be adapted to this task.

38.6.1
Endovascular Interventions

CTA is well suited to follow-up examinations after endovascular interventions, especially after implantation of endovascular stents (iliac, renal, or aortic stents) (RUBIN et al. 1994b; BRINK 1997; POSTMA et al. 1997). CTA proved to be equivalent to arteriography for evaluation of the luminal diameter and the outflow of stents. CTA is superior to arteriography for imaging the position of the stent in relation to

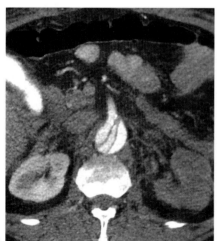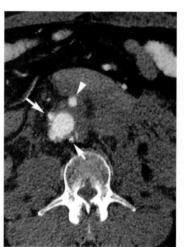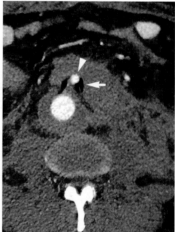

a,b   c

Fig. 38.18. Postoperative bleeding in a patient with an aortic dissection and malperfusion of the left kidney. An infrarenal aortic straight graft and a bypass graft (*arrowhead*) from the iliac artery to the left renal artery was inserted. CTA demonstrates postoperative air inclusions and small hyperdense Teflon patches (*arrows*) that were used to strengthen the suture sites

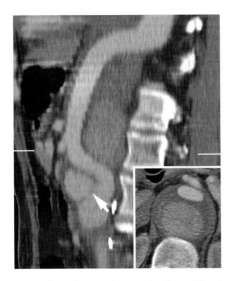

Fig. 19. Perigraft perfusion after repair of an abdominal aortic aneurysm: a graft was inserted into the aortic lumen and sutured to the wall proximally and distally ('graft inclusion' technique). A dehiscence of the distal anastomosis (*arrow*) has led to a perigraft perfusion with compression of the graft but no retroperitoneal hemorrhage

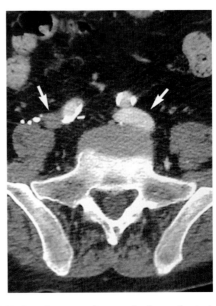

Fig. 38.20. Arteriovenous shunt at the femoral arterial puncture site: rapid unilateral filling of the left iliac vein can be noted. The iliac veins are indicated by arrows

the vessel course and to branching arteries (Rubin et al. 1994b). Reformats perpendicular to the stent show neo-intimal hyperplasia to best advantage. The efficiency of CTA for detection of extrinsic luminal compression, occlusion of aneurysms and displacement of intimal flaps is evident (Broeders et al. 1998).

Complications of angiographic interventions such as dissection, hemorrhage, vascular occlusion and arteriovenous shunting can be detected with CT angiography. Femoral arteriovenous fistulae lead to a typical early enhancement of the ipsilateral iliac vein and the inferior vena cava due to early perfusion with contrast-enhanced blood (Fig. 38.20).

After implantation of an aortic stent graft, CTA is the method of choice for follow-up (Fig. 38.21). CTA can demonstrate primary or secondary perigraft leaks (Broeders et al. 1998; White et al. 1998). These are most often due to persistent perfusion of a lumbar artery, the inferior mesenteric artery or an accessory renal artery (Fig. 38.22a). Perfused vessels can best be visualized using interactive cine viewing of axial sections. Displacement of the graft, dislocation of one leg of a Y-graft, stenosis of the graft lumen or even retroperitoneal hemorrhage are severe complication of the intervention that may require surgical repair (Fig. 38.22b). They can be best appreciated on axial images and multiplanar reformats.

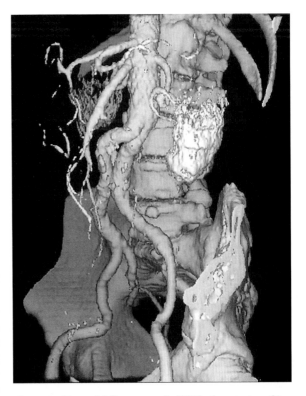

Fig. 38.21. Normal follow-up study (SSD) after stent grafting of an abdominal aortic aneurysm (AAA)

a 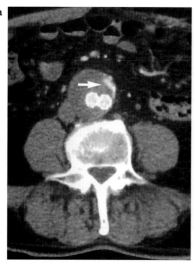 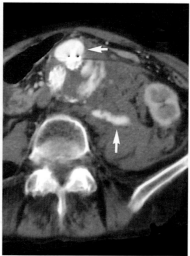 b

Fig. 38.22a, b. Complications after stent grafting of AAA: **a** small perigraft endoleak due to a perfused inferior mesenteric artery (*arrow*); **b** massive hemorrhage due to aortic rupture in another patient with dislocation of the distal leg of a bifurcated stent graft and a resulting endoleak (*short arrows*)

38.6.2
Abdominal Bypass Grafts

CTA can easily demonstrate patency after abdominal bypass grafts for revascularization of the renal or visceral arteries (MULLIGAN et al. 1992). Aneurysms or stenoses of the proximal and distal anastomoses can best be seen on multiplanar reformats. Bending of straight grafts may lead to membrane-like stenoses. These can best be appreciated on SSD or VRT. If no specific attention is paid to these findings, they can easily be missed.

38.7
Pelvic Arteries

Pelvic arteries are usually examined in combination with peripheral arteries, requiring a large volume to be covered. Although there are some reports in the literature (RICHTER et al. 1994; LAWRENCE et al. 1995; RAPTOPOULOS et al. 1996, RIEKER et al. 1997), this imaging task exceeds the volume that can be covered by CTA with reasonable spatial resolution and contrast volume if single-row detectors are used. Hence, indications for CTA of pelvic arteries are limited to the pre- and post-therapeutic assessment (RICHTER et al. 1994b). CTA is especially helpful after a nondiagnostic color Doppler exam and if arterial DSA does not allow for a transfemoral approach (bilateral grafts). MIP images excellently display arterial calcifications and may thus alter the interventional procedure (Richter et al. 1994b).

With the advent of multirow detectors, CTA of the whole abdomen, including the peripheral arteries of the leg, will become possible. Spatial resolution is excellent, with similar advantages over arteriography to those of MRA: vessels with a slow perfusion that are opacified late may be missed on DSA but are reliably demonstrated with MRA or new CTA techniques. Overlying veins and contrast timing may become a problem, although there are no hard data available yet.

38.8
Visceral Arteries

38.8.1
Anatomic Variants

Anatomic variants of the arterial supply of the upper abdominal organs occur in up to 50% of patients. The arterial phase of biphasic spiral CT examinations prior to partial liver resection or liver transplantation provides sufficient angiographic information for reliable assessment of anatomy and variants of hepatic arterial supply and accompanying arteriosclerotic changes in the visceral arteries (WINTER et al. 1995a, b). These examinations may serve as a preoperative splanchnic vascular mapping that reduces the need for additional risky, costly and time-consuming arteriograms.

The following constellations should alert the radiologist to the presence of a displaced visceral or an accessory hepatic artery:

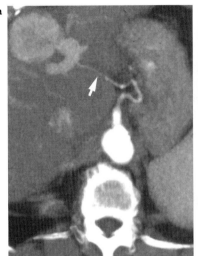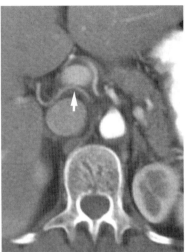

Fig. 38.23a, b. Anomalies of the hepatic arterial supply: an accessory / displaced left hepatic artery (*arrow*) running superior to the hepatic hilum and anterior to the caudate lobe (**a**), and an accessory / displaced right hepatic artery (*arrow*) running posterior to the portal vein (**b**)

1. A separate origin of branches of the celiac artery directly from the aorta.
2. An artery that runs between the caudate lobe and the left liver lobe cranial to the liver hilum: this is due to a displaced or accessory left hepatic artery that directly originates from the left gastric artery (Fig. 38.23a).
3. An artery posterior to the portal vein: this is due to a displaced or accessory right hepatic artery (Fig. 38.23b). Following the vessel in a proximal direction will allow for a discrimination between an origin directly from the celiac artery, from the SMA, from the aorta, or an early branching of the hepatic artery.
4. A displaced common hepatic or celiac artery can be suspected if there is a large and early right-sided branching vessels of the SMA. The vessel then runs posterior to the postal vein.

Accessory renal arteries occur in some 25% of the population. Most of these arteries arise from the aorta between the level of the superior mesenteric artery and the aortic bifurcation. An iliac or high aortic origin is exceedingly rare. As for the hepatic arteries, axial sections are the primary diagnostic mode. Thin-slab MIP may improve anatomic orientation. Only with dedicated thinly collimated CTA scans will SSD be able to depict smaller vessels. The display technique of choice is VRT: even tiny vessels can be demonstrated and high-quality images are obtained.

38.8.2
Tumor Involvement

In patients with abdominal tumors (e.g., pancreatic carcinoma) the preoperative assessment of vascular involvement is essential for planning the further treatment. Typical patterns are changes in diameter or a 'pad' effect on the surface of a vessel indicating tumor adherence (ZEMAN et al. 1994a; YOSHIMI et al. 1995) that may be demonstrated by 3D models of the vascular structures. Intraluminal filling defect, contour irregularities and resulting variations of vessel diameter are direct signs for tumor infiltration. If they are not present infiltration and adhesion may be impossible to differentiate. VRT is able to further improve display of findings (SMITH et al. 1998), although the primary axial data set still is the most essential diagnostic mode.

38.8.3
Aneurysms

Aneurysms of the aortic side branches are occasional incidental findings during CT angiography or the arterial phase of a biphasic examination of the upper abdomen. They are frequently associated with arteriosclerosis and with aortic aneurysms. Renal artery aneurysms are often congenital and are accompanied by stenoses. CTA can be used for preoperative assessment of the spatial relationship of aneurysm and branching vessels.

Large saccular aneurysms are easily detected already on axial images. Small aneurysms and fusi-

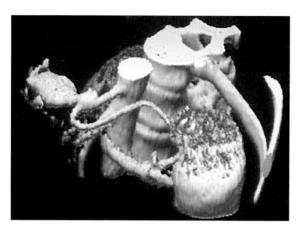

FFig. 38.24. Large aneurysm of the common hepatic artery with a second smaller aneurysm at the celiac bifurcation. The latter was missed on angiography owing to a suboptimum position of the catheter

form dilatations can be missed more easily. Aneurysms can have a calcified wall or wall-adherent thrombi. Large aneurysms may lead to compression effects. In renal aneurysms, the spatial relation to side branches and associated stenoses have to be described (cf. Fig. 38.26).

Thin-slab MIP are well suited for demonstrating simple aneurysms of celiac branches. 3D reconstructions (SSD, VRT) are better suited if the findings become more complex (Fig. 38.24) (HOWLING et al. 1997; NGHIEM and JEFFREY 1998; SOUDACK et al. 1999). They are especially important for planning of surgical reconstruction of the vasculature.

38.8.4
Celiac and Mesenteric Stenoses

A stenosis of the origin of the celiac artery is a relatively frequent incidental finding that is mainly caused by diaphragmatic compression by the median accurate ligament of the diaphragm (KOPECKY et al. 1997; DURE SMITH et al. 1998). Typical is a U-shaped celiac artery that is compressed by the diaphragm at the level of the aortic hiatus. This finding can best be appreciated on axial sections (oval shape of the compressed proximal portion of the celiac artery) and on lateral thin-slab MIP. The findings are accentuated during inspiration – which is used for almost all CT examinations of the upper abdomen.

Stenoses of the celiac artery (CA), superior mesenteric artery (SMA, cf. Fig. 38.8) or inferior mesenteric artery (IMA) become symptomatic if there is insufficient collateralization via the anastomosis of

Riolan (SMA/IMA) or gastroduodenal collaterals (CA/SMA). Abdominal angina is, thus associated by an increased frequency of combined stenoses of two vessels or tandem stenoses within one vessel.

Acute bowel ischemia should not be seen as an indication for CTA, although bowel wall edema or intestinal pneumatosis serves as an indirect CT sign and large occlusions may be visualized. Limitations of spatial resolution may mean that small occlusions are not detected. Since fast intervention is required, DSA appears to be the superior diagnostic method for this indication.

For the diagnosis of chronic ischemia with involvement of the main arteries color duplex sonography may be less costly and noninvasive. CTA is less accurate in detecting the less frequent peripheral stenoses. Since the presence of calcifications can be easily assessed, CTA is a potent imaging modality prior to operative revascularization.

38.8.5
Liver Transplantation

Malperfusion due to stenosis or occlusion of the hepatic artery, parenchymal damage, concomitant problems with the portal vein, and abscesses can all be evaluated with a biphasic liver CT that uses a thinly collimated protocol (3-mm collimation) for the arterial phase.

38.9
Renal Arteries

38.9.1
Renovascular Hypertension

Renal artery stenosis accounts for less than 5% of cases with arterial hypertension. Since treatment of renal artery stenosis may eliminate the need for antihypertensive medication, or reduce the amount needed, early detection of the disease is important. Since there is a very low prevalence of renal artery stenoses in the hypertensive population, a preselection based on clinical parameters (Table 38.3) is necessary to increase the prevalence of disease in the examined patient group. This way, the absolute amount of false-positive examinations is reduced. CTA can then be cost-effectively used as a screening tool (NELEMANS et al. 1998).

Table 38.3. Clinical symptoms of renal artery stenosis

Severe hypertension in a young patient
Unstable hypertension with hypertensive crises
Disrupted circadian rhythm
Rapid increase in blood pressure over a few months
Deterioration of hypertension after successful drug therapy
An insufficient response to a multi-drug regimen
Increase in renal retention parameters after angiotensin-
    converting enzyme inhibitors

38.9.2
Quantification of Stenoses

While detection of stenoses is reliably possible with CTA, quantification is hampered by partial volume effects (renal arteries run parallel or obliquely relative to the scan plane). The degree of stenosis is therefore estimated by classifying them according to a 4-point scale:

Grade I: 0–50%, nonsignificant
Grade II: 50–70%, hemodynamically significant
Grade III: 70–<100%, high-grade stenosis
Grade IV: 100%, occlusion

A post-stenotic dilatation of the renal artery suggests a significant stenosis rather than a nonsignificant stenosis or an occlusion (RUBIN et al. 1994a). Other collateral signs include a decreased size of one kidney, a delayed cortical enhancement (relative to the contralateral side) and a thinning of the renal cortex (Fig. 38.25) (BERG et al. 1998). Delayed enhancement should rely on the comparison of CT numbers of both kidneys at the same level relative to the z-axis (Fig. 38.26) and not relative to the anatomy.

Diagnosis of arterial occlusion relies on anatomy only: at least for a small portion of the renal artery, no opacified lumen must be detected on cross-sectional images or MIP. Almost always there is some degree of distal enhancement of the occluded renal artery due to collateral circulation (Fig. 38.25).

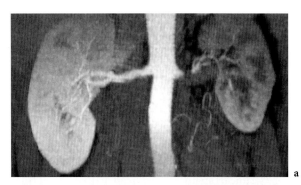
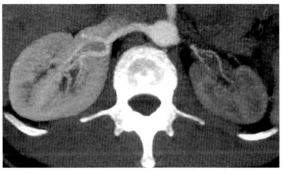

Fig. 38.25a, b. Occlusion of the left renal artery with retroperitoneal collaterals seen best on thin-slab MIP: **a** curved MIP of 7-mm width parallel to the course of the renal arteries; **b** axial oblique MIP of 20-mm width parallel to both renal arteries. Note the decreased size, the delayed cortical enhancement and the thinning of the cortex of the left kidney

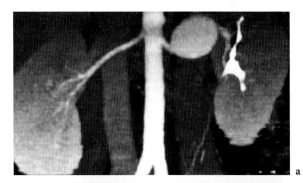
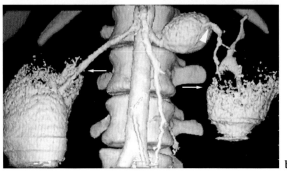

Fig. 38.26a,b. Large fusiform renal artery aneurysm. There is a stenosis of the renal artery as it leaves the aneurysm (*arrowhead*). This stenosis cannot be appreciated on the MIP (**a**) owing to superimposition of the contrast-enhanced aneurysm; only the post-stenotic dilatation is visible. The SSD (**b**) directly demonstrates the stenosis. Note that there is delayed parenchymal enhancement of the left kidney: the parenchyma exceeds the chosen threshold earlier (at a higher z-position) on the right side (*small arrows*)

Occlusion therefore must not be misinterpreted as a high-grade stenosis (GALANSKI et al. 1993). Post-stenotic dilatation is not present in cases of occlusion. Depending on the size of the postocclusive segment of the renal artery and the concomitant damage to the renal parenchyma, surgical revascularization may be considered.

Calcified hard plaques have to be distinguished from soft plaques that are hypodense and lie within the vascular lumen (Fig. 38.27). Proximal renal artery (truncal) stenoses have been distinguished from pseudotruncal ones that are caused by atheromatous plaques within the aorta and not within the renal arteries (KAATEE et al. 1996).

A second imaging plane (e.g., coronal or sagittal MIP or reformats) is necessary in most cases, since eccentric stenoses are possible. However, on MIP or multiplanar reformats, diaphragmatic movements during the scan may simulate stenoses, occlusions (Fig. 38.28) or aneurysmatic dilatation of vessels. It is therefore necessary to check for movement artifacts at the level of a suspected stenosis (discontinuities or deformation of the renal contours).

CTA is superior to arteriography for the quantification of eccentric stenoses (plaques at the anterior or posterior arterial wall) and for the discrimination between hard and soft plaques (probability of successful dilatation; Fig. 38.27). CTA is suited to the demonstration of accessory vessels or an atypical anterior origin of renal arteries. In cases in which a stenosis may be superimposed by other vessels such as the aorta or aneurysmatic dilatations (Fig. 38.26), CTA may be used to determine the optimum projection for subsequent renal angiography (VERSCHUYL et al. 1997). Intrarenal stenoses cannot be reliably detected but stenoses that are suited for interventional therapy can be found with sufficient accuracy.

38.9.3
Display Modes

CTA has been proven to be an excellent screening procedure for renal artery stenosis if CTA evaluation includes not only MIP or SSD images but also the primary transaxial data set. In a recent update (80 patients, 198 arteries) of our previous series (GALANSKI et al. 1993, 1994; OLBRICHT et al. 1996), we were able to demonstrate all accessory renal arteries (30 patients) using supraselective DSA as the gold standard (PROKOP et al. 1997a). We found a negative predictive value for significant stenosis (≥50%) of 97%. The sensitivity for the detection of any renal artery stenosis was 95%, while it was 99% for the detection of significant stenoses (≥50%). Over- or undergrading occurred only by one grade. The specificity was 93–95%.

In a series of 62 arteries, RUBIN et al. (1994a) found a sensitivity of 93% and a specificity of 83% when the diagnosis was based on MIPs, and a sensitivity of 59% and a specificity of 82% when the diagnosis was based on SSD images. Stenosis was accurately graded by MIPs in 80% and in only 55% by SSD. These findings underline the fact that diagnosis of CTA should include the primary data set and use 3D reconstructions as useful adjunct. HALPERN et al. (1995) showed that SSD is not suited for grading of renal artery stenosis: a threshold difference of 50 HU (80->130 HU) resulted in a vessel diameter alteration of 22%.

Hard and soft plaques are best evaluated on axial images and multiplanar reformats parallel and perpendicular to the vessel course. There is software available that semiautomatically tracks the vessel course. MIPs are most suitable for the presentation of findings. Not only antero-posterior views but also caudo-cranial projections may be helpful (Fig. 38.29).

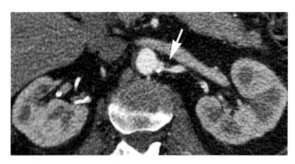

Fig. 38.27. CTA allows for a distinction between hard and soft plaques (*arrow*), and is superior to DSA for quantifying eccentric stenoses due to plaques at the anterior or posterior circumference of the renal arteries

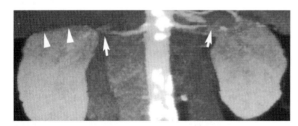

Fig. 38.28. Pseudo-occlusion (*arrow*) of both renal arteries due to breathing. Note that the breathing artifacts lead to irregular contours and flattening of the kidneys (*arrowheads*)

Evaluation of CTA relies on MIP with the thinnest possible subvolume to exclude as many overlying structures as possible. Findings are checked using an interactive cine display of axial sections and interactive multiplanar reformats. Instead of MIP, VRT may be used with the additional advantage that the course of the vessels can be demonstrated to better advantage.

38.9.4
Living Renal Donors

CTA is sufficient for preoperative evaluation of the anatomy of renal donors. SSD was superior to axial images in demonstrating perihilar branches (RUBIN et al. 1995). CTA also provides information about the presence of accessory or retroaortic renal veins. This information may be crucial as more explantation procedures are performed in a minimally invasive way using endoscopic techniques (FIGUEROA et al. 1997; PLATT et al. 1997; DACHMAN et al. 1998; SMITH et al. 1998). Here, CTA is superior over DSA in providing all the necessary preoperative information in one exam (RUBIN et al. 1995; FIGUEROA et al. 1997) and is at least equivalent to MRA (TOKI et al. 1998; TSUDA et al. 1998).

38.9.5
Ureteropelvic Junction Obstruction

With the advent of minimally invasive procedures, the precise preinterventional planning and selection of suitable patients become important. Ureteropelvic junction obstruction is usually treated with pyeloplasty. New endourologic procedures use balloon incision endopyelotomy to incise and dilate the obstructed region. This minimally invasive technique offers good success rates with shorter hospitalization, lower cost, and lower morbidity (HERTS 1998). The number of complications in these patients, however, may increase with the presence of vessels that cross at the level of the ureteropelvic junction. CTA provides an excellent visualization of vessels crossing anterior or posterior to the ureteropelvic junction and can substitute for more expensive techniques such as the combination of intravenous urography and intraarterial angiography (RUBIN 1996; HIRAYAMA et al. 1996; LEE et al. 1997; SIEGEL et al. 1997; NAKADA et al. 1998). If demanded by the local urologist, a post-contrast abdominal radiograph can be obtained after CTA.

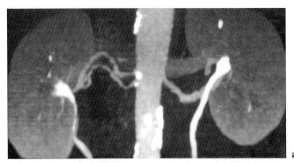

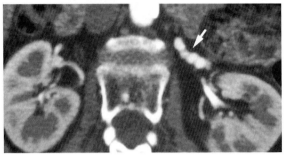

Fig. 38.29. Fibromuscular dysplasia: the MIP only demonstrates contour irregularities but does not allow for a definitive diagnosis of fibromuscular dysplasia (**a**). An axial oblique reformat excellently displays the membrane-like multiple stenoses (*arrows*) (**b**)

38.10
Conclusion

CTA is a minimally invasive problem-solving tool for many questions that concern vascular pathology in the abdomen. With a single examination, very often all questions relevant for diagnosis and patient management can be answered. Only few patients require further diagnostic work-up. CTA therefore is a powerful and cost-effective tool for vascular imaging that is especially suited for critically ill patients. CTA is readily available. Examination technique can be standardized and is simpler than that of competing technologies such as arterial DSA, Doppler ultrasound and contrast-enhanced MRA. Intraarterial DSA can be avoided as a primary diagnostic tool for most indications. MRA or Doppler ultrasound should be preferred in young patients due to the radiation exposure of CT, and in patients with severely impaired renal function due to the large amount of contrast agents necessary to provide optimum results.

With future multislice detectors for CT, near-isotropic imaging will be possible, with CTA providing an excellent spatial resolution in all directions. This technique can be expected to overcome many of the present limitations of CTA: accessory arteries will be displayed to better advantage, peripheral run-off angiographies will become possible within one run from the celiac axis down to the calves, the load of contrast media can be reduced and scan time (and thus, motion artifacts) will be further decreased.

References

Armon MP, Wenham PW, Whitaker SC, Gregson RH, Hopkinson BR (1998) Common iliac artery aneurysms in patients with abdominal aortic aneurysms. Eur J Vasc Endovasc Surg 15:255–257

Armon MP, Whitaker SC, Gregson RH, Wenham PW, Hopkinson BR (1998) Spiral CT angiography versus aortography in the assessment of aortoiliac length in patients undergoing endovascular abdominal aortic aneurysm repair. J Endovasc Surg 5:222–227

Balm R, Stokking R, Kaatee R, Blankensteijn JD, Eikelboom BC, van Leeuwen MS (1997) Computed tomographic angiographic imaging of abdominal aortic aneurysms: implications for transfemoral endovascular aneurysm management. J Vasc Surg 26:231–237

Berg MH, Manninen HI, Vanninen RL, Vainio PA, Soimakallio S (1998) Assessment of renal artery stenosis with CT angiography: usefulness of multiplanar reformation, quantitative stenosis measurements, and densitometric analysis of renal parenchymal enhancement as adjuncts to MIP film reading. J Comput Assist Tomogr 22:533–540

Blankensteijn JD, Lindenburg FP, Van der Graaf Y, Eikelboom BC (1998) Influence of study design on reported mortality and morbidity rates after abdominal aortic aneurysm repair. Br J Surg 85:1624–1630

Bluemke DA, Chambers TP (1995) Spiral CT angiography: an alternative to conventional angiography. Radiology 195:317–319

Brink JA (1997) Spiral CT angiography of the abdomen and pelvis: interventional applications. Abdom Imaging 22:365–372

Broeders IA, Blankensteijn JD, Olree M, Mali W, Eikelboom BC (1997) Preoperative sizing of grafts for transfemoral endovascular aneurysm management: a prospective comparative study of spiral CT angiography, arteriography, and conventional CT imaging. J Endovasc Surg 4:252–261

Broeders IA, Blankensteijn JD, Eikelboom BC (1998) The role of infrarenal aortic side branches in the pathogenesis of endoleaks after endovascular aneurysm repair. Eur J Vasc Endovasc Surg 16:419–426

Cochran ST, Krasny RM, Danovitch GM, Rajfer J, Barbaric ZM, Wilkinson A, Rosenthal JT (1997) Helical CT angiography for examination of living renal donors. AJR Am J Roentgenol 168:1569–1573

Costello P, Gaa J (1995) Spiral CT angiography of abdominal aortic aneurysms. Radiographics 15:397–406

Dachman AH, Newmark GM, Mitchell MT, Woodle ES (1998) Helical CT examination of potential kidney donors. AJR Am J Roentgenol 171:193–200

Dorffner R, Thurnher S, Youssefzadeh S, Winkelbauer F, Holzenbein T, Polterauer P, Lammer J (1997) Spiral CT angiography in the assessment of abdominal aortic aneurysms after stent grafting: value of maximum intensity projections. J Comput Assist Tomogr 21:472–477

Dorros G, Parodi J, Schonholz C, Jaff MR, Diethrich EB, White G, Mialhe C, Marin ML, Stelter WJ, White R, Coppi G, Bergeron P (1997) Evaluation of endovascular abdominal aortic aneurysm repair: anatomical classification, procedural success, clinical assessment, and data collection. J Endovasc Surg 4:203–225

Dure Smith P, Bloch RD, Fymat AL, Chang P, Hammond PG (1998) Renal artery entrapment by the diaphragmatic crus revealed by helical CT angiography. AJR Am J Roentgenol 170:1291–1292

Errington ML, Ferguson JM, Gillespie IN, Connell HM, Ruckley CV, Wright AR (1997) Complete pre-operative imaging assessment of abdominal aortic aneurysm with spiral CT angiography. Clin Radiol 52:369–377

Figueroa K, Feuerstein D, Principe AL (1997) A comparison of three-dimensional spiral computed tomoangiography with renal angiography in the live-donor work-up. J Transplant Coord 7:195–198

Fitzgerald EJ, Spence LD (1996) Pre-operative computed tomography in abdominal aortic aneurysms. Postgrad Med J 72:484–486

Galanski M, Prokop M, Chavan A, Schaefer CM, Jandeleit K, Nischelsky JE (1993) Renal arterial stenoses: spiral CT angiography. Radiology 189:185–192

Galanski M, Prokop M, Chavan A, Schaefer C, Jandeleit K, Olbricht C (1994) Leistungsfähigkeit der CT-Angiographie beim Nachweis von Nierenarterienstenosen. Rofo Fortschr Geb Roentgenstr Neuen Bildgeb Verfahr 161: 519–525

Gomes MN, Davros WJ, Zeman RK (1994) Preoperative assessment of abdominal aortic aneurysm: the value of helical and three-dimensional computed tomography; Discussion. J Vasc Surg 20:367–375; 375–376

Halpern EJ, Wechsler RJ, DiCampli D (1995) Threshold selection for CT angiography shaded surface display of the renal arteries. J Digit Imaging 8:142–7

Heinemann MK, Buehner B, Schaefers HJ, Jurmann MJ, Laas J, Borst HG (1994) Malperfusion of the thoracoabdominal vasculature in aortic dissection. J Card Surg 9:748–755

Herts BR (1998) Helical CT and CT angiography for the identification of crossing vessels at the ureteropelvic junction. Urol Clin North Am 25:259–269

Hirayama K, Kobayashi M, Yamaguchi N, Iwabuchi S, Gotoh M, Inoue C, Yamada S, Ebata H, Ishida H, Koyama A (1996) A case of renovascular hypertension associated with neurofibromatosis. Nephron 72:699–704

Holland BR, Freyschmidt J, Neumann S (1995) Spiral CT of ruptured abdominal aneurysms. Eur Radiol 5 [Suppl]:252 (SS 1258)

Howling SJ, Gordon H, McArthur T, Hatfield A, Lees WR (1997) Hepatic artery aneurysms: evaluation using three-dimensional spiral CT angiography. Clin Radiol 52:227–230

Kaatee R, Beek FJ, Verschuyl EJ, v d Ven PJ, Beutler JJ, van Schaik JP, Mali WP (1996) Atherosclerotic renal artery stenosis: ostial or truncal? Radiology 199:637–640

Kaatee R, Beek FJ, de Lange EE, van Leeuwen MS, Smits HF, van der Ven PJ, Beutler JJ, Mali WP (1997) Renal artery stenosis: detection and quantification with spiral CT angiography versus optimized digital subtraction angiography. Radiology 205:121–127

Koehler A, Prokop M, Heinemann M, Galanski M (1994) Spiral CT angiography in acute or chronic aortic dissection. Radiology 193(P):352

Kopecky KK, Stine SB, Dalsing MC, Gottlieb K (1997) Median arcuate ligament syndrome with multivessel involvement: diagnosis with spiral CT angiography. Abdom Imaging 22:318–320

Lacquet JP, Lacroix H, Nevelsteen A, Suy R (1997) Inflammatory abdominal aortic aneurysms. A retrospective study of 110 cases. Acta Chir Belg 97:286–292

Lawrence JA, Kim D, Kent KC, Stehling MK, Rosen MP, Raptopoulos V (1995) Lower extremity spiral CT angiography versus catheter angiography. Radiology 194:903–908

Lee JY, Chung JW, Kim SH, Cho SW, Park JH (1997) Proximal ureter obstruction caused by a lower polar renal artery: demonstration with spiral CT angiography. J Comput Assist Tomogr 21:641–642

Marcus CD, Ladam Marcus VJ, Gausserand FM, Menanteau BP (1997) CT angiography of aortoiliac disease with volumetric rendering technique. AJR Am J Roentgenol 168:1619–1620

Marin ML, Parsons RE, Hollier LH, Mitty HA, Ahn J, Parsons RE, Temudom T, D'Ayala M, McLaughlin M, DePalo L, Kahn R (1998) Impact of transrenal aortic endograft placement on endovascular graft repair of abdominal aortic aneurysms. J Vasc Surg 28:638–646

May J, White GH, Yu W, Waugh RC, Stephen MS, Harris JP (1996) Results of endoluminal grafting of abdominal aortic aneurysms are dependent on aneurysm morphology. Ann Vasc Surg 10:254–261

Moritz JD, Rotermund S, Keating DP, Oestmann JW (1996) Infrarenal abdominal aortic aneurysms: implications of CT evaluation of size and configuration for placement of endovascular aortic grafts. Radiology 198:463

Mulligan SA, Koslin DB, Berland LL (1992) Duplex evaluation of native renal vessels and renal allografts. Semin Ultrasound CT MR 13:40–52

Nakada SY, Wolf JS Jr, Brink JA, Quillen SP, Nadler RB, Gaines MV, Clayman RV (1998) Retrospective analysis of the effect of crossing vessels on successful retrograde endopyelotomy outcomes using spiral computerized tomography angiography. J Urol 159:62–65

Napel S, Marks MP, Rubin GD, Dake MD, McDonnell CH, Song SM, Enzmann DR, Jeffrey RB Jr (1992a) CT angiography with spiral CT and maximum intensity projection. Radiology 185:607–610

Napel S, Marks MP, Rubin GD, Dake MD, McDonnell CH, Song SM, Enzmann DR, Jeffrey RB Jr (1992b) CT angiography with spiral CT and maximum intensity projection. Radiology 185:607–610

Nelemans PJ, Kessels AG, De Leeuw P, De Haan M, van Engelshoven J (1998) The cost-effectiveness of the diagnosis of renal artery stenosis. Eur J Radiol 27:95–107

Nghiem HV, Jeffrey RB Jr (1998) CT angiography of the visceral vasculature. Semin Ultrasound CT MR 19:439–446

Olbricht CJ, Galanski M, Chavan A, Prokop M (1996) Spiral CT angiography – can we forget about arteriography to diagnose renal artery stenosis? Nephrol Dial Transplant 11:1227–1231

O'Neill JA Jr, Berkowitz H, Fellows KJ, Harmon CM (1995) Midaortic syndrome and hypertension in childhood. J Pediatr Surg 30:164–171

Park JH, Chung JW, Lee KW, Park YB, Han MC (1997) CT angiography of Takayasu arteritis: comparison with conventional angiography. J Vasc Interv Radiol 8:393–400

Platt JF, Ellis JH, Korobkin M, Reige K (1997) Helical CT evaluation of potential kidney donors: findings in 154 subjects. AJR Am J Roentgenol 169:1325–1330

Postma CT, Thien T (1997) Treatment of ostial renal-artery stenoses with vascular endoprostheses. N Engl J Med 337:132–133

Pozniak MA, Balison DJ, Lee FT Jr, Tambeaux RH, Uehling DT, Moon TD (1998) CT angiography of potential renal transplant donors. Radiographics 18:565–587

Prokop M, Schaefer CM, Leppert A, Galanski M (1993) Spiral CT angiography for diagnosis and follow up of chronic aortic dissection. Radiology 189(P):112

Prokop M, Schaefer-Prokop C, Koehler A, Galanski M (1994) Artifacts in CT angiography. Radiology 193(P):379

Prokop M, Schaefer-Prokop C, Galanski M (1997a) Spiral CT angiography of the abdomen. Abdom Imaging 22:143–153

Prokop M, Shin HO, Schanz A, Schaefer-Prokop CM (1997b) Use of maximum intensity projections in CT angiography: a basic review. Radiographics 17:433–451

Raptopoulos V, Rosen MP, Kent KC, Kuestner LM, Sheiman RG, Pearlman JD (1996) Sequential helical CT angiography of aortoiliac disease. AJR Am J Roentgenol 166:1347–1354

Richter CS, Biamino G, Ragg C, Felix R (1994) CT angiography of the pelvic arteries. Eur J Radiol 19:25–31

Rieker O, Düber C, Neufang A, Pitton M, Schweden F, Thelen M (1997) CT angiography versus intraarterial digital subtraction angiography for assessment of aortoiliac occlusive disease. AJR Am J Roentgenol 169:1133–1138

Rubin GD (1996) Spiral (helical) CT of the renal vasculature. Semin Ultrasound CT MR 17:374–397

Rubin GD, Dake MD, Napel SA, McDonnell CH, Jeffrey RB Jr (1993) Three-dimensional spiral CT angiography of the abdomen: initial clinical experience. Radiology 186:147–152

Rubin GD, Dake MD, Napel S, Jeffrey RB Jr, McDonnell CH, Sommer FG, Wexler L, Williams DM (1994a) Spiral CT of renal artery stenosis: comparison of three-dimensional rendering techniques. Radiology 190:181–189

Rubin GD, Dake MD, Semba CP, Napel SA, Jeffrey RB (1994b) Helical CT angiography for evaluation of endovascular interventions. Radiology 193(P):379

Rubin GD, Alfrey EJ, Dake MD, Semba CP, Sommer FG, Kuo PC, Dafoe DC, Waskerwitz JA, Bloch DA, Jeffrey RB (1995) Assessment of living renal donors with spiral CT. Radiology 195:457–462

Rubin GD, Beaulieu CF, Argiro V, et al (1996) Perspective volume rendering of CT and MR images: applications for endoscopic imaging. Radiology 199:321–330

Rubin GD, Paik DS, Johnston PC, Napel S (1998) Measurement of the aorta and its branches with helical CT. Radiology 206:823–829

Satta J, Laara E, Reinila A, Immonen K, Juvonen T (1997) The rupture type determines the outcome for ruptured abdominal aortic aneurysm patients. Ann Chir Gynaecol 86:24–29

Schumacher H, Eckstein HH, Kallinowski F, Allenberg JR (1997) Morphometry and classification in abdominal aortic aneurysms: patient selection for endovascular and open surgery. J Endovasc Surg 4:39–44

Siegel CL, McDougall EM, Middleton WD, Brink JA, Quillin SP, Teefey SA, Wolf JS Jr, Clayman RV (1997) Preoperative assessment of ureteropelvic junction obstruction with endoluminal sonography and helical CT. AJR Am J Roentgenol 168:623–626

Smith PA, Ratner LE, Lynch FC, Corl FM, Fishman EK (1998) Role of CT angiography in the preoperative evaluation for laparoscopic nephrectomy. Radiographics 18:589–601

Sommer T, Fehske W, Holzknecht N, et al (1996) Aortic dissection: a comparative study of diagnosis with spiral CT. Multiplanar transesophageal echocardiography, and MR imaging. Radiology 199:347–352

Soudack M, Gaitini D, Ofer A (1999) Celiac artery aneurysm: diagnosis by color Doppler sonography and three-dimensional CT angiography. J Clin Ultrasound 27:49–51

Stella A, Gargiulo M, Faggioli GL, Bertoni F, Capello I, Brusori S, D'Addata M (1993) Postoperative course of inflammatory abdominal aortic aneurysms. Ann Vasc Surg 7:229–238

Toki K, Takahara S, Kokado Y, Ichimaru N, Wang J, Tsuda K, Narumi Y, Nakamura H, Okuyama A (1998) Comparison of CT angiography with MR angiography in the living renal donor. Transplant Proc 30:2998–3000

Tsuda K, Murakami T, Kim T, Narumi Y, Takahashi S, Tomoda K, Takahara S, Okuyama A, Oi H, Nakamura H (1998) Helical CT angiography of living renal donors: comparison with 3D Fourier transformation phase contrast MRA. J Comput Assist Tomogr 22:186–193

Udekwu PO, Gurkin B, Oller DW (1996) The use of computed tomography in blunt abdominal injuries. Am Surg 62:56–59

Van Hoe L, Baert AL, Gryspeerdt S, Marchal G, Lacroix H, Wilms G, Mertens L (1996) Supra- and juxtarenal aneurysms of the abdominal aorta: preoperative assessment with thin-section spiral CT. Radiology 198:443–448

Verschuyl EJ, Kaatee R, Beek FJ, Patel NH, Fontaine AB, Daly CP, Coldwell DM, Bush WH, Mali WP (1997) Renal artery origins: best angiographic projection angles. Radiology 205:115–120

Walter F, Henrot P, Blum A, Hirsch JJ, Beot S, Guillemin F, Boccaccini H, Regent D (1998) Valeur comparative de l'angio-IRM, du scanner helicoidal et de l'angiographie numerisee dans le bilan preoperatoire des anevrismes de l'aorte abdominale. J Radiol 79:529–5539

White GH, May J, Waugh RC, Chaufour X, Yu W (1998) Type III and type IV endoleak: toward a complete definition of blood flow in the sac after endoluminal AAA repair. J Endovasc Surg 5:305–309

Williams DM, Lee DY, Hamilton BH, Marx MV, Narasimham DL, Kazanjian SN, Prince MR, Andrews JC, Cho KJ, Deeb GM (1997) The dissected aorta: percutaneous treatment of ischemic complications -principles and results. J Vasc Interv Radiol 8:605–625

Winter TC III, Nghiem HV, Freeny PC, Hommeyer SC, Mack LA (1995a) Hepatic arterial anatomy: demonstration of normal supply and vascular variants with three-dimensional CT angiography. Radiographics 15:771–780

Winter TC III, Freeny PC, Nghiem HV, et al (1995b) Hepatic arterial anatomy in transplantation candidates: evaluation with three-dimensional CT arteriograms. Radiology 195:363–370

Winter TC III, Nghiem HV, Schmiedl UP, Freeny PC (1996) CT angiography of the visceral vessels. Semin Ultrasound CT MR 17:339–351

Yoshimi F, Hasegawa H, Koizumi S, Amemiya R, Ono H, Kobayashi H, Matsueda K, Itabashi M (1995) Application of three-dimensional spiral computed tomographic angiography to pancreatoduodenectomy for cancer. Br J Surg 82:116–117

Zeman RK, Davros WJ, Bermann P, et al (1994a) Three-dimensional models for abdominal vasculature based on helical CT: usefulness in patients with pancreatic neoplasms. AJR Am J Roentgenol 162:1425–1429

Zeman RK, Silverman PM, Berman PM, Weltman DI, Davros WJ, Gomes MN (1994b) Abdominal aortic aneurysms: evaluation with variable-collimation helical CT and overlapping reconstruction. Radiology 193:555–560

Zeman RK, Berman PM, Silverman PM, Davros WJ, Cooper C, Kladakis AO, Gomes MN (1995) Diagnosis of aortic dissection: value of helical CT with multiplanar reformation and three-dimensional rendering. AJR Am J Roentgenol 164:1375–1380

Abdominal Vessels:
Role of CT Angiography and Controversies

39 The Case for Doppler Sonography

R. Kubale

CONTENTS

39.1 Introduction 443
39.2 Doppler and Color-coded Doppler Sonography Techniques 443
39.2.1 Continuous Wave and Pulsed Wave Doppler 443
39.2.2 Color-coded Duplex Sonography 444
39.2.3 Contrast-enhanced CCDS 444
39.3 Applications of CCDS in the Abdomen 444
39.3.1 Aorta and Iliac Arteries 444
39.3.2 Renal Arteries 445
39.3.3 Celiac and Mesenteric Vessels 445
39.3.4 Portal Venous System and Liver 446
39.3.5 Inferior Vena Cava, Renal and Gonadal Veins 448
29.4 Advantages and Outlook 448
References 448

39.1
Introduction

Traditional first diagnostic procedure for abdominal arteries was selective angiography. Due to its drawbacks of patients exposure to ionizing radiation and nephrotoxicity of contrast media several other modalities were applied for assessment of abdominal vessels. First attempts were made with Doppler and duplex sonography that had been used mainly for examinations in cardiology and peripheral vessels (Satomura et al. 1959; Müller et al. 1971; Pourcelot et al. 1971; von Reutern et al. 1976; Taylor et al. 1985; Seitz and Kubale 1987; Widder 1995; Arning 1996). With the introduction of color coded duplex sonography (CCDS) and improvement of scanners with better sensitivity and moving artifact filters abdominal vessels became accessible to CCDS evaluation (Ralls et al. 1988; Grant et al. 1989; Bluth et al. 1990; Wolff and Fobbe 1993).

R. Kubale, MD; Institut für Radiologie und Nuklearmedizin, Ringstrasse 62–64, D-66953 Pirmasens, Germany

39.2
Doppler and Color-coded Doppler Sonography Techniques

Sonographic techniques for vascular assessment are generally divided in those using gray-scale alone and those based upon the Doppler effect. The Doppler effect is the phenomenon of observed changes in the frequency of energy wave transmission when motion occurs between the source of transmission and the observer. Red blood cells circulating in vessels act as moving receivers and sources of scattered ultrasound waves forming the basis for the Doppler equation

$$fd = \frac{2*fo*\cos(\alpha)*v}{c}$$

where f_d represents the Doppler frequency shift, f_o the transducer frequency, α the angle of insonation, v the velocity of scatterers in a given direction and c the propagation of ultrasound in the medium (e.g. liver: 1540 cm/s).

39.2.1
Continuous Wave and Pulsed Wave Doppler

First applications were based on continuous wave (CW) Doppler transducers, transmitting and receiving ultrasonic signals continuously. On the contrary pulsed wave (PW) Doppler has a single crystal emitting pulses of bursts of ultrasound energy, giving the chance of depth selective measurements without mixing the flow information of all vessels within the Doppler beam. Analysis of the Doppler signal is done by spectral analysis yielding an spectrum of constituent frequencies and corresponding amplitudes of the signal. A combination of parameters enables evaluation of mean and maximum flow velocities, turbulence and indicies of resistance describing the distal vascular bed (Seitz and Kubale 1986; Widder 1995).

39.2.2
Color-coded Duplex Sonography

Color-coded duplex sonography (CCDS) automatically displays color-coded flow information superimposed on all or selected portions of the gray-scale image giving information about morphology and hemodynamics in one picture. Each pixel of color represents motion. Flow is indicated by colors like "red" or "blue" representing the direction of blood flow towards or away from the transducer (Fig. 39.1). Hue of color can be used for encoding the average Doppler shift frequency at each pixel so, as the Doppler frequency increases, the color moves from a simple "red" towards "orange" or "yellow" ("velocity mode") or for encoding the amount of moving corpuscles as saturation of color ("power or intensity mode"). Later method has the methodological advantage of being more sensitive and nearly angle independent (Fig. 39.2). High quality images of abdominal vessels mandates a good signal-to-noise ratio in a short breath-hold acquisition. Optimizing velocity range, wall filters (reducing noise of low frequencies coming from wall movements) , moving/flash artifact suppression, resolution and sensitivity of color enables depicting angiography-like pictures that can be documented as "vessel stripes" or in a 3D fashion ("work in progress").

Color or flow voids in the lumen and additional measurements of velocities and resistance indices calculated by parameters of the Doppler spectrum in a given "sample volume" are the basis for depicting occlusions and stenoses, or physiological and pathological changes of blood flow.

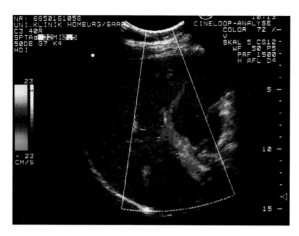

Fig. 39.1. Liver with portal vein and hepatic artery (color-coded Duplex sonography, CCDS). View from lateral, intercostal with liver, portal vein and hepatic artery. Flow towards the transducer is coded *red*, flow away from the transducer is shown in *blue*

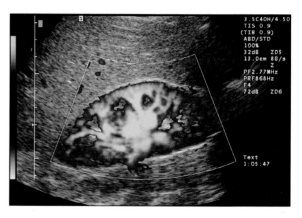

Fig. 39.2. Longitudinal scan showing perfusion of the right kidney (power or intensity Doppler). Longitudinal view with liver and right kidney. The amount of moving corpuscles are coded *orange* showing a normal perfusion without segmental infarcts

39.2.3
Contrast-enhanced CCDS

Due to absorption and overlying structures in 10–25% of patients flow-coded images of good quality. This can be overcome by sonographic contrast media, which when injected into a vessel are able to enhance the Doppler signal intensity. The concept of using contrast material was first conceived by GRAMIAK (1968). Ultrasonic contrast is based on microbubbles of gas or particles that are highly reflective (review in NANDA et al. 1997). Attempts have been made to produce contrast media that can be injected into a peripheral vein and circulate throughout the body passing the lungs and capillary system while still maintaining their ability to enhance ultrasound signals. Special techniques like "second harmonic imaging" (BURNS et al. 1992) are helpful for detecting parenchymal perfusion.

39.3
Applications of CCDS in the Abdomen

39.3.1
Aorta and Iliac Arteries

Although conventional gray-scale sonography is a well established modality for screening and follow-up of aortic aneurysms (KREMER et al. 1984) assessment of stenoses and occlusions needs additional information: Conventional duplex sonography was once considered promising in the diagnosis of stenoses of aortic and pelvic arteries but it was time consuming and had difficulties relating to tortuosity and calcifications (SEITZ and KUBALE 1987). With the advent of CCDS examination time could be significantly reduced. Low echogenic thrombi in the lumen, flow disturbances caused by stenoses or fistula and occlusions can easily be detected by CCDS within minutes in up to 95% of patients (KUBALE 1995).

CCDS is particularly useful in aortic aneurysms (Fig. 39.3) and dissections. The patency of the lumen and its relationship to aortic branches as well as re-entry tears are easily identified (TARTARINI et al. 1988; BLUTH et al. 1990). Analysis of the vessel wall and delineation of thrombus is possible in slim patients or in thick patients using newer techniques like "tissue harmonic imaging" (THI) reducing overall system noise. For detecting the thoracic part of aneurysms as well as entry and re-entry in thick patients MRA or CTA are necessary.

39.3.2
Renal Arteries

Arterio-venous parenchymal fistulas for example as a result of biopsy or congenital malformations can be recognized on CCDS by localized flow turbulence at the site of fistula. Additionally marked increase in flow velocities of the supplying artery and decrease of resistance index are helpful to confirm the diagnosis (TAKEBAYASHI et al. 1991).

Stenoses of the renal artery are characterized by a flow elevation of more than 180 cm/s and/or a difference of intrarenal resistance measurements of 0.05 between both sides (BREITENSEHER et al. 1992; SCHWERCK et al. 1994; for review see KRUMME et al. 1996). Although the accuracy for detection of renal artery stenosis is reported high with values for sensitivity and specificity ranging between 85 and 100%. CCDS is still controversial as a screening method, whereas proximal stenoses are detected reliably, it is difficult to detect stenoses in the central and distal third of the artery. Indirect criteria much as differences in resistance indices are helpful in unilateral disease, but they are limited in bilateral involvement of the arteries.

CCDS is of greatest value in detection of renal artery occlusion. If segmental and interlobular arteries are seen, occlusion is unlikely. Nonvisualization of intrarenal vessels even after application of contrast media may warrant emergency angiography including possible thrombolytic treatment depending on the clinical situation. Using contrast media it is possible to depict even segmental and subsegmental infarction (Fig. 39.4).

CCDS is extremely helpful in kidney transplants for diagnosis early acute vascular occlusions and high-grade stenosis. It has already replaced scintigraphy in nearly all clinical centers. Increase of resistance indices indicates acute rejection of vascular type or tubular necrosis.

39.3.3
Celiac and Mesenteric Vessels

Since several years Duplex sonography and CCDS have been used for evaluation of celiac trunk and superior mesenteric artery (SAM) diseases

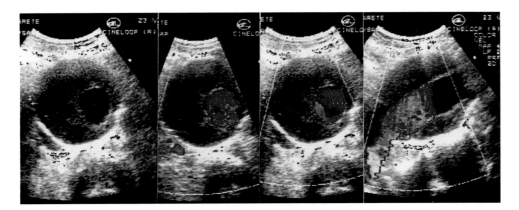

Fig. 39.3. Aneurysm of the abdominal aorta with partial thrombosis (CCDS). Gray-scale image and color-coded transverse and longitudinal scans showing a 5.2×4.8 cm aneurysm of the abdominal aorta with thrombus formation and eccentric flow in CCDS

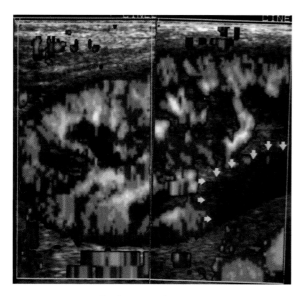

Fig. 39.4. Segmental infarction of a transplant kidney due to an occluded aberrant artery. Longitudinal view of the transplant kidney with a segmental loss of flow due to an occlusion of an accessory small aberrant artery

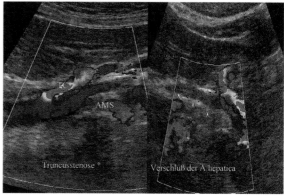

a,b

Fig. 39.5a, b. Stenosis and occlusion of celiac trunk and hepatic artery (CCDS). a Longitudinal scan with laminar flow in the aorta and superior mesenteric artery. Flow increase immediately distally to the origin of celiac trunk associated with jet phenomenon and aliasing. Doppler measurements showed a peak flow velocity of more than 420 cm/s (normal <140 cm/s). b Transverse scan in a second patient showing celiac trunk and aorta. Loss of flow signals in the hepatic artery (>>>) due to vascular occlusion confirmed at angiography

(ALDOORI et al. 1985; JÄGER et al. 1986; KUBALE 1988; FLINN et al. 1990; MONETA et al. 1991; MOSTBECK et al. 1992). Thanks to technical improvement inferior mesenteric artery as well as first and even second order branches of SMA can reliably be assessed.

Aneurysms of intestinal arteries and malformations are easily seen and reported increasingly giving radiologists the chance for elective embolization (FRANZEN et al. 1989; ENDRESS et al. 1989; KUBALE et al. 1992; JUNEWICK et al. 1993).

Although CCDS still has limited importance for the diagnosis of acute intestinal ischemia, it is most valuable as a screening tool in patients with chronic intestinal ischemia, nonspecific abdominal pain and bruits. Stenoses are characterized by flow elevation or vibration artifacts. Complete lack of flow is indicates an occlusion (Fig. 39.5). Correlative studies show sensitivity and specificity ranges of 89 to 98% (KUBALE et al. 1987; MOSTBECK et al. 1992). Depicting collaterals is helpful in distinguishing relevant stenoses from incidental findings without clinical relevance. CCDS already has replaced angiography for the postinterventional follow-up of transplantation, bypass procedures, stents and dilatation (SEGEL et al. 1986; LIM et al. 1989).

Several authors reported promising preliminary results in patients with Crohn's disease, colitis or celiac diseases (KATHREIN et al. 1990, GIOVAGNORIO et al. 1998; VAN-OOSTAYEN et al. 1998). There is an in-

crease of flow signals correlating with the grade of inflammation in Crohn's disease. Quantification of flow measurements are helpful in monitoring effects of medicaments (KUBALE et al. 1987; LILLY et al. 1989). Lack of decrease of the resistance index after a test meal seems to be an effective way to express severity of celiac disease and to document its regression after diet therapy (GIOVAGNORIO et al. 1998).

Mesenteric veins are visible in more than 94% including their first order branches. Thrombi are characterized by an increased vessel volume and complete or partial loss of flow. Early depiction of thrombi and its noninvasive repeatability were helpful to change therapeutic management from operation to anticoagulation. Routine application already has reduced lethality of mesenteric vein thromboses significantly (KUBALE 1996).

39.3.4
Portal Venous System and Liver

Due to its increasing sensitivity CCDS has been shown to give a quick, easy and cheap overview over the splenoportal system, depicting all clinical relevant pathologies including aneurysms, fistula and stenoses as well as complete or partial thromboses (LAFORTUNE et al. 1987; SEITZ and KUBALE 1987; JABRA and TAYLOR 1991; HERBETKO et al. 1992).

Aneurysms or ectasias of the portal vein are characterized by a color-filled sack adjacent to the vessel (Fig. 39.6). They can be differentiated from arterial aneurysm by a slow, only slightly turbulent flow. AV-malformations are characterized by high flow signals with or without confetti-like vibration artifacts with a constant high amplitude spectrum. Indirect signs are enlarged feeding arteries with increased flow as well as an arterial signal in the vein. Even rare malformations as congenital portocaval shunts are depicted increasingly by CCDS (Kubale et al. 1987; Jabra and Taylor 1991; Tanaka et al. 1992).

First attempts had been made to use gray-scale or B-scan sonography for depicting thromboses and tumor thrombi: Although intraluminal echoes on the gray-scale image are helpful for detecting thromboses and tumor-thrombi, they support but do not definitively establish the diagnosis of a clot because acute thrombosis is often anechoic or even hypoechoic. Duplex Doppler or CCDS confirms the

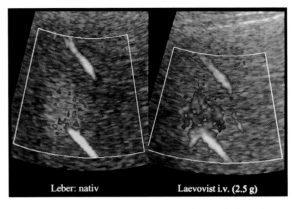

Leber: nativ   Laevovist i.v. (2.5 g)

Fig. 39.7. CCDS of liver hemangioma before and after administration of contrast medium. Hemangioma with feeding vessel before (**a**) and after application of 2.5 g/l Levovist (**b**)

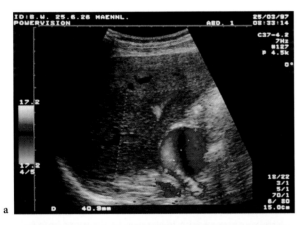

a

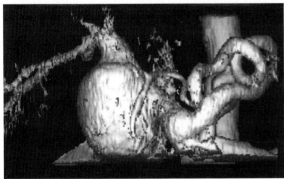

b

Fig. 39.6a, b. CCDS and 3D-CTA of an aneurysm of the portal vein. View from lateral intercostal showing an ectasia of the portal vein in CCDS (**a**) being confirmed by CTA with 3D reconstruction (**b**). Even after follow-up of more than 12 years no significant increase of diameter or complications were seen

diagnosis by showing complete loss of flow or delineation of partial thrombus (Seitz and Kubale 1987; Tessler et al. 1991). Cavernous transformation is characterized by numerous collaterals with hepatopetal flow associated with collaterals in the lesser omentum and gallbladder varices. Budd-Chiari syndrome can be diagnosed by loss of flow in the hepatic veins and collateral pathways delineated by CCDS. Other collaterals that are detectable by CCDS are enlarged paraumbilical, left gastric and coronary veins, retroperitoneal, spleno-renal and spleno-retroperitoneal veins.

In cirrhotic patients CCDS can depict enlarged tortuous arteries in the liver according to the angiographic pattern of corkscrew arteries with slow or even reverse flow in the portal vein. Finding portal venous collaterals can prompt the diagnosis of portal hypertension or reinforce it when already clinically suspected. Measurements of flow and flow direction is helpful for follow-up measurements in cirrhotic patients. They can give insight into various diseases even in diffuse parenchymal disease (Bolondi et al. 1991; Seitz and Kubale 1987). However very slow flow in the portal system can lead to false positive results of occlusion. Application of contrast media can help depicting flow in obese patients, showing tumor blood supply (Fig. 39.7) or giving pathophysiological parameter like appearance time of contrast for further differentiation of parenchymal diseases (Albrecht et al. 1999). Analysis of tumor vascularization remains still controversial (Tanaka et al. 1990; Cosgrove 1996).

Follow-up measurements after transplantation or TIPPS implantation are essential showing complications early enough for treatment.

39.3.5
Inferior Vena Cava, Renal and Gonadal Veins

In more than 91% of patients the inferior vena cava (IVC) and renal veins are well displayed with conventional CCDS techniques. Normal vessels are characterized by complete filling of the lumen with color. Depiction of thrombi, invasion of tumor and congenital malformations are easily seen. Additional reports describe thrombi in ovarian and even in adrenal veins (BARAN and FRISCH 1987; BAKA et al. 1989).

49.4
Advantages and Outlook

Noninvasiveness, low cost and lack of nephrogenic toxicity coupled with high diagnostic accuracy for the abdominal aorta and iliac arteries, and for the portal venous system had driven the popularity of CCDS for depicting aneurysms, fistula, stenoses and occlusions.

Complete or incomplete portal vein thromboses of various etiologies are reliably detectable by CCDS. For the portal venous system nearly all questions can be answered by CCDS alone. Additional application of CTA or MRA is helpful for depicting complex malformations and getting anatomical overview especially in obese patients.

In acute arterial intestinal ischemia, angiography is still the method of first choice. However CCDS gains increasing importance for depicting stenoses and occlusions especially in chronic intestinal ischemia. With modern therapeutic options of angioplasty and stenting also in mesenteric arteries, CCDS is helpful to select and prepare patients for the interventional procedure. In mesenteric venous disease CCDS is superior to angiography, so that the latter is seldom necessary. In unclear cases and complex malformations, or in renal artery disease the combination of CCDS and CTA is sufficient in most cases and replaces angiography.

New techniques like "Tissue harmonic imaging" (THI) uses subtraction algorithms in which two impulses with a 180 degree delay are subtracted, leaving only signals with nonlinear properties. This method can be used for reducing background and scattering signals effectively. With the widespread use of new ultrasound scanners with improved sensitivity and application of contrast media abdominal vessels will be observed even more accurately. In conclusion CCDS is a feasible approach for depicting diseases of abdominal vessels and its importance is increasing.

References

Albrecht T, Bloomley MJK, Cosgrove DO, Taylor-Robinson SD, Jayaram V, Eckersley R, Urbank A, Butler-Barnes J, Patel N (1999) Non-invasive diagnosis of hepatic cirrhosis by transmit-time analysis of an ultrasound contrast agent. Lancet 353:1579--1583

Aldoori MI, Qamar MI, Read AE, Williamson RC (1985) Increased flow in the superior mesenteric artery in dumping syndrome. Br J Surg 72:389–390

Arning C (1996) Farbkodierte Duplexsonographie der hirnversorgenden Arterien. Thieme, Stuttgart

Baka JJ, Lev-Toaff AS, Friedman AC, Radecki PD, Caroline DF (1989) Ovarian vein thrombosis with atypical presentation: role of sonography and duplex Doppler. Obstet Gynecol 73:887–889

Baran GW, Frisch KM (1987) Duplex Doppler evaluation of puerperal ovarian vein thrombosis. AJR Am J Roentgenol 149:321–322

Bluth EI, Murphey SM, Hollier LH, Sullivan MA (1990) Color flow Doppler in the evaluation of aortic aneurysms. Int Angiol 9:8–10

Bolondi L, Bassi SL, Gaiani S, Zironi G, Benzi G, Santi V, Barbara L (1991) Liver cirrhosis: changes in Doppler waveform of hepatic veins. Radiology 178:513–516

Breitenseher M, Kainberger F, Huebsch P, Trattnig S, Baldt M, Barton P, Karnel F (1992) Screening von Nierenarterienstenosen. Erste Ergebnisse zur Aussagekraft der Farbdopplersonographie. Rofo Fortschr Rontgenstr Neuen Bildgeb Verfahr 156:228–231

Cosgrove DO (1996) Echo enhancement of the liver vasculature to improve the diagnosis of tumours using colour Doppler ultrasound. Eur J Ultrasound 4:177–184

Endress C, Kling GA, Medrazo BL (1989) Diagnosis of hepatic artery aneurysm with portal vein fistula using image-directed Doppler ultrasound. J Clin Ultrasound 17:206–208

Flinn WR, Rizzo RJ, Park JS, Sandager GP (1990) Duplex scanning for assessment of mesenteric ischemia. Surg Clin North Am 70:99–107

Fransen H, Kubale R, Wurche KD, Kalaehne A (1989) Nichtinvasive Diagnostik von Milzarterienaneurysmata. Fortschr Rontgenstr 151:532–535

Giovagnorio F, Picarelli A, diGiovambattista F, Mastracchio A (1998) Evaluation with Doppler sonography of mesenteric blood flow in celiac disease. AJR Am J Roentgenol 171:629–632

Gramiak R, Shah PM (1968) Echocardiography of the aortic root. Invest Radiol 3:356–366

Grant EG, Perrella R, Tessler FN, Lois J, Busuttil R (1989) Budd-Chiari syndrome: the results of duplex and color Doppler imaging. AMJ Am J Roentgenol 152:377–381

Herbetko J, Grigg AP, Buckley AR, Phillips GL (1992) Venoocclusive liver disease after bone marrow transplantation: findings at duplex sonography. AMJ Am J Roentgenol 158:1001–1005

Jabra AA, Taylor GA (1991) Ultrasound diagnosis of congenital intrahepatic portosystemic venous shunt. Pediatr Radiol 21:529–530

Jäger K, Bollinger A, Valli C, Ammann R (1986) Measurement of mesenteric blood flow by duplex scanning. J Vasc Surg 3:462–469

Junewick JJ, Grant TH, Weiss CA, Piano G (1993) Celiac artery aneurysm: color Doppler evaluation. J Ultrasound Med 12:355–357

Kathrein H, Dzien A, Schuhmayer R, Judmaier G, Braunsteiner H Diagnose von Änderungen des Blutflusses in der Arteria mesenterica inferior bei entzündlichen Darmerkrankungen mit der Duplexsonographie. Vasa [Suppl] 30:129–132

Kremer H, Weigold B, Dobrinski W, Schreiber M, Zöllner N (1984) Sonographische Verlaufsbeobachtungen von Bauchaortenaneurysmen. Klin Wochenschr 62:1120–1125

Krumme B, Blum U, Schwerdtfeger E, Flugel P, Hollstin F, Schollmeyer P, Rump LC (1999) Diagnosis of renovascular disease by intra- and extrarenal Doppler scanning. Kidney Int 50:1288–1292

Kubale R (1988) Mesenteriale Gefäße. In: Seitz KH, Kubale R (eds) Duplexsonographie der abdominellen und retroperitonealen Gefäße. VCH, Weinheim

Kubale R (1995) Aorta and symmetric branches. In: Wolf KH (ed) Color Doppler sonography. Thieme, Stuttgart

Kubale R (1996) Diagnostic problems of mesenteric veins. Annual Meeting of the Radiological Society of North America, Chicago, 29 November to 4 December 1996

Kubale R, Vonnahme F-J, Broelsch C, Burdelski W (1987) Der kongenitale portokavale Shunt – eine seltene Variante. Ultraschall Klin Prax [Suppl] 1:8

Kubale R, Omlor G, Walter P, Thiel R, Defreyne L, Gebhard J, Kramann B (1992) Sonographic appearance, differential diagnostic and therapeutical aspects of non-aortic aneurysms. J Ultrasound Med 11:62

Lafortune M, Patriquin H, Pomier G, Huet PM, Weber A, Lavoie P, Blanchard P, Breton G (1987) Hemodynamic changes after portosystemic shunts: use of Duplex sonography in 43 patients. AJR Am J Roentgenol 149:701–706

Lafortune M, Madore F, Patriquin H, Breton G (1991) Segmental anatomy of the liver: a sonographic approach to the Couinaud Nomenclature. Radiology 181:443–448

Lilly MP, Harward TR, Flinn WR, Blackburn DR, Astleford PM, Yao JS (1989) Duplex ultrasound measurement of changes in mesenteric flow velocity with pharmacologic and physiologic alteration of intestinal blood flow in man. J Vasc Surg 9:18–25

Lim GM, Jeffrey RB, Tolentino CS (1989) Pancreatic pseudoaneurysm. Monitoring the success of transcatheter embolization with duplex sonography. J Ultrasound Med 8:643–646

Moneta GL, Yeager RA, Dalman R, Antonovic R, Hall LD, Porter JM (1991) Duplex ultrasound criteria for diagnosis of splanchnic artery stenosis or occlusion. J Vasc Surg 14:511–520

Mostbeck G, Mallek R, Gebauer A, Tschollakoff D (1992) Duplex-Sonographie und farbkodierte Duplex-Sonographie viszeraler Gefäße bei abdominellen Erkrankungen. Wien Klin Wochenschr 104:227–233

Müller HR (1971) Direktionale Doppler-Sonographie der A. frontalis medialis. EEG-EMG 2:24–32

Nandar NC, Schlieff R, Goldberg BB (1997) Advances in echo imaging using contrast enhancement. Kluwer, Dordrecht

Pourcelot L (1971) Nouveau débitmètre sanguin à effet Doppler. In: Ultrasonographia Media (Wien) :125–130

Ralls PW, Mayekawa DS, Lee KP, Colletti PM, Johnson MB, Halls JM (1988) Gallbladder wall varices: diagnosis with color flow Doppler sonography. J Clin Ultrasound 16:595–598

Satomura S (1959) Study of the flow patterns in peripheral arteries by ultrasound. J Acoust Soc Jap 15:151–154

Schwerck WB, Restrepo IK, Stellwaag M, Klose KJ, Scade-Brittinger C (1994) Renal artery stenosis: grading with image directed Doppler US. Evaluation of renal resistive index. Radiology 190:785–790

Segel MC, Zajko AB, Bowen A, Skolnick ML, Bron KM, Penkrot RJ, Slasky BS, Starzl TE (1986) Doppler ultrasound as a screening for hepatic artery thrombosis after liver transplantation. Transplantation 41:539–541

Seitz KH, Kubale R (1987) Duplexsonographie der abdominellen und retroperitonealen Gefäße. VCH, Weinheim

Takebayashi S, Aida N, Matsui K (1991) Arteriovenous malformations of the kidneys: diagnosis and follow-up with color Doppler sonography in six patients. AMR Am J Roentgenol 157:991–995

Tanaka S, Kitamura T, Fujita M, Nakanishi K, Okuda S (1990) Color Doppler flow imaging of liver tumors. AMJ Am J Roentgenol 154:509–514

Tanaka S, Kitamura T, Fujita M, Iishi H, Kasugai H, Nakanishi K, Okuda S (1992) Intrahepatic venous and portal venous aneurysms examined by color Doppler flow imaging. J Clin Ultrasound 20:89–98

Tartarini G, Bertoli D, Baglini R, Balbarini A, Mariani M (1988) Diagnosis of aortic dissection by color-coded Doppler. J Nucl Med Allied Sci 32:127–130

Taylor KJW, Burns PN, Woodcock JP, Wells PNT (1985) Blood flow in deep abdominal and pelvic vessels. Radiology 154:495–498

Tessler FN, Gehring BJ, Gomes AS, Perrella RR, Ragavendra N, Busuttil RW, Grant EG (1991) Diagnosis of portal vein thrombosis: value of color Doppler imaging. AJR Am J Roentgenol 157:293–296

van-Oostayen JA, Wasser MN, Griffioen G, van-Hogezand RA, Lamers CB, de-Roos A (1998) Diagnosis of Crohn's ileitis and monitoring of disease activity: value of Doppler ultrasound of superior mesenteric artery flow. Am J Gastroenterol 93:88–91

VonReutern GM, Büdingen HJ, Freund HJ (1976) Diagnose und Differenzierung von Stenosen und Verschlüssen der A. carotis mit der Doppler-Sonographie. Arch Psychiatr Nervenkr 222:191–207

Widder B (1995) Doppler- und Duplexsonographie der hirnversorgenden Gefäße. Springer, Berlin Heidelberg New York

40 The Case for CT Angiography

M. Prokop

CONTENTS

40.1 Introduction *451*
40.2 Impact on Patient Management
     and Cost Effectiveness *451*
40.2.1 Abdominal Aortic Aneurysms *451*
40.2.2 Dissection *452*
40.2.3 Renal Arteries *452*
40.2.4 Visceral Arteries *452*
40.2.5 Postoperative Controls *453*
40.3 Potential Disadvantages of CTA *453*
40.3.1 Contrast Load *453*
40.3.2 Radiation Exposure *453*
40.3.3 3D Editing Procedures *453*
40.3.4 z-Axis Resolution *454*
40.3.5 Flow Information *454*
40.4 Advantages over Arterial DSA *454*
40.5 Advantages over MRA *455*
40.6 Advantages over Color Duplex Sonography *455*
40.7 Conclusions *456*
     References *456*

40.1
Introduction

For abdominal examinations, arterial DSA is being replaced by less invasive techniques, such as CTA, MRA, and color-coded duplex sonography. All techniques may be used as primary diagnostic modalities, but as yet, CT angiography appears to be the most cost-effective technique for many indications and the least dependent on the skills of individual examiners.

40.2
Impact on Patient Management and Cost Effectiveness

For most diagnostic questions regarding the abdominal aorta and visceral arteries, CTA has maximum impact on patient management and can rule

M. PROKOP, MD; Allgemeines Krankenhaus der Stadt Wien, Universitätsklinik für Radiodiagnostik, Abteilung Radiologie für konservative Fächer, A-1090 Vienna, Austria

out disease, determine which patients require follow-up, and give the information necessary for therapy planning (BLUEMKE and CHAMBERS 1995). For many indications, sensitivity and specificity compare favorably with those of color Doppler (HALPERN et al. 1998) and are similar to high-end MRA techniques (WALTER et al. 1998). CTA has the advantage that it solves clinical problems and rarely creates new ones.

Reimbursement for CT has fallen dramatically over the past years, as has the cost of new equipment. The cost of a CT scanner may be similar to that of a high-end ultrasound machine and is generally less, by a factor of 2–4, than the cost of a MR scanner that supplies images of comparable quality.

A diagnostic test is cost effective if it solves a clinical problem with lower costs than other techniques. This means it has to rule out disease, detect disease and direct patient management. At the same time the new questions that may result as a consequence of the test should not generate significantly more costs.

Few cost-effectiveness studies are available as yet. For the evaluation of renal artery stenoses, a Dutch group showed that protocols including CTA were cost effective while protocols that included MRA were not (NELEMANS et al. 1998). Given a similar diagnostic performance of CTA and MRA for most other applications in the abdomen, one can deduct that CTA will often be cost effective while MRA is still too expensive.

40.2.1
Abdominal Aortic Aneurysms

CTA has almost completely eliminated arterial angiography or DSA for the primary diagnostic workup of aortic aneurysms (BLUEMKE and CHAMBERS 1995; BROEDERS et al. 1997; ERRINGTON et al. 1997). In general, all diagnostically relevant questions can be answered with CTA, with a sensitivity and specificity that is close to 100% (ERRINGTON et al. 1997). Because of the short time the patient has to remain on the table, CTA is the method of choice for evaluating acutely ill patients. It gives a comprehensive overview of all therapeutically relevant findings. Compared with MRA, access to the patient is always easily possible. Thus, even critically ill patients can be examined as long as they are hemodynamically stable.

For use in the chronic patient, CTA and MRA are in direct competition (WALTER et al. 1998). Since radiation exposure is not a major issue in the patient group with AAA, CTA remains the most cost effective and versatile technique for the diagnostic workup and therapy planning for AAA. There is only one remaining indication for angiography: preoperative localization of the origin of the anterior spinal artery in patients with thoraco-abdominal grafting and increased risk for spinal cord damage.

Ultrasound may be able to detect aneurysms, but it rarely allows for reliable determination of the relationship between the renal and visceral arteries and the aneurysm. Thus, further work-up will be necessary in most instances. In the acute setting, ultrasound may detect intra- or retroperitoneal hemorrhage and thus may be an excellent tool for selecting candidates for surgery. Since there are many other critical questions that cannot be answered in this situation, most patients will still go on to CT anyway.

40.2.2
Dissection

CTA is less invasive and yields more therapeutically relevant information than arterial DSA in most cases of acute aortic dissection (SOMMER et al. 1996; ZEMAN et al. 1995). It demonstrates collateral findings, such as hypoperfusion of abdominal organs or swelling of bowel walls, that cannot be assessed so well by DSA. In chronic aortic dissection, CTA competes with MRA. In terms of time requirements and cost-effectiveness, CTA still appears superior. Ultrasound may have a role in follow-up, but it rarely contributes to the management of the acute patient. The main limiting factor for ultrasound is the need for round-the clock availability of an experienced examiner.

40.2.3
Renal Arteries

Since there is a very low prevalence of renal artery stenoses in the hypertensive population, a prese-

lection based on clinical parameters is necessary. With a specificity of some 95% for CTA, too many superfluous DSA examinations would be indicated if every hypertensive patient were screened with CTA. In a preselected population, however, CTA can be used as a screening tool (NELEMANS et al. 1998). A normal CTA virtually excludes the presence of a significant stenosis that requires therapy (KAATEE et al. 1997). There is excellent sensitivity for the detection of hemodynamically relevant renal artery stenoses given optimized scan protocols (>95%). CTA also provides important additional information for the interventional radiologist, such as the presence of mural thromboses or an atypical anterior origin of a renal artery (VERSCHUYL et al. 1997).

CTA, however, is competing with contrast-enhanced MRA and Doppler ultrasound. These techniques may yield similarly good results in the hands of experienced examiners, although Doppler ultrasound appears somewhat inferior and more dependent on patient-related factors (HALPERN et al. 1998). Intraarterial DSA can be avoided as a primary diagnostic tool for renal artery stenosis. However, in a tertiary care setting in which there is a high likelihood that the patient will have a renal artery stenosis, one should consider going directly to intraarterial DSA and be prepared for an intervention within the same session.

CT has found its place as a standard tool to preoperatively evaluate living renal donors (COCHRAN et al. 1997; TOKI et al. 1998). It is superior to angiography for the detection of accessory veins and is especially helpful if laparoscopic surgery is planned. CTA is an excellent tool for the preoperative work-up before laparoscopic nephrectomy for various types of diseases (SMITH et al. 1998). CTA can help in the planning of minimally invasive surgery for repair of ureteropelvic junction obstruction (BRINK 1997). For this indication, CTA is able to detect crossing vessels that may complicate surgery.

40.2.4
Visceral Arteries

For the visceral arteries, color Doppler is the technique of choice for many indications (SOUDACK et al. 1999). CTA, however, can be performed as a part of the preoperative work-up of patients for liver and pancreatic tumors and there provides all therapeutically relevant information without extra cost (WINTER et al. 1995; YOSHIMI et al. 1995). The same holds true for MRA, although MRA is rarely performed as part of an abdominal work-up for liver tumors while it has become standard in the evaluation of pancreatic cancer.

40.2.5
Postoperative Controls

In the postoperative or postinterventional setting, CTA's main rival is ultrasound. As long as the vascular territory can be visualized easily, ultrasound appears to be more cost-effective. In patients that are difficult to examine with ultrasound, CTA is the technique of choice. In patients who have undergone implantation of vascular stents or grafts CTA appears to be the standard noninvasive technique for follow-up and detection of complications (BRINK 1997; BROEDERS et al. 1998).

40.3
Potential Disadvantages of CTA

40.3.1
Contrast Load

CT angiography requires large volumes of intravenous contrast material (100–150 ml). The total iodine load varies between 30 g and 50 g. This may become a problem in patients with impaired renal function, because further impairment may be possible, and the need for hemodialysis may arise. However, adequate hydration prior to contrast administration significantly improves tolerance of iodinated contrast material. Under these conditions, CTA can safely be performed even in patients with moderately reduced renal function. In hemodialysis patients with total lack of urine excretion, iodine load is not an issue since renal function cannot be damaged further. In the presence of severe renal damage with residual urine excretion CTA should not be performed and other imaging modalities such as MRA or color Doppler are to be preferred. This patient group, however, is relatively small.

High flow rates of 4–5 ml/s are helpful, although not mandatory, especially when the abdominal aorta is being evaluated. For this indication, flow rates as low as 2 ml/s may suffice. While some radiologists feel uneasy about using higher flow rates, the approach is safe, and paravasations are rare (far below 1%).

40.3.2
Radiation Exposure

The second major drawback of CTA is that it is an X-ray technique that leads to significant radiation exposure compared with a conventional chest radiograph. With dedicated CTA protocols patient exposure can be substantially reduced (often by a factor of 3 or more) compared with standard CT examinations. When comparing CTA and intraarterial DSA, the radiation exposure with DSA depends heavily on technical factors such as angiography equipment, use of pulsed fluoroscopy and the skill of the examiner. In DSA, radiation exposure grows with each additional run and projection angle. Thus, the more complex an examination or anatomic situation is, the more radiation is administered. In CTA, only one scan is performed, and arbitrary viewing angles can be reconstructed from the three-dimensional data set. Thus, CTA is inherently superior in complex situations, and may even help the investigator to optimize a subsequent DSA, as it can indicate the optimum projection angle for DSA. Since many patients in whom abdominal CTA is performed are old or have an unfavorable prognosis of their underlying disease, the additional radiation-induced risk can be neglected. Especially in life-threatening situations in which CTA has maximum impact on further therapy (helps establish the correct diagnosis and determine the further course of therapy), the dose aspect is of limited importance. Radiation exposure becomes important, however, for young patients with a benign prognosis, such as fibromuscular dysplasia of the renal arteries, in whom MRA or color Doppler should be preferred.

40.3.3
3D Editing Procedures

Similar to MRA, image presentation in CTA is based mainly on 3D visualization techniques (MIP, surface displays or VRT), while image interpretation is based more on the actual 2D data set. Bones and opacified vessels have similar CT numbers. Thus, skeletal structures have to be removed prior to MIP reconstruction. This editing has been a tedious and time-consuming effort. With newer software, however, editing is much simplified and a lot faster. Especially helpful are algorithms that allow separation of structures by clicking on the aorta (include) and the vertebrae (exclude). These watershed algorithms markedly simplify editing and speed up evaluation.

Presently, a lot of work is being directed at further simplification of editing and automation of the measurements of the aorta and its side branches.

40.3.4
z-Axis Resolution

In CTA, optimum spatial resolution is limited to the transaxial (xy) plane (pixel size 0.5–0.8 mm). The z-axis resolution is lower, depending on the scan range that has to be covered. Overlapping image reconstruction, however, partially compensates for the lower z-axis resolution. Newer CT scanners with more than one detector or faster rotation speed will allow for improved spatial resolution over extended scan ranges. This improvement grows proportionally with the amount of detector arrays and allows for almost isotropic imaging with multislice CT scanners.

Since the first applications of spiral (helical) CT for imaging of the vascular system, the technique has seen rapid technological improvement. The first commercially available scanners allowed for a scan duration of only 24 s, and only had older raw data interpolation algorithms (360° LI) with unfavorable slice sensitivity profiles available. The pitch factor (the ratio between table feed per rotation and slice collimation) had to be chosen equal to or less than 1; that is to say the table feed could not exceed the chosen slice thickness. At present, subsecond scanners with rotation times of 0.5 s and split detector systems with two detector rows are on the market. Scan times of 70 s and more are possible. In addition, raw data interpolation has been improved, which results in much narrower slice sensitivity profiles and allows for an increase in pitch factor from 1 to 2 and more.

New subsecond scanners with multiple detector rows are currently being developed by various manufacturers: these will allow for near-isotropic imaging of the aorta and renal arteries within time periods as small as 10–15 s.

40.3.5
Flow Information

CT angiography is a morphological technique that does not allow for functional measurements such as flow direction, flow rates or pressure gradients. Since, in the vast majority of situations, flow in the arterial system in the abdomen is antegrade, information about flow direction is seldom necessary for an accurate diagnosis. It is not yet clear whether such an information improves clinical decision making, although could be helpful in the renal arteries. Noninvasive measurement of pressure gradients is not possible.

40.4
Advantages over Arterial DSA

CT angiography is minimally invasive and only requires an intravenous contrast medium injection. In DSA local complications may occur in 5–10% of cases, with severe complications in 0.5–2%. In CTA, the risk of local complications such as hematoma is negligible. Contrast medium paravasation, the only major complication due to the intravenous access, can be managed conservatively in most instances.

There is less preparation (no sterile environment), a shorter time requirement for patient and staff, and generally much less patient discomfort than in DSA. CTA can always safely be performed as an outpatient procedure. Costs for the hospital and the patient are significantly lower with CTA.

In CTA, one scan can be used to reconstruct as many viewing angles as are necessary to solve the diagnostic question. In arterial DSA, each addition series means a longer examination time, more contrast medium load, and a higher radiation dose.

The biggest diagnostic advantage of CTA is that is a cross-sectional imaging technique: vascular wall and lumen can be simultaneously visualized. CTA is thus superior to DSA for the display of soft tissue organs, thrombi, wall calcification, intimal flaps and inflammatory disease (ZEMAN et al. 1995). For the planning of interventions (expected success rate, primary stenting), it may be important to know whether a stenosis is caused by a hard plaque or a soft plaque, or whether a stenosis is ostial or pseudotruncal (i.e. actually within a mural aortic thrombus). In intraarterial DSA, the anterior origin of vessels may be obscured by aorta. CTA may help in determining the optimum projection angle, and thus may improve the accuracy of DSA for the demonstration of ostial renal artery stenoses that might otherwise be undetected because of suboptimum projections (VERSCHUYL et al. 1997). In the rare event that two vessels originate directly within the same scan plane, DSA may not be able to separate them and lead to the suspicion of a single origin.

Since each CTA examination is an ordinary contrast-enhanced CT in the arterial phase, at the same time all CT information about surrounding tissues and parenchymal organs is available. This may help detect other unrelated diseases, but also disease that account for the patient's symptoms (such as the presence of adrenal tumors or renal parenchymal disease in suspected renovascular hypertension).

Since CTA provides a 3D data volume of the vascular territory examined, precise measurements of distances and volumes become possible. Measurements are no longer subject to projection effects. Even mural thrombi can be included in the measurements if necessary.

40.5
Advantages over MRA

The main advantages of CTA over MRA are cost and availability. Since almost all new CT scanners have spiral capability, CTA can be performed on any of these scanners. The cost of the equipment is still lower than for MR, by a factor of 2–4. The cost for contrast medium varies widely from country to country, but generally the cost of contrast medium required for one CTA study is less than for MRA. This difference becomes even wider when double-dose protocols are used for Gd-enhanced MRA.

One problem with MRA remains the relatively uncomfortable situation for most patients: quite a few have attacks of claustrophobia or at least suffer as a result of lying in the narrow tube in which the examination is performed. The limited space for the patient and problems with metallic material cause problems for acutely ill patients. There is less direct access, and specialized equipment is necessary to help the patient in the case of an emergency. Therefore, one should carefully weigh the risks of performing an MR examinations in a situation where a less problematic examination, CT, can answer all the questions.

CTA is a simple technique that is easy to learn. With the use of standardized protocols, there are few sources of error. Thus, the diagnostic results are consistent from patient to patient.

CTA is able to directly distinguish between calcified and noncalcified plaques. It thus provides information that is valuable for the planning of angioplasty procedures. Using MIP displays, the extent of the vascular calcifications can be easily demonstrated. In patients with vascular stent grafts, the stent, intimal proliferation and the vessel lumen can be directly demonstrated.

MRA in the abdomen usually acquires coronal slices. Image quality on antero-posterior projections in MRA is often better than in most CTA examinations. This, however, has no influence on patient management. Problems may occur if an (unexpected) abnormality lies outside the chosen slab. It may either be missed or not be properly displayed. Since subtraction techniques are often used in contrast-enhanced MRA, there is very limited information about the soft tissues of the abdomen. In cases in which this information might become crucial (ruptured aneurysms, tumors), MRA has to be combined with other sequences. 'One-stop shopping' is possible in this way, but the exam becomes rather lengthy (>30 min instead of <15 min).

MRA has the potential to provide time-resolved images at the cost of spatial resolution. This may prove helpful if the venous phase also has to be visualized. In the vast majority of cases, no advantage in terms of therapy-relevant information can be expected for the common indications.

MRA, however, should be considered as a primary diagnostic tool in young patients (radiation exposure of CTA) and in patients with marked renal impairment (iodine load).

40.6
Advantages Over Color Duplex Sonography

CTA is highly reproducible and simple to learn. Color-coded duplex sonography requires a skilled examiner who has had extensive training in the technique and is prepared to perform a significant number of examinations per week in order to stay well trained.

Ultrasound can be an excellent examination tool for the vascular structures of the abdomen. It is generally considered a less costly examination than CTA, MRA or DSA. However, there are several points that stand against this: good examinations require high-tech equipment to ensure consistent visualization of the vascular territory of interest. High-end ultrasound machines currently cost about the same as a standard middle-class (1-s) CT scanner. Costs for the radiological department depend on whether the examination is performed by a radiologist or a technologist. However, time requirements for a thorough examination, for example of the renal arteries, are quite extensive, ranging between 30 min and 1 h. CTA is much less time consuming: the time the patient has to remain on the table is in the order of 10–15 min, and may be even less given optimum organization (preprogrammed scan protocols, RIS–CT interface for direct input of patient data). The time needed to evaluate an examination depends on the diagnostic question (simple for the aorta, more complex for the renal arteries) and on the requirement for 3D image representations. Here, new editing and display equipment has dramatically reduced time requirements (e.g., 2–3 min for the renal arteries).

There is a significant proportion of patients in whom the examination will not yield sufficient results because of adiposity, bowel gas or other factors. Here the examination produces costs but is otherwise useless. The same holds true in patients with uncertain results. Other examinations are necessary before a clinical conclusion can be drawn. This proportion of patients can be reduced with the injection of ultrasound contrast agents. The cost of these agents is very similar to those for CTA, so why not perform CTA at the start?

Ultrasound thus creates significant costs for a hospital or a health care provider, while still not being able to solve all diagnostically relevant questions (e.g., presence of accessory renal arteries in patients with AAA or renovascular hypertension). The reimbursement for ultrasound is very variable, depending on the local situation in each country. Usually, however, it is substantially lower than with CTA.

Diagnostically, anatomy can sometimes not be visualized directly, and indirect (functional) parameters (Doppler spectrum) are included to achieve diagnostic results. These indirect parameters may be helpful in the majority of cases, but they are less reliable than direct signs of vascular disease. In CTA there is no need for indirect signs, although these are often also available (parenchymal contrast enhancement and other collateral signs).

In CTA and MRA, with their 3D capacity, there is a better overview over anatomic and pathologic vascular structures. Presentation is much easier with these techniques. Ultrasound is therefore inherently inferior in all preoperative or preinterventional situations in which there is a need for 3D planning or for an anatomic overview of the vascular situation.

In the case of acute aortic rupture, aneurysms and hematoma may be detected with ultrasound but it is generally difficult to define the relationship of the aneurysm to the renal arteries. The examination takes too long; there are problems with documentation; and nobody wants to press hard on the abdomen of one of these patients just to get an optimum image quality in the ultrasound examination. In aortic dissection, organ malperfusion can be visualized only in optimum cases without the use of intravenous ultrasound contrast. The superior mesenteric artery is usually less of a problem, but involvement of the renal arteries and the pelvic arteries is often impossible to determine.

Visceral arteries are well visualized in their proximal portions, but more distal portions are hard to evaluate. Again, however, there are collateral signs, such as bowel wall edema.

Color-coded duplex ultrasound appears to be best suited to young, slim patients and all situations in which there is a dedicated question that can be easily answered with ultrasound. Examples are the venous system, occlusion of the hepatic artery after orthotopic liver transplantation, stenoses of the proximal visceral arteries, and suspected fibromuscular dysplasia.

40.7
Conclusions

In summary, CT angiography is an excellent diagnostic tool for most applications concerning the abdominal aorta and the renal and visceral arteries. The actual cost of CTA for the hospital or practice depends on the frequency of examinations, the complexity of the particular indications (radiologist's time), reimbursement, and process optimization (standardized scanning and evaluation protocols). In general, CTA is cost effective and has maximum impact on patient management. It is rare for any further examinations to be necessary, as most problems can be definitively solved. CTA helps in decisions on the intervention necessary and in the assessment of patient risk. It is easily performed and can rely on standardized protocols. In young patients or patients with impairment of the renal function, however, preference should be given to other diagnostic techniques.

References

Bluemke DA, Chambers TP (1995) Spiral CT angiography: an alternative to conventional angiography. Radiology 195:317–319

Brink JA (1997) Spiral CT angiography of the abdomen and pelvis: interventional applications. Abdom Imaging 22:365–372

Broeders IA, Blankensteijn JD, Olree M, Mali W, Eikelboom BC (1997) Preoperative sizing of grafts for transfemoral endovascular aneurysm management: a prospective comparative study of spiral CT angiography, arteriography, and conventional CT imaging. J Endovasc Surg 4:252–261

Broeders IA, Blankensteijn JD, Eikelboom BC (1998) The role of infrarenal aortic side branches in the pathogenesis of endoleaks after endovascular aneurysm repair. Eur J Vasc Endovasc Surg 16:419–426

Cochran ST, Krasny RM, Danovitch GM, Rajfer J, Barbaric ZM, Wilkinson A, Rosenthal JT (1997) Helical CT angiography for examination of living renal donors. AJR Am J Roentgenol 168:1569–1573

Errington ML, Ferguson JM, Gillespie IN, Connell HM, Ruckley CV, Wright AR (1997) Complete pre-operative imaging assessment of abdominal aortic aneurysm with spiral CT angiography. Clin Radiol 52:369–377

Halpern EJ, Rutter CM, Gardiner GA Jr, Nazarian LN, Wechsler RJ, Levin DB, Kueny Beck M, Moritz MJ, Carabasi RA, Kahn MB, Smullens SN, Feldman HI (1998) Comparison of Doppler US and CT angiography for evaluation of renal artery stenosis. Acad Radiol 5:524–532

Kaatee R, Beek FJ, de Lange EE, van Leeuwen MS, Smits HF, van der Ven PJ, Beutler JJ, Mali WP (1997) Renal artery stenosis: detection and quantification with spiral CT angiography versus optimized digital subtraction angiography. Radiology 205:121–127

Nelemans PJ, Kessels AG, De Leeuw P, De Haan M, van Engelshoven J (1998) The cost-effectiveness of the diagnosis of renal artery stenosis. Eur J Radiol 27:95–107

Rieker O, Duber C, Neufang A, Pitton M, Schweden F, Thelen M (1997) CT angiography versus intraarterial digital subtraction angiography for assessment of aortoiliac occlusive disease. AJR Am J Roentgenol 169:1133–1138

Smith PA, Ratner LE, Lynch FC, Corl FM, Fishman EK (1998) Role of CT angiography in the preoperative evaluation for laparoscopic nephrectomy. Radiographics 18:589–601

Sommer T, Fehske W, Holzknecht N, et al (1996) Aortic dissection: a comparative study of diagnosis with spiral CT, multiplanar transesophageal echocardiography, and MR imaging. Radiology 199:347–352

Soudack M, Gaitini D, Ofer A (1999) Celiac artery aneurysm: diagnosis by color Doppler sonography and three-dimensional CT angiography. J Clin Ultrasound 27:49–51

Toki K, Takahara S, Kokado Y, Ichimaru N, Wang J, Tsuda K, Narumi Y, Nakamura H, Okuyama A (1998) Comparison of CT angiography with MR angiography in the living renal donor. Transplant Proc 30:2998–3000

Verschuyl EJ, Kaatee R, Beek FJ, Patel NH, Fontaine AB, Daly CP, Coldwell DM, Bush WH, Mali WP (1997) Renal artery origins: best angiographic projection angles. Radiology 205:115–120

Walter F, Henrot P, Blum A, Hirsch JJ, Beot S, Guillemin F, Boccaccini H, Regent D (1998) Valeur comparative de l'angio-IRM, du scanner hélicoïdal et de l'angiographie numérisée dans le bilan préoperatoire des anevrismes de l'aorte abdominale. J Radiol 79:529–539

Winter TC III, Nghiem HV, Freeny PC, Hommeyer SC, Mack LA (1995) Hepatic arterial anatomy: demonstration of normal supply and vascular variants with three-dimensional CT angiography. Radiographics 15:771–780

Yoshimi F, Hasegawa H, Koizumi S, Amemiya R, Ono H, Kobayashi H, Matsueda K, Itabashi M (1995) Application of three-dimensional spiral computed tomographic angiography to pancreatoduodenectomy for cancer. Br J Surg 82:116–117

Zeman RK, Berman PM, Silverman PM, Davros WJ, Cooper C, Kladakis AO, Gomes MN (1995) Diagnosis of aortic dissection: value of helical CT with multiplanar reformation and three-dimensional rendering. AJR Am J Roentgenol 164:1375–1380

41 The Case for MR Angiography

S.G. Rühm, J.F. Debatin

CONTENTS

41.1   Introduction *459*
41.2   MR Angiography – Techniques *459*
41.2.1 Conventional MRA *459*
41.2.2 Contrast-enhanced 3-D MRA *459*
41.3   Applications in the Abdomen *460*
41.3.1 Aorta *460*
41.3.2 Renal Arteries *461*
41.3.3 Celiac and Superior Mesenteric Arteries *462*
41.3.4 Portal Venous System *462*
41.3.5 Renal Veins/Inferior Vena Cava *463*
41.4   Advantages Over CT *463*
41.5   Outlook for MRA in the Abdomen *463*
        References *464*

41.1
Introduction

For the assessment of the abdominal vasculature, conventional angiography is being increasingly challenged as the 'gold standard'. Limitations of conventional angiography include invasiveness with the associated risk of iatrogenic injuries, patient and personnel exposure to ionizing radiation, nephrotoxicity of the contrast media used, and the projectional nature of the images collected. These limitations have given rise to the development of MR-angiography (MRA).

41.2
MRA Techniques

Since the early days of magnetic resonance imaging (MRI), the inherent motion sensitivity of the MR experiment has been exploited for noninvasive vascular imaging giving rise to both 'black blood' and

S.G. Rühm, MD; Institute of Diagnostic Radiology, University Hospital Zurich, Rämistrasse 100, CH-8091 Zurich, Switzerland
J.F. Debatin, MD; Institute of Diagnostic Radiology, University Hospital Zurich, Rämistrasse 100, CH-8091 Zurich, Switzerland

'bright blood' MRA. While black blood techniques, based on signal voids within vessels containing flowing spins, can confirm vessel patency, they remain of limited use in the assessment of vascular morphology (Herfkens et al. 1983).

41.2.1
Conventional MRA

Bright blood MRA techniques are generally divided into those influenced by the effect of blood flow onto the signal amplitude (time of flight, TOF) and those based upon the flow effect on phase (phase contrast, PC) (Dumoulin and Hart 1986; Edelman et al. 1989). Both TOF-MRA and PC-MRA sequences have been employed for the morphologic evaluation of the abdominal vasculature. While they were proven to be most valuable in the assessment of the portal and systemic venous systems, attempts to use these techniques for assessing the renal arteries (Debatin et al. 1991) remained limited by a variety of unsolved technical challenges, including in-plane dephasing, overestimation of stenoses, and long data acquisition times.

PC-MRI also offers the possibility of mapping blood flow velocities and volumes over time (Pelc et al. 1991). The integration of fast data acquisition strategies has enhanced the technique's applicability throughout the abdominal arterial system (Debatin et al. 1994, 1996). Measurement accuracy has been improved by enabling breathheld data acquisition, thereby eliminating the corrupting influence of respiratory motion (Debatin et al. 1994). Shortening of data acquisition times also reduces temporal averaging.

41.2.2
Contrast-Enhanced 3D MRA

The implementation of stronger and faster gradient systems has laid the foundation for the most promising form of MRA yet: ultrafast contrast-enhanced 3D MRA (LEUNG et al 1996; PRINCE et al. 1993). No longer based on flow effects, this technique overcomes most of the limitations inherent in conventional flow-sensitive MRA by relying upon the T1-shortening effects of paramagnetic contrast within the vessels under consideration (PRINCE et al. 1993). Hence, arterial contrast is based on the difference in T1 relaxation between blood and surrounding tissue. As a result, problems associated with slow flow and turbulence-induced signal voids are overcome. Large 3D volumes can be acquired with the imaging plane oriented along the long axis of the vessels of interest (LEUNG et al. 1996; PRINCE et al. 1993). The technique's striking success in the clinical arena is reflected by its rapid integration into routine clinical imaging protocols in centers throughout the world.

High quality of 3D MRA image sets of the abdominal vasculature mandates a breathheld data acquisition strategy (PRINCE et al. 1995a, 1996). This can be achieved with high-performance gradient systems, which allow a reduction in imaging times such that an entire 3D data set can be sampled within a comfortable breath-hold interval lasting less than 30 s (PRINCE et al. 1993). For optimal image quality the repetition time (TR) should be reduced to 3–7 ms and the time to echo (TE) to about 1–3 ms (PRINCE et al. 1995a). Future improvements in gradient switching capabilities will probably reduce the minimum achievable TR and TE further. A flip angle of 30–50° has been shown to provide optimal results (PRINCE et al 1993, 1995a).

The spatial resolution should be maximized within the limits of the breath-holding capabilities of a given patient by adjusting the matrix size and number of slices and by using a rectangular field of vision (FOV). The incorporation of zero-filling routines in all three axes can further enhance spatial resolution. To minimize imaging time further, the sampling bandwidth can be increased at the cost of a slight relative reduction in the signal-to-noise ratio (SNR). Finally, acquisition times can be shortened with partial Fourier methods.

Timing of the contrast medium application must be chosen to ensure the presence of a high concentration of contrast material within the vessels of interest during acquisition of the central portion of k-space, which is responsible for the contrast-defining low spatial frequency image information. Poor timing of the contrast bolus results in insufficient signal within the vessel of interest if the bolus arrives too late, and venous/background overlap if the bolus arrives too early. To determine the contrast travel time from the venous access site to the vascular region of interest, a bolus-timing acquisition should be performed prior to the acquisition of the 3D MRA data set (HANY et al. 1997a).

Gadolinium-based contrast agents are characterized by a most favorable safety profile. The lack of nephrotoxicity permits their use even in patients with renal insufficiency (NIENDORF et al. 1991). A dose of 0.2 mmol per kg body weight has been shown to provide diagnostic image quality of most arterial regions for most 3D MRA applications (HANY et al. 1998a). 3D MRA images are best interpreted on an independent workstation with 3D reconstruction capabilities. In addition to perusal of the original sections, diagnoses should be based on a combination of maximum intensity projection (MIP) images and interactive 3D multiplanar reformations (MPR). The MPR technique permits cross-sectional visualization of the vessels in any plane (Fig. 41.1). Venous overlap can effectively be compensated for and the course of tortuous vessels can easily be reconstructed.

41.3
Applications in the Abdomen

41.3.1
Aorta

3D MRA is well suited to the morphological assessment of the abdominal aorta. All major pathologies, including dissections and aneurysms, are well depicted (HANY et al. 1997b; PRINCE et al. 1995a,b, 1996). The technique is fast and combines the advantages of luminal opacification, similar to conventional contrast angiography, with cross-sectional information.

3D MRA is particularly useful in aortic dissections. Multiplanar reformations locate sites of intimal perforation and of aortic branch vessel involvement (PRINCE et al. 1996). In addition, patency of the false lumen and entry and re-entry tears are easily identified. Homogeneous enhancement of all blood-filled spaces also makes contrast-enhanced 3D MRA well suited to the assessment of abdominal aortic aneurysms. The 3D image set provides exact topographic information on the aneurysmal lumen and also on its relationship to branch vessels. Important preoperative information on associated disease of the renal arteries and their relationship to the proxi-

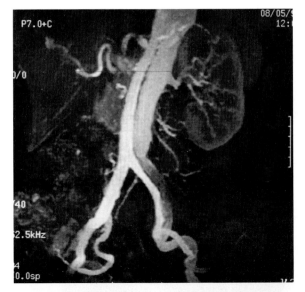

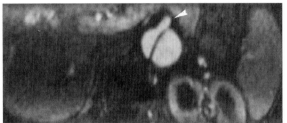

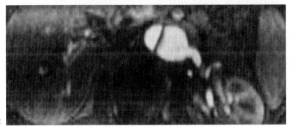

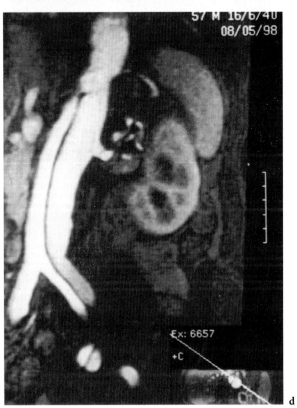

Fig. 41.1a–d. A 57-year-old male patient with dissection of the abdominal aorta. **a** The 3D MR-angiographic MIP (maximum intensity projection) image demonstrates the extent of the dissection into the left common iliac artery. Note the enhancement of both true and false lumen. **b–d** Multiplanar reformations are necessary, however, to identify the origin of the visceral and renal arteries. **b** Axial reformatted image showing the superior mesenteric artery (*arrowhead*) arising from the smaller true lumen. **c** Axial and **d** oblique coronal reformations demonstrate the origin of the left renal artery from the larger false lumen (**c, d**). The right kidney has been surgically removed

mal neck of the aneurysm can easily be obtained from multiplanar reformations. To permit analysis of the abdominal aortic wall and facilitate the delineation of thrombosed regions, it is useful to acquire a T1-weighted sequence after the administration of contrast medium. Enhancement of the aortic wall is indicative of an inflammatory aneurysm. Compared with conventional catheter angiography, 3D MRA has been found to be 100% sensitive and specific regarding the detection and characterization of aortic aneurysmal and occlusive disease (HANY et al. 1997b). Contrast-enhanced 3D MRA is particularly helpful in assessing the abdominal aorta in patients with Leriche syndrome (Fig. 41.2). Both the afferent and the efferent arteries are well delineated.

41.3.2 Renal Arteries

Breath-hold contrast-enhanced 3D MRA holds considerable promise for renal artery screening, because it is a fast, robust, non-operator-dependent, noninvasive technique and can be performed on patients with renal insufficiency. The accuracy of the technique in detection of renal artery stenosis is high, with reported sensitivity and specificity values ranging between 85% and 100% and between 93% and 98%, respectively (HANY et al. 1997c; KAUFMANN et al. 1994; PRINCE 1994; SNIDOW et al. 1996). The technique provides image quality sufficient to detect even small accessory renal arteries, with a detection rate of 100% (ATKINSON and EDELMANN 1991).

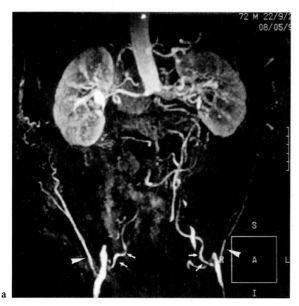

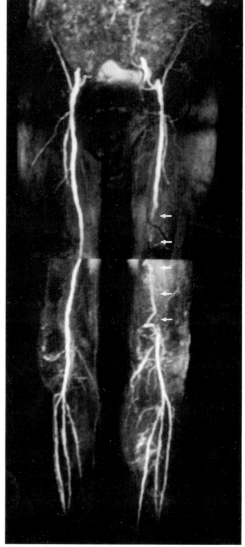

Fig. 41.2a, b. Leriche syndrome. **a** MIP image of 3D contrast-enhanced MRA displays complete occlusion of the infrarenal aorta with bilateral reconstitution of blood flow via mesenteric vessels, deep iliac circumflex (*arrowheads*) and inferior epigastric arteries (*arrows*) in the common femoral arteries. **b** 3D MRA of the runoff vessels which was obtained in the same sitting. A long-distance occlusion (*arrows*) of the superficial femoral artery in the adductory canal with reconstitution via collaterals at the level of the popliteal artery is depicted

41.3.3
Celiac and Superior Mesenteric Arteries

Breath-hold contrast-enhanced 3D MRA can provide a comprehensive morphological assessment of the celiac and superior mesenteric arteries. Recently, MEANEY et al. (1997) reported promising preliminary results in patients with suspected chronic mesenteric ischemia, with sensitivity and specificity values of 100% and 95%, respectively. The authors concluded that 3D contrast-enhanced MRA is accurate in the evaluation of the origins of the mesenteric and celiac arteries, though too low in image resolution for reliable assessment of the inferior mesenteric artery.

41.3.4
Portal Venous System

Beyond displaying normal anatomy, conventional TOF- and PC-MRA has been shown to provide insight into various pathologies, including portal vein stenosis and partial or complete thrombosis. Collateral vessels are well depicted. Furthermore, the sensitivity to flow direction allows differentiation of hepatopetal from hepatofugal flow (FINN et al. 1993; HANY et al. 1998b; HUGHES et al. 1996; LI et al. 1994; MEANEY et al. 1997; SILVERMAN et al. 1991). The ability to depict the portal venous system in both the axial and the coronal plane is particularly helpful in the planning of a transjugular intrahepatic portosystemic shunt (TIPS) procedure (BURKART and JOHNSON 1995). Analysis of portal venous morphology can be complemented by assessing flow characteristics with the aid of PC techniques. Besides permitting accurate quantitation of hypo- or hyperdynamic portal venous flow conditions (BURKART et al. 1993; GAA et al. 1997), PC measurements can be used to determine the effect induced by such therapeutic interventions as TIPS placement on mean portal venous flow (MEANEY et al. 1997). Accurate PC flow measurements of the azygous venous system can also be obtained, providing a quantitative measure for collateral flow volume (RUBIN et al. 1992).

Recently, contrast-enhanced 3D MRA has also been evaluated for imaging the portal venous system (FINN et al. 1991). The portal venous anatomy is seen during the portal venous and equilibrium phases of abdominal arterial 3D contrast-enhanced MRA examinations. Thus, assessment of the portal vein can be added to a study of the abdominal arterial system without the need for additional contrast medium.

41.3.5
Renal Veins/Inferior Vena Cava

Similar to the portal venous system, both the renal veins and the inferior vena cava (IVC) are well displayed with conventional MRA techniques. Depiction of bland and tumor thrombus within the renal veins or the IVC has been shown to be better with MRA than with CTA (THOMSEN et al. 1993). MR also makes it possible to differentiate between a benign and a malignant thrombus based on the enhancement profiles following administration of intravenous paramagnetic contrast: a malignant thrombus enhances, while a bland thrombus does not.

41.4
Advantages Over CTA

The similarities between CTA and contrast-enhanced 3D MRA make a comparison of these two particular techniques most interesting:
1. Compared with iodinated contrast media, paramagnetic contrast agents are considerably safer. Gadolinium-based agents have been shown to be non-nephrotoxic and can even be used in patients with renal failure. In addition, allergic reactions occur less frequently.
2. With proper contrast timing, only the arterial vessels contain signal. Both bone and calcium remain dark. Another difference from CTA is that

no effort is required to cut out high-density structures such as bone or calcium, which might obscure the reconstructed vascular anatomy. Therefore, 3D MRA reconstruction times are shorter.
3. Contrast-enhanced 3D-MRA does not expose the patient to ionizing radiation. This is a particular advantage in the assessment of young patients and of patients requiring frequent follow-ups.
4. The data acquisition plane of 3D MRA can be adjusted to fit the anatomy of the vascular territory under consideration. The ability to acquire the data in the coronal or sagittal plane allows the use of a larger field of view and consequent depiction of more of the vascular territory.

In addition, it is important to note that conventional TOF-MRA and PC-MRA are also still available. They do not require any contrast medium at all and will continue to play an important part in the assessment of the portal and systemic venous systems. Furthermore, MRA offers functional information by virtue of the PC flow-mapping techniques. This aspect is increasing in importance as the medical community learns to integrate functional and morphological data.

41.5
Outlook for MRA in the Abdomen

Owing to the development and quick implementation of contrast-enhanced 3D MRA techniques, the future of abdominal MRA in the clinical environment looks very bright. 3D MRA provides data that have applications beyond mere screening for disease; the image quality is sufficient to permit therapeutic planning. The technique is easy to use. The images are interpreted in a similar way to those yielded by conventional angiography, so that most radiologists are familiar with the technique.

Noninvasiveness, the 3D nature of the data sets allowing reformations in any desired plane, relatively low cost and lack of contrast medium toxicity coupled with high diagnostic accuracy will drive up the popularity of contrast-enhanced 3D MRA within the medical community. In the abdomen it will undoubtedly surpass other noninvasive techniques, such as color-coded Doppler or CT angiography. The characteristics of contrast-enhanced 3D MRA that have been outlined here stand to increase the number of referrals for vascular assessments well beyond current levels.

References

Atkinson DJ, Edelman RR (1991) Cineangiography of the heart in a single breath hold with a segmented turboFLASH sequence. Radiology 178:357–360

Burkart DJ, Johnson CD (1995) Upper abdominal phase-contrast MR angiography: comparison of cine and non-cine techniques. Radiology 195:101–105

Burkart DJ, Johnson CD, Ehman, RL, Weaver AL, Ilstrup DM (1993) Evaluation of portal venous hypertension with cine phase-contrast MR flow measurements: high association of hyperdynamic portal flow with variceal hemorrhage. Radiology 188:643–648

Debatin JF, Spritzer CE, Grist TM (1991) Imaging of the renal arteries: value of MR angiography. AJR Am J Roentgenol 157:981–990

Debatin JF, Ting RH, Wegmüller H, Sommer FG, Fredrickson JO, Brosnan TJ, Bowman BS, Myers BD, Herfkens RJ, Pelc NJ (1994) Renal artery blood flow: quantification with phase contrast imaging with and without breath-holding. Radiology 190:371–378

Debatin JF, Zahner B, Meyenberger C, Romanowski B, Schöpke W, Marincek B, Fuchs WA (1996) Cine-Pc M_r quantitation of azygous blood flow in volunteers and patients with portal hypertension before and after TIPS. Hepatology 24:1109–1115

Dumoulin CL, Hart HR (1986) Magnetic resonance angiography. Radiology 161:717–720

Edelman RR, Wentz KU, Mattle H, Zhao B, Liu C, Kim D, Laub G (1989) Projection arteriography and venography: initial clinical results with MR. Radiology 172:351–357

Finn JP, Edelman RR, Jenkins RL et al (1991) Liver transplantation: MR angiography with surgical validation. Radiology 179:265–269

Finn JP, Kane RA, Edelman RR et al (1993) Imaging of the portal venous system in patients with cirrhosis: MR angiography vs duplex Doppler sonography. AJR Am J Roentgenol 161:989–994

Gaa J, Laub G, Georgi M (1997) Breath-hold three-dimensional gadolinium-enhanced dual-phase MR angiography of the abdomen: first clinical results. In: Oudkerk M, Edelman RR (eds) High-power gradient MR-imaging. (Advances in MRI II) Blackwell Science, Berlin Vienna, pp 334–339

Hany TF, McKinnon GC, Leung DA, Pfammatter T, Debatin JF (1997a) Optimization of contrast timing for breathhold 3D MR angiography. J Magn Reson Imaging 7:552–557

Hany TF, Debatin JF, Leung DA, Pfammatter T (1997b) Evaluation of the aortoiliac and renal arteries with breath-hold contrast-enhanced 3D MR angiography: comparison with conventional angiography. Radiology 204:357–362

Hany TF, Pfammatter T, Schmidt M, Leung DA, Debatin JF (1997c) Ultraschnelle, kontrastverstärkte 3 D MR Angiographie der Aorta und Nierenarterien in Apnoe. Rofo Fortschr Geb Roentgenstr Neuen Bildgeb Verfahr 166:397–405

Hany TF, Schmidt M, Davis CP, Goedhe SC, Debatin JF (1998a) Evaluation of 4 different post- processing techniques in the evaluation of contrast-enhanced 3D MR angiography. AJR Am J Roentgenol (in press)

Hany TF, Schmidt M, Schoenenberger AW, Debatin JF (1998b) Contrast enhanced 3D MRA of the splanchnic vasculature

before and after caloric stimulation. Invest Rad 9:682–686

Herfkens RJ, Higgins CB, Hricak H (1983) Nuclear magnetic resonance imaging of atherosclerotic disease. Radiology 148:161–166

Hughes LA, Hartnell GG, Finn JP et al. (1996) Time-of-flight MR angiography of the portal venous system: value compared with other imaging procedures. AJR Am J Roentgenol 166:375–378

Kaufmann JA, Geller SC, Petersen MJ, Cambria RP, Prince MR, Waltman AC (1994) MR imaging (including MR angiography) of abdominal aortic aneurysms: comparison with conventional angiography. AJR Am J Roentgenol 163:203–210

Leung DA, McKinnon GC, Davis CP, Pfammatter T, Krestin GP, Debatin JF (1996) Breathheld contrast-enhanced 3D MR angiography. Radiology 201:569–571

Li KC, Whitney WS, McDonnell CH et al (1994) Chronic mesenteric ischemia: evaluation with phase-contrast cine MR imaging. Radiology 190:175–179

Meaney JFM, Prince MR, Nostrant TT, Stanley JC (1997) Gadolinium-enhanced MR angiography of the visceral arteries in patients with suspected chronic mesenteric ischemia. J Magn Reson Imaging 7:171–176

Niendorf HP, Haustein J, Cornelius I, Alhassan A, Clauss W (1991) Safety of gadolinium-DTPA: extended clinical experience. Magn Reson Med 22: 222–228

Pelc NJ, Herfkens RJ, Shimakawa A, Enzmann DR (1991) Phase contrast cine magnetic resonance imaging. Magn Reson Q 7:229–254

Prince MR (1994) Gadolinium-enhanced MR aortography. Radiology 191:155–164

Prince MR, Yucel EK, Kaufmann JA, Harrison DC, Geller SC (1993) Dynamic gadolinium-enhanced three dimensional abdominal MR arteriography. J Magn Reson Imaging 3:877–881

Prince MR, Narasimhan DL, Stanley JC (1995a) Breath-hold gadolinium-enhanced MR angiography of the abdominal aorta and its major branches. Radiology 197:785–792

Prince MR, Narasimham DL, Stanley JC, Wakefield TW, Messina LM, Zelenock GB, Jacoby WT, Marx MV, Williams DM, Cho KJ (1995b) Gadolonium-enhanced magnetic resonance angiography of abdominal aortic aneurysms. J Vasc Surg 21:656–669

Prince MR, Narasimhan DL, Jacoby WT (1996) Three-dimensional gadolinium-enhanced MR angiography of the thoracic aorta. Am J Roentgenol 166:1387–1397

Rubin DL, Herfkens RJ, Pelc NJ, Jeffrey RB (1992) MR measurement of portal blood flow in chronic liver disease: application to predicting clinical outcome (abstract). Society of Magnetic Resonance in Medicine, Berkeley

Silverman PM, Patt RH, Garra BS et al (1991) MR imaging of the portal venous system: value of gradient-echo imaging as an adjunct to spin-echo imaging. AJR Am J Roentgenol 157:297–302

Snidow JJ, Johnson MS, Harris VJ, Margosian PM, Aisen AM, Lalka SG, Cikrit DF, Trerotola SO (1996) Three-dimensional gadolinium-enhanced MR angiography for aortoiliac inflow assessment plus renal artery screening in a single breath hold. Radiology 198:725–732

Thomsen C, Ståhlberg F, Henriksen O (1993) Quantification of portal venous blood flow during fasting and after a standardized meal_–_a MRI phase-mapping study. Eur Radiol 3:242–247

42 Synthesis

C.D. BECKER

CONTENTS

42.1   Advantages of CTA   465
42.2   Drawbacks of CTA   466
42.3   Conclusions   467
        References   467

Owing to rapid technical development of non-invasive vascular imaging modalities, the role of conventional catheter angiography with the digital subtraction technique (DSA) has decreased considerably. Despite its superior resolution, DSA is now increasingly being limited to selected diagnostic indications and is mainly performed in the context of intravascular interventional procedures, thus allowing avoidance of catheter-related side effects and complications in diagnostic studies. As the above discussions have shown, controversy still exists over the respective roles of CT angiography (CTA), magnetic resonance angiography (MRA), and Doppler ultrasonography (US). The diagnostic key elements for imaging of the abdominal vessels are summarized in Table 42.1. The choice of the most appropriate angiographic technique depends not only on the suspected pathology, but also on a variety of technical and logistic parameters. These include the patient's general condition (hemodynamic stability, mobility, monitoring requirements, renal function, ability to cooperate), local availability of imaging modalities and experienced operators, and the need for examining other, extraabdominal, regions at the same time. Some important features determining the usefulness of CTA in comparison with MRA and US are addressed below.

42.1
Advantages of CTA

All diagnostic criteria except flow direction and flow velocity can be evaluated with CTA. CT is also the technique of choice for the detection of calcified plaque, active contrast medium extravasation, and secondary, ischemic changes in abdominal organs. An abdominal CTA study can be accomplished in 10–15 min. Vessels in additional body regions, e.g., the thoracic aorta, may be examined at the same time if needed. Patient monitoring is possible throughout the procedure. Standardized protocols make it possible to obtain consistent diagnostic information, although adequate reconstruction images require patient cooperation. The diagnostic information obtained with CTA is not limited to vessels but may also be used for diagnostic evaluation of secondary perfusion changes in the organs in the body region concerned. DSA remains unchallenged by CTA for demonstration of stenosis and thromboembolic occlusion of the peripheral vascular territories. However, bowel ischemia may present with uncharacteristic clinical findings and may be only one of many possible diagnoses. Abdominal CT is therefore often performed in the course of the diagnostic work-up. Careful examination technique and meticulous reading of arterial and venous phase CT

Table 42.1. Diagnostic key elements for imaging of the abdominal vessels

Complete delineation of normal arteries, systemic veins, veins of portal system, anatomic variants
Presence and degree of stenosis
Vessel occlusion
Localization and measurement of aneurysm
Thrombus, calcified and noncalcified plaques
Dissection and involvement of side branches
Vessel rupture / acute hemorrhage
Hemodynamic changes: flow velocity, flow direction, collateral circulation
Perivascular changes: hematoma, tumor, perfusion changes/ infarction

C.D. BECKER, MD; Department of Radiology, Division of Diagnostic and Interventional Radiology, Geneva University Hospital, 24, Rue Micheli-du-Crest, CH-1211 Geneva 14, Switzerland

images may allow visualization of thromboembolic occlusion of major visceral arteries and veins along with signs of ischemia (e.g., lack of perfusion, bowel wall thickening). The specificity of contrast-enhanced axial CT for the detection of acute mesenteric ischemia using cross-sectional images has been reported to be 90% and the sensitivity, 64% (TAOUREL et al. 1996). The diagnostic value of maximum intensity and multiplanar reconstruction images in the context of ischemia remains to be proven, however.

MRA has recently gone through a phase of rapid technical development. In patients who can cooperate appropriately, contrast-enhanced MRA now yields superb angiographic images; maximum intensity projections obtained from coronal or sagittal 3D data sets acquired with gadolinium chelate enhancement are often superior to those obtained with CTA. Nonetheless, important advantages of CTA over MRA include lower cost of both equipment and contrast material, better availability, higher acquisition speed, superiority in detection of calcifications, and ability to obtain more comprehensive evaluation of the entire abdomen. MRA is generally limited by claustrophobia and metallic implants and is also less practical than CTA in critically ill patients.

US enables detection of many vascular abdominal pathologies. However, a complete abdominal Doppler study takes considerably longer than CTA, since each vessel needs to be analyzed and documented individually. This remains true even if contrast materials for enhancement of flow signals are being used. Precise and complete evaluation of the intraabdominal vessels, especially in the emergency situation, requires considerable operator expertise. If image quality is impaired by bowel gas or obesity, important questions may remain unanswered even by an experienced operator. Although the investment costs for US are lower than those for CT, this advantage may be outweighed by the physician time required by US. There are currently too few data available to prove the cost effectiveness of CT in the major clinical settings. On the basis of the good diagnostic performance of CTA in the context of many diseases, however, we can assume that CTA compares favorably with both US and MRA for many indications (ETTORE et al. 1997; PROKOP et al. 1997a, b).

42.2
Drawbacks of CTA

Fast acquisitions with narrow collimation require high performance of the X-ray generator, tube and detector system. The need for intermittent tube cooling reduced the performance of CTA considerably earlier, although this has been solved with the latest generation of scanners. Although considerable progress is currently being made in the field of image processing, multiplanar rendering of 2D and 3D images is still quite time consuming, and the routine use of CTA requires adequate staffing with qualified medical or technical personnel. An understanding of the structures displayed is an important prerequisite for image reconstruction, since superposition of arteriosclerotic plaques or bony structures with opacified vessel lumina may create artifacts and confusion. This is clearly a disadvantage compared with MRA. Unlike US and, to a lesser degree, MRA, CTA cannot provide flow information but is limited to morphologic information. US is therefore the method of choice for obtaining hemodynamic information.

Side effects of and contraindications to iodinated contrast material are a major drawback of CTA. Chronic vascular disease may be associated with impaired renal function, and CTA is therefore often inappropriate in patients with suspected renal artery stenosis. Contrast-enhanced MRA is the technique of choice for display of vascular morphology in these situations and should be used whenever possible. The reported sensitivity for the detection of renal artery stenosis of more than 50% is 93–100%, while the associated specificity varies from 98% to 94% (DONG et al. 1998; STEFFENS et al. 1997). In centers with good local expertise and availability, MRA may also be preferable for a variety of other indications, e.g., subacute or chronic aortic dissection or vessel analysis in the context of abdominal tumor staging.

Radiation exposure is another significant drawback of CTA. Therefore, repeat studies, e.g., monitoring of the hepatic artery after liver transplantation, of portosystemic shunts after TIPS or surgical procedures, or of vessels after thrombolytic therapy, should be performed with US whenever possible. If US cannot provide the necessary diagnostic information, preference should be given to MRA for selective noninvasive morphologic evaluation of vascular territories. For similar reasons, MRA is preferable to CTA in children.

42.3
Conclusions

Its ability to provide comprehensive and consistent diagnostic information makes CTA appropriate for the majority of clinical situations in which an acute vascular abdominal pathology is suspected, and it is also very well suited to preoperative or preinterventional studies of the abdominal vessels, particularly the aorta and the major systeme and portal venous structures. The need for relatively high doses of contrast material and radiation exposure are inherent drawbacks of CTA and may be a point in favor of MRA on the long term. Although the availability of MRA is still limited in many institutions, it yields excellent technical and diagnostic results and is playing an expanding part in subacute and elective situations, because nephrotoxicity is often an issue in patients with vascular disease. US remains unchallenged for hemodynamic studies. Since CTA provides no information on the direction and velocity of flow, US can be used as a complementary method to CTA. Owing to the radiation exposure it involves, CTA should be avoided for serial follow-up studies and in children whenever possible.

References

Dong Q, Schoenberg SO, Carlos RC, Prince MR (1998) Renal MR angiography. Semin Intervent Radiol 15:163–178

Ettore GC, Francioso G, Garribba AP et al (1997) Helical CT angiography in gastrointestinal bleeding of obscure origin. AJR Am J Roentgenol 168:727

Prokop M, Shin HO, Schaefer-Prokop CM (1997a) Use of maximum intensity projections in CT angiography: basic review. Radiographics 17:433

Prokop M, Schaefer-Prokop CM, Galanski M (1997) Spiral CT angiography of the abdomen. Abdom Imaging 22:143

Steffens JC, Link J, Grassner J et al (1997) Contrast- enhanced k- space centered breath-hold MR angiography of the renal artery and abdominal aorta. J Magn Reson Imaging 7:617–622

Taourel PG, Deneuville M, Pradel JA, Régent DA, Bruel JM (1996) Acute mesenteric ischemia: diagnosis with contrast -enhanced CT. Radiology 199:632

Special Topics

43 Helical CT in Patients with Abdominal Trauma

H. Genghis Khan and C.D. Becker

CONTENTS

43.1 Introduction *471*
43.2 Impact of Scanning Speed *471*
43.3 Helical CT Examination Technique *472*
43.4 Detection and Localization of Active
     Intra-abdominal Haemorrhage *472*
43.5 Splenic Injury *473*
43.6 Liver Injury *474*
43.7 Injury to the Diaphragm *475*
43.8 Gastrointestinal Injuries *476*
43.9 Renal Injury *476*
43.10 Applications of Helical CT in Clinical
      Trauma Research *477*
      References *478*

43.1 Introduction

Imaging of acute trauma has been influenced fundamentally by the advent of helical CT. The role of CT in the diagnostic work-up and management of trauma patients is currently being reassessed, and it is likely to increase in the future. The purpose of this chapter is to review the impact of helical CT on clinical imaging of the patient with acute abdominal trauma.

43.2 Impact of Scanning Speed

During the 1980s, contrast-enhanced CT with the dynamic incremental scanning technique became well accepted for examination of trauma patients, because it enables complete imaging of multiple body regions and organ systems in a single examination with consistent, acceptable image quality. The drawback of this technique is that approximately 20–30 min is required for image acquisition alone. Therefore, it has often been difficult to balance the benefit of a CT examination against the risk inherent in a delay in going to the operating theatre in the case of a rapidly developing, life-threatening situation. Analysis of a large series of abdominal trauma patients undergoing diagnostic work-up including CT has shown that the risk of complications attributable to the delay caused by performing CT is not at all negligible (Davis et al. 1990). The general consensus in the literature has so far been that the use of CT should be restricted to patients who are haemodynamically stable on admission or who have been completely stabilized haemodynamically after resuscitation. This has been recognized as a major limitation in the early diagnostic work-up of the acutely and severely traumatized patient (Gay and Sistrom 1992; Shuman 1997; Becker et al. 1998a,b).

Helical CT makes it possible to scan the entire abdomen within approximately 30 s and to examine multiple body regions within a few minutes (Fishman and Spiral 1996; Pretorius and Fishman 1995). Time for image acquisition and reconstruction is thus no longer a concern, and patient turnaround time mainly depends on the logistics involved in transferring, repositioning and monitoring. Therefore, provided that the CT scanner is situated relatively close to the emergency room, the operating room and the angiography suite, the indications for CT in trauma patients may now be expanded. Because all images can be viewed on-line by the radiologist immediately after acquisition the speed of the diagnostic process is further enhanced. Although in clinical practice the image quality is often impaired in the setting of acute trauma by artefacts due to motion, respiration, metallic monitoring devices, instruments and other foreign bodies, the acquisition speed and artefact suppression algorithms implemented in modern helical scan-

H.G.Khan; Department of Radiology, Division of Diagnostic and Interventional Radiology, Geneva University Hospital, 24, Rue Micheli-du-Crest, CH-1211 Geneva 14, Switzerland
C.D. Becker; Department of Radiology, Division of Diagnostic and Interventional Radiology, Geneva University Hospital, 24, Rue Micheli-du-Crest, CH-1211 Geneva 14, Switzerland

ners greatly improve the overall diagnostic quality of images.

In our department, we have seen indications for CT in acute trauma patients expand gradually with the build-up of experience with two modern helical scanners over the past few years. Helical CT is now being used for the initial diagnostic work-up of many patients with severe, multiple trauma even while resuscitation is continued; as a matter of fact suspected acute intra-abdominal haemorrhage is no longer considered as a general contraindication to the use of CT.

43.3
Helical CT Examination Technique

Although a standard CT protocol is important in the setting of trauma, the examination needs to be tailored to the patient's condition. If the patient's condition permits, 250–500 ml of water-soluble oral contrast material (2–5%) is administered via the nasogastric tube in the emergency department and an additional 250 ml in the CT suite immediately before scanning. Additional administration of rectal contrast material is an option in patients with pelvic trauma or a suspected colon injury. Typical helical scanning parameters are 5- to 8-mm collimation, 1–2 pitch and 5- to 8-mm reconstruction thickness (SHUMAN 1997; BECKER et al. 1998a). In a patient with abdominal trauma, CT should always cover the entire volume from the lung base to the symphysis pubis. Preliminary scanning before administration of intravenous contrast material may sometimes facilitate image interpretation, but is not recommended routinely as it also increases the radiation dose significantly. An automated single-phase bolus injection of 130–180 ml of intravenous iodinated contrast material (60–75%) is given at 2–4 ml/s; nonionic contrast material is preferable to ionic contrast material as it reduces the risk of vomiting with subsequent aspiration. A standard scan delay of 70–90 s may be used, but a longer delay may be preferable in patients with significant arterial hypotension, in order to avoid artefacts in the early parenchymal phase or to avoid missing extravasation of contrast material. Repeat, delayed scanning may be necessary for better demonstration of the distribution of extravasated contrast material from the blood vessels, parenchymal organs, gastrointestinal tract or urinary system. All images should be viewed immediately by the radiologist at the workstation with appropriate window settings. Depending on the ques-

tions that need to be answered, additional acquisitions may then be performed and two-dimensional or three-dimensional reconstructions can be obtained if necessary.

43.4
Detection and Localization of Active Intra-abdominal Haemorrhage

Demonstration and quantification of free intra-abdominal blood with CT is helpful but of only limited diagnostic value, as the mere presence of blood in an anatomical compartment at the moment of a single CT examination gives no information on the presence and severity of active bleeding. Detection and localization of acute intra-abdominal haemorrhage is one of the major challenges in the early diagnostic work-up of acutely and severely traumatized patients, as it is very helpful in haemostasis accomplished by means of transarterial embolization or surgery. Demonstration of active haemorrhage or of expansion of a haematoma over time are also relevant as criteria for grading the severity of blunt injuries to the parenchymal abdominal organs according to the surgical organ injury scale (OIS) (MOORE et al. 1989, 1990, 1995). With dynamic incremental scanning in the past, the diagnosis of active haemorrhage resulting from parenchymal organs often depended on indirect signs rather than direct visualization of extravasation of contrast material, although increasing attention has also been given in the recent literature to signs of active haemorrhage (JEFFREY et al. 1991). Helical CT can demonstrate even small amounts of extravasated contrast material in the peritoneal cavity or retroperitoneum, and may also show vascular injuries (Figs. 43.1–43.4). A second acquisition may be obtained after a short delay to investigate the distribution of extravasated contrast material. The ability to detect active bleeding with helical CT may be considered a major diagnostic improvement, as it enables a focused therapeutic approach to either radiological transcatheter embolization or trauma surgery (SHUMAN 1997; FISHMAN and SPIRAL 1996). In a prototype project, a helical CT scanner has been combined with a digital angiography unit in the same suite within the emergency department to allow transarterial embolization procedures on the same table. This set-up, although costly, probably makes optimal use of the speed provided by the helical scanning technique (CAPASSO et al. 1996).

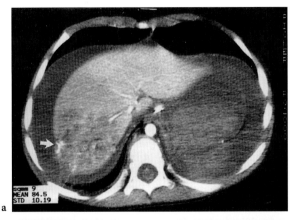

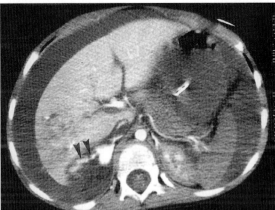

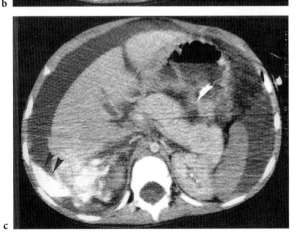

Fig. 43.1a–c. Active haemorrhage from blunt hepatic and adrenal injuries. **a, b** Early phase after contrast injection: **a** contrast medium extravasation at the surface of the liver *(arrow)*. heterogeneous perfusion of right hepatic lobe due to extensive parenchymal contusion; **b** contrast medium extravasation from the right adrenal gland *(arrowheads)*. **c** Delayed phase demonstrates accumulation of contrast material in the peritoneal cavity and retroperitoneum *(arrowheads)*

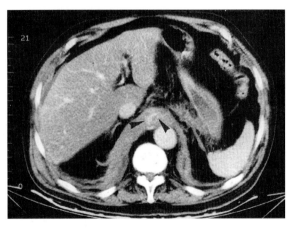

Fig. 43.2 Active haemorrhage following blunt injury of the diaphragm. Extravasation of contrast material is seen within the muscular portion of the diaphragm, anterior to the aorta *(arrowheads)*. Note thickening of the diaphragmatic as a result of haematoma

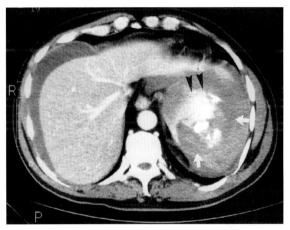

Fig. 43.3 Active haemorrhage from the spleen following blunt splenic rupture. A major accumulation of extravasated contrast material is seen within the spleen and adjacent to the splenic hilum *(black arrowheads)*. Enhancemant of the splenic parenchyma is reduced *(with arrows)* Note hyperdense haematoma arround the spleen

43.5
Splenic Injury

The important role of CT in the detection and characterization of blunt splenic injuries has been well documented in the literature. Grading systems that are similar to the surgical OIS and scores based on the extent of capsular or parenchymal laceration and haematoma and the degree of haemoperitoneum at the time of admission have been proposed by some investigators as instruments that

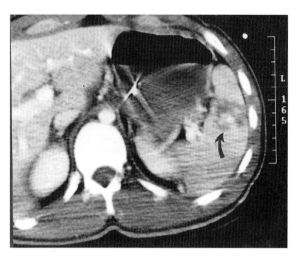

Fig. 43.4. Blunt splenic injury: intraparenchymal "contrast blush" without free contrast medium extravasation. According to newer observations, presence of this sign indicates that nonsurgical management is unlikely to be successful. Splenectomy was considered necessary in this case

could be useful in predicting the outcome (SHUMAN 1997; BECKER et al. 1994, 1998a; FEDERLE et al. 1998; GAVANT et al. 1997). Although it is generally accepted that severe (grade 4–5) injuries usually require surgical repair, CT-based grading of splenic injuries has not so far been found sufficiently reliable as a means of identifying injuries that can be successfully treated conservatively (BECKER et al. 1998a). So far, the identification of those patients who are at risk of developing delayed splenic rupture and those who are not remains a particular diagnostic challenge.

With the increasing use of helical CT scanners, attention has recently been directed at the visualization of active extravasation of contrast material from the splenic parenchyma (BECKER et al. 1994; FEDERLE et al. 1998) (Fig. 43.3). According to these studies, it appears that the presence of active haemorrhage from the spleen, the appearance of an intraparenchymal "contrast blush" or the demonstration of an intrasplenic arterial pseudoaneurysm are useful CT criteria indicating the need for surgery or catheter embolization even if destruction of the splenic parenchyma is only moderate, i.e. grade 2–3 (Fig. 43.4) (FEDERLE et al. 1998; GAVANT et al. 1997). Further data are now needed to determine whether absence of contrast medium extravasation on a properly performed contrast-enhanced helical CT study in the presence of an injury graded 2–3 allows the prediction that conservative treatment will be successful.

Although the acquisition speed of helical CT greatly improves the detection of active haemorrhage and reduces streak artefacts caused by respiratory motion, it does also have some pitfalls owing to flow artefacts. These are of particular importance in the spleen. In the early parenchymal phase enhancement is normally heterogeneous and may thus prevent detection of an injury. Although a scan delay of 70 s usually results in a homogeneous enhancement of the spleen, this may not be the case in a trauma victim with arterial hypotension. Because perfusion defects in the parenchymal phase do not always indicate vascular injury or contusion but can also be due to transient local hypoperfusion in a hypotensive state, repeat scanning may become necessary in such a situation.

The distinction between intrasplenic and subcapsular haematoma and perisplenic free blood is often difficult, because density differences may be subtle. In this context, the improved image quality obtained with helical CT increases diagnostic confidence (Fig. 43.5).

43.6
Liver Injury

Helical CT is well suited to delineation of the presence, extent, and location of blunt injuries of the hepatic parenchyma and the demonstration of active intra- or extrahepatic bleeding (Fig. 43.6) (SHUMAN 1997; BECKER et al. 1998a; NUNEZ et al. 1996a).

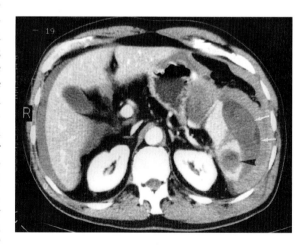

Fig. 43.5. Blunt splenic fracture: perisplenic intraperitoneal blood, a subcapsular splenic haematoma (*white arrows*), and intrasplenic haematoma (*black arrow*) can be clearly distinguished

Various patterns of injuries may be distinguished and classified, including capsular tear, intra-parenchymal laceration or fracture, subcapsular or intraparenchymal haematoma, and partial devascularization as a result of parenchymal contusion (Figs. 43.6, 43.7). Currently, even extensive parenchymal damage of the liver following blunt trauma is usually managed conservatively when helical CT shows no active haemorrhage and the patient is haemodynamically stable and does not require laparotomy for extrahepatic injuries (BECKER et al. 1996, 1998a). Delayed hepatic rupture is a very rare complication of conservative treatment. It is nonetheless important in the initial diagnostic work-up to identify injuries of the major intra- and perihepatic vessels or lesions of the biliary system that require surgical or radiological intervention. Fractures near the course of the central hepatic veins or the inferior vena cava are of particular interest to the surgeon who performs exploratory laparotomy, since major haemorrhage can occur when the liver is mobilized in the presence of a laceration of a major central vein. Periportal blood is sometimes the only sign of liver injury in cases of major trauma. Disruption of the portal triad can occur, resulting in the formation of a false aneurysm or a posttraumatic arterioportal fistula within a week of trauma (BECKER et al. 1996). These lesions can be readily demonstrated by CT and can then be treated definitively by transcatheter embolization. Owing to the dual blood supply of the liver, local disturbances of arterial and portal flow with subsequent compensatory perfusion phenomena are commonly observed after major hepatic trauma. The resulting parenchymal perfusion heterogeneities may be difficult to distinguish from direct devascularization if only a single acquisition is made in a relatively early phase of contrast enhancement. Repeat scanning in a later vascular phase can often clarify such situations.

43.7
Injury to the Diaphragm

Although major traumatic lesions of the diaphragmatic crura are usually readily visualized on transverse CT sections (Fig. 43.2), rupture of the diaphragmatic dome, which often occurs on the left side, is missed in approximately one-third of cases on initial CT evaluation with routine transverse sections (MURRAY et al. 1996). Early diagnosis of dia-

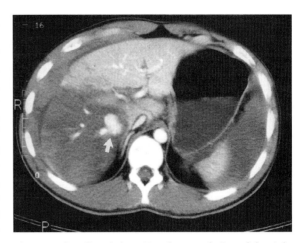

Fig. 43.6. Blunt liver injury. Note hypoperfusion of the right lobe and intraparenchymal contrast extravasation, indicating rupture of a major intrahepatic venous branch (*arrow*). Surgery revealed laceration of a hepatic vein

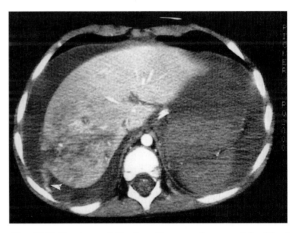

Fig. 43.7. Rupture of the hepatic capsule caused by blunt trauma, active bleeding (*arrow*)

phragmatic rupture is essential, because herniation of gastrointestinal organs may not only result in compression atelectasis of the adjacent lung but may also result in strangulation of the herniated organs. The advantage of helical CT scanning is that volumetric acquisition makes it possible to perform high-quality 2D sagittal reformations, thus improving the visibility of traumatic lesions and of any herniation of intra-abdominal structures into the chest. The usefulness of the reformatted images has recently been shown experimentally and clinically (ISRAEL et al. 1996a,b). Optimal acquisition parameters for 2D reformatting in the case of suspected diaphragmatic rupture include 3-mm collimation with pitch 1–1.5. Oral contrast material is very helpful in this context as it facilitates the detection of visceral herniation.

43.8
Gastrointestinal Injuries

Although CT has long been considered insensitive to injuries of the gastrointestinal tract, recent studies based on examinations with modern CT equipment have shown that CT allows the detection of blunt gastrointestinal injuries with a high sensitivity provided that appropriate scanning protocols are used and meticulous attention is given to the often subtle diagnostic findings (BECKER et al. 1998a; SHERCK et al. 1994; HAGIWARA et al. 1995; RIZZO et al. 1989; MIRVIS et al. 1992; CASEY et al. 1995; DOWE et al. 1997). Detection of the CT signs of gastrointestinal trauma requires images of optimal resolution, and helical CT is the technique best suited to providing the necessary image quality in the often difficult conditions encountered in trauma patients. Signs indicating full-thickness bowel perforation include discontinuity of the gastrointestinal wall and spillage of contrast material or luminal contents into the peritoneal cavity or retroperitoneum, and free extraluminal, extraperitoneal or intraperitoneal air. There is a second group of indirect CT signs: a 'sentinel clot' adjacent to a loop of bowel, visualization of contrast medium extravasation originating from a mesenteric vessel, focal thickening of the wall of the small bowel (>3 cm) and intramesenteric fluid or haematoma, and a "streaky" appearance of the mesenteric fat (Fig. 43.8). Finally, unexplained free fluid localized between the mesenteric loops should be carefully sought, as it may sometimes be the only sign indicating a traumatic lesion of the bowel or mesentery. Mesenteric vascular injury may lead to bowel necrosis by way of ischaemia, which may become visible due to intramural gas collections (Fig 43. 9).

Our recent review of the literature indicates that the overall sensitivity of CT for the detection of blunt gastrointestinal tract injuries is as high as 85%–95% (BECKER et al. 1998a). On the basis of experience at our institution, we concur with these observations. It appears logical that the increasing use of helical CT and the resulting improvements in overall image quality have a favourable impact on the detection of the often subtle diagnostic findings seen in blunt gastrointestinal injuries. It is therefore mandatory for the radiologist to review all CT images closely for the above-mentioned signs so as to alert the surgeon to the possibility of a gastrointestinal injury.

43.9
Renal Injury

CT is regarded as the imaging method of choice in the evaluation of blunt renal trauma, as it provides both morphological and functional information that would otherwise require several different modalities, e.g. ultrasound, intravenous urography or even arteriography (SHUMAN 1997; BECKER et al. 1998a; MILLER and McANINCH 1995; BRETAN et al. 1986;

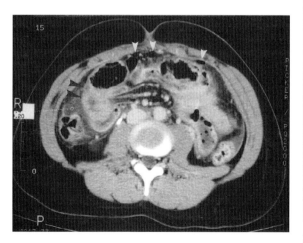

Fig. 43.8. Blunt bowel injury. Helical CT demonstrates thickening of a small bowel loop owing to haematoma (*black arrowheads*) and pneumoperitoneum (*white arrowheads*), indicating perforation

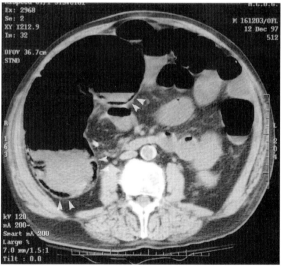

Fig. 43.9. Posttraumatic infarction of ascending colon caused by blunt injury. Following injury of branches of the superior mesenteric artery, the ascending colon is distended and there is intramural gas (*white arrowheads*). At laparotomy, partially necrotic colon was resected

FANNEY et al. 1990; NUNEZ et al. 1996b). Helical CT acquisition enables visualization of the entire kidneys during the same phase of contrast enhancement. It also minimizes breathing misregistration artefacts, thus facilitating multiplanar reconstructions, which are increasingly used for optimal display of the relationship of the parenchyma and the hilar vessels and the proximal collecting system, especially if kidney-sparing surgery is envisaged. Because renal enhancement is quite heterogeneous owing to intense corticomedullary differentiation during the standard early parenchymal phase, a second helical acquisition with the same parameters is best done after a 3-min delay. This will also give valuable additional information regarding the renal collecting system, the ureters, and the urinary bladder.

The clinical role of CT has become enhanced by the current trend toward conservative treatment of blunt renal trauma. Approximately 80% of blunt renal injuries may be considered minor, and these heal spontaneously (MILLER and MCANINCH 1995; BRETAN et al. 1986). These include lesions such as contusions (seen on CT as ill-defined perfusion defects), superficial lacerations, segmental renal ischaemic infarcts (seen as segmental perfusion defects), and subcapsular or perirenal haematoma. Helical CT avoids the well-known misregistration artefacts that can mimic perirenal haematoma on conventional CT. Major renal injuries include deep lacerations with injury of the renal pelvis, vascular injury with partial or complete renal devascularization, and the so-called shattered kidney. In the haemodynamically unstable patient with blunt retroperitoneal trauma, CT provides very helpful information on the morphological extent of renal injury, the status of vascularization, and the site of active bleeding (Fig. 43.10).

Using a dual-phase acquisition, helical CT is well suited to distinguishing between contrast medium extravasation from the renal pelvis and active haemorrhage, as in the presence of the latter contrast medium appears before the renal collecting system is opacified. In addition, premature opacification of the veins or the inferior vena cava on dynamic studies may herald the presence of an arteriovenous fistula. Owing to shunting within an arteriovenous fistula, the enhancement of the parenchyma distal to the fistula may be reduced. Pseudoaneurysms present with dense but short-lived (arterial-phase) enhancement (BECKER et al. 1998b). When diagnosed with CT, such lesions are now usually treated successfully with transarterial embolization.

43.10 Applications of Helical CT in Clinical Trauma Research

Two-dimensional and three-dimensional image reconstruction based on volumetric image acquisition with helical CT may become increasingly helpful for research purposes in the future. Simple applications include measurements of the precise volume of devascularization and the subsequent development of necrosis or healing. While these are being used widely as routine clinical procedures, more complex tools are currently being developed. At our institution, research is directed toward studying the injury mechanisms in renal trauma using a biomedical approach with computer-simulated kidney models. In a first step, a 2D finite element model of the kidney with normal hydrostatic pelvic pressure was used to

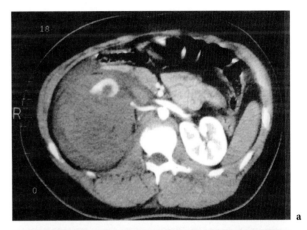

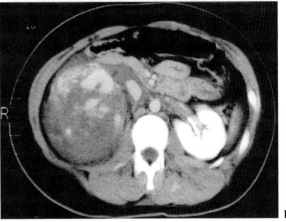

Fig. 43.10a, b. Blunt renal injury with arterial disruption, major parenchymal laceration, and retroperitoneal haematoma. **a** Early-phase image shows arterial disruption and residual perfusion of a small anterior segment of the right kidney. **b** Delayed-phase image shows diffuse active extravasation of contrast material into the retroperitoneum

demonstrate that injury to the kidney is caused by the combined effects of impact force and the reaction of the inner, liquid-filled compartment (SCHMIDLIN et al. 1996). Recently, volume rendering of image data acquired with helical CT has been used to introduce the true 3D, in vivo geometry of the human kidney into the model, thereby enabling the generation of much more realistic 2D or 3D finite element models (Fig. 43.11). Stress and injury patterns produced by various finite element simulations were quite similar to those observed in clinical practice. These on-going investigations suggest that bending fields in the outer portion of the renal parenchyma play a part in the injury patterns seen after blunt renal trauma (SCHMIDLIN et al. 1998).

Summary. The impact of helical CT in the setting of acute abdominal trauma is threefold. Fast helical image acquisition increases safety, thus allowing to expansion of the range of indications for CT. Detection and localization of active haemorrhage is greatly enhanced and may guide therapeutic decisions. The improved overall image quality obtained with modern helical CT technique greatly facilitates the detection of subtle diagnostic signs in difficult general imaging conditions. In addition, the image processing capacity of helical CT scanners enables the radiologist to employ multiplanar reformatting in the diagnostic process and also offers new tools for trauma research.

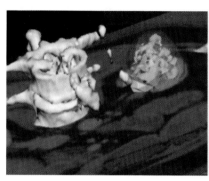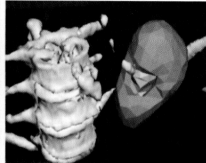

Fig. 43.11a, b. 3-Dimensional renderings from a volumetric, helical data acquisition, demonstrating the surface of the kidney. Such image models are used at our institution to study trauma mechanisms. (Courtesy of the Laboratory of Functional and Multidimensional Imaging, University Hospital of Geneva)

References

Becker CD, Spring P, Glättli A, Schweizer W (1994) Blunt splenic trauma in adults: can CT findings be used to determine the need for surgery? AJR Am J Roentgenol 162:343–347

Becker CD, Gal I, Baer HU, Vock P (1996) Blunt hepatic trauma in adults: correlation of CT injury grading with outcome. Radiology 201:215–222

Becker CD, Mentha G, Terrier F (1998a) Blunt abdominal trauma in adults: role of CT in the diagnosis and management of visceral injuries. 1. Liver and spleen. Eur Radiol 8:553–562

Becker CD, Mentha G, Schmidlin F, Terrier F (1998b) Blunt abdominal trauma in adults: role of CT in the diagnosis and management of visceral injuries. 2. Gastrointestinal tract and retroperitoneal organs. Eur Radiol 8:772–780

Bretan PN, McAninch JW, Federle MP, Jeffrey RB Jr (1986) Computerized tomographic staging of renal trauma : 85 consecutive cases. J Urol 136:561–565

Capasso P, Trotteur G, Flandroy P, Dondelinger RF (1996) A combined CT and angiography suite with a pivoting table. Radiology 199:561–563

Casey LR, Vu D, Cohen AJ (1995) Small bowel rupture after blunt trauma: CT signs and their sensitivity. Emerg Radiol 2:90–95

Davis JW, Hoyt DB, Mackersie RC, McArdle MS (1990) Complications in evaluating abdominal trauma: diagnostic peritoneal lavage versus computerized axial tomography. J Trauma 30(12):1506–1509

Dowe MF, Shanmuganathan K, Mirvis SE, Steiner RC, Cooper C (1997) CT findings of mesenteric injury after blunt trauma: implications for surgical intervention. AJR Am J Roentgenol 168:425–428

Fanney DR, Casillas J, Murphy B (1990) CT in the diagnosis of renal trauma. Radiographics 10:29–40

Federle MP, Courcoulas AP, Powell M, Ferris JV, Peitzman AB (1998) Blunt splenic injury in adults: clinical and CT criteria for management, with emphasis on active extravasation. Radiology 206:137–142

Fishman EK (1996) Spiral CT: applications in the emergency patient. Radiographics 16:943

Gavant ML, Schurr M, Flick P, Croce MA, Fabian T, Gold R (1997) Predicting clinical outcome of nonsurgical management of blunt splenic injury: using CT to reveal abnormalities of splenic vasculature. AJR Am J Roentgenol 168:207–212

Gay SB, Sistrom CL (1992) Computed tomographic evaluation of blunt abdominal trauma. Radiol Clin North Am 30:367–388

Hagiwara A, Yukioka T, Satou M, Yoshii H, Yamamoto S, Matsuda H, Shimazaki S (1995) Early diagnosis of small intestine rupture from blunt abdominal trauma using computed tomography: significance of the streaky density within the mesentery. J Trauma 38(4):630–633

Israel RS, Mayberry JC, Primack SL (1996b) Diaphragmatic rupture: use of helical CT scanning with multiplanar reformations. AJR 167:1201–1203

Israel RS, McDaniel PA, Primack SL, Salmon CL, Fountain RTL, Koslin DB (1996a) Diagnosis of diaphragmatic trauma with helical CT in a swine model. AJR Am J Roentgenol 167:637–641

Jeffrey RB Jr, Cardoza JD, Olcott EW (1991) Detection of active intraabdominal arterial hemorrhage: value of dynamic contrast-enhanced CT. AJR Am J Roentgenol 156:725–729

Miller KS, McAninch JW (1995) Radiographic assessment of renal trauma: our 15-year experience. J Urol 154:352–355

Mirvis SE, Gens DR, Shanmuganathan K (1992) Rupture of the bowel after blunt abdominal trauma: diagnosis with CT. AJR 159:1217–1221

Moore EE, Shackford SR, Pachter HL et al (1989) Organ injury scaling: spleen, liver, and kidney. J Trauma 29:1664–1666

Moore EE, Cogbill TH, Malangoni MA, Jurkovich GJ, Champion HR, Gennarelli TA, McAninch JW, Pachter HL, Shackford SR, Trafton PG (1990) Organ injury scaling II: pancreas, duodenum, small bowel, colon, rectum. J Trauma 30(11):1427–1429

Moore EE, Cogbill TH, Jurkovich GJ, Shackford SR, Malangoni MA, Champion HR (1995) Organ injury scaling: spleen and liver (1994 revision). J Trauma 38(3):323–324

Murray JG, Caoili E, Gruden JF, Evans SJJ, Halvorsen RA, Mackersie RC (1996) Acute rupture of the diaphragm due to blunt trauma: diagnostic sensitivity and specificity of spiral CT. AJR Am J Roentgenol 166:1035–1039

Nunez DB Jr, Wester JD, Lentz K (1996a) Helical computed tomography evaluation of liver injuries: trial of dual phase imaging. Emerg Radiol 3:20

Nunez DB, Becerra JL, Fuentes D (1996b) Traumatic occlusion of the renal artery: helical CT diagnosis. AJR Am J Roentgenol 167:777–778

Pretorius ES, Fishman EK (1995) Spiral CT of upper abdominal trauma. Emergency Radiol 2:285

Rizzo MJ, Federle MP, Griffith BG (1989) Bowel and mesenteric injury following blunt abdominal trauma. Radiology 173:143

Schmidlin FR, Schmid P, Kurtyka T, Iselin CE, Graber P (1996) Force transmission and stress distribution in a computer-simulated model of the kidney: An analysis of the injury mechanisms in renal trauma. J Trauma 40(5):791–796

Schmidlin F, Farshad M, Bidaut L et al (1998) Biomedical analysis and clinical treatment of blunt renal trauma. Swiss Surg (in press)

Sherck J, Shatney C, Sensaki K, Selivanov V (1994) The accuracy of computed tomography in the diagnosis of blunt small-bowel perforation. Am J Surg 168:670–675

Shuman WP (1997) CT of blunt abdominal trauma in adults. Radiology 205:297–306

44 Spiral CT of the Paediatric Abdomen: Technique and Applications

H. Tschäppeler

CONTENTS

44.1   Introduction   *481*
44.2   Technical Parameters   *481*
44.3   Clinical Aspects   *482*
44.3.1 Radiation Dose   *482*
44.3.2 Breathing Strategies   *482*
44.3.3 Sedation   *482*
44.3.4 Intravenous Contrast Medium   *483*
44.3.5 Bowel Opacification   *484*
44.4   Clinical Indications   *484*
44.5   Pitfalls   *489*
44.6   Conclusions   *489*
        References   *490*

44.1
Introduction

Helical or spiral CT has rapidly become the standard for quality scanning not only in adults but also in children (FRUSH and DONNELLY 1998; SIEGEL and LUKER 1995; WHITE 1996). The use of spiral scanning is a new challenge, as new protocols have had to be established, but new capabilities are available. The benefits of the new technology are of great importance in children; the two general advantages of spiral CT are more rapid scanning and volume acquisition of data, as there is continuous data sampling during rotation of the tube/detector system while the table moves at a constant, preset velocity:

– The spiral technique reduces the scanning time and allows a much more rapid completion of the exam. It decreases motion artefacts even when scans of the paediatric abdomen are performed without suspended respiration; thus the faster scanning reduces the need for sedation or anaesthesia. Furthermore, the short scanning time op-

H. TSCHÄPPELER, MD; Department of Diagnostic Radiology, Section of Paediatric Radiology, Inselspital, CH-3010 Bern, Switzerland

timizes peak contrast enhancement of vascular structures even when smaller volumes of intravenous contrast media are used. A further reduction in scan time (and radiation dose) is possible without any significant decrease in diagnostic accuracy when the pitch is increased.

– Volume data acquisition allows retrospective image reconstruction for any desired slice position along the *z*-axis: reconstruction of overlapping slices becomes possible, which results in an increased lesion detection without increasing radiation exposure to the paediatric patient. Movement artefacts may be "cut out" by the volume data set; this helps to save time and, more importantly, reduces radiation exposure, as repeat scans are no longer necessary. Furthermore, multiplanar reconstructions generated from the volumetric spiral data help display complex anatomic relationships and are much appreciated by the clinicians. These (unlimited) reformations are performed once the patient has left the scanner without the potential difficulty encountered with magnetic resonance imaging (necessity of deciding while the patient is still in the scanner whether one more sequence will add worthwhile information).

44.2
Technical Parameters

Protocols for spiral CT are more complex than those for the conventional technique: in addition to mA, kV, collimation thickness and field of view, the reconstruction algorithm for spiral CT, pitch and image spacing must be specified. Collimation and table speed vary with the age of the patient, the area of interest and the clinical indication for the examination. Generally in older children 8 mm collimation is used, while for small children and for detailed examinations of smaller structures the collimation is 2–4 mm. For an abdominal survey a pitch of 2:1 may be sufficient with a 180° linear interpolation. Detection of small lesions or delineation of small anatomic areas is performed using a pitch of 1:1; many centres have chosen a compromise and routinely use a pitch of 1.5:1.

Whenever 3-D or multiplanar reconstructions are planned, overlapping slices should be obtained.

Usually the patient is scanned from the dome of the liver to the iliac crests; if the pelvis has to be included as a continuation of the abdominal CT the examination is extended to the pubic symphysis.

Although common protocols provide an adequate imaging approach to the major diagnostic problems, ultimately individualized protocols are needed to answer particular clinical questions (WHITE 1996).

44.3
Clinical Aspects

44.3.1
Radiation Dose

In children the effective dose delivered by CT is higher, and organs or tissues are more radiosensitive than in adults (HUDA et al. 1997); spiral CT allows a dose reduction compared with the conventional incremental technique. This is partly due to improved detector technology, which allows exposure adjustment both before and during scanning. In fact it is still the radiologist's responsibility to ensure appropriate application of exposure parameters; larger dose reductions are feasible with individualized selection of milliampere setting and pitch. Whenever spatial resolution is not the main issue, protocols for paediatric patients should have much lower milliampere settings than those for adults; the appropriate adjustments that will still allow sufficient diagnostic information have to be determined (APPLEGATE et al. 1997).

Another possible way of reducing the radiation dose is adjusting the pitch: doubling the pitch reduces exposure by 50%. Increasing the pitch by increasing the table speed not only reduces the dose, but also increases coverage (at the expense of poorer z-axis resolution). Comparison of various pitches revealed no subjective difference in quality when a pitch of 1.5 : 1 (dose reduction of one third) was used instead of a pitch of 1 : 1 (VADE et al. 1996). Whenever possible the highest pitch should be applied; at the same time collimation should be reduced and overlapping reconstructions used.

Another potential mechanism for dose reduction is the avoidance of recuts because there is the ability for retrospective reconstruction of images at any desired position including intermediate slices (HUDA et al. 1997).

There is a caveat: in spite of identical kV and mA settings it is necessary to be aware of significant differences in absorbed dose delivered by equipment from different manufacturers; the equipments vary in tube geometry and beam filtration, for example.

44.3.2
Breathing Strategies

In cooperative children older than 7 years a single spiral scan may be obtained with breath-holding (during 20–30 s); previous coaching improves the success rate of suspended inspiration. Children younger than 7 years are generally not able to hold their breath, but with quiet and regular breathing acceptable to good image quality may be achieved.

44.3.3
Sedation

There is no controversy over the tenet that avoiding any kind of sedation is most desirable, as there is a definite incidence of adverse events in children sedated for imaging procedures. The spiral technique, which allows faster scanning, is less susceptible for motion artefacts and reduces sedation requirements in children younger than 6 years (WHITE 1995). Infants less than 18 months old are sedated with oral chloral hydrate (50–100 mg/kg) at a dose not exceeding 2000 mg. Older children are given pentobarbital sodium i.v.; a dose of 2.5 mg/kg is given initially over 1–2 min. If needed, an additional dose of 1.25 mg/kg may be given 1–2 min after the first dose and may be repeated up to a maximum dose of 6 mg/kg or 200 mg. Every child undergoing sedation must be monitored carefully during and after the examination, which needs proper equipment and personnel trained in paediatric resuscitation and cardiorespiratory support (EGELHOFF et al. 1996). Children older than 6 years usually cooperate after explanation of the procedure and verbal reassurance; often the presence of a parent in the CT suite helps to comfort the child. If sedation is planned or necessary the patient should receive no solid food for 6 h, otherwise for 3 h, prior to the study; this precaution may reduce the risk of aspiration after vomiting caused by i.v. bolus injection of the contrast medium.

44.3.4
Intravenous Contrast Medium

Spiral CT improves the ability to depict various phases of vessel and organ enhancement with quicker and more extensive coverage of target areas after intravenous contrast medium administration. However owing to the faster acquisition time the approach to administration of the intravenous contrast medium has to be adapted, especially for abdominal CT. New protocols specifying the route and site of contrast medium administration, injection rates and delay times are necessary (WHITE 1996).

Safe placement of the largest possible gauge intravenous plastic catheter or butterfly needle prior to the child's arrival in the CT suite is very desirable, in order to avoid any agitation associated with the procedure immediately before CT.

Nonionic low-osmolar contrast medium is the standard for the paediatric age group (iodine content 280–320 mg/ml). The volume to be administered varies in relation to the size of the patient and is scaled to the weight of the child; a reliable dose is 2 ml/kg body weight, the maximum dose being 120 ml. In children weighing less than 20 kg the dose of contrast medium may be increased up to 3 ml/kg.

Venous access in children can be central or peripheral. In smaller children peripheral access is more commonly achieved in the hands with small-gauge devices, e.g. 23-G or even 25-G butterfly catheters. In older children the antecubital fossa is the common peripheral access. More and more paediatric patients with chronic disease are having a multilumen or subcutaneous port placed to provide long-term access. Today peripherally inserted central venous catheters are used routinely in children as well as in adults. Improved device technology allows sufficient opacification; however, if peripherally inserted central venous catheters have small lumens and/or are made of softer materials this raises questions about safety.

There are two options for contrast medium administration: with either peripheral or central venous access manual or power injection is feasible. Manual injection has been the traditional method since contrast-enhanced CT has been performed; however relatively high pressures can be generated, which exceed the manufacturer's recommendations (25–50 psi). Pressure during manual injection can be

reduced by using larger calibre catheters and syringes with a capacity of more than 30 ml. A consequence of spiral CT in adults is more extensive use of power injectors; in future, with the increasingly frequent reports on the safety of power injection in children as well this technique will be routinely used both for peripheral and for central venous catheters (KASTE and YOUNG 1996). Power injection through peripheral catheters has a low frequency of complications. Whenever appropriate patient monitoring during the injection is provided and the peripheral venous catheter or butterfly needle is in a stable intraluminal position power injection is possible. The maximum rate for a needle size of 24 G is 0.7 ml/s, for 22 G it is 1 ml/s, for 20 G it is 1.5–2 ml/s and for 18 G it is 2.0 ml/s or more (ROCHE et al. 1996). There are concerns about the use of power injectors with peripherally inserted central catheters. A recent in vitro study (RUESS et al 1997) included measurements of the pressures generated using power injection; using a large 7.0-F double lumen catheter, rates of 2.0 ml/ s could be achieved before the manufacturer's threshold pressure was reached. Much slower rates of less than 0.4 ml/s for 4.2-F and 3.0-F catheters could be applied before threshold pressures were reached; two 4.2-F peripherally inserted central catheters ruptured with a rate of only 0.2.ml/s. On the other hand, the complication rate of power injection through central venous catheters was 0.4% (KASTE and YOUNG 1996) and did not differ from the rate in adults. At present there are no absolute contraindications for use of power injection in children; however, the technique has to be meticulous and low flow rates of 0.3–0.8 ml/s should be applied (FRUSH and DONNELLY 1998).

In children the intensity of maximal tissue enhancement is not significantly influenced by the injection rate; slow rates, such as 0.5 ml/s, may provide good to excellent hepatic enhancement (ROCHE et al. 1996). On the other hand one of the most important and critical aspects of paediatric abdominal spiral CT is timing of initiation of scanning after contrast administration. It depends on a variety of factors: target organ, phase of enhancement desired according to the clinical indication; variables in paediatric patients: gauge of catheter, site of intravenous access, amount of contrast medium and rate of delivery; interpatient variability including status of hydration, cardiovascular and/or metabolic status (WHITE 1996). Available recommendations are based on empiric observations: the correct setting of the delay is preferably referred to the completion of contrast medium injection rather than to the time of its initiation; a too early beginning of the scan should be avoided. There is general agreement that scanning should begin after all contrast medium has been administered (Siegel and Luker 1995) or up to 20 s after completion of contrast medium injection (Ruess et al. 1998). As all the investigations cited were performed with a predetermined rate of administration, these recommendations may be less reliable for manual injection with an uncertain or unknown rate.

Use of bolus tracking makes predictions about the initiation of scanning unnecessary. In a series of children younger than 10 years scan quality was better with bolus tracking (Frush and Bisset 1996): fewer early enhancement artefacts in the spleen, improved nephrographic phase, higher and more consistent hepatic enhancement. However, there are disadvantages of this technique, including the increased radiation at the selected region of interest, failure of correct tracking if there is patient movement, expense of the software; use of bolus tracking in children is not mandatory, but it is useful for optimizing standard CT examinations or for CT angiography in small children (Frush and Donnelly 1998).

Noncontrast reference images are not obtained on a routine basis, as for many paediatric radiologists the additional radiation is not justifiable; however, there are clinical indications for preliminary noncontrast scanning: evaluation of potential calcifications within a visceral organ or an abdominal tumour (e.g. neuroblastoma), and possible calculi. Recently unenhanced spiral CT was advocated as a reasonably priced, rapid and accurate imaging method for use in (adult) patients with acute abdominal pain (Mindelzun and Jeffrey 1997).

44.3.5
Bowel Opacification

Administration of oral contrast medium helps to differentiate bowel structures, as in children there is the usual paucity of mesenteric and retroperitoneal fat. However the utility of mandatory bowel opacification in all paediatric abdominal CT patients is controversial. Its benefits are not always greater than the disadvantages; therefore the advantages and disadvantages should be considered on a case-by-case basis (Donnelly 1997). There is a potential risk of aspiration (Donnelly et al. 1998), though a recent study (Lim-Dunham et al. 1997) did not demonstrate any harm or injury to patients receiving oral contrast medium; however, children with acute ab-

domen and suffering from nausea and vomiting often have poor tolerance of its administration. In patients with abdominal trauma detection of bowel injury is largely independent of oral contrast medium; bowel-wall thickening, mesenteric infiltration, and peritoneal fluid, the most sensitive signs of bowel trauma (Bulas et al. 1989), are seen as well without oral contrast medium; many paediatric trauma centres do not routinely administer oral contrast medium. Furthermore, intraluminal bowel opacification may obscure intravenous bowel-wall enhancement and even decrease CT sensitivity for some diseases [e.g. bowel wall inflammation (Jabra et al. 1994)]. On the other hand there are definite indications, for which bowel opacification is mandatory: for example, evaluation of abscess, circumscribed fluid collection, pseudocyst.

Both dilute barium and dilute (1–2%) water-soluble iodine-based oral contrast medium can be used. If the child refuses to drink, it can be given through a naso-gastric tube. The amount to be given depends on the child's age: the total amount for infants is 200–300 ml; for young children up to 5 years, 350–500 ml; for older children, 500–800 ml. The first administration comprises about two thirds of the total amount given 45–60 min before the examination, and the second volume is given about 15 min before the scan. Rectal contrast medium administration is useful for pelvic CT examinations.

44.4
Clinical Indications

At many institutions abdominal spiral CT is routinely performed to evaluate blunt trauma. In haemodynamically stable children it is the most reliable method, providing complete information on the morphological and functional integrity of an abdominal organ (Figs. 44.1–44.4). Debate continues on the matter of specific indications for CT studies in paediatric abdominal trauma patients, as a broad palette of indications for CT (e.g. suspicion of abdominal trauma, impossibility of clinical evaluation of the abdomen) results in a low percentage of documented abdominal injury. Recent prospective studies (Neish et al.. 1998; Ruess et al. 1997) showed that there was an overall gain in terms of diagnostic certainty; CT information influenced initial management decisions, considerably changing the level of intensity of care (the percentage of cases with decreased intensity of care being much higher than the

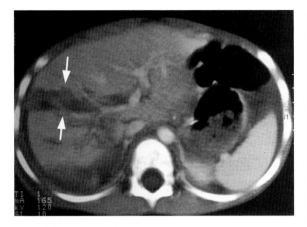

Fig. 44.1. Fracture of the liver (*arrows*) and intrahepatic haematoma in an 8-year-old boy; extension from the surface to the hilum; haemascos

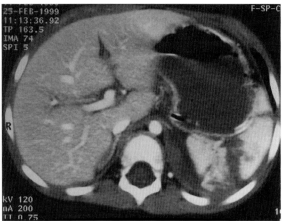

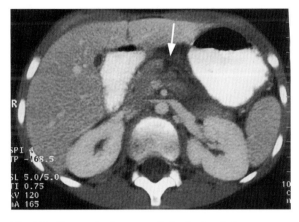

Fig. 44.2. Traumatic fracture of the body of the pancreas (*arrow*) in a 6-year-old boy. Parenchymal hypodensities between body and tail of pancreas; small amount of peripancreatic fluid

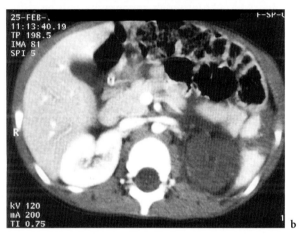

Fig. 44.3a, b. Simultaneous splenic and renal injuries in a 2-year-old boy: **a** disrupted spleen with multiple fragments; **b** absent perfusion of the left kidney due to vascular pedicle injury (subintimal flap and vascular thrombosis); peri- and pararenal haematoma

percentage with increased intensity). But expectations that CT would have a major effect on decisions on which children should undergo laparotomy for solid organ injury have been disappointed. The CT appearance of liver, spleen, or kidney injury does not correlate with the need for operative intervention. The need for therapeutic laparotomy is still based primarily on clinical signs of haemodynamic instability or on continuous blood transfusion requirements. However, CT did affect the decision on whether to perform surgery in most children with documented hollow viscus injury. On the other hand, normal findings on abdominal CT were strongly predictive of a favourable clinical follow-up not requiring any operative intervention. Thus, the question of the overall economic effect of CT information in paediatric trauma has yet to be answered by further studies. These should also include investi-

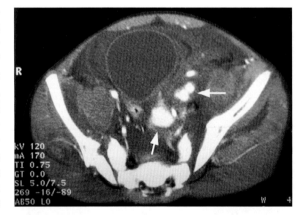

Fig. 44.4. Pelvic injury in a 9-year-old boy: acute and active bleeding with extravasation of contrast material (*arrows*); significant intrapelvic haematoma

gation of the specific role of ultrasound, which in experienced hands is a very valuable tool.

Spiral technical parameters are: slice thickness 5–8 mm, pitch 1.5:1 or even 2:1; and contrast medium dose 2 ml/kg body weight; it is important not to begin to scan too soon after the completion of contrast medium administration (minimum delay 10 s), as incomplete opacification of the liver, spleen (mottled appearance of the parenchyma) and the renal medulla may seriously interfere with correct interpretation of the findings. Precontrast series and oral contrast material are not mandatory.

Abdominal abscess (primary or postoperative) is another, well-established and rewarding indication (Figs. 44.5, 44.6); though sonography will be sufficient in many cases of appendicitis or "simple" abscesses, spiral CT is superior in outlining a complex or multiloculated abscess; furthermore CT-guided drainage is an established method and obviates surgical intervention in selected patients. A precontrast series is desirable, and bowel opacification is mandatory; the contrast series is accomplished with a slice thickness of 4–8 mm and a pitch of 1.5:1.

Diagnostic procedures for evaluation of an abdominal neoplasm such as nephroblastoma (Fig. 44.7), neurogenic tumour (Fig. 44.8), rhabdomyosarcoma (Fig. 44.9) and malignant lymphoma include a wide range of modalities; the main goal is to confirm the lesion and to characterize and to stage it. Essential criteria for the selection of a method are its potential diagnostic information (and accuracy) and whether it is invasive (which involves evaluation of radiation exposure, duration of the examination, need of sedation to perform it). In this respect, the diagnostic radiation from spiral CT delivered to chil-

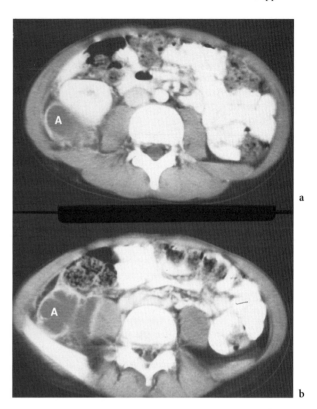

Fig. 44.6. a Right-sided posterior pararenal abscess (*A*) in a 10-year-old boy, who underwent lithotomy. b Its caudad extent is in the lower pararenal space (*A*); internal septations and thickened, enhancing wall

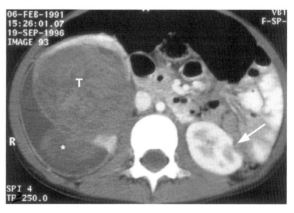

Fig. 44.7. Right-sided nephroblastoma (*T*) in a 5-year-old boy. Spread beyond the pseudocapsule (*). Small (histologically proven) cortical tumour of the left kidney (*arrow*)

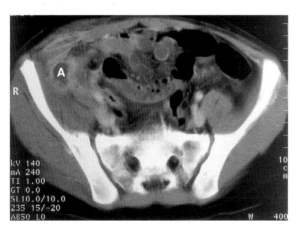

Fig. 44.5. An 11-year-old girl with postoperative abscess (*A*) within the right lower quadrant and the abdominal wall; thickened abscess wall with strong contrast-enhancement

dren undergoing radiation therapy should be relativized; furthermore, spiral CT of the abdomen is achieved much faster than MRI, probably with less discomfort for the child.

The ability to reconstruct the volumetric data at overlapping arbitrary intervals helps to define the exact site of origin of a retroperitoneal mass. Opti-

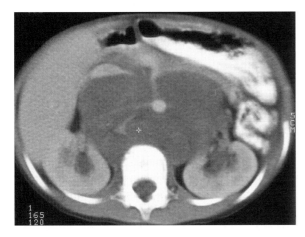

Fig. 44.8. Former retroperitoneal neuroblastoma, histologically transformed after nonsurgical treatment into a ganglioneuroma: huge retroperitoneal, scarcely enhancing masses with encasement of the great vessels; slight obstruction of both kidneys (8-year-old girl)

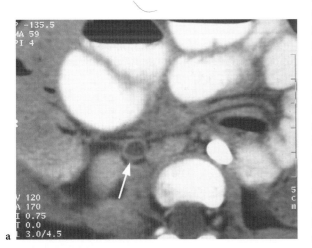

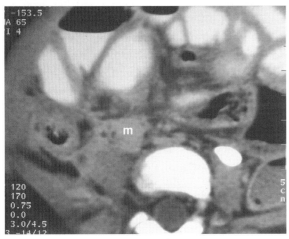

Fig. 44.9a, b. Local recurrence of a retroperitoneal rhabdomyosarcoma in a 4-year-old boy: **a** dilated right ureter filled with noncontrasted urine (*arrows*); **b** slightly enhancing, roundish mass (*m*), complete obstruction of the ureter

mal vascular enhancement after intravenous contrast medium demonstrates the presence or absence of vascular invasion (e.g. vascular encasement by neuroblastoma) as well as venous compression or thrombosis (e.g. by nephroblastoma); multiplanar reconstruction, especially in the coronal plane, shows intraspinal invasion.

Whenever chest CT is mandatory for staging purposes (to detect pulmonary metastases or mediastinal lymphadenopathy), it can be performed during the same procedure and without taking significantly more time. For this latter indication it is preferable to begin with the thoracic, contrast-enhanced examination: the chest scan delay is about 80% of the contrast injection time (dosage: 2 ml/kg); using a pitch of 1.5:1 the dome of the liver is reached after approximately 15 s; the effective delay between the end of the injection and the initiation of the abdominal scan provides adequate contrast enhancement of the abdomen. The paediatric patient benefits from the rapid completion of a comprehensive examination. Often CT is required for planning of radiation therapy.

Spiral CT examination of the paediatric liver is useful in detecting focal parenchymal abnormalities (Figs. 44.10, 44.11): primary neoplasm, metastases, abscess; it helps to define vascular and biliary pathology (e.g. portal vein thrombosis, Budd-Chiari syndrome, trauma). There is a dual vascular supply to the liver: (1) the hepatic artery, which is the source of blood flow for most pathologic lesions of the parenchyma and (2) the portal vein, which is the dominant source (about 70%) of enhancement for the normal hepatic parenchyma. As the intravenous contrast medium diffuses rapidly from the intravascular compartment into the interstitial space and enters both the normal parenchyma and pathologic lesions, the latter may be obscured during this equilibrium phase (SILVERMAN et al. 1998). For optimal lesion detection it is therefore essential to scan the liver during peak portal vein / parenchymal enhancement, that is to say before onset of the equilibrium (LUKER et al. 1996). Using a contrast medium dose of 2 ml/kg body weight the peak hepatic enhancement threshold is greater than 35 HU in more than 80% of children (RUESS et al. 1998). Despite the lower peak values than in adult patients, diagnostic quality is adequate. Though there is significant interpatient variability, approximate peak times may be defined (ROCHE et al. 1996): using power injection of contrast material (2 ml/kg) a scan start time about 10 s after completion of injection results in adequate contrast-enhanced spiral CT of the liver,

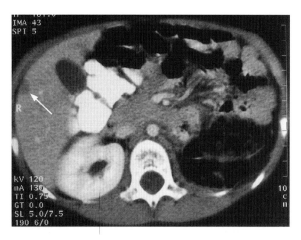

Fig. 44.10. Follow-up examination 6 months after left-sided nephrectomy because of nephroblastoma in a 4-year-old girl. Small peripheral hepatic metastasis (*arrow*)

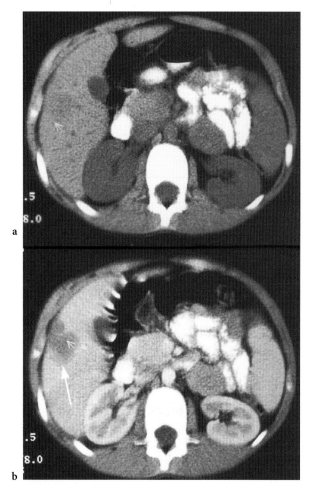

Fig. 44.11a, b. Hepatic abscess in a 9-year-old girl. **a** Before i.v. contrast; **b** after i.v. contrast: slight enhancement of the wall, the abscess remains hypointense (*arrow*)

which is completed within 10–16 s. Single-phase contrast-enhanced CT is usually sufficient in children, with the exception of those with suspected haemangioma, in whom multiphasic examination helps to establish the diagnosis.

Biliary disease in children is not as common as in adults; the majority of paediatric biliary pathology is congenital (e.g. choledochal cyst, atresia), syndromic (Caroli disease, lithiasis) or acquired (post-inflammatory, posttraumatic). Both CT- and MR-cholangiography are compelling methods for evaluation of the biliary system; they are of rather limited value especially in smaller children because the structures are so tiny and because small children are not yet able to hold their breath.

Collimation varies with patient size from 4 mm to 8 mm; the pitch is 1:1; reconstructions are performed every 4–8 mm. The use of overlapping axial images may further improve the overall detection rate (URBAN et al. 1993).

Splenic abnormalities in children include congenital and systemic diseases, trauma or infection, all of which are promptly and well evaluated by spiral CT (Figs. 44.3, 44.12). However, there is the unique feature of early enhancement artefacts; they occur frequently when spiral CT is performed during the arterial phase of contrast enhancement, as they are rate dependent (FRUSH and DONNELLY 1998). The artefacts are uncommon with a rate less than 1 ml/s and delayed beginning of scanning. Therefore, knowledge of the rate and time of initiation of scanning is crucial to help distinguish artefacts from subtle parenchymal abnormalities.

Spiral CT of the paediatric gastrointestinal tract has two major foci: appendicitis and detection of bowel wall inflammation or injury. Because the paucity of fat can limit the detection of appendicitis, use of oral and intravenous contrast material may be necessary (FRIEDLAND and SIEGEL 1997). Specific patterns of bowel wall enhancement after optimized intravenous contrast bolus help in detection of inflammatory or injured bowel without wall thickening, thus decreasing the dependence on administration of oral contrast material (DONNELLY 1997).

The most frequent pathology of the paediatric pancreas (SIEGEL and SIVIT 1997) is trauma (Fig. 44.2); early identification of transection and/or other ductal injury is essential. Optimal timing of contrast enhancement is of the utmost importance for detection of small areas of trauma. As peak enhancement of the pancreas occurs before that of the liver, slightly earlier scanning helps to improve diagnostic accuracy; furthermore, the use of oral con-

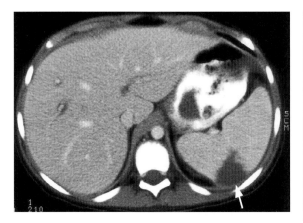

Fig. 44.12. Splenomegaly with segmental infarction (*arrow*) in a 14-year-old boy with known acute lymphatic leukaemia

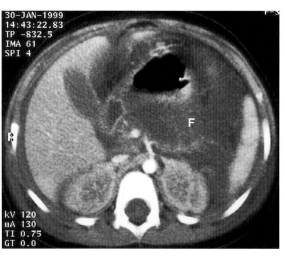

Fig. 44.13. Acute, necrotizing pancreatitis in a 5-year-old girl; no obvious trauma. Widespread necrosis without enhancing parenchymal structures of the pancreatic body and tail; huge peri- and prepancreatic fluid accumulation (*F*); no definite pseudocyst formation. Thrombosis of splenic vein

trast medium is mandatory as in children there is hardly any surrounding fat. Similar techniques are appropriate for the evaluation of inflammatory (Fig. 44.13) or neoplastic disease, both of which are much more uncommon in children than in adults.

The spectrum of diseases of the kidneys and adrenal glands includes trauma (Fig. 44.3) and (malignant) mass lesions (Fig. 44.7), which are usually large at the time of diagnosis. Though a survey technique (collimation up to 8 mm, pitch of 1.5:1 or even 2:1) may be sufficient for its primary evaluation, a more subtle technique is appropriate for the detection of small lesions (e.g. contralateral disease in nephroblastoma, regional lymph node involvement), using a collimation of 4 mm and a pitch of 1:1. Multiphase imaging of the kidneys may be necessary: cortical imaging is performed during rapid administration of contrast medium, and the nephrographic phase coincides with the portal venous phase. As in adults, renal and/or ureteral calculi can be demonstrated by nonenhanced CT and overlapping reconstructions, thus obviating the need for intravenous urography.

The complementary method of choice for imaging paediatric intrapelvic disease is MR. However, pelvic CT is often performed as a continuation of the (thoraco)-abdominal scan, and the examination is extended to the pubic symphysis (Fig. 44.4). If simultaneous opacification of the iliac vessels is needed, another rapid contrast material administration is required (dosage 1 ml/kg).

There has been little investigation of abdominal CT angiography, and there are currently no routine vascular applications in children; especially in small children the amount of intravenous contrast medium that can be administered is limited; they have little ability to hold their breath; small-gauge needles

and remote access sites prevent rapid injection. Therefore, predictable timing for CT angiography is difficult. The unique complexities of paediatric CT angiography are only now beginning to be addressed; prospective comparative studies of paediatric CT and MR angiography are not yet available.

44.5
Pitfalls

As spiral CT of the abdomen is completed very rapidly, the early arterial enhancement of the splenic parenchyma is heterogeneous and creates a mottled appearance, which may mimic laceration (after trauma) or neoplastic infiltration. A similar phenomenon occurs during the cortical contrast phase, resulting in insufficient opacification of the renal medulla and collecting system. For clarification in equivocal cases delayed images may be necessary (Herts et al. 1993).

44.6
Conclusions

Spiral CT produces images faster than the conventional technique. The potential decrease in the dose of radiation delivered, the fact that fewer children require sedation, and the improved image quality brought about by the decreased frequency of motion-induced artefacts are the major practical advantages. Overlapping reconstructions increase the diagnostic accuracy, and high-quality multiplanar reconstructions contribute to a visualization much appreciated by the clinicians. However, careful attention to intravenous contrast medium administration is mandatory to obtain optimal abdominal images.

References

Applegate KE, Dardinger JT, Lieber MS, Herts BR, Davros WJ, Baker ME (1997) Helical CT in pediatrics: comparison of image quality between low dose techniques using a solid state detector and conventional techniques with xenon detector (abstract). Radiology 205 (P):515

Bulas DI, Taylor GA, Eichelberger MR (1989) The value of CT in detecting bowel perforation in children after blunt abdominal trauma. AJR Am J Roentgenol 153:561–564

Donnelly LF (1997) Commentary: oral contrast medium administration for abdominal CT-reevaluating the benefits and disadvantages in the pediatric patient. Pediatr Radiol 27:770–772

Donnelly LF, Frush DP, Frush KS (1998) Aspirated contrast material contributing to respiratory arrest in a pediatric trauma patient. AJR Am J Roentgenol 171:471–473

Egelhoff JC, Ball WS, Koch BL, Parks TD (1997) Safety and efficacy of sedation in children using a structured sedation program. AJR Am J Roentgenol 168:1259–1262

Friedland GA, Siegel MJ (1997) CT appearance of acute appendicitis in childhood. AJR Am J Roentgenol 168:439–442

Frush DP, Bisset GS III (1996) Spiral abdominal CT evaluation of children: optimizing enhancement with a bolus-tracking technique (abstract). Radiology 203: (P)136

Frush DF, Donnelly LF (1998) Helical CT in children: technical considerations and body applications. Radiology 209:37–48

Herts BR, Einstein DM, Paushter DM (1993) Spiral CT of the abdomen: artifacts and potential pitfalls. AJR Am J Roentgenol 161:1185–1190

Huda W, Atherton JV, Ware DE, Cumming WA (1997) An approach for the estimation of effective radiation dose at CT in pediatric patients. Radiology 203:417–422

Jabra AA, Fishman EK, Taylor GA (1994) CT findings in inflammatory bowel disease in children. AJR Am J Roentgenol 162:975–979

Kaste SC, Young CW (1996) Safe use of power injectors with central and peripheral venous access devices for pediatric CT. Pediatr Radiol 26:499–501

Lim-Dunham JE, Narra J, Benya EC, Donaldson JS (1997) Aspiration after administration of oral contrast material in children undergoing abdominal CT for trauma. AJR Am J Roentgenol 169:1015–1018

Luker GD, Siegel MJ, Bradley DA, Baty JD (1996) Hepatic spiral CT in children: scan delay time-enhancement analysis. Pediatr Radiol 26:337–340

Mindelzun RE, Jeffrey RB (1997) Unenhanced helical CT for evaluating acute abdominal pain: a little more cost, a lot more information. Radiology 204:43–45

Neish AS, Taylor GA, Lund DP, Atkinson CC (1998) Effect of CT information on the diagnosis and management of acute abdominal injury in children. Radiology 206:327–331

Roche KJ, Genieser NB, Ambrosino NM (1996) Pediatric hepatic CT: an injection protocol. Pediatr Radiol 26:502–507

Ruess L, Bulas DI, Rivera O, Markle BM (1997) In-line pressures generated in small-bore central venous catheters during power injection of CT contrast media. Radiology 203:625–629

Ruess L, Sivit CJ, Eichelberger MR, Gotschall CS, Taylor GA (1997) Blunt abdominal trauma in children: impact of CT on operative and nonoperative management. AJR Am J Roentgenol 169:1011–1014

Ruess L, Bulas DI, Kushner DC, Silverman PM, Fearon TC (1998) Peak enhancement of the liver in children using power injection and helical CT. AJR Am J Roentgenol 170:677–681

Siegel MJ, Luker G (1995) Pediatric applications of helical (spiral) CT. Radiol Clin North Am 33:997–1022

Siegel MJ, Sivit CJ (1997) Pancreatic emergencies. Radiol Clin North Am 35:815–830

Silverman PM, Kohan L, Ducic I, Javadis S, Meyer C, Sharma N, Cooper C, Zeman RK (1998) Imaging of the liver with helical CT: a survey of scanning techniques. AJR Am J Roentgenol 170: 149–152

Urban BA, Fishman EK, Kuhlman JE et al (1993) Detection of focal hepatic lesions with spiral CT: comparison of 4- and 8- mm interscan spacing. AJR Am J Roentgenol 160:783–785

Vade A, Demos TC, Olson MC, Subbaiah P, Turbin RC, Vickery K, Carrigan K (1996) Evaluation of image quality using 1:1 pitch and 1.5:1 pitch helical CT in children: a comparative study. Pediatr Radiol 26:891–893

White KS (1995) Reduced need for sedation in patients undergoing helical CT of the chest and abdomen. Pediatr Radiol 25:344–346

White KS (1996) Helical/spiral CT scanning: a pediatric radiology perspective. Pediatr Radiol 26:5–14

45 Interventional Procedures

M. Grossholz, N. Howarth

CONTENTS

45.1   Introduction *491*
45.2   Diagnostic Procedures *492*
45.2.1 Indications and Contraindications *492*
45.2.2 Preparation of the Patient *492*
45.2.3 Biopsy Needles and Preparation Techniques *492*
45.2.4 Fine-needle Biopsy Techniques for Cytological
        Evaluation *492*
45.2.5 Core Biopsy Techniques for Histological
        Evaluation *494*
45.2.6 Technical Considerations and Guidance
        Systems *496*
45.2.7 Complications *497*
45.2.8 Biopsies of Specific Organs and Body Regions *497*
45.3   Therapeutic Procedures *504*
45.3.1 Materials and Techniques *505*
45.3.2 Complications *507*
45.3.3 Drainage of Liver Abscesses and Liver Cysts *507*
45.3.4 Drainage of the Gallbladder *508*
45.3.5 Interventional Procedures During Pancreatitis *508*
45.3.6 Enteric, Abdominal Cavity and Retroperitoneal
        Abscesses *509*
45.3.7 Alcohol Treatment of Hepatocellular Carci
        noma *509*
45.3.8 Neurolysis *513*
45.3.9 Sclerotherapy of Lymphoceles *514*
Appendix A   Diameters of Needles and Catheters *514*
Appendix B   Manufacturers *514*
              References *514*

45.1
Introduction

Aspiration biopsies have been reported since the early nineteenth century. The last 100 years of development of the technology of X-ray applications has witnessed a slow and sporadic perfection, acceptance and general application of percutaneous, radiographically guided biopsies (Hopper 1995). In addition to advances in such radiographic equip-

M. Grossholz, MD; Hôpital de la Tour, CH-1217 Meyrin, Switzerland
N. Howarth, MD; Department of Radiology, University Hospital of Geneva, CH-1211 Geneva 14, Switzerland

ment as the roentgenoscope and, in the 1950s, the TV fluoroscope, the widespread use of percutaneous biopsy techniques required technical advances and the development of expertise among pathologists to enable them to process and interpret small cyto- and histopathological specimens. In the last two decades, computer tomography (CT) and ultrasonography (US) have mainly been used to guide percutaneous biopsy and drainage procedures. The first CT-guided biopsy was reported in 1975 (Alfidi et al. 1975). The choice of imaging technique depends on technical considerations, the operator's training and conditions related to the patient. However, whenever a lesion can be clearly demonstrated by US, this technology should be selected. US guidance often allows more rapid and more accurate procedures than does CT guidance, mainly because of its real-time capabilities (Sheafor et al. 1998). Biopsies and therapeutic procedures under control of magnetic resonance imaging (MRI) are still undergoing investigation and are restricted to centers with special equipment.

The option of percutaneous access for diagnostic and therapeutic procedures is a great advantage for the patient. Spiral CT technology offers fast image control and reduces the duration of an intervention and therefore the risk of complications. The development of new cutting needles has enabled extraction of tissue specimens with a diameter allowing histological examination, without an increase in risk for the patient. The biopsy generally hastens the diagnosis. Furthermore, it can often be performed in an outpatient setting, thereby lowering health costs (Rimm et al. 1997; Silverman et al. 1998). The patient may be able to work the following day. Even in children, radiologically guided cutting needle biopsy should replace open biopsy in most cases (Chesney et al. 1996; Somers et al. 1993).

The percutaneous therapeutic procedures make it possible to avoid surgery. They may be attempted for patients either as temporizing or definitive therapy. Often performed to treat postsurgical complications, they can replace repeated surgery in some critically ill patients. They lower the risks with a shorter length of procedure, often with no need for general anesthesia (Lambiase et al. 1992; van Sonnenberg et al. 1984, 1991).

In this chapter, diagnostic and therapeutic procedures will be discussed separately, even though there is some overlap, especially with regard to patient preparation.

45.2
Diagnostic Procedures

45.2.1
Indications and Contraindications

In general terms, a diagnostic biopsy in the abdomen can be considered indicated for the following purposes: (1) to specify the cell type of a neoplastic mass to allow planning of the therapeutic regimen in primary or secondary tumors of the liver, kidneys, pancreas, adrenal glands, spleen or retroperitoneal lymph nodes; (2) to perform staging of a known neoplasm; (3) to characterize a lymphoma; and (4) to prove or exclude the presence of viable or recurrent tumor after therapy. A patient with gastrointestinal wall thickening, if this is not accessible by endoscopy, can also be referred for percutaneous biopsy.

There are three relative contraindications to percutaneous biopsy. The first is low coagulation factors; critical values are 50–60% reduction in prothrombin time and thrombocytes below 100,000/µl. If a biopsy or drainage procedure is nevertheless necessary, an appropriate transfusion can be carried out. Noncooperation of the patient can be another contraindication; in such a case, sedation and standby anesthesiology are helpful. The third contraindication is a lesion that is not safely accessible – the main problem is that of major vessels, which may cause important bleeding if injured.

45.2.2
Preparation of the Patient

The patient is asked to fast for at least 4 h. The coagulation status has to be checked; 1 week prior to the procedure is sufficient for patients without a known coagulation disorder. For a patient with known hepatic cirrhosis or known iatrogenic or other coagulation disorders, the status must be verified 24 h before the examination and transfusion of suitable blood products organized if necessary.

Written informed consent is obtained from all patients, if possible the day before.

After the procedure, the patient should stay in a day clinic facility for 4–6 h for observation. Heart rate and blood pressure are checked every 30 min during the first 2 h after the intervention, and then hourly. If the needle has penetrated the pleura a chest X-ray is obtained after 4 h.

45.2.3
Biopsy Needles and Preparation Techniques

Two main types of biopsy needles are available: fine needles for cytological aspiration and needles of larger caliber for histological sampling. Needle diameter is expressed in gauge (see Appendix A). The diameter in gauge corresponds to the maximum number of needles that can be introduced into a standard tube. For example, twenty-two 22-gauge (G) needles can be placed into the standard tube (the diameter of which is 0.71 cm). The diameter in gauge is the outer diameter of the needle and not the diameter of its lumen.

If possible, the tissue sample should provide enough material to carry out bacteriological, chemical and immunohistochemical investigations in addition to the histological examination. The combination of histological and cytological examinations of biopsy specimens maximizes the diagnostic yield and sensitivity for detecting malignancy (Dusenberg et al. 1995; Tikkakoski et al. 1993; Tsang et al. 1995). In our experience, sometimes the cytological evaluation only provides the definitive diagnosis of malignancy. Aspiration for cytological evaluation remains the only choice if the lesion is very small (less than 1 cm in diameter) or if the access is dangerous with major vessels close to the needle's pathway. In this case, a small needle is preferable to reduce the risk of a bleeding complication (Gazelle et al. 1992). For puncture of cystic lesions, a small needle caliber is normally sufficient. For thick mucoid cystic lesions, from which it can be very difficult to obtain material through a 20-G needle, an 18-G or 16-G needle is usually necessary.

45.2.4
Fine-needle Biopsy Techniques for Cytological Evaluation

All needle types have an outer thin wall cannula and an inner stylet. They are available with centimeter graduation and plastic stoppers.

For cytological aspiration, two main different types of needle can be used. Chiba needles (Cook, William Cook Europe, 4632-Bjaeverskov, Denmark) (Fig. 45.1) are available in different diameters ranging from 18 G to 26 G, with different lengths. With the smaller needle diameters (20 G or thinner) severe complications are very rare. Deep lesions can be punctured safely. One disadvantage is the flexibility of the fine needles, which can be distorted by the passage through different tissues. It is preferable to biopsy the lesion with a "one-shot " direct puncture rather than proceeding by controlled steps.

The second needle type is the Franseen needle (Cook, William Cook Europe), which has a trephine tip. This needle is available in sizes of 18 G to 22 G. The end is very sharp and effectively acts as a cutting needle, even often yielding an adequate histological specimen. These two needle types, with their different needle lengths, are normally sufficient for virtually every type of fine-needle biopsy.

There are other types of needle, for example the hybrid Westcott needle (Becton Dickinson and Company, Franklin Lakes, NJ 07417) (Fig. 45.2), which is very small (up to 24 G) and has an acute beveled cutting tip. It also has a side notch, to obtain a tissue specimen. However, the quantity of material is often only sufficient for cytological analysis. For superficial lesions, a simple needle for intramuscular injections or a spinal 20-G to 22-G needle is sufficient (DAHNERT 1992). Needles with an acute bevel are superior to flat beveled needles.

The different needle tips are demonstrated in Fig. 45.3.

Some authors favor the theory that no aspiration is necessary and that the to-and-fro motion and tor-

sion of the needle within the lesion yields an adequate sample (FAGELMAN and CHESS 1990; SAVAGE et al. 1995). We believe, with other authors, that good aspiration is mandatory (HOPPER et al. 1992, 1996; HUEFTLE and HAAGA 1986; KINNEY et al. 1993; KREULA et al. 1990). With a 10- to 20-ml syringe filled with approximately 1 ml of saline solution, the operator can achieve a vacuum respectively of 10–20 ml free handed. Special devices such as a syringe with an in-built stopper (Fig. 45.4) or a metal holder for the syringe (Cook, William Cook Europe) can be helpful. The special handle on the holder, due to its improved configuration, is easier to pull and can therefore make it possible to achieve constant suction (Fig. 45.5). Sampling size increases with the number of passes, a change in needle direction and the amplitude of excursion in lesions larger than 3 - 4 mm (KREULA 1990). After positioning the needle tip within the lesion, the operator maintains suction whilst the needle is advanced and rotated. Different parts of the lesion should be punctured in a star-like

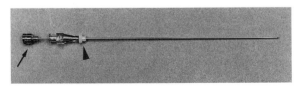

Fig. 45.1. Chiba needle (Cook) with inner stylet (*arrow*) and moveable plastic stopper (*arrowhead*)

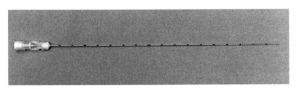

Fig. 45.2. Westcott needle (Becton Dickinson) with centimeter graduation

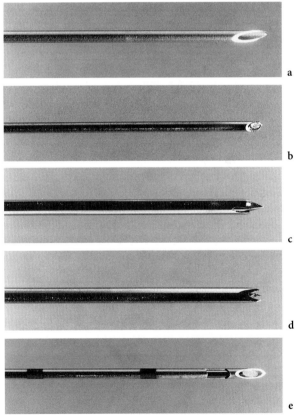

Fig. 45.3a–e. Magnification of different needle tips. **a** Needle for intramuscular injections; **b** Chiba needle (Cook); **c** two-part Chiba needle with end-notch (Cook); **d** Franseen needle with trepine (Cook); **e** Westcott needle with side-notch (Becton Dickinson)

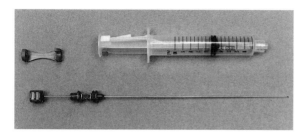

Fig. 45.4. End-cut biopsy needle (Otto, Angiomed) with inner stylet, plastic stopper and syringe with in-built stopper

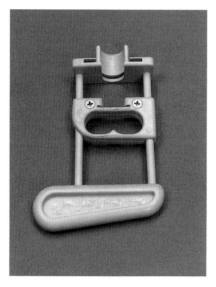

Fig. 45.5. Handle (Cook) for use in insertion of a 20-ml syringe: a sustained vacuum can easily be achieved

manner and the suction maintained as the needle is withdrawn. When blood is aspirated suction should be discontinued. The specimen is smeared on glass slides and fixed with 95% ethanol. If the operator is not experienced with the smearing technique it is preferable to place the specimen in a preservative solution in a sterile tube and to send it to the cytology laboratory. Sometimes tissue core biopsies can be obtained with flexible 20-G or 22-G needles.

A cytological diagnosis can be obtained in almost 82–90% of patients after two passes of a fine needle (BROWN et al. 1993; DAHNERT et al. 1992), with increases of 8% with the third pass, 6% with the fourth pass, 2% with the fifth pass, and 1% with the sixth pass (DAHNERT et al. 1992).

Accuracy of diagnosis depends on both the cytopathologist and the quality of the biopsy material. The need for the presence of a cytopathologist during the procedure is controversial. A study conducted during percutaneous fine-needle aspiration

biopsy of the lung with a meta-analysis of the literature concluded that an accurate diagnosis was more likely when a cytopathologist was present. If the biopsy was inappropriate, additional biopsy specimens were obtained (AUSTIN and COHEN 1993). Other studies showed no statistically significant improvement in accuracy or reduction in number of needle passes or inadequate specimens when immediate cytological evaluation was performed (WARD et al. 1994). Even with a negative immediate evaluation of the smears by the cytopathologist, the cell-block analysis of the aspirate remaining after the smears are made can increase the diagnostic accuracy in up to 14% of the patients (BROWN et al. 1993).

45.2.5
Core Biopsy techniques for Histological Evaluation

For histological sampling, needles with cutting surfaces yield a cylinder of tissue, which can be examined as a histological specimen. Below a diameter of 20 G it is usually difficult to obtain sufficient material. We prefer, if possible, to use at least an 18-G needle, as from this size onward it is nearly always possible to obtain sufficient material for histological analysis.

Two principal systems are available, a gun system with an end-notch (Fig. 45.6a) (Autovac, Angiomed, Karlsruhe, Germany) and a system with a side-notch of Tru-Cut type (Fig. 45.6b) (Somatex, Berlin, Germany; Temno, Bauer Medical, Clearwater, FL 34620; Bard, C.R. Bard, Covington, GA 30209).

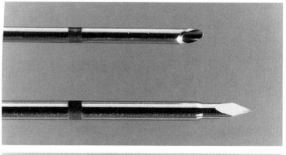

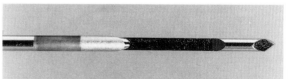

Fig. 45.6. Magnification of the tips of **a** an end-notch needle and its coaxial needle (Autovac, Angiomed) and **b** a side-notch system (Temno, Bauer Medical)

The end-notch systems exist as automated biopsy devices, which create a set amount of suction by employing a locking syringe or a Vacutainer automatic biopsy gun with 15-G to 18-G needles (Fig. 45.7). In comparison with the side-notch biopsy gun, the end-notch biopsy guns perform equivalently, but in a significant number of biopsy attempts no tissue is obtained (HOPPER et al. 1995a). This probably occurs because the specimen is not cut automatically by the end of the biopsy gun.

Tru-Cut-type needles have an outer cutting cannula and an inner stylet containing a 1.5-cm long side-notch. After insertion, the cutting cannula is slid over the inner component, slicing the specimen and holding it for retrieval. The Tru-Cut type can be used manually (Somatex) (Fig. 45.8) or with automated devices (Temno, Bauer Medical; Bard). The hand-held Tru-Cut needles require some training, but for the experienced operator they are a cheap and efficient tool. Nevertheless, the automated biopsy device seems to provide more diagnostic specimens than the manual or conventional needles (HOPPER 1993a, b).

The automated device exists in a form for single use (Temno, Bauer Medical; Medi-tech) (Fig. 45.9a, b). It is very easy to handle, but relatively cumbersome and sometimes difficult to install with the patient in the gantry of the CT scanner. A stopper on the calibrated shaft of the needle can be adjusted to the depth of the lesion.

Other biopsy guns have a reusable metal component (e.g. the Bard biopsy gun) (Fig. 45.10). The handle can be attached once the needle is in position and the gun is activated by pushing a button. The

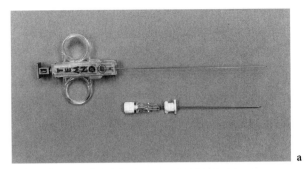

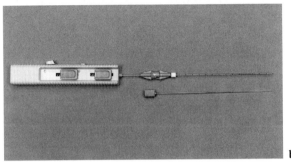

Fig. 45.9a, b. Automated Tru-Cut needles (a Temno, b Medi-Tech) and their coaxial needles

stylet is driven forward by pulling the gun's trigger. This system is easier to handle in the gantry, because the needle is light and the heavy metal gun is installed outside the gantry just before the biopsy is performed.

To avoid several needle pathways with the rather large caliber, a coaxial system can be employed. A larger cannula with a stylet is placed at the margin of the lesion to be punctured, the stylet is withdrawn and the biopsy needle is inserted. Now several biopsies can be achieved by angling the more rigid outer cannula in different directions. The coaxial technique can be employed for fine-needle and core biopsies (BANKOFF and BELKIN 1989; FREDERICK et al. 1989; HOPPER et al. 1995a, b; JEFFREY 1988; MOULTON and MOORE 1993). However, SHEIMAN et al. (1998), in a review of different technical causes for inconclusive results from CT-guided core biopsies, identified the coaxial technique as having significantly less conclusive results than the paraxial method.

The biopsy material is sent to the pathology laboratory in a 10% buffered formalin solution, and there it is fixed and stained in the standard fashion for histological examination. One exception is the biopsy of suspected lymphomas, where an unfixed, fresh specimen should be obtained for immunohistochemical analysis. A touch preparation for cytol-

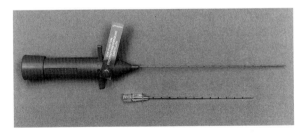

Fig. 45.7. End-cut needle biopsy gun and its coaxial needle (Autovac, Angiomed). Both have centimeter graduation

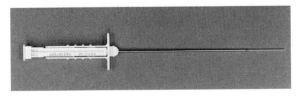

Fig. 45.8. Needle of Tru-Cut type for manual use

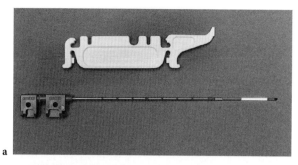

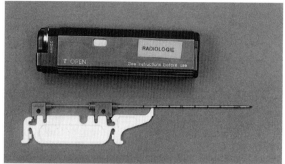

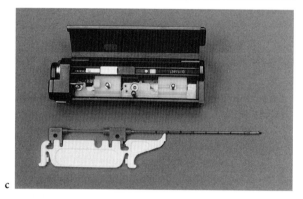

Fig. 45.10a–c. Biopsy gun with a metal part (Bard). **a** The needle is shown detached. When it is positioned in the lesion it is attached to the metal component (**b** in closed, **c** in opened position)

ogy of the core biopsy can be performed, which may offer a rapid diagnosis from a single core biopsy sample. Carefully performed, the touch preparation method preserves the core material for subsequent permanent fixation and sectioning (HAHN et al. 1995).

45.2.6
Technical Considerations and Guidance Systems

The diagnostic study is reviewed to select the best approach and position of the patient. The patient is positioned within the CT scanner, in such a manner that the lesion is accessible along the shortest and safest pathway. The supine position is preferred, except for paravertebral or deep retroperitoneal lesions. If necessary, the gantry is tilted and the patient is turned into an oblique position. Series of scans are performed at the preselected level, with a radio-opaque wire or grid on the patient's skin, and distance and angles are measured. Depending on the situation of the lesion, oral, rectal and/or intravenous contrast media are administered beforehand. The depth from the skin to the anterior and posterior margins of the lesions is measured. The entry point is marked with a water-resistant felt-tip pen, the marker is removed, and the skin is cleansed and draped under sterile conditions. After superficial and deep local anesthesia, a small skin incision is performed and the needle is inserted to the premeasured depth. Images are obtained to verify the needle position. With spiral CT, it is preferable to perform a short spiral scan of three to five images. In this way, the needle localization can be obtained during the same breath-hold, without respiratory misregistration (SILVERMAN et al. 1992), and the time required to identify the needle tip is reduced.

The tandem needle technique is an elegant method of placing several needles into one lesion, each needle sequentially positioned with the same inclination and depth (FERRUCI and WITTENBERG 1978).

Whenever a lesion is obscured behind bowel loops or the kidney, spleen, or retroperitoneal colon, is near great vessels or is only accessible via a lung, a saline injection along the needle pathway may be used to displace the organ to be avoided and thus gain safe access for a biopsy or a drainage procedure. The needle is advanced to the margin of the organ to be displaced. A maximum of 120–150 ml of physiological saline solution is injected in 10-ml to 20-ml aliquots via a connecting tube to avoid displacement of the needle. Control scans are performed and the needle advanced step by step towards the lesion to be biopsied. One major disadvantage may be patient discomfort (LANGEN et al. 1995).

Experienced operators aim at the lesion directly, if necessary with gantry-tilt and triangulation techniques (HUSSAIN 1996; HUSSAIN et al. 1994; VAN SONNENBERG et al. 1981; YANKELEVITZ et al. 1993; YUEH et al. 1989). Guidance systems may help in the performance of some biopsies and drainage procedures, for example with stereotactic instruments or light- or laser-guidance systems, which can be installed in the CT room (FREDERICK et al. 1985; JACOBI et al. 1999; MIAUX et al. 1995; PERELES et al.

1998) . These facilities may make the biopsy procedure easier, especially for less experienced operators. In addition, the experienced operator may find these devices helpful for small, hard-to-reach targets (JACOBI et al. 1999; PERELES et al. 1998). There are now systems available that hold a biopsy gun in the CT gantry and mechanically aid insertion of the needle tip (Bard CT guide system) (BROWN et al. 1995).

However, whichever method is used, be it the single-needle free-hand technique, a coaxial needle system (BANKOFF and BELKIN 1989; FREDERICK 1989; HOPPER et al. 1995a, b; JEFFREY 1988; MOULTON and MOORE 1993), guidance by simple geometric calculation or sophisticated guidance systems (BROWN et al. 1995; FREDERICK et al. 1985; JACOBI et al. 1999; MIAUX et al. 1995; PERELES et al. 1998), the needle must be placed accurately, the biopsy must proceed safely and the success rate must be high.

45.2.7
Complications

Discrete hemorrhage along the pathway of the needle after a biopsy is found in nearly 30% of cases and depends on the needle size (GAZELLE et al. 1992; SHEETS et al. 1991; YANKASKAS et al. 1986). It is important to place the patient on the side of the puncture for several hours after a biopsy of the liver or spleen, to prevent bleeding. A pneumothorax may occur after a transpleural puncture. This complication can be managed with placement of a small-caliber catheter attached to a one-way chest drain valve (GURLEY et al. 1998). A chest X-ray should always be performed 4 h after a transpleural puncture. Peritonitis, biliary and urinary leakage are very rare complications reported in the literature and in our own experience and can be avoided by careful planning.

SMITH (1991), who reviewed the literature reports of about 156,000 fine-needle biopsies, found a 0.031–0.006% death rate and 23 cases of malignant seeding in needle tracts, predominantly from pancreatic carcinoma. Amongst 33 deaths related to biopsies, 22 were due to hemorrhage. Four patients died of sepsis following a biopsy procedure. Liver biopsies were the most frequent cause of bleeding complications: amongst 21 deaths from liver biopsies, 17 were due to hemorrhage, 11 occurring in patients with primary liver tumors, 2 in patients with hemangioma and 2 with angiosarcoma. The predominant cause of death

in pancreatic biopsies was pancreatitis (5 of 6 patients). Pancreatitis was more frequent in patients without a pancreatic tumor. As hemorrhage may occur immediately after biopsy or be delayed, postintervention observation is mandatory.

45.2.8
Biopsies of Specific Organs and Body Regions

45.2.8.1
Liver

Biopsies of large cores of hepatic tissue in diffuse hepatic disease are generally performed without imaging; nevertheless, significant complications occur after large core hepatic biopsies in 10–17% of cases. Hemorrhage mainly occurs in patients with coagulopathy (GAZELLE et al. 1992; SHEETS 1991). The advantages of image-guided biopsy soon became obvious, with higher yields of diagnostic specimen, especially for focal lesions (HA et al. 1991; HAAGA and VANEK 1979). Biopsy techniques under CT guidance have been well described in the literature (BERNARDINO 1984; GAZELLE and HAAGA 1989; GERVAIS et al. 1996; HARTER et al. 1983; LJUNG and GELLER 1998; MARTINO et al. 1984; MUELLER et al. 1981; WELCH et al. 1989; ZORNOZA et al. 1980). Biopsy needles can be directed accurately into lesions, even when deeply situated (Fig. 45.11). Necrotic lesions have to be sampled both at their periphery and their center. A biopsy of a presumed benign lesion has to be performed in the center of the lesion, but also in the normal liver to permit a histological comparison (Fig. 45.12). Cystic lesions can be punctured and treated in the same session, with injection of cytotoxic drugs such as 94% alcohol or Aethoxysclerol® (active principle: polidocanol 600; see Appendix B) (Kreussler, Wiesbaden, Germany). Occasionally, it may be difficult to target a hypervascular lesion, which is only seen in the arterial phase and not on the precontrast images or in the portal phase. Vascular landmarks can be used to locate the region to be biopsied. In some cases the lesion is better seen with US. Cutting needle biopsies for histological analysis provide a higher yield than aspiration biopsies (GAZELLE and HAAGA 1989; MARTINO et al. 1984; WELCH et al. 1989). The complication rate varies from 0.83% to 1.167% (BERNARDINO 1984; GAZELLE and HAAGA 1989; SHEETS et al. 1991; SMITH 1991; WELCH et al. 1989; YANKASKAS et al. 1986). Hemorrhage, sepsis, fistula formation, car-

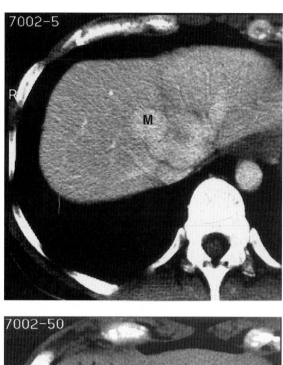

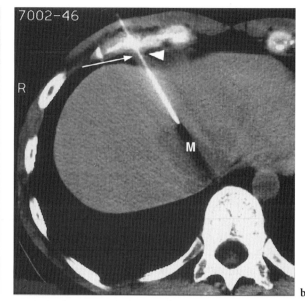

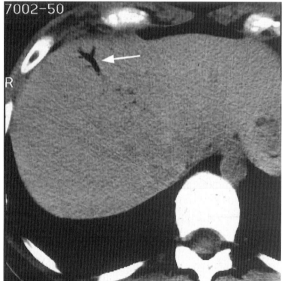

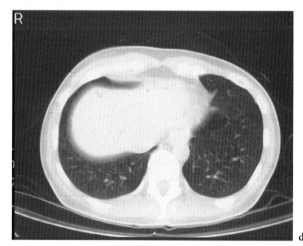

Fig. 45.11a–d. Liver biopsy of a focal nodular hyperplasia of segments VIII and IV (a--c *m*) with an 18-G automatic Tru-Cut needle (b *arrow*). Injection of physiologic saline solution (*arrowhead*) along the needle pathway to avoid pneumothorax. Presence of air probably in a portal vein (c *arrow*). d After biopsy there is no pneumothorax

cinoid crisis, tumour seeding along the needle path and death have been described (ISHII et al. 1998; SMITH 1991).

To prevent hemorrhage after percutaneous transhepatic liver biopsy in patients with diffuse liver disease, with or without coagulopathy or ascites, needle tract embolization with gelatin sponge can be performed (SMITH et al. 1996). The biopsy is performed with a cutting needle placed through a 10-cm-long vascular sheath. Gelatin sponge is then introduced into the biopsy tract through the vascular sheath. This procedure has a relatively high complication rate related both to the severity of the coagulopathy and operator experience.

CT-guided percutaneous transpulmonary liver biopsy is a safe and effective method for a biopsy of a lesion near the diaphragm (GERVAIS et al. 1996). The main advantage is its directness. The lesion can be rapidly targeted, fewer needle course adjustments may be needed, and both the length of the procedure and the risk of hemorrhage may be limited. Nevertheless, the radiologist must minimize unnecessary passes to correct for inaccurate needle positioning in order to decrease the risk of pneumothorax. A diag-

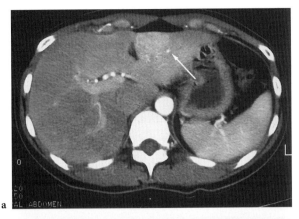

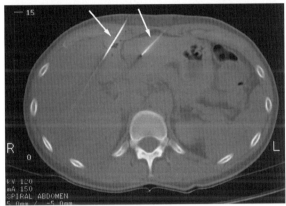

Fig. 45.12. **a** In a young patient with no liver history a hypervascular liver mass in segment III (*arrow*) was found, presumed to be benign. **b** A biopsy of the lesion (*left arrow*) and the surrounding healthy liver (*right arrow*) was performed with a tandem technique. At histology, the tumor was found to be focal nodular hyperplasia

that core biopsies are appropriate for assessing the degree of fibrosis or cirrhosis (IAMURA et al. 1993). For lesion evaluation, the 18-G automated side-cutting needle showed no statistically significant difference in the diagnostic accuracy for lesions of different pathology and size (range 0.7–3 cm, average size 2.3±0.7 cm). The biopsy specimen was sufficient for diagnosis in 98.5% (HA et al. 1991; YU et al. 1998). Smaller liver lesions (1.5 cm or less) are better targeted with US-guided biopsy (MIDDLETON et al. 1997).

A special problem is that of hypervascular hepatic lesions such as hepatocellular carcinoma, hemangioma or hypervascular hepatic metastases. Biopsy with an 18-G side-notch automatic needle has been shown to be safe in cirrhotic patients with suspected hepatocellular carcinoma provided that the length of interposing liver parenchyma along the needle track is at least 1 cm (CH YU et al. 1997). The larger the caliber of the needle, the greater the absolute blood loss. However, to obtain the same amount of diagnostic tissue more passes are needed with the smaller caliber needles. Therefore, the use of larger needles may be more efficient despite the greater amount of blood loss, because more tissue can be recovered and because fewer passes are required (PLECHA et al. 1997). Evaluation of the histological subtype of hepatocellular carcinoma may be essential because the subtype may affect treatment planning. Sclerosing, poorly differentiated and undifferentiated hepatocellular carcinomas respond poorly to percutaneous ethanol injection therapy, while early, small (less than 2 cm in diameter), hepatocellular carcinomas are usually well differentiated and can be successfully treated with percutaneous ethanol injection. Tumor vascularity in early and sclerosing hepatocellular carcinomas is poorly developed. These tumor types do not respond to transcatheter arterial embolization. However, hypervascularity is observed in most frank hepatocellular carcinomas with a good response to transcatheter arterial embolization (YAMASHITA et al. 1995).

Hemangiomas are associated with an increased risk of hemorrhage (SOLBIATI et al. 1985; TAAVITSAINEN et al. 1990). However, even core biopsies with 18-G needles are safe if a cuff of normal hepatic parenchyma is interposed between the capsule and the margins of the hemangioma (HEILO and STENWIG 1997).

A rare complication of liver biopsy is a carcinoid crisis, which has been described after fine-needle aspiration biopsy of hepatic metastases (BISSONNETTE et al. 1990).

nostic accuracy of 93% was found in a large series (WELCH et al. 1989).

A biopsy-induced pneumothorax should be aspirated if it is larger than one third of the lung area. This can be achieved safely and easily with a percutaneous catheter or a needle with a soft sheath on the CT table (YANKELEVITZ et al. 1996). Only 30% of patients treated by immediate aspiration had a recurrence of their pneumothorax requiring chest tube placement, which can be done as an outpatient procedure (GURLEY et al. 1998).

Perihepatic ascites does not have any statistically significant effect on the major or minor complication rate of image-guided percutaneous hepatic biopsy, irrespective of the needle type used, the number of passes made or the type of imaging modality employed (LITTLE et al. 1996; MURPHY et al. 1988).

Comparison between wedge and needle biopsy samples performed during open surgery showed

45.2.8.2
Spleen

Biopsy of the spleen can be performed as a staging procedure in patients with malignant lymphomas (CAVANNA et al. 1992; LINDGREN et al. 1985), for etiologic diagnosis in patients with diffuse splenomegaly, or to evaluate splenic lesions (CARAWAY and FANNING 1997; SILVERMAN et al. 1993a). Whereas the diagnostic yield is rather low in diffuse splenomegaly (LISHNER et al. 1996), a directed biopsy in suspected malignancy can even replace splenectomy (LINDGREN et al. 1985). Splenic biopsy can be performed with fine-needle aspiration biopsy or core biopsy with an 18-G needle. The major complication is hemorrhage, in up to 12.5% with the core biopsy method (LINDGREN et al. 1985), which can then require transfusion or even splenectomy.

45.2.8.3
– Pancreas

Percutaneous pancreatic biopsy is performed to rule out pancreatic malignancy, especially when the clinician is confronted with the differential diagnosis of chronic pancreatitis. Usually performed preoperativly (ELVIN et al. 1990; HALL-CRAGES and LEES 1986) (Fig. 45.13), it is sometimes also used after surgery, when intraoperative sampling could not be achieved safely. However, when intraoperative fine-needle aspiration biopsy is feasible it has a sensitivity of 100% (BLANDUMARA et al. 1995).

Small needles (20–22 G) are often used to penetrate vertically through abdominal wall, stomach, and intervening bowel (BRANDT et al. 1993; GRAHAM et al. 1994; HALL-CRAGGS and LEES 1986; LERMA et al. 1996; DELMASCHIO et al. 1991) (Fig. 45.14). The inconvenience of needle deflection when passing through different tissues must be considered. Larger needle size does not seem to produce a higher rate of complications (BALEN et al.1994; BRANDT 1993; ELVIN 1990; KARLSON 1996). Tandem needle and coaxial techniques can be used. Histological samples with biopsy guns of 18 G have an accuracy of 70–95%. Complications are uncommon but do occur: sepsis, hematomas, spread of pancreatic carcinoma, and pancreatitis in 0–3% of cases (MUELLER et al. 1988), and pseudoaneurysms have also been reported.

Pancreatic biopsy can be performed under CT or US guidance (BRANDT et al. 1993; DELMASCHIO et al. 1991; KARLSON et al. 1996; MAHONEY et al. 1993). DELMASCHIO et al. (1991) found CT guidance supe-

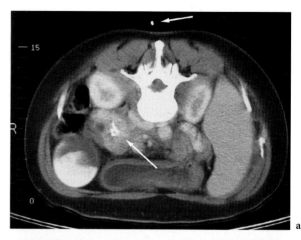

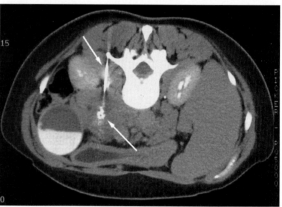

Fig. 45.13a, b. A calcified mass of the head of the pancreas is found with CT (*lower arrows*). **a** Marker for the planned biopsy (*upper arrow*). **b** The biopsy is achieved using an 18-gauge core biopsy needle (*upper arrow*) with the patient in the prone position. Histology revealed a neuroendocrine tumor (extraadrenal pheochromocytoma)

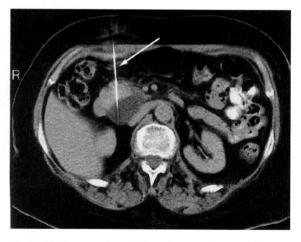

Fig. 45.14. Biopsy and aspiration of a mucoid cyst of the pancreas (*c*) with a 19-G fine needle (*arrow*). The needle passes through the head of the pancreas. No pancreatitis or hemorrhage occurred after the biopsy

rior to US guidance for fine-needle aspiration, while BRANDT et al. (1993) found a higher accuracy for US-guided biopsy, which was between 85% and 95%. The higher accuracy of US may be explained by the continuous real-time sonographic guidance of the needle into the hypoechoic area of the pancreas. The radiologist can guide the needle tip directly into the mass. Conversely, with CT, this continuous monitoring is not available, and the mass becomes less apparent after passage of the initial bolus of intravenous contrast material.

Accuracy is higher with larger masses (larger than 3 cm) and larger needle size (16–19 G: 92%; 20–22 G: 85%). Needle passage through gastrointestinal tract, including the colon, is usually safe. Use of even a thin, 21-G or 22-G needle can nevertheless result in a major complication.

Core biopsy of pancreas transplants can be achieved safely, though not without a risk of hemorrhage (AIDEYAN et al. 1996).

45.2.8.4
Kidneys

Renal biopsies for both focal lesions and diffuse disease are mostly guided by US (COZENS et al. 1992; MAHONEY et al. 1993; NYMAN et al. 1997; TUNG et al. 1992), and only in the case of failure are they guided by CT. The trend is to use a needle size between 16 G and 18 G (COZENS et al. 1992; MAHONEY et al. 1993; MOSTBECK et al. 1989) and an automatic core biopsy system (BURSTEIN et al. 1993; COZENS et al. 1992; MAHONEY et al. 1993). Renal transplant biopsy should be performed under imaging guidance

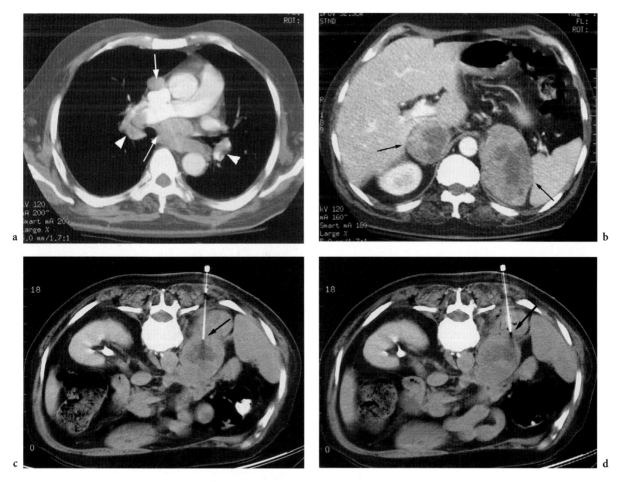

Fig. 45.15a–d. This patient presented with **a** pulmonary emboli and hilar (*arrowheads*), mediastinal (*arrows*), cerebral (not shown) and **b** bilateral adrenal masses (*arrows*), which were thought to be metastatic lung cancer. A biopsy of the left adrenal mass was achieved with the patient in the prone position. **c** One biopsy was performed in the central hypodense necrotic region (*arrow*) and **d** a second in the peripheral solid region of the tumor (*arrow*). Histology revealed a papillary carcinoma of the kidney

(Mahoney et al. 1993) to lower the complication rate. Posterior renal lesions are best punctured in the prone position (Fig. 45.15). The major complication is hemorrhage.

45.2.8.5
Pelvis and Intestine

The uterus and the prostate are not target organs for CT biopsy. Solid ovarian tumors and cystic tumors are better treated with laparoscopic procedures, except perhaps in young patients with negative tumor markers. A puncture with aspiration of the cystic content, followed by injection of a tissue toxic drug such 94% alcohol or Aethoxysclerol, can be achieved.

Presacral masses are encountered after abdominoperineal resection for colorectal carcinoma. Latero-pelvic masses in contact with the internal obturator muscle are seen with prostate or bladder carcinoma. The presacral region can be reached simply and safely by a transgluteal approach avoiding the sciatic nerve (Butch et al. 1985) (Fig. 45.16). For latero-pelvic masses, a posterior approach is also preferable, to avoid intestinal and vascular structures, especially the external iliac vessels. However, in large pelvic masses, an anterior approach is also feasible (Fig. 45.18).

Intestinal wall thickening, which cannot be biopsied by endoscopic methods, can be aspirated with a fine needle from 22G to 20 G. The biopsy can be performed under US or CT guidance (Bree et al. 1991; Carson et al. 1998). It is a simple and safe procedure. Diagnostic failure may occur with lymphoma, because of small sample size (Fig 45.17).

45.2.8.6
Retroperitoneum (Lymph Nodes and Adrenal Glands)

Image-guided needle biopsy should be first procedure performed for the diagnosis of lymphoma, except in easily accessible superficial neck, inguinal, and axillary nodal sites for which image-guidance is not needed (Quinn et al. 1995). Immunochemical and flow cytometric techniques have greatly enhanced the diagnostic capabilities of needle biopsy procedures in the diagnosis and subtyping of lymphoma (Sneige et al. 1990), which is important for treatment. Different needle types and sizes have been used to establish the diagnosis of lymphoma. Some series have used fine-needle aspiration biopsy (Fisher et al. 1997; Leong and Stevens 1996; Oyen

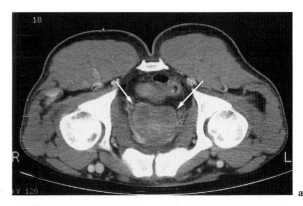

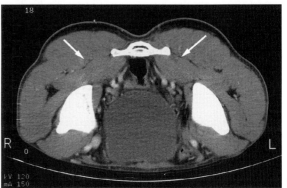

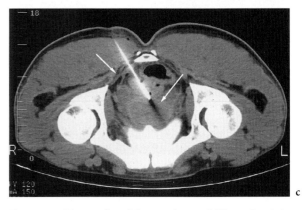

Fig. 45.16. a Biopsy of a pelvic mass (*arrows*). The patient is in the prone position. b The biopsy is performed below the piriform muscle (*arrows*). c The Tru-Cut biopsy needle passes lateral to the coccyx through the sacroiliac ligament (*small arrow*) into the mass (*arrow*). Histology revealed a peritoneal mesothelioma

et al. 1994; Sneige et al. 1990; Stewart et al. 1998), and others have used core biopsy needles (Quinn et al. 1995). Samples from fine needles are just as likely as larger needles to enable tumor grading and treatment (Silverman et al. 1994). However, the distinction between low- and intermediate-grade lymphoma may not be possible on the basis of cytological features only (Fisher et al. 1998; National Cancer Institute 1982). Therefore, if architectural

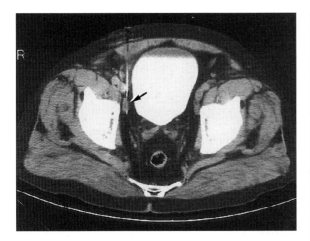

Fig. 45.17. Biopsy of an external iliac lymph node with a 20-G automated core biopsy needle (*arrow*). The patient was thought to have recurrent lymphoma, but no tumor was found at histology

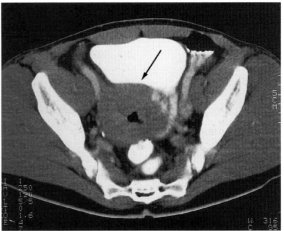

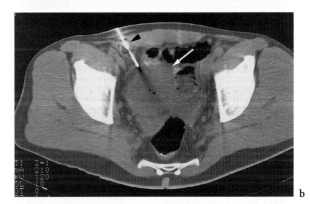

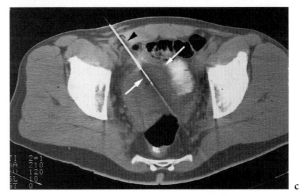

Fig. 45.18. a Mass in the pelvic region with a diameter of 8 cm (*arrow*). A central hypodense region of air density is visible. b, c The biopsy is performed by an anterior approach with a core biopsy needle (*black arrowheads*). The needle is advanced into the tumor (*arrows*). Histology revealed a mesenchymal sarcoma.

studies are necessary to distinguish the type of lymphoma, large core biopsies may be necessary (CAFFERTY et al. 1990). In order to obtain sufficient tissue, we therefore prefer to use core biopsy needles routinely. Targeting the lesion is just as easy as with fine needles, and the complication rate is not significantly higher (Fig. 45.21).

The biopsy material is sent to the pathology laboratory in a 10% buffered formalin solution and is fixed and stained there in the standard fashion for histological examination. Immunochemical studies can be performed on the paraffin-fixed specimen, but it is better also to send a specimen in normal saline, so that immunochemical studies and cytogenic studies are possible, or a cell suspension can be produced for flow cytometry and characterization of DNA surface markers.

Most adrenal biopsies are performed in patients with lung cancer and adrenal masses (Fig. 45.20) (SILVERMAN et al. 1993b; WELCH et al. 1994), but they are also performed in patients with melanoma, colon carcinoma and lymphoma or other neoplasms that can metastasize to the adrenal glands. Incidental adrenal masses are often found in nononcological patients, and these are rarely malignant (BERNARDINO et al. 1985). To avoid performing unnecessary biopsies, we have adopted the following strategy: adrenal masses, that have an attenuation of less than 18 HU on unenhanced CT images are considered as adenomas (CASOLA et al. 1987; MIYAKE et al. 1995). Although a threshold value for the diameter of an adrenal mass is not an accurate criterion because there is overlap between malignant and nonmalignant masses when the mass is small, a size over 3.5–4 cm should be considered malignant until proven otherwise (KOROBKIN et al. 1996b). Even in patients with lung cancer, the low attenuation of adrenal masses on unenhanced CT images can discriminate a benign adrenal tumor from a metastasis (MACARI et al.

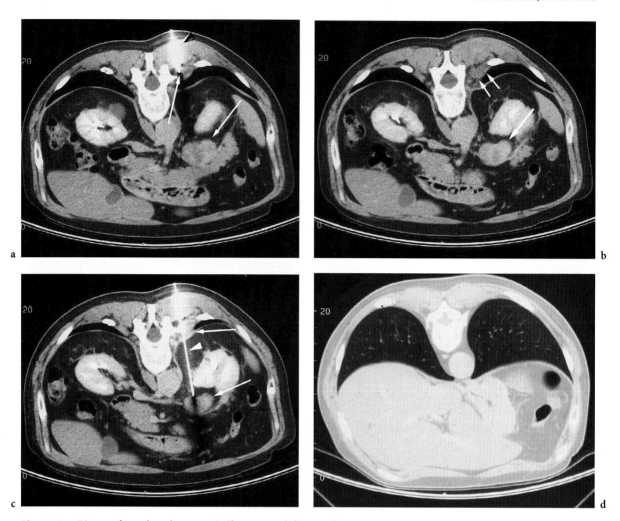

Fig. 45.19. a Biopsy of an adrenal metastasis (*lower arrow*) from melanoma. **b** Physiological saline solution is injected in the extrapleural space (*small arrows*) to avoid injury to the lung parenchyma. **c** The biopsy is performed with a Franseen 18-G needle (*arrowhead*). **d** After the biopsy no pneumothorax was seen

1998). If an unenhanced CT has not been performed, delayed scans, either early-delayed at 15 min (Boland 1997) or late-delayed at 60 min (Korobkin et al. 1996a), can be obtained to measure the washout of the contrast material. Threshold values around ≤24 HU on 15-min delayed scans (Boland et al. 1977) or ≤30 HU on 60-min delayed scans (Korobkin et al. 1996a) seem to be characteristic of benign lesions (Fig. 45.20).

A posterior, a right-lateral transhepatic or a left-lateral transsplenic, or an anterior transpancreatic approach can be chosen. We prefer a posterior pathway with the patient prone, possibly with an artificial widening of the paravertebral space with injection of physiologic saline solution (Karampekios et al. 1998; Langen et al. 1995) (Fig. 45.19). Fine-needle biopsy (20–22 G) is used if organs such as liver, spleen or pancreas are to be passed through. Never-

theless, a fine needle does not prevent complications (Mody et al. 1995). If the access route avoids the liver, spleen or pancreas, and the lesion is large (>2 cm), we prefer a core biopsy.

Pneumothorax is a possible complication with the posterior approach, as is hemorrhage of the liver, kidney or spleen (Mody et al. 1995). In addition, pancreatitis has been described after a transpancreatic approach (Kane et al. 1991).

45.3
Therapeutic Procedures

In the early days of percutaneous abscess drainage (PAD), only drainage of unilocular abscesses with an

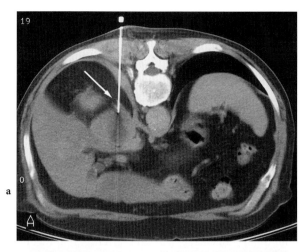

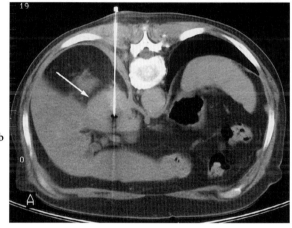

Fig. 45.20a, b. Adrenal metastasis from lung cancer. **a** A biopsy gun is used with a coaxial technique. The coaxial needle is advanced to the outer margin of the tumor (*arrow*). **b** The biopsy needle is inserted into the coaxial needle and advanced into the tumor (*arrow*). Histology revealed an undifferentiated carcinoma compatible with a pulmonary origin

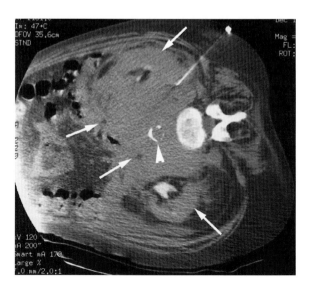

obvious access route and no communications, fistulae or complicating factors was performed (VAN SONNENBERG et al. 1991). Today PAD is performed in critically ill patients either before surgery, as a temporizing act or postoperatively, to evacuate postoperative fluid collections. PAD of multiple and multilocular abscesses with or without communication and deep-seated collections with overlying structures can be attempted (VAN SONNENBERG et al. 1991; LAMBIASE et al. 1992). CT can locate an abscess accurately and show its relationship to adjacent organs and peritoneal spaces.

In addition, drainage of noninfected fluid collections can be achieved with or without injection of sclerosing drugs, in order to damage the secretory surface. Therapeutic injections of sclerosant drugs can also be performed for treatment of certain liver tumors or for neurolysis of splanchnic nerves in patients with intractable pain.

45.3.1
Materials and Techniques

External catheter diameter is expressed in French (F) or Charrière (Ch) (see Appendix A). One French (or Charrière) corresponds to 1/3 mm. Catheter diameters from 5 F to 30 F are available, with or without a double lumen for flushing. Internal retention mechanisms such as a locking pigtail, inflatable balloons or wings can be used. The locking pigtail best prevents dislodgment (CHAN et al. 1996). We prefer pigtail catheters with side-holes (Fig. 45.22, 45.23). The pigtail shape prevents perforation of the wall abscess. Drainage catheters must be of sufficient caliber: for thin, nonviscous fluid, catheters from 7 F to 10 F may be suitable. For viscous fluid collections, 12- to 20 F catheters are recommended. Sump catheters irrigated with sterile physiologic saline solution can help liquefy viscous contents. Administration of urokinase in abscesses with thick fluid or which have septa or are multilocular may be of benefit to decrease the viscosity of any purulent material (PARK et al. 1993). No bleeding complications or change in coagulation parameters are encountered (LAHORRA et al. 1993). In most cases it is safe to ad-

Fig. 45.21. Biopsy of a retroperitoneal mass (*arrows*) surrounding a calcified aorta (*arrowhead*), infiltrating the left kidney (*upper arrow*) and displacing the right kidney (*lower arrow*). The biopsy is performed with a 16-G automatic Tru-Cut needle. Histology revealed an aggressive non-Hodgkin lymphoma

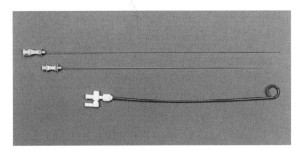

Fig. 45.22. Pigtail catheter (Otto B, Angiomed), which is inserted by a trocar technique. The catheter has three coaxial inner cannulae: one with a blunt end to hold the pigtail straight, and two with sharp ends. One of the sharp cannulae is hollow, allowing simultaneous suction during insertion. The catheter can also be used for the Seldinger technique

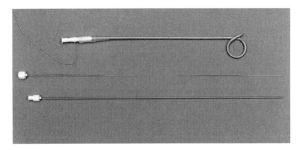

Fig. 45.23. Pigtail catheter with a locking thread (Navarre), which is inserted by a trocar technique

minister 5000 IU of urokinase per centimeter of abscess diameter every 8 h for 3 days through the percutaneous drainage catheter without risk of hemorrhage. However, some patients with CNS disorders (tumors, vascular problems), coagulopathy, hepatic failure, pregnancy, or abscesses in the spleen, pancreas, or interloop area should be excluded (LAHORRA et al. 1993). In interloop abscesses it is uncertain whether urokinase would prevent closure of enteric fistulas.

Depending on the localization of the abscess, a trocar or Seldinger technique can be used. Superficial abscesses, with no overlying organs or bowel loops, can be drained rapidly with the trocar technique. After skin cleansing, draping, local anesthesia, and a small skin incision, a "one-shot" direct puncture of the abscess is performed. This is feasible with up to 12- to 14-F catheters. If a larger catheter is required or if deeply located collections are to be targeted the Seldinger technique should be employed. This consists in a multiple step procedure, with the insertion initially of a sheathed 20- to 22-G needle. To displace overlying bowel loops or organs, the injection of physiological saline solution along the needle pathway can be used (KARAMPEKIOS et al.

1998; LANGEN et al. 1995). A guidewire of at least 0.035 inch is inserted into the abscess. The tract is dilated with dilators of increasing size to reach the catheter diameter, which is then inserted over the guide wire (Fig. 45.24). Attention has to be paid to the length of the tract to be dilated, meaning the distance from the skin to the center of the abscess. A marker (e.g., steri-strip) should be fixed to the dilators, to avoid perforation of the opposite wall of the abscess. The guide wire is then removed. The abscess is aspirated to dryness by manual suction. Specimens are sent for appropriate biochemical and microbiological analysis. Aerobic and anaerobic cultures are recommended for abdominal abscesses and biliary drainage, but not after percutaneous nephrostomy, unless the patient has a urinary tract malignancy or has had previous urinary instrumentation (MALDEN et al. 1995). After evacuation of the abscess, the catheter is secured to the skin. We prefer a suture to the skin over adhesive devices attached to the skin, as we have seen several catheter dislocations with adhesive devices.

Occasionally, symptoms of sepsis with shivering may occur during the drainage procedure; therefore, a broad spectrum antibiotic should be administered 1–2 h beforehand.

The interventional radiology team should perform the follow-up catheter care. If there is a problem with the catheter, adjustments may be necessary. Clinical colleagues and nursing personal generally appreciate the radiologist's participation (VAN SONNENBERG et al. 1991).

PAD can treat the patient effectively, often with no further medical treatment after the catheter has been withdrawn. PAD may also be performed as a temporizing procedure, to improve the patient's condition prior to surgery. PAD can be palliative if abscesses are complicating a severe underlying illness. PAD may fail, however, particularly if the ongoing

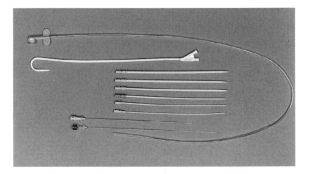

Fig. 45.24. A double-lumen catheter (Gastrotop sump drainage set, Angiomed) with biopsy needle, guidewire and dilators for use with Seldinger technique

sepsis cannot be stopped by drainage (LAMBIASE et al. 1992).

The clinical response to the drainage of the abscess should be immediate, with a fall in temperature within 24 h. Catheter drainage can require 15–30 days; patients with enteric communications may have a longer course, even up to 130 days (VAN SONNENBERG et al. 1991).

45.3.2
Complications

Complications are hemorrhage, pleural effusion, infection of a sterile collection, sepsis, catheter dislodgment and fistula formation. Failure is usually due to a viscous content, with material too thick to be drained even by the larger catheters.

45.3.3
Drainage of Liver Abscesses and Liver Cysts

Liver abscesses may either be drained with catheter insertion in the manner described above or treated by single or multiple needle aspirations. Needles of varying caliber are used, from 16 G to 22 G according to the size of the abscess. This percutaneous needle aspiration technique with injection of antibiotics into the abscess cavity and simultaneous intravenous antibiotic therapy seems to be a valid alternative to prolonged catheter drainage for the treatment of a pyogenic liver abscess (GIORGIO et al. 1995). Percutaneous needle aspiration can be repeated every 3–7 days in an out-patient setting. A 98% cure rate has been reported (GIORGIO et al. 1995). However, other authors have favored catheter drainage over needle aspirations, with a success rate of 60% with needle aspiration and 100% with catheter drainage in a randomized patient group (RAJAK et al. 1998). Duration of drainage is longer with an intrahepatic biliary communication, but with a comparable cure rate (63%) to that obtained in the case of abscesses without a biliary communication (68%) (DO 1991).

Drainage of amebic abscesses should only be performed exceptionally. In general, medical treatment is sufficient (RALLS et al. 1987). One exception is when it is necessary to differentiate pyogenic from amebic abscesses, although diagnosis is rarely possible from examination of amebic abscesses' content and a core biopsy of the wall may be necessary (VAN SONNENBERG et al. 1985). Other reasons are pain, imminent rupture, a left lobe abscess with risk of

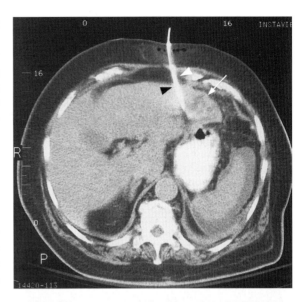

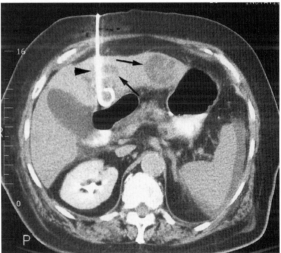

Fig. 45.25. Drainage of two amebic abscesses (*arrows*) of the left lobe of the liver with a 12-F pigtail catheter (*arrowheads*)

perforation into the thorax, pregnancy, false negative serology, a need for therapy before the serologic results are available and abscesses greater than 8–10 cm in diameter (VAN SONNENBERG et al. 1985, 1991) (Fig. 45.25).

Hepatic cysts can be divided into three categories: congenital solitary cysts, polycystic liver disease and *Echinococcus granulosus* cysts. Symptomatic congenital solitary cysts and cysts in polycystic liver disease can be treated with single-session percutaneous drainage and sclerotherapy. The sclerosing agents used are alcohol, tetracycline and doxycycline. Success rates vary from 85% to 97% (TIKKAKOSKI et al. 1996; VAN SONNENBERG et al. 1994).

Percutaneous needle aspiration of hydatid cysts

has long been discouraged because of the fear of potential complications, such as anaphylactic shock
and the spread of daughter cysts. Cyst aspiration is
described with 19-G to 22-G needles and drainage
with 5-F to 8-F catheters, with subsequent injection
of hypertonic (20%) saline. Only mild allergic reactions such as temporary pruritus were encountered
(BRET et al. 1988; KHUROO et al. 1991; MUELLER et al.
1985).

45.3.4
Drainage of the Gallbladder

Cholecystitis is normally an indication for surgery,
especially if there is underlying cholelithiasis. However, percutaneous drainage of the gallbladder is
performed in critically ill patients who present a
high anesthetic risk for surgery. In acalculous cholecystitis, percutaneous drainage may be the definitive
therapy (BOLAND et al. 1994b; VAN OVERHAGEN et
al. 1996). Patients in the intensive care unit have an
increased risk of developing cholecystitis, sometimes presenting with unexplained sepsis and otherwise nonspecific clinical and radiological symptoms
(BOLAND et al. 1994a). US or CT can guide percutaneous drainage. A transhepatic catheter route is not
mandatory; the transperitoneal route is not associated with a higher complication rate (GARBER et al.
1994).

For decompression of a dilated biliary tract, CT is
not often used. This intervention is usually performed under fluoroscopic or US guidance.

45.3.5
Interventional Procedures During Pancreatitis

Different fluid collections can be observed during
the course of acute pancreatitis, which may be
diffuse or well localized, infected or sterile, of
heterogeneous soft-tissue density or of fluid attenuation. More than 50% of acute fluid collections resolve spontaneously. Infected collections or pseudocysts can be referred for percutaneous drainage
(BALTHAZAR et al. 1994). Peripancreatic collections
with heterogeneous and partly soft tissue density,
thick necrotic pancreatic tissue and hemorrhagic
high-attenuation collections should not be drained
percutaneously (BALTHAZAR et al. 1994). Surgical
necrosectomy or angiographic embolization of a
bleeding vessel may be required. However, abscesses
in the course of acute pancreatitis or infected necro-

tizing pancreatitis should be considered for percutaneous drainage (FREENY et al. 1988, 1998).

Pseudocysts smaller than 5 cm often resolve
spontaneously. Infected pseudocysts and cysts larger
than 5 cm that are causing pain and gastrointestinal
or biliary tract obstruction should be treated with
percutaneous drainage (VAN SONNENBERG et al.
1989). High cure rates reaching 90% can be achieved
in infected and noninfected pseudocysts. Octroide
acetate (Sandostatin, Novartis Pharma Schweiz,
Bern, Switzerland) (see Appendix B) administered
s.c. in doses increasing progressively from 50 to
1,000 µg three times a day is effective in decreasing
the secretion from a pancreatic pseudocyst
(D'AGOSTINO et al. 1993). A direct route is preferable
for successful drainage. The optimal location is
where the fluid collections are largest and in contact
with the parietal peritoneum. The external catheter
is preferred to endoscopic drainage into the stomach, because of the absent risk of catheter migration,
the easy exchange if necessary, the possibility of
daily monitoring of the fluid output and its appearance and the capability for irrigation.

Communications with the gastrointestinal tract
or pancreatic duct can be detected by injecting contrast material through the drainage catheter.

A small 7- to 9-F catheter is adequate to drain
clear fluid collections and noninfected pseudocysts.
Infected pseudocysts, abscesses and liquefied necrotic tissue are better drained with large double-lumen sump catheters (12–16 F). For highly viscous
collections, catheter size may be increased to 20–30
F. More than one catheter can be used, if necessary.
Evacuation of the various sites and widespread irrigation across the collection should be obtained. Infected and necrotic tissue should be evacuated as
much as possible (BALTHAZAR et al. 1994; TANAKA et
al. 1991). A general rule is not to remove the catheter
until the cyst has collapsed and the communication
with the pancreatic duct has closed.

In infected necrotizing pancreatitis, sepsis can be
controlled in 74% of patients and 47% of patients
cured without surgery (FREENY et al. 1998). Infected
diffuse pancreatic fluid collections benefit from percutaneous drainage with a 65% cure rate (FREENY et
al. 1988). Finally, pancreatic abscesses can be cured
in 86% of cases (TANAKA et al. 1991) (Fig. 45.26).

45.3.6
Enteric, Abdominal Cavity and Retroperitoneal Abscesses

Abscesses are a frequent complication of Crohn's disease. Radiologically guided catheter drainage can either cure the patient or achieve a temporizing effect. Subsequently, elective surgery with a single-stage intestinal resection and primary anastomosis can be performed in most cases. Rarely, enterocutaneous fistulas secondary to drainage are encountered. Intestinal communications generally close during drainage (CASOLA et al. 1987; LAMBIASE et al. 1988; SAFRIT et al. 1987).

Periappendiceal abscesses can be treated by percutaneous drainage with simultaneous antibiotic therapy. A success rate of up to 90% has been described (JEFFREY et al. 1987). Communication between the abscess and the base of the cecum or the appendix is seen in up to 44% of cases. They close with drainage within 14 days. In addition, children can be successfully treated with percutaneous drainage (JAMIESON et al. 1997). In critically ill patients, temporization improves their clinical condition, and elective surgery can be performed, avoiding surgery for abscess drainage and thereby reducing the length of hospital stay and health costs (VAN SONNENBERG et al. 1987) (Fig. 45.27).

Diverticular abscesses benefit particularly from the temporization achieved with percutaneous drainage, which obviates surgical abscess drainage and permits a single operation with resection of the sigmoid colon and primary anastomosis. Surgery can be performed within 10 days of drainage (MUELLER et al. 1987; NEFF et al. 1987). Depending on the localization, the access to sigmoid abscesses can be anterior (Fig. 45.28), transrectal (GAZELLE et al. 1991), transvaginal, or posterior with a transgluteal (BUTCH et al. 1986; RYAN et al. 1998) or paracoccygeal route (LONGO et al. 1993). A disadvantage of the transgluteal approach is the risk of injury to the sciatic plexus or blood vessels. The access route must be inferior to the piriform muscle at the level of the sacrospinous ligament (Fig. 45.16). Using this approach, postsurgical lower pelvic abscesses or tubo-ovarian abscesses can be drained.

Percutaneous drainage of subphrenic abscesses can be achieved with an angled subcostal approach, under US or CT guidance (MUELLER et al. 1986). The transpleural access is associated only with a slight increase in complication rate, mainly from pneumothorax, with a success rate similar to that of extrapleural drainage. No subsequent empyema has been reported (McNICHOLAS et al. 1995).

Percutaneous drainage of renal and perirenal abscesses alone was curative in 67% of patients as determined by resolution of signs and symptoms or follow-up CT (DEYVE et al. 1990); 27% of patients demonstrated improvement of signs, but required surgery for the underlying causes of the perirenal abscess. For these patients nephrectomy was performed for poorly functioning or nonfunctioning kidney, for removal of a renal cell carcinoma and for loculated abscess that could not drained adequately percutaneously (DEYOE et al. 1990).

Intra- or retroperitoneal hematoma evacuation should only be attempted if the hematoma has undergone complete liquefaction and can be aspirated; with clotted blood, the risk of introducing infection is high. However, decompression is sometimes necessary, especially in the psoas muscles (VAN SONNENBERG et al. 1991).

45.3.7
Alcohol Treatment of Hepatocellular Carcinoma

Percutaneous ethanol injection (PEI) can be proposed to patients with hepatocellular carcinoma (HCC), either alone or in combination with transcatheter intraarterial chemoembolization (TACE) (TANAKA et al. 1991). We treat a single nodule with a diameter of less than 3 cm with PEI alone. A single nodule between 3 and 5 cm and up to three lesions less than 3 cm across are treated with a combination of TACE and PEI. Nodules larger than 5 cm are treated either with TACE alone or with systemic chemotherapy, or not at all (BECKER et al. 1997; PALMA 1998). Recently, a combined therapy with a single TACE followed by PEI in larger tumors (3–8 cm in diameter) was reported to have an overall survival rate (Kaplan-Meier method) of 47% at 5 years (LENCIONI et al. 1998).

The formula: $V(ml) = {}^4/_3 \, \Pi \, [0.5 + r \, (cm)]^3$ gives the volume V required for injection into the nodule, where r is the radius of the nodule (Becker et al. 1997). The alcohol is injected over several sessions (for example between 10 and 20 ml per session), but a high-dose single-shot PEI with 16–120 ml in one session also seems promising, with survival rates similar to those obtained with conventional PEI and even better than those after surgery (Giorgio et al. 1998).

The nodule is punctured under either US or CT guidance, depending on the lesion conspicuity with each of these techniques. A 21-G needle of the Chiba type (Sterylab, Milan, Italy) is used, which is closed

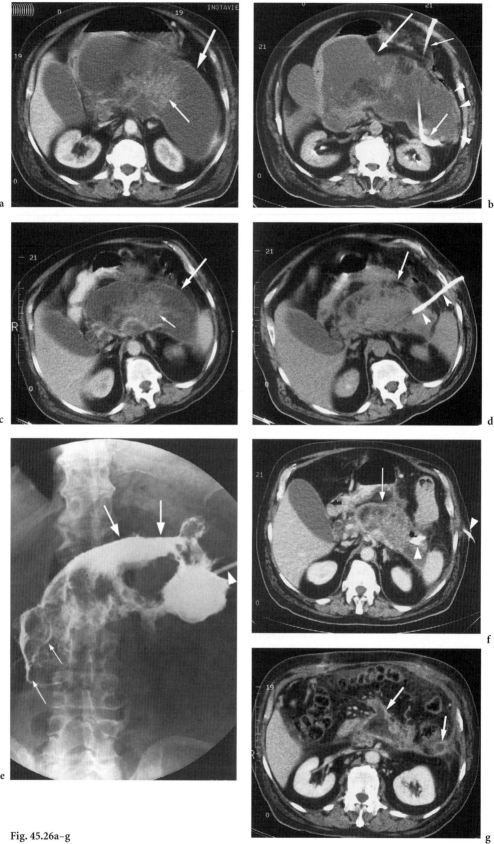

Fig. 45.26a–g

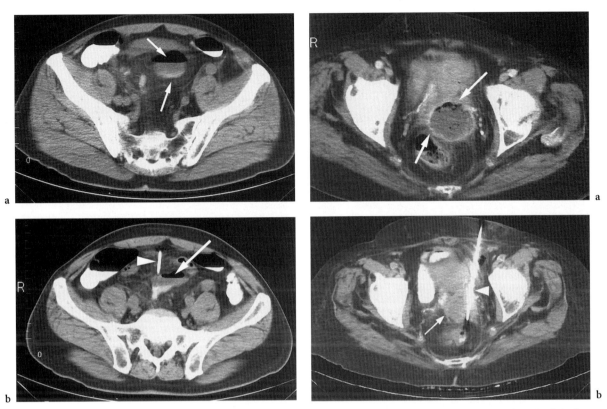

Fig. 45.27. A central pelvic collection is shown, filled with contrast medium by an intestinal fistula (*arrows*). The patient was thought to have a recurrence of Crohn's disease, but no thickening of the small bowel was seen. Drainage was achieved with a 12-F pigtail single-lumen catheter by a trocar technique (*arrowhead*). This was a temporizing procedure. At surgery, a fistula from appendicitis was found

Fig. 45.28. Abscess (*arrows*) from acute diverticulitis (*arrows*), drained with a 12-F single-lumen pigtail catheter by a trocar (*arrowhead*) technique

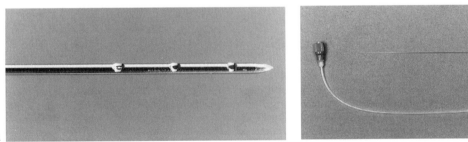

Fig. 45.29. a Magnification of the needle used for percutaneous ethanol injection (PEI) (Sterylab) of intrahepatic malignant lesions, showing the three side-holes and the blind-ending tip of the needle. b The full needle with a plastic tube

◁ Fig. 45.26a–g. Patient with necrotizing pancreatitis. **a, b** A large fluid collection (*large arrow*) is shown surrounding the remaining vascularized pancreas (**a** *small arrow*). First a 14-F double-lumen sump catheter is inserted (**b** *small arrow*). On the left side the collection was in contact with the splenic flexure of the colon (**b** *arrowheads*). **c, d** Ten days later the collection (*large arrow*) is smaller but the patient has a raised temperature. The remaining pancreas can be seen (*small arrow*). A second drainage with a 14-F double lumen catheter is performed (*arrowheads*). **e** Fistulography performed via the catheter (*arrowhead*) shows outline of the collection (*arrows*) and subsequent filling of the pancreatic duct (*small arrows*), demonstrating the communication between the pancreatic duct and the collection. The patient was treated with octroide and the catheter left in place. **f** Fourteen days later the fluid collection (*arrow*) has diminished and has developed a pseudocapsule. The catheter remains in place (*arrowheads*). **g** Two months later, a smaller but persisting collection is shown to the left of the head of the pancreas (*left arrow*) and along the left anterior pararenal space (*right arrow*). The patient was asymptomatic by this time

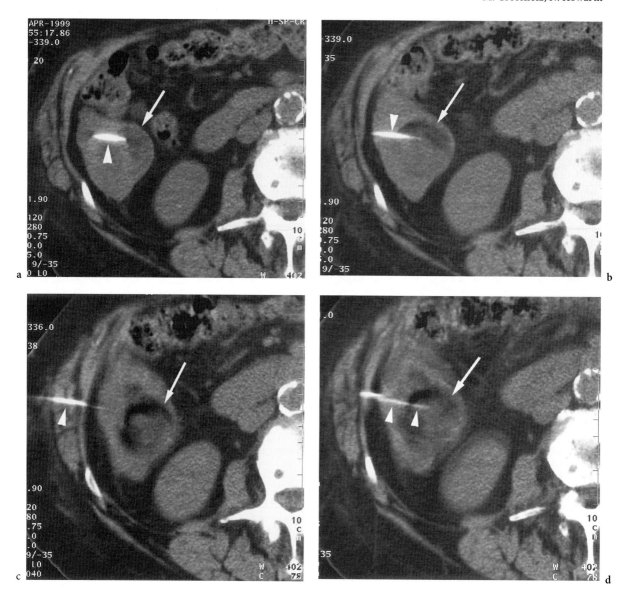

Fig. 45.30a–d. Hepatocellular carcinoma (*arrow*) in a cirrhotic liver treated by injection of 94% alcohol. A needle (*arrowheads*) with side-holes over a length of 1.2 cm is inserted into the lesion with the side-holes in the middle of the lesion. After verifying the needle localization (**a**), alcohol is progressively injected (**b–d**). The distribution of the very hypodense alcohol is well demonstrated within the encapsulated tumor (**d**). A total of 50 ml alcohol was injected. At the end of the injection, small traces of alcohol can be seen around the tumor capsule, demonstrating extravasation of the alcohol. This procedure is performed with stand-by anesthesia

at its tip but has side-holes over up to 1.2 cm from the tip, permitting improved diffusion of the alcohol into the lesion (Fig. 45.29). If blood is aspirated after the needle is positioned in the lesion the needle position must be corrected. We prefer to have stand-by anesthesia because accidental diffusion of the alcohol to the liver capsule, especially during treatment of a superficial nodule, is very painful and effective analgesia is mandatory. The alcohol is injected with very light pressure up to the volume required. The diffusion of the alcohol is best controlled with CT. Complications are rare and consist in hemorrhage, infection of necrotic tumor and "chemical" portal vein thrombosis, which is usually reversible (BECKER et al. 1997) (Fig. 45.30).

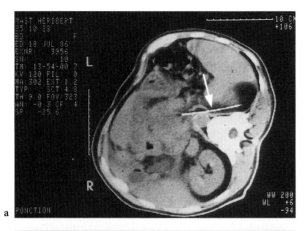

a

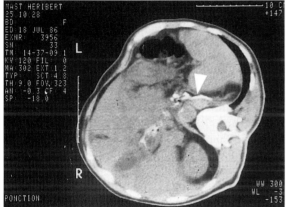

b

Fig. 45.31. Patient with pancreatic carcinoma. Percutaneous sclerotherapy of the celiac ganglion from a posterior approach. The needle is in position anterior to the aorta (*arrow*). A total of 20 ml of absolute alcohol mixed with 2 ml of contrast medium has been injected (*arrowhead*). By courtesy of Dr. H. Hauser, Hôpital de la Tour, Geneva

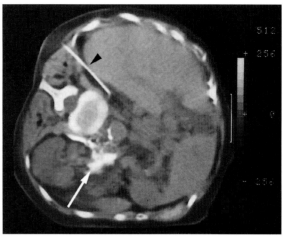

Fig. 45.32. Patient with pancreatic carcinoma. Percutaneous sclerotherapy of the celiac ganglion with a bilateral posterior approach. The needle (*arrowhead*) is in position in the paravertebral region. Injection of 20 ml of absolute alcohol bilaterally. To improve visualization, the alcohol is mixed with 2 ml contrast medium (*arrow*). By courtesy of Dr. H. Hauser, Hôpital de la Tour, Geneva

45.3.8
Neurolysis

Celiac ganglion block is used for intractable back or upper abdominal pain, especially in patients with pancreatic neoplasms or chronic pancreatitis, but also with other upper abdominal tumors associated with severe pain. The celiac artery indicates the position of the celiac ganglia. The sympathetic nerves are found along the antero-lateral surface of the upper abdominal aorta. The celiac block can be performed under fluoroscopic, CT, US or endosonographic guidance (GIMENEZ et al. 1993; LEE et al. 1993; WIERSEMA and WIERSEMA 1996).

Either a posterior or an anterior approach can be chosen (ROMANELLI et al. 1993; LEE et al. 1993). Preliminary thin-section scans (5 mm) are performed to identify the celiac and superior mesenteric arteries.

For the anterior and posterior approach, one or two needles are placed just anterior to the diaphragmatic crus at or between the levels of the celiac and superior mesenteric arteries, and 18–22 ml of 94% alcohol, which can be mixed with 2–3 ml of contrast medium, is injected through each needle if two needles are used, or 40 ml is injected if a single-needle approach is chosen.

For the anterior approach, one or two 20-G needles are chosen, because of the high probability of puncturing the stomach or the pancreas to reach the celiac ganglia.

For the posterior approach, the patient is placed prone on the CT-table. One or two 18-G or 20-G needles are inserted. Care must be taken not to injure the kidney. The prone position is less comfortable for patients with severe abdominal pain, however (LEE et al. 1993).

Persistent improvements in pain scores have been reported for 79–88% of patients, with a higher improvement score for patients with pancreatic carcinoma (WIERSEMA and WIERSEMA 1996). The mean daily analgesic usage fell by 58% (ROMANELLI et al. 1993) (Figs. 45.31, 45.32).

The complications reported were hemorrhage, aortic dissection and diarrhea.

45.3.9
Sclerotherapy of Lymphoceles

Treatment of postoperative lymphoceles can be achieved by opening a window in the wall of the lymphocele using endoscopic techniques or by percutaneous drainage, with alcohol sclerotherapy (SAWHNEY et al. 1996; ZUCKERMAN and YEAGER 1997). After drainage of the lymphocele, absolute alcohol (10–100 ml) is instilled one to three times a day and aspirated after 30 min. This procedure is repeated three times a week for a median 19–30 days (SAWHNEY et al. 1996; ZUCKERMAN and YEAGER 1997). The success rate is 94–100%.

Appendix A: Diameters of Needles and Catheters

Gauge (G)	External diameter (mm)	(in.)	Charrière (Ch)/ French (F)	External diameter (mm)
35	0.13	0.005	1	0.33
34	0.18	0.007	2	0.67
33	0.20	0.008	3	1.00
32	0.23	0.009	4	1.33
31	0.25	0.010	5	1.67
			6	2.00
30	0.30	0.012	7	2.33
29	0.33	0.013	8	2.67
28	0.36	0.014	9	3.00
27	0.41	0.016	10	3.33
26	0.46	0.018		
			11	3.67
25	0.51	0.020	12	4.00
	0.53	0.021	13	4.33
24	0.56	0.022	14	4.67
23	0.64	0.025	15	5.00
22	0.71	0.028	16	5.33
21	0.81	0.032	17	5.67
			18	6.00
20	0.89	0.035	19	6.33
	0.97	0.038	20	6.67
19	1.07	0.042		
18	1.27	0.050	21	7.00
17	1.50	0.059	22	7.33
16	1.65	0.065	23	7.67
			24	8.00
15	1.83	0.072	25	8.33
14	2.11	0.083	26	8.67
13	2.41	0.095	27	9.00
12	2.77	0.109	28	9.33
11	3.05	0.120	29	9.67
			30	10.00
10	3.40	0.134		
9	3.76	0.148	32	10.67
8	4.19	0.165	34	11.33
7	4.57	0.180	36	12.00
6	5.16	0.203	38	12.67
			40	13.33
			45	15.00

Appendix B: Manufacturers

Needle for intramuscular injection: Temno Europe N.V., B-3030 Leuven, Belgium

Angiomed, Wachhausstrasse 6, D-76227 Karlsruhe, Germany

Sterylab s.p.a., Via Togliatti, I-20017 RHO-Milan, Italy

Cook, William Cook Europe A/S, 4632-Bjaeverskov, Denmark

Bard, C.R. Bard, Inc. Covington, GA 30209, USA

Navarre Biomedical, Ltd., 2645 Fernbrook Lane N, Plymouth, MN 55447, USA

Somatex, Postfach 420620, D-12066 Berlin, Germany

Becton Dickinson and Company, Franklin Lakes, NJ 07417, USA

Temno, Bauer Medical, Inc., Clearwater, FL 34620, USA

Medi-tech, Boston Scientific Corporation, 480 Pleasant Street, Watertown, MA 02172, USA

Kreussler, Rheingaustr. 87–93, D-65203 Wiesbaden, Germany

Novartis Pharma Schweiz, Bern, Switzerland

References

Aideyan OA, Schmidt AJ, Trenckner SW, Hakim NS, Gruessner RWG, Walsh JW (1996) CT-guided percutaneous biopsy of pancreas transplants. Radiology 201:825–828

Alfidi RJ, Haaga J, Meaney TF, MacIntyre WJ, Gonzalez L, Tarar R, Zelch MG, Boller M, Cook SA, Jelden G (1975) Computed tomography of the thorax and abdomen; a preliminary report. Radiology 117:257–264

Austin JH, Cohen MB (1993) Value of having a cytopathologist present during percutaneous fine-needle aspiration biopsy of the lung: report of 55 cancer patients and metaanalysis of the literature. AJR Am J Roentgenol 160:175–177

Balen FG, Little A, Smith AC, Theis BA, Abrams KR, Houghton J, Hatfield AR, Christopher R, Russell G, Lees WR (1994) Biopsy of inoperable pancreatic tumors does not adversely influence patient survival time. Radiology 193:753–755

Balthazar EJ, Freeny PC, van Sonnenberg E (1994) Imaging and intervention in the acute pancreatitis. Radiology 193:297–306

Bankoff MS, Belkin BA (1989) Percutaneous fine needle aspiration biopsy using a modified coaxial technique. Cardiovasc Intervent Radiol 12:43–44

Becker C, Grossholz M, Mentha G, Roth A, Giostra E, Schneider PA, Terrier F (1997) Ablation of hepatocellular carcinoma by percutaneous ethanol injection: imaging findings. Cardiovasc Intervent Radiol 20:204–210

Bernardino ME (1984) Percutaneous biopsy. AJR Am J Roentgenol 142:41–45

Bernardino ME, Walther MM, Phillips VM, Graham SD Jr, Sewell CW, Gedgaudas-McClees K, Baumgartner BR,

Torres WE, Erwin BC (1985) CT-guided adrenal biopsy: accuracy, safely, and indications. AJR Am J Roentgenol 144:67–69

Bissonnette RT, Gibney RG, Berry BR, Buckley AR (1990) Fatal carcinoid crisis after percutaneous fine-needle biopsy of hepatic metastasis: case report and literature review. Radiology 174:751–752

Blandamura S, Costantin G, Nitti D, Boccato P (1995) Intraoperative cytology of the pancreatic masses. A 10 year experience. Acta Cytol 39:23–27

Boland GW, Lee MJ, Leung J, Mueller PR (1994) Percutaneous cholecystostomy in critically ill patients: early reponse and final outcome in 82 patients. AJR Am J Roentgenol 163:339–342

Boland GW, Lee MJ, Mueller PR, Dawson SL, Gaa J, Lu DS, Gazelle GS (1994) Gallstones in critically ill patients with acute calculous cholecystitis treated by percutaneous cholecystostomy: nonsurgical therapeutic options. AJR Am J Roentgenol 162:1101–1103

Boland GW, Hahn PF, Pena C, Mueller PR (1997) Adrenal masses: characterization with delayed contrast-enhanced CT. Radiology 202:693–696

Brandt KR, Charoneau JW, Stephens DH, Welch TJ, Goellner JR (1993) CT- and US-guided biopsy of the pancreas. Radiology 187:99–104

Bree RL, McGough MF, Schwab RE (1991) CT- or US-guided fine needle aspiration biopsy in gastric neoplasms. J Comput Assist Tomogr 15:565–569

Bret PM, Fond A, Bretagnolle M, Valette PJ, Thiesse P, Lambert R, Labadie M (1988) Percutaneous aspiration and drainage of hydatid cysts in the liver. Radiology 168:617–620

Brown KT, Fulbright RK, Avitabile AM, Bashist B (1993) Cytologic analysis in the fine-needle aspiration biopsy: smears vs cell block. AJR Am J Roentgenol 161:629–631

Brown KT, Getrajdman GI, Botet JF (1995) Clinical trial of the Bard guide system. JVasc Interv Radiol 6:405–410

Burstein DM, Korbet SM, Schwartz MM (1993) The use of the automatic core biopsy system in percutaneous renal biopsies: a comparative study. Am J Kidney Dis 22:545–552

Butch RJ, Wittenberg J, Mueller PR, Simeone JF, Meyer JE, Ferrucci JT Jr (1985) Presacral masses after abdominoperineal resection for colorectal carcinoma: the need for needle biopsy. AJR Am J Roentgenol 144:309–312

Butch RJ, Mueller PR, Ferrucci JT Jr, Wittenberg J, Simeone JF, White EM, Brown AS (1986) Drainage of pelvic abscesses through the greater sciatic foramen. Radiology 158:487–491

Cafferty LL, Katz RL, Ordonez NG, Carraso CH, Cabanillas FR (1990) Fine needle aspiration diagnosis of intra-abdominal and retroperitoneal lymphomas by a morphologic and immunocytochemical approach. Cancer 65:72–77

Caraway NP, Fanning CV (1997) Use of fine-needle aspiration biopsy in the evaluation of the splenic lesions in a cancer center. Diagn Cytopathol 16:312–316

<referenCarson BW, Brown JA, Cooperberg PL (1998) Ultrasonographically guided percutaneous biopsy of gastric, small bowel, and colonic abnormalities: efficacy and safety. J Ultrasound Med 17:739–742

Casola G, van Sonnenberg E, Neff CC, Saba RM, Withers C, Emarine CW (1987) Abscesses in Crohn's disease: percutaneous drainage. Radiology 163:19–22

Cavanna L, Civardi G, Fornari F, Di Stasi M, Sbolli G, Buscarini E, Vallisa D, Rossi S, Tansini P, Buscarini L (1992) Ultrasonically guided percutaneous splenic tissue core biopsy in patients with malignant lymphomas, Cancer 69:2932–2936

Chan KK, D'Agostino HB, Carillo AF, O'Laoide R, Vasconcellos-vieira M (1996) Drainage catheters: in vitro comparison of internal retention mechanisms. Radiology 199:579–581

Chesney DS, Brouhard BH, Cunningham RJ (1996) Safety and cost effectiveness of pediatric percutaneous renal biopsy. Pediatr Nephrol 10:493–495

Ch Yu S, Metreweli C, Lau WY, Leung WT, Liew CT, Leung NW (1997) Safety of percutaneous biopsy of hepatocellular carcinoma with 18 gauge automated needle. Clin Radiol 52:907–911

Cozens NJ, Murchison JT, Allan PL, Winney RJ (1992) Conventional 15 G needle technique for the renal biopsy compared with ultrasound-guided spring-loaded 18 G needle biopsy. Br J Radiol 65:594–597

D'Agostino HB, van Sonneberg E, Sanchez RB, Goodacre BW, Villaveiran RG, Lyche K (1993) Treatment of pancreatic pseudocysts with percutaneous drainage and octroide. Work in progress. Radiology 187:685–688

Dahnert WF, Hoagland MH, Hamper UM, Erozan YS, Peirce JC (1992) Fine-needle aspiration biopsy of abdominal lesions: diagnostic yield for different needle tip configurations. Radiology 185:263–268

DelMaschio A, Vanzulli A, Sironi S, Castrucci M, Mellone R, Staudacher C, Carlucci M, Zerbi A, Parolini D, Faravelli A, et al (1991) Pancreatic cancer versus chronic pancreatitis: diagnosis with CA 19-9 assessment, US, CT, and CT-guided fine-needle biopsy. Radiology 178:95–99

Deyoe LA, Cronan JJ, Lanbiase RE, Dorfman GS (1990) Percutaneous drainage of renal and perirenal abscesses: results in 30 patients. AJR Am J Roentgenol 155:81–83

Do H, Lambiase RE, Deyoe L, Cronan JJ, Dorfman GS (1991) Percutaneous drainage of hepatic abscesses: comparison of results in abscesses with and without intrahepatic biliary communication. AJR Am J Roentgenol 157:1209–1212

Dusenberg D, Ferris JV, Thaete FL, Carr BI (1995) Percutaneous ultrasound-guided needle biopsy of hepatic mass lesions using a cytohistologic approach. Comparison of two needle types. Am J Clin Pathol 104:583–587

Elvin A, Andersson T, Scheibenpflug L Lindgren PG (1990) Biopsy of the pancreas with a biopsy gun. Radiology 176:677–679

Fagelman D, Chess Q (1990) Nonaspiration fine-needle cytology of the liver. A new technique for obtaining diagnostic samples. AJR Am J Roentgenol 155:1217–1219

Ferruci JT Jr, Wittenberg J (1978) CT Biopsy of abdominal tumors: aids for lesion localization. Radiology 129:739–744

Fisher AJ, Paulson EK, Sheafor DH, Simmons CM, Nelson RC (1997) Small lymphnodes of the abdomen, pelvic and retroperitoneum: usefulness of sonographically guided biopsy. Radiology 205:185–190

Fisher RI, Miller TP, Grogan TM (1998) New REAL clinical entities. Cancer J Sci Am 4 [Suppl 2]:5–12

Frederick PR, Brow TH, Miller MH, Bahr AL, Taylor KH (1985) A light-guidance system to be used for CT-guided biopsy. Radiology 154:535–536

Frederick PR, Miller MH, Bahr AL, Longson FW (1989) Coaxial needles for repeated biopsy sampling. Radiology 170:273–274

Freeny PC, Lewis GP, Traverso LW, Ryan JA (1988) Infected pancreatic fluid collections: percutaneous catheter drainage. Radiology 167:435–441

Freeny PC, Hauptmann E, Althaus SJ, Traverso LW, Sinanan M (1998) Percutaneous CT-guided catheter drainage of infected acute necrotizing pancreatitis: techniques and results. AJR Am J Roentgenol 170:969–975

Garber SJ, Mathieson JR, Cooperberg PL, MacFarlane JK (1994) Percutaneous cholecystostomy: safety of the transperitoneal route. J Vasc Interv Radiol 5:295–298

Gazelle GS, Haaga JR (1989) Guided percutaneous biopsy of intraabdominal lesions. AJR Am J Roentgenol 153:929–935

Gazelle GS, Haaga JR, Stellato TA, Gaudere MW, Plecha DT (1991) Pelvic abscesses: CT-guided transrectal drainage Radiology 181:49–51

Gazelle GS, Haaga JR, Rowland DY (1992) Effect of needle gauge, level of anticoagulation, and target organ bleeding associated with aspiration biopsy. Work in progress. Radiology 183:509–513

Gervais DA, Gazelle GS, Lu DSK, Hahn PF, Mueller PR (1996) Percutaneous transpulmonary CT-guided liver biopsy: a safe and technically easy approach for the lesions located near the diaphragm. AJR Am J Roentgenol 167:482–483

Gimenez A, Martinez-Noguera A, Donoso L, Catala E, Serra R (1993) Percutaneous neurolysis of the celiac plexus via the anterior approach with sonographic guidance. AJR Am J Roentgenol 161:1061–1063

Giorgio A, Tarantino L, Mariniello N, Francica G, Scala E, Amoroso P, Nuzzo A, Rizzatto G (1995) Pyogenic liver abscesses: 13 years of experience in percutaneous needle aspiration with US guidance. Radiology 195:122–124

Giorgio A, Tarantino L, Mariniello N, de Stefano G. Perrota A, Aloisio V, Voza A, Finizia L, Alaia A, Del Viscovo L (1998) Percutaneous ethanol injection under general anesthesia for hepatocellular carcinoma: 3-year survival in 112 patients. Eur J Ultrasound 8:201–206

Graham RA, Bankoff M, Hediger R, Shaker HZ, Reinhold RB (1994) Fine-needle aspiration biopsy of pancreatic ductal adenocarcinoma: loss of accuracy with small tumors. J Surg Oncol 55:92–94

Gurley MB, Richli WR, Waugh KA (1998) Outpatient management of pneumothorax after fine-needle aspiration; economic advantages for the hospital and the patient. Radiology 209:717–722

Ha HK, Sachs PB, Haaga JR, Abdul-Karim F (1991) CT-guided liver biopsy: an update. Clin Imaging 15:99–104

Haaga JR, Vanek J (1979) Computed tomographic guided liver biopsy using the Meninghini needle. Radiology 133:405–408

Hahn PF, Eisenberg PJ, Pitman MB, Gazella GS, Mueller PR (1995) Cytopathologic touch preparations (imprints) from core needle biopsies: accuracy compared with that of the fine-needle aspirates; AJR Am J Roentgenol 165:1277–1279

Hall-Craggs MA, Lees WR (1986) Fine-needle aspiration biopsy: pancreatic and biliary tumors. AJR Am J Roentgenol 147:399–403

Harter LP, Moss AA, Goldberg HI, Gross BH (1983) CT-guided fine-needle aspirations for diagnosis of benign and malignant disease. AJR Am J Roentgenol 140:363–367

Heilo A, Stenwig AE (1997) Liver hemangioma: US guided 18-gauge core-needle biopsy. Radiology 204:719–722

Hopper KD (1995) Percutaneous, radiographically guided biopsy: a history. Radiology 196:329–333

Hopper KD, Abendroth CS, Sturtz KW, Matthews YL, Shirk SJ (1992) Fine-needle aspiration biopsy for cytopathologic analysis: utility of syringe, automated guns, and the nonsuction method. Radiology 185:819–824

Hopper KD, Abendroth CS, Sturtz KW, Matthews YL, Shirk SJ, Stevens LA (1993a) Blinded comparison of biopsy needles and automated devices in vitro. 1. Biopsy of diffuse hepatic disease. AJR Am J Roentgenol 161:1293–1297

Hopper KD, Abendroth CS, Sturtz KW, Matthews YL, Shirk SJ, Stevens LA (1993b) Blinded comparison of biopsy needles and automated devices in vitro. 2. Biopsy of medical renal disease. AJR Am J Roentgenol 161:1299–1301

Hopper KD, Abendroth CS, Sturtz KW, Matthews YL, Hartzel JS, Potok PS (1995a) CT percutaneous biopsy guns: comparison of end-cut and side-notch devices in cadaveric specimens. AJR Am J Roentgenol 164:195–199

Hopper KD, Abendroth CS, TenHave TR, Hartzel J, Savage CA (1995b) Multiple fine-needle biopsies using a coaxial technique: efficacy and a comparison of three methods. Cardiovasc Intervent Radiol 18:307–311

Hopper KD, Grenko RT, TenHave TR, Hartzel J, Sturtz KW, Savage CA (1995c) Percutaneous biopsy of the liver and kidney by using coaxial technique: adequacy of the specimen obtained with three different needles in vitro. AJR Am J Roentgenol 164:221–224

Hopper KD, Grenko RT, Fisher AI, TenHave TR (1996) Capillary versus aspiration biopsy: effect of needle size and length on the cytopathological specimen quality. Cardiovasc Intervent Radiol 19:341–344

Hueftle MG, Haaga JR (1986) Effect of suction on biopsy sample size. AJR Am J Roentgenol 147:1014–1016

Hussain S (1996) Gantry angulation in CT-guided percutaneous adrenal biopsy. AJR Am J Roentgenol 166:537–539

Hussain S, Santos-Ocampo RS, Silverman SG, Seltzer SE (1994) Dual-angled CT-guided biopsy. Abdom Imaging 19:217–220

Iamura H, Kawasaki S, Bandai Y, Sanjo K, Idezuki Y (1993) Comparison between wedge and needle biopsies for the evaluating the degree of the cirrhosis. J Hepatol 17:215–219

Ishii H, Okada S, Okusaka T, Yoshimori M, Nakasuka H, Shimada K, Yamasaki S, Nakanishi Y, Sakamoto M (1998) Needle tract implantation of hepatocellular carcinoma after percutaneous ethanol injection. Cancer 82:1638–1642

Jacobi V, Thalhammer A, Kirchner J (1999) Value of a laser guidance system for CT interventions: a phantom study. Eur Radiol 9:137–140

Jamieson DH, Chait PG, Filler R (1997) Interventional drainage of appendiceal abscesses in children. AJR Am J Roentgenol 169:1619–1622

Jeffrey RB Jr (1988) Coaxial technique for CT-guided biopsy of deep retroperitoneal lymph nodes. Gastrointest Radiol 13:271–272

Jeffrey RB Jr, Tolentino CS, Federle MP, Laing FC (1987) Percutaneous drainage of periappendiceal abscesses: review of 20 patients. AJR Am J Roentgenol 149:59–62

Kane NM, Krobkin M, Francis IR, Quint LE, Cascade PN (1991) Percutaneous biopsy of left adrenal masses: prevalence of pancreatitis after anterior approach. AJR Am J Roentgenol 1157:777–780

Karampekios S, Hatjidakis AA, Drositis J, Gourtsoyiannis N (1998) Artificial paravertebral widening for percutaneous CT-guided adrenal biopsy. J Comput Assist Tomogr 22:308–310

Karlson BM, Forsman CA, Wilander E, Skogseid B, Lindgren PG, Jacobson G, Rastad J (1996) Efficiency of percutaneous core biopsy in pancreatic tumor diagnosis. Surgery 120:75–79

Khuroo MS, Zargar SA, Mahajan R (1991) Echinococcus granulosus cysts in the liver: management with percutaneous drainage. Radiology 180:141–145

Kinney TB, Lee MJ, Filomena CA, Krebs TL, Dawson SL, Smith PL, Raafat N, Mueller PR (1993) Fine-needle biopsy: prospective comparison of aspiration versus nonaspiration techniques in the abdomen. Radiology 186:549–552

Korobkin M, Brodeur FJ, Francis IR, Quint LE, Dunnick NR, Goodsitt M (1996a) Delayed enhanced CT for differentiation of benign from malignant adrenal masses. Radiology 200:737–742

Korobkin M, Brodeur FJ, Yutzy GG, Francis IR, Quint LE, Dunnick NR, Kazerooni EA (1996b) Differentiation of adrenal adenomas from nonadenomas using CT attenuation values. AJR Am J Roentgenol 166:531–536

Kreula J (1990) Effect of sampling technique on specimen size in fine needle aspiration biopsy. Invest Radiol 25:1294–1299

Kreula J, Virkkunen P, Bondestam S (1990) Effect of suction on specimen size in fine-needle aspiration biopsy. Invest Radiol 25:1175–1181

Lahorra JM, Haaga JR, Stellato T, Flanigan T, Graham R (1993) Safety of intracavitary urokinase with percutaneous abscess drainage. AJR Am J Roentgenol 160:171–174

Lambiase RE, Cronan JJ, Dorfman GS, Paolella LP, Haas RA (1988) Percutaneous drainage of abscesses in patients with Crohn disease AJR Am J Roentgenol 150:1043–1045

Lambiase RE, Deyoe L, Cronan JJ, Dorfman GS (1992) Percutaneous drainage of 335 consecutive abscesses: results of primary drainage with 1-year follow-up. Radiology 184:167–179

Langen HJ, Jochims M, Günther RW (1995) Artificial displacement of kidneys, spleen, and colon by injection of physiologic saline and CO_2 as an aid to percutaneous procedures: experimental results. J Vasc Interv Radiol 6:411–416

Lee MJ, Mueller PR, van Sonnenberg E, Dawson SL, D'Agostino H, Saini S, Cats AM (1993) CT-guided celiac ganglion block with alcohol. AJR Am J Roentgenol 161:633–636

<reference>Lencioni R, Paolicchi A, Moretti M, Pinto F, Armillotta N, Di Giulio M, Cicorelli A, Donati F, Cioni D, Bartolozzi C (1998) Combined transcatheter arterial chemoembolization and percutaneous ethanol injection for the treatment of large hepatocellular carcinoma: local therapeutic effect and long term survival rate. Eur Radiol 8:439–444

Leong AS, Stevens M (1996) Fine-needle aspiration biopsy for the diagnosis of lymphoma: a perspective. Diagn Cytopathol 15:352–357

Lerma E. Musulen E, Cuatrecasas M, Martinez A, Montserrat E, Prat J (1996) Fine needle aspiration cytology in pancreatic pathology. Acta Cytol 40:683–686

Lindgren PG, Hagberg H, Eriksson B, Glimelius B, Magnusson A, Sundstrom C (1985) Excision biopsy of the spleen by ultrasonic guidance. Br J Radiol 58:853–857

Lishner M, Lang R, Hamlet Y, Halph E, Steiner Z, Radnay J, Ravid M (1996) Fine needle aspiration biopsy in patients with diffusely enlarged spleens. Acta Cytol 40:196–198

Little AF, Ferris JV, Dodd GD III, Baron RL (1996) Image-guided percutaneous hepatic biopsy: effect of ascites on the complication rate. Radiology 199:79–83

Ljung BM, Geller DA (1998) Fine-needle aspiration techniques for biopsy of deep-seated impalpable targets: a primer for radiologists. AJR Am J Roentgenol 171:325–328

Longo JM, Bilbao JI, deVilla VH, Iglesias A, Pueyo J, Lecumberri FJ, Cienfuegos JA (1993) CT-guided paracoccygeal drainage of pelvic abscesses. J Comput Assist Tomogr 17:909–914

Macari M, Rofsky NM, Naidich DP, Megibow AJ (1998) Non-small cell lung carcinoma: usefulness of unenhanced helical CT of the adrenal glands in an unmonitored environment. Radiology 209:807–812

Mahoney MC, Racadio JM, Merhar GL, First MR (1993) Safety and efficacy of kidney transplant biopsy: Tru-Cut needle vs sonographically guided Biopty gun. AJR Am J Roentgenol 160:325–326

Malden ES, Picus D, Dunagan WC (1995) Anaerobic culture yield in interventional radiologic drainage procedures. J Vasc Interv Radiol 6:933–937

Martino CR, Haaga JR, Bryan PJ, LiPuma JP, El Yousef SJ, Alfidi RJ (1984) CT-guided liver biopsies: eight years' experience. Work in progress. Radiology 152:755–757

McNicholas MM, Mueller PR, Lee MJ, Echeverri J, Gazelle GS, Boland GW, Dawson SL (1995) Percutaneous drainage of subphrenic fluid collections that occur after splenectomy: efficacy and safety of transpleural versus extrapleural approach. 165:355–359

Miaux Y, Guermazi A, Gossot D, Bourrier P, Angoulvant D, Khairoune A, Turki C, Bouche E (1995) Laser guidance system for CT-guided procedures. Radiology 194:282–284

Middleton WD, Hiskes SK, Teefey SA, Boucher LD (1997) Small (1.5 cm or less) liver metastases: US-guided biopsy. Radiology 205:729–732

Miyake H, Takaki H, Matsumoto S, Yoshida S, Maeda T, Mori H (1995) Adrenal nonhyperfunctioning adenoma and nonadenoma: CT attenuation value as discriminative index. Abdom Imaging 20:559–562

Mody MK, Kazerooni EA, Korobkin M (1995) Percutaneous CT-guided biopsy of adrenal masses: immediate and delayed complications. J Comput Assist Tomogr 19:434–439

Mostbeck GH, Wittich GR, Derfler K, Ulrich W, Walter RM, Herold C, Haller J, Tscholakoff D (1989) Optimal needle size for renal biopsy: in vitro and in vivo evaluation. Radiology 173:819–822

Moulton JS, Moore PT (1993) Coaxial percutaneous biopsy technique with automated biopsy devices: value in improving accuracy and negative predictive value. Radiology 186:515–522

Mueller PR, Wittenberg J, Ferrucci JT Jr (1981) Fine-needle aspiration biopsy of abdominal masses. Semin Roentgenol 16:52–62

Mueller PR, Dawson SL, Ferrucci JT Jr, Nardi GL (1985) Hepatic echinococcal cyst: successful percutaneous drainage. Radiology 155: 627–628

Mueller PR, Simeone JF, Butch RJ, Saini S, Stafford SA, Vici LG, Soto-Rivera C, Ferrucci JT Jr (1986) Percutaneous drainage of subphrenic abscess: a review of 62 patients. AJR Am J Roentgenol 147:1237–1240

Mueller PR, Saini S, Wittenberg J, Simeone J, Hahn PF, Steiner E, Dawson SL, Butch RJ, Stark DD, Ottinger LW, et al (1987) Sigmoid diverticular abscesses: percutaneous drainage as an adjunct to surgical resection in 24 cases. Radiology 164:321–325

Mueller PR, Miketic LM, Simeone JF, Silverman SG, Saini S, Wittenberg J, Hahn PF, Steiner E, Forman BH (1988) Severe acute pancreatitis after percutaneous biopsy of the pancreas. AJR Am J Roentgenol 151:493–494

Murphy FB, Barefield KP, Steinberg HV, Bernardino ME (1988) CT- or sonography-guided biopsy of the liver in the presence of ascites: frequency of complications. AJR Am J Roentgenol 151:485–486

National Cancer Institute (sponsor) (1982) Study of classifications of non-Hodgkin's lymphoma: summary and description of a working formulation for clinical usage. The non-Hodgkin's lymphoma pathologic classification project. Cancer 49:2112–2135

Neff CC, vanSonnenberg E, Casola G, Wittich GR, Hoyt DB, Halasz NA, Martini DJ (1987) Diverticular abscesses: percutaneous drainage. Radiology 163:15–18

Nyman RS, Cappelen-Smith J, al Suhaibani H, Alfurayh O, Shakweer W, Akhtar M (1997) Yield and complications in percutaneous renal biopsy. A comparison between ultrasound-guided gun-biopsy and manual techniques in native and transplant kidneys. Acta Radiol 38:431–436

Oyen RH, Van Poppel HP, Ameye FE, Van de Voorde WA, Baert AL, Baert LV (1994) Lymph node staging of localized prostatic carcinoma with CT and CT-guided fine-needle aspiration biopsy: prospective study of 285 patients. Radiology 190:315–322

Palma LD (1998) Diagnostic imaging and interventional therapy of hepatocellular carcinoma. Br J Radiol 71:808–818

Park JK, Kraus FC, Haaga JR (1993) Fluid flow during percutaneous drainage procedures: an in vitro study of the effects of fluid viscosity, catheter size and adjunctive urokinase. AJR Am J Roentgenol 160:165–169

Pereles FS, Baker M, Baldwin R, Krupinski E, Unger EC (1998) Accuracy of CT biopsy: laser guidance versus conventional freehand techniques. Acad Radiol 5:766–770

Plecha DM, Goodwin DW, Rowland DY, Varnes ME, Haaga JR (1997) Liver biopsy: effects of needle caliber on bleeding and tissue recovery. Radiology 204:101–104

Quinn SF, Sheley RC, Nelson HA, Demlow TA, Wienstein RE, Dunkley BL (1995) The role of percutaneous needle biopsies in the original diagnosis of lymphoma: a prospective evaluation. J Vasc Interv Radiol 6:947–952

Rajak CL, Gupta S, Jain S, Chawla Y, Gulati M, Suri S (1998) Percutaneous treatment of liver abscesses: needle aspiration versus catheter drainage. AJR Am J Roentgenol 170:1035–1039

Ralls PW, Barnes PF, Johnson MB, De Cock KM, Radin DR, Halls J (1987) Medical treatment of hepatic amebic abscess: are rare need for percutaneous drainage. Radiology 165:805–807

Rimm DL, Stastny JF, Rimm EB, Ayer S, Frable WJ (1997) Comparison of the cost of the fine-needle aspiration and open surgical biopsy as methods for obtaining a pathologic diagnosis. Cancer 81:51–56

Romanelli DF, Beckmann CF, Heiss FW (1993) Celiac plexus block: efficacy and safety of the anterior approach. AJR Am J Roentgenol 160:497–500

Ryan JM, Murphy BL, Boland GW, Mueller PR (1998) Use of the transgluteal route for percutaneous abscess drainage in acute diverticulitis to facilitate delayed surgical repair. AJR Am J Roentgenol 170:1189–1193

Safrit HD, Mauro MA, Jacques PF (1987) Percutaneous abscess drainage in Crohn's disease. AJR Am J Roentgenol 148:859–862

Savage CA, Hopper KD, Abendroth CS, Hartzel JS, TenHave TR (1995) Fine-needle aspiration biopsy versus fine-needle capillary (nonaspiration) biopsy: in vivo comparison. Radiology 195:815–819

Sawhney R, D'Agostino HB, Zinck S, Rose SC, Kinney TB, Oglevie SB, Stapakis JC, Fishbach TJ (1996) Treatment of postoperative lymphoceles with percutaneous drainage and alcohol sclerotherapy. J Vasc Interv Radiol 7:241–245

Sheafor DH, Paulson EK, Simmons CM, DeLong DM, Nelson RC (1998) Abdominal percutaneous interventional procedures: comparison of CT and US guidance. Radiology 207:705–710

Sheets PW, Brumbaugh CJ, Kopecky KK, Pound DC, Filo RS (1991) Safety and efficacy of a spring-propelled 18-gauge needle for US-guided liver biopsy. J Vasc Interv Radiol 2:147–149

Sheiman RG, Fey C. McNicholas M, Raptopoulos V (1998) Possible causes of inconclusive results on CT-guided thoracic and abdominal core biopsies. AJR Am J Roentgenol 170:1603–1607

Silverman JF, Geisinger KR, Raab SS, Stanley MW (1993) Fine needle aspiration biopsy of the spleen in the evaluation of neoplastic disorders. Acta Cytol 37:158–162

Silverman SG, Bloom DA, Seltzer SE, Tempany CM, Adamus DF (1992) Needle-tip localization during CT-guided abdominal biopsy: comparison of conventional and spiral CT. AJR Am J Roentgenol 159:1095–1097

Silverman SG, Mueller PR, Pinkney LP, Koenker RM, Seltzer SE (1993) Predictive value of image-guided adrenal biopsy: analysis of results of 101 biopsies. Radiology 187:715–718

Silverman SG, Lee BY, Mueller PR, Cibas ES, Seltzer SE (1994) Impact of positive findings at image-guided biopsy of lymphoma on the patient care: evaluation of clinical history, needle size, and pathologic findings on biopsy performance. Radiology 190:759–764

Silverman SG, Deuson TE, Kane N, Adams DF, Seltzer SE, Phillips MD, Khorasani R, Zinner MJ, Holman BL (1998) Percutaneous abdominal biopsy: cost-identification analysis. Radiology 206:429–435

Smith EH (1991) Complication of percutaneous abdominal fine-needle biopsy. Radiology 178:253–258

Smith TP, Mcdermott VG, Ayoub DM, Suhocki PV, Stackhouse DJ (1996) Percutaneous transhepatic liver biopsy with tract embolization. Radiology 198:769–774

Sneige N, Dekmezian RH, Katz RL, Fanning TV, Lukeman JL, Ordonez NF, Cabanillas FF (1990) Morphologic and immunocytochemical evaluation of 220 fine-needle aspirates of malignant lymphoma and lymphoid hyperplasia. Acta Cytol 34:311–322

Solbiati L, Livraghi T, De Pra L, Ierace T, Masciadri N, Ravetto C (1985) Fine-needle biopsy of hemangioma with sonographic guidance AJR Am J Roentgenol 144:471–474

Somers JM, Lomas DJ, Hacking JC, Coleman N, Broadbent VA, Dixon AK (1993) Radiologically-guided cutting needle biopsy for suspected malignancy in childhood. Clin Radiol 48:236–240

Stewart CJ, Duncan JA, Farquharson M, Richmond J (1998) Fine needle aspiration cytology diagnosis of malignant lymphoma and reactive lymphoid hyperplasia. J Clin Pathol 51:197–203

Taavitsainen M, Airaksinen T, Kreula J, Paivansalo M (1990) Fine-needle aspiration biopsy of liver hemangioma. Acta Radiol 31:69–71

Tanaka K, Okazaki H, Nakamura S, Endo O, Inoue S, Takamura Y, Sugiyama M, Ohaki Y (1991) Hepatocellular carcinoma: treatment with combination therapy of transcatheter arterial embolization and percutaneous ethanol injection. Radiology 179:713–717

Tikkakoski T, Paivansalo M, Siniluoto T, Hiltunen S, Typpo T, Jartti P, Apaja-Sarkkinen M (1993) Percutaneous ultrasound-guided biopsy. Fine needle biopsy, cutting biopsy, or both? Acta Radiol 34:30–34

Tikkakoski T, Makela JT, Leinonen S, Paivansalo M, Merikanto J, Karttunen A, Siniluoto T, Kairaluoma MI (1996) Treatment of symptomatic congenital hepatic cysts with single-session percutaneous drainage and ethanol sclerosis: technique and outcome. J Vasc Interv Radiol 7:235–239

Tsang P, Greenebaum E, Starr G, Brunetti J, Garfinkel R, Austin JH (1995) Image-directed percutaneous biopsy with large-core needles. Comparison of cytologic and histologic findings. Acta Cytol 39:753–758

Tung KT, Downes MO, O'Donnell PJ (1992) Renal biopsy in diffuse renal disease – experience with 14-gauge automated biopsy gun. Clin Radiol 46:111–113

Van Overhagen H, Meyers H, Tilanus HW, Jeekel J, Lameris JS (1996) Percutaneous cholecystostomy for patients with acute cholecystitis and an increased surgical risk. Cardiovasc Intervent Radiol 19:72–76

van Sonnenberg E, Wittenberg J, Ferrucci JT, Mueller PR, Simeone JF (1981) Triangulation method for percutaneous needle guidance: the angled approach to upper abdominal masses. AJR Am J Roentgenol 137:757–761

van Sonnenberg E, Mueller PR, Ferrucci JT Jr (1984) Percutaneous drainage of 250 abdominal abscesses and fluid collections. I. Results, failures, and complications. Radiology 151:337–341

van Sonnenberg E, Mueller PR, Schiffmann HR, Ferrucci JT Jr, Casola G, Simeone JF, Cabrera OA, Gosink BB (1985) Intrahepatic amebic abscesses: indications for and results of percutaneous catheter drainage. Radiology 156:631–635

van Sonnenberg E, Wittich GR, Casola G, Neff CC, Hoyt DB, Polansky AD, Keightley A (1987) Periappendiceal abscesses: percutaneous drainage. Radiology 163:23–26

van Sonnenberg E, Wittich GR, Casola G, Brannigan TC, Karnel F, Stabile BE, Varney RR, Christensen RR (1989) Percutaneous drainage of infected and noninfected pancreatic pseudocysts: experience in 101 cases. Radiology 170:757–761

van Sonnenberg E, D'Agostino HB, Casola G, Halasz NA, Sanchez RB, Goodacre BW (1991) Percutaneous abscess drainage: current concepts. Radiology 181:617–626

van Sonnenberg E, Wroblicka JT, D'Agostino HB, Mathieson JR, Casola G, O'laoide R, Cooperberg PL (1994) Symptomatic hepatic cysts: percutaneous drainage and sclerosis. Radiology 190:387–392

van Sonnenberg E, Wittich GH, Chon KS, D'Agostino HB, Casola G, Easter D, Morgan RG, Walser EM, Nealon WH, Goodrace B, Stabile BE (1997) Percutaneous radiologic drainage of pancreatic abscesses. AJR Am J Roentgenol 168: 979–984

Ward SC, Carey BM, Chalmers AG, Sutton J (1994) The role of immediate cytological evaluation in CT-guided biopsy. Clin Radiol 49:531–534

Welch TJ, Sheedy PF, Johnson CD, Johnson CM, Stephens DH (1989) CT-guided biopsy: prospective analysis of 1000 procedures. Radiology 171:493–496

Welch TJ, Sheedy PF II, Stephens DH, Johnson CM, Swensen SJ (1994) Percutaneous adrenal biopsy: review of a 10-year experience. Radiology 193:341–344

Wiersema MJ, Wiersema LM (1996) Endosonography-guided celiac plexus neurolysis. Gastrointest Endosc 44:656–662

Yamashita Y, Matsukawa T, Arakawa A, Hatanaka Y, Urata J, Takahashi M (1995) US-guided liver biopsy: predicting the effect of interventional treatment of hepatocellular carcinoma. Radiology 196:799–804

Yankaskas BC, Staab EV, Craven MB, Blatt PM, Sokhandan M, Carney CN (1986) Delayed complications from fine-needle biopsies of solid masses of the abdomen. Invest Radiol 21:325–328

Yankelevitz DF, Henschke CI, Davis SD (1993) Angulated needle placement in CT-guided percutaneous needle biopsy of the thorax. Clin Imaging 17:124–125

Yankelevitz DF, Davis SD, Henschke CI (1996) Aspiration of a large pneumothorax resulting from transthoracic needle biopsy. Radiology 200:695–697

Yu SC, Lau WY, Leung WT, Liew CT, Leung NW, Metreweli C (1998) Percutaneous biopsy of the small hepatic lesions using an 18 gauge automated needle. Br J Radiol 71:621–624

Yueh N, Halvorsen RA Jr, Letourneau JG, Crass JR (1989) Gantry tilt technique for CT-guided biopsy and drainage. J Comput Assist Tomogr 13:182–184

Zornoza J, Wallace S, Ordonez N, Lukeman J (1980) Fine-needle aspiration biopsy of the liver. AJR Am J Roentgenol 134:331–334

Zuckerman DA, Yeager TD (1997) Percutaneous ethanol sclerotherapy of postoperative lymphoceles. AJR Am J Roentgenol 169:433–437

46 New Contrast Media for Liver CT

A. Spinazzi, X. Fouillet

CONTENTS

46.1   Introduction *521*
46.2   Liver-specific Agents *522*
46.2.1 RES Cell Imaging Agents *522*
46.2.2 Hepatocyte-directed Contrast Agents *523*
46.2.3 Limitations of Purely Liver-specific Agents *524*
46.2.4 Dual Extracellular-fluid- and
        Liver-specific Agents *524*
46.2.5 Blood Pool Radiopaque Agents *526*
46.3   Conclusions *527*
        References *527*

46.1
Introduction

The detection of focal liver lesions is the most important challenge in liver imaging: its success or failure can have major clinical consequences, especially in patients with liver cancer. However, the liver is a soft tissue radiodensity organ, and tumors within it, especially subcentimeter nodules, can have a similar radiodensity to normal tissue, which may lead to their presence going undetected on computed tomographic (CT) images (Baron 1994; Small et al. 1994).

To increase the inherent contrast differences between the liver and the lesion in CT imaging, exogenous pharmaceutical compounds are often needed. To be effective, these compounds must increase the differences in density between lesion and liver by reaching predominantly the normal liver or predominantly the focal liver lesion, but not both (Baron 1994).

The most widely available agents today, such as iopamidol or iohexol, are targeted to the extracellular fluid space (Bourin et al. 1994). They distribute freely and rapidly into the interstitial compartment and go both to the lesion and to the normal liver parenchyma in approximately equal degrees. To be effective, imaging of the liver with these compounds must be based on the vascular phase of their kinetics and on exploitation of differences in blood flow between the two tissues (Baron 1994). Since the imaging window is quite narrow, their use must be optimized in terms of iodine content and volume, rate of injection and length of delay between the start of contrast injection and that of image acquisition.

However, even with adequate techniques of contrast medium administration and despite recent advances in CT techniques, such as volumetric CT scanning in spiral or helical geometry, the sensitivity of CT for detection of small hepatic tumors is still unsatisfactory (Baron 1994; Heiken et al. 1989). This is of particular importance when we consider that aggressive surgical techniques, which have constituted significant therapeutic advances in the management of hepatocellular carcinoma (HCC) and liver metastases, and recent significant advances in nonsurgical tumor-reductive approaches have greatly increased the need for accurate detection and localization of tumor nodules. New contrast media, such as the purely liver-specific agents, the "dual" extracellular-fluid-specific and liver-specific agents, and the intravascular agents, may meet this need, especially coupled with the recent technical developments in CT imaging, such as faster scan times, higher resolution and multiple detector technology.

Strategies for developing liver-specific contrast media to improve rates of liver lesion detection have focused on targeting either the reticuloendothelial system (RES) or the hepatocytes. Particulate contrast media that are cleared from the circulation by the liver-resident macrophages (i.e., Kupffer cells) provide an attractive approach for detecting liver cancer. Since it is uncommon for liver malignancies to exhibit Kupffer cell activity, tumors would not be expected to enhance following the administration of RES-cell-targeted contrast agents, and would therefore appear as areas of decreased density. The hepa-

A. Spinazzi, MD; Division of Medical and Regulatory Affairs, Bracco S.p.A., Via Egidio Folli, 50, I-20134 Milan, Italy
X. Fouillet, PhD; Safety Assessment, Bracco Research SA, 31, route de la Galaise, CH-1228 Plan-les-Ouates, Geneva, Switzerland

tocyte-directed strategies, on the other hand, are based either on the hepatobiliary pathway or on a biochemical rationale, whereby naturally occurring compounds known to be stored or metabolized in the hepatocytes serve as carriers for the radiological moiety. Hepatocyte-directed contrast agents are expected to increase the contrast between liver parenchyma and tumor nodules, which are devoid of functioning hepatocytes.

Amongst the more interesting new compounds are the dual agents which, along with the liver-specific distribution and enhancement, can also be used as extracellular fluid agents for bolus dynamic CT imaging for both liver and extrahepatic abdominal organs.

Finally, another promising approach to contrast-enhanced CT of the abdomen involves looking to significantly prolong the vascular phase of contrast media kinetics by the use of contrast agents that are able to produce selective and prolonged opacification of the vascular compartment (the so-called intravascular or blood pool contrast agents). These agents are expected to permit the best assessment of lesion hemodynamics.

As yet none of the liver-specific, dual or blood-pool agents for CT imaging has reached the market. The aim of this paper is to give an overview of the major lines of research and development of new CT contrast agents.

46.2
Liver-specific Agents

46.2.1
RES Cell Imaging Agents

RES cells are located mainly in the liver (Kupffer cells), with additional phagocytic cells present in decreasing quantities in the spleen, bone marrow, and lungs. Several X-ray contrast agents targeted specifically to these cells are currently undergoing development. All these agents are radiopaque particles of 2 μm or less, which are able to traverse the pulmonary bed safely and to be available for phagocytosis. In the liver, the Kupffer cells rapidly clear these particulate agents from the blood. Increased liver lesion conspicuity is based on the absence of Kupffer cell activity in almost all space-occupying lesions, the only exception being the benign hepatocyte-derived solid lesions, such as focal nodular hyperplasia and adenoma.

RES cell imaging agents that have undergone clinical investigations in patients include emulsions of iodinated esters of poppyseed oil (EOE-13) and perfluoroctylbromide.

Following intravascular infusion, colloidal EOE-13 emulsion clears rapidly from the blood and accumulates in RES cells (VERMESS 1984). Problems related to product sterilization, deiodination following intravascular administration with liberation of free iodine, and a relatively high incidence (3.6%) of serious adverse reactions, including fever and shaking chills at 2–4 h after infusion have, however, precluded further development of this agent (MILLER et al. 1984; VERMESS 1984).

Emulsions of radiopaque perfluorocarbons have been used in animal models for angiography, in which they have been shown to increase X-ray attenuation in a variety of organs (LONG et al. 1980). More recent clinical studies have shown that perfluoroctylbromide, also used as an ultrasound contrast agent, is able to increase the X-ray attenuation of liver and spleen. Unfortunately, it also produces severe side effects, which significantly limits its use for CT imaging (BEHAN et al. 1993; BRUNETON et al. 1989).

A number of other research attempts have been reported, but the contrast agents involved have never reached the stage of clinical testing. They range from micro-barium sulfate particles (ISHIKAWA and MUNECHIKA 1987), nanoparticles of ethyl ester derivatives of diatrizoic, iothalamic or iodipamic acid (VIOLANTE et al 1980a, b; LEE et al. 1995) and iodinated starch particles (COHEN et al. 1981), to the more sophisticated micelles of block copolymers of polyethylene glycol and polylysine as carriers of inorganic iodine (TRUBETSKOY et al. 1997) and biodegradable particles based on a prodrug ester design of metrizoic acid (LEANDER et al. 1993) or the biodegradable ioxilan-carbonate particles (LI et al. 1994, 1996a, b).

Kupffer cell imaging agents based on liposome-encapsulated X-ray contrast agents certainly provide a more attractive approach. The liposomes used for intravenous administration of contrast media are small spherical unilamellar vesicles with an average diameter in the range of 0.2–2 μm. These small vesicles have a membrane which, similarly to normal cell membranes, is constituted of a bilayer of phospholipids associated with cholesterol. The water-soluble contrast agent is entrapped within the vesicle, while the external milieu is composed either of a buffer or of a solution of the same iodinated contrast agent as present inside the vesicle.

523

The idea of targeting water-soluble iodinated contrast agents to the liver and the spleen using liposomes was proposed at the beginning of the 1980s (McKaness and Hou 1980; Havron et al. 1981; Rozenberg et al. 1983, Ryan et al. 1984; Zherbin et al. 1982, 1983; Jendrasiak et al. 1985; Aliiakparov et al. 1981; Khason et al. 1982; Henze et al. 1989), and techniques for preparing the contrast-carrying liposomes by micro-emulsion procedures were published in the mid-1980s (Cheng et al. 1987; Zalutsky et al. 1987; Seltzer et al. 1988; Seltzer 1988). Thereafter, all major pharmaceutical companies operating in the field of diagnostic imaging very rapidly began to prepare their own liposome formulations using their newest proprietary low-osmolar contrast agents. Iomeprol-carrying liposomes (Bracco), prepared by an extrusion procedure through polycarbonate membranes (Musu et al. 1988) and evaluated in a model of chemically induced liver tumors in rats, were shown to permit precise localization of very small hepatocellular carcinomas (Fouillet et al. 1995). Iotrolan-carrying vesicles (Schering) were prepared by the interdigitation-fusion procedure and were evaluated for biodistribution and imaging in rats and dogs (Seltzer et al. 1991). Iopromide liposomes (Schering) prepared by ethanol evaporation, lyophilization and resuspension have been found to provide contrast in the liver and spleen of rats and rabbits (Krause et al. 1991, 1993; Sachse et al. 1993) and, more recently, primates (Schmiedl et al. 1995). Ioxaglate-liposomes (Guerbet) (Revel et al. 1990) and iodixanol-liposomes (Nycomed) (Leander 1996) have been evaluated as hepatosplenic contrast agents in rabbits.

Thus far, however, only the iodixanol-liposomes have been tested in non-patient volunteers (Leander et al. 1998). Although the slow infusion of 70 mg and 100 mg encapsulated iodine/kg produced a marked and stable enhancement of hepatic and splenic tissues for approximately 3 h, the further development of this agent has been curtailed owing to a dose-dependent incidence in adverse events, particularly changes in leukocyte counts and increase in body temperature.

46.2.2
Hepatocyte-directed Contrast Agents

Another strategy for liver-specific delivery is based on the synthesis of known compounds that are taken up and metabolized or excreted by the hepatocytes and can be used as carriers for the radiopaque moiety to selectively enhance the normal liver parenchyma. Amphophils, for example, are bile acid mimics, which are taken up into the hepatocytes via specific transport pathways (Anelli et al. 1997). The hydrophobic modification of tri-iodinated organic media further favors the liver uptake by promoting plasma protein binding while concomitantly reducing renal excretion. As recently shown, the synthesis of hydrophobic and amphophilic diatrizoate derivatives leads to molecules with high liver distribution (Ranganathan et al. 1998). Further preclinical testing on these compounds is ongoing.

Lanthanide metal ions coupled with hepatocyte-directed ligands (BOPTA, EOB-DTPA) may also serve as liver-specific contrast media. Using dysprosium as the X-ray absorbing element and EOB-DTPA as the ligand, a net increase in CT liver attenuation of 20--30 HU has been demonstrated in animal models (Schumann-Giamperi et al. 1998). The enhancement in CT attenuation was stable for about 60 min and adequate for the detection of liver lesions as small as 5 mm in size in rabbits into which a VX2 tumor had been implanted 14 days before imaging.

Polyiodinated triglycerides (ITG, University of Wisconsin and Molecular Biosystems) have been assembled into the core of synthetic chylomicron remnants for specific targeting of normal hepatocytes via a receptor-mediated uptake pathway (Weichert et al. 1994). These micro-emulsions have been shown to enhance the detection of small hepatic tumors in both rats and rabbits (Weichert et al. 1994; Ivancev et al. 1989; Longino et al. 1996).

Other hepatocyte-specific contrast agents (FP 736--03 and FP 736--04, Pharmacia and Upjohn) are oil-in-water emulsions containing iodinated ethyl esters of linoleic acid and cholesterol, which amplifies the hepatocyte uptake (Bergman 1997; Bergman et al. 1997, 1998; Magnusson et al. 1998). FP 736--04 has been tested in healthy male volunteers. Following administration of the emulsion by slow (0.05 ml/kg per min) intravenous infusion, a dose-dependent increase in liver enhancement was observed, albeit with wide individual variations. At the highest dose (2 ml/kg), the increase in attenuation was shown to be greater than 20 HU for approximately 120 min. However, all patients dosed with the 2.0 ml/kg dose and five of six patients to whom the next lower dose (1.75 ml/kg) was administered suffered from adverse events (sore throat, headache, rhinitis, skin reactions).

46.2.3
Limitations of Purely Liver-specific Agents

The major problem that would significantly limit the clinical use of purely liver-specific agents is their lack of specificity in differentiating the nature of the space-occupying lesions demonstrated. Moreover, the blood clearance of the liver-specific agents results in the visualization of intrahepatic vascular structures as low-density areas in delayed CT studies. Therefore, a CT study with a liver-specific agent should always follow a dynamic CT investigation with an extracellular fluid agent.

The adverse side effects and the need to increase the exposure of patients to X-rays and contrast material, combined with the poor tolerance shown by the purely liver-specific agents in non-patient and patient volunteers has led to the further development of these agents being halted.

The goal is now to perform both dynamic imaging and liver-specific imaging with one agent. Since the contrast preparation would have to be injected as a rapid intravenous bolus ($\geq$2 ml/s), the liver-specific component would need to be very well tolerated and safe. The increase in CT attenuation should be at least comparable to that obtainable with purely extracellular fluid agents during the dynamic investigation, and the increase in liver-lesion contrast should be comparable to that obtainable with purely liver-specific agents on static, delayed, liver-specific imaging.

46.2.4
Dual Extracellular-fluid- and Liver-specific Agents

These agents are liposome formulations that contain the nonionic monomer iomeprol both free in solution and entrapped within liposomal vesicles. Thanks to the free iomeprol content (300 mg iodine/ml), the product is suitable for both conventional and spiral dynamic bolus contrast-enhanced CT imaging. It thus fulfills the full diagnostic potential of any iodinated extracellular-fluid agent currently available in the marketplace. Additionally, the iomeprol-containing liposomes are taken up by the RES cells, mostly by the Kupffer cells in the liver, where they remain for hours and increase CT attenuation (Fig. 46.1). The progressive washout of free iomeprol from malignancies, which are devoid of Kupffer cells, leads to a progressive decrease in the CT attenuation of lesions and to a progressive increase in liver-lesion contrast, thus improving lesion conspicuity on delayed images.

The first of these agents, BR21 (Bracco), a sterile, pyrogen-free suspension of iomeprol-containing liposomes in a solution of free iomeprol, has already been tested in non-patient male volunteers (SPINAZZI et al. 1998). In BR21, the liposomes are 0.4-μm unilamellar vesicles in which the membrane is made up of a phospholipid bilayer and in which both the internal phase and the external phase is iomeprol 320 (a solution of 650 mg iomeprol per ml containing 320 mg iodine). The total lipid (phospholipids plus cholesterol) concentration of the suspension is about 20 mg/ml. Approximately 40 mg I/ml is

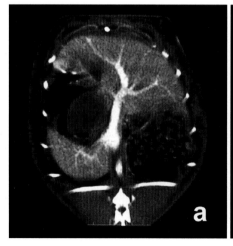 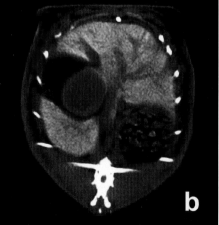

Fig. 46.1. CT in a rabbit **a** 30 s and **b** 30 min after injection of iomeprol-liposomes

entrapped within the liposomal vesicles, while 280 mg I/ml is present in the external phase.

A study in non-patient volunteers has been conducted to assess the tolerability, the safety and the pharmacokinetics of single ascending doses of BR21 (0.5 up to 2.5 ml/kg) and to compare them with placebo (0.9% physiological saline). Following rapid bolus injection (2 ml/s), maximum blood concentrations of iomeprol were measured at the first sampling time of 2 min after administration. Thereafter, blood concentrations declined rapidly in a triphasic manner, corresponding to a distribution phase, with mean half-life of 0.12–0.22 h, a fast-elimination phase, with mean half-life 1.2–1.5 h, and a slow-elimination phase, with mean half-life of 4.1–4.5 h. The entire pharmacokinetic data showed linear kinetics over the range of dose levels tested. Renal excretion of iomeprol from BR21 was rapid and was essentially complete 24 h after dosing.

The distribution and fast-elimination phases of iomeprol in BR21 make the compound suitable for dynamic CT studies. The slow-elimination phase describes the clearance from a deep compartment that might be the RES.

BR21 has been shown to be well tolerated and safe in the first clinical tests. Single intravenous bolus (2 ml/s) injections up to a dose level of 2.5 ml/kg did not cause any significant changes in vital signs, laboratory parameters and ECG parameters. All the observed adverse events were mild and rapidly self-resolving. The most frequent adverse event was a mild sensation of warmth, which was due to the slight hyperosmolality of the preparation (about 560 mosmol/kg). There was no difference in the incidence of adverse events between BR21 and matched volumes of physiologic saline.

The tolerability and the safety profile following the rapid bolus injection of this iomeprol-liposome preparation was then much more satisfactory than that reported previously for the infusion of the iodixanol-liposomes (LEANDER et al. 1998). This difference may be explained by the different liposomes used in the two preparations. The reduction of the potential side effects after injection of liposomes is a major challenge for pharmaceutical companies. The reaction of the RES cells, mainly the liver Kupffer cells and the splenic macrophages, which release into the bloodstream the eicosanoids and other cell mediators responsible for inducing hypotension, headache and fever, can be reduced by appropriate tuning of the physico-chemical characteristics of the liposomes, such as their average diameter, the phospholipids to cholesterol ratio and the chemical composition of the lipids.

Studies are currently under way to evaluate the contrast-enhancing ability of BR21 in patients with focal liver disease.

Two other dual enhancers (BR23 and BR24) have been tested in rabbits, rats and cynomolgus monkeys and compared with the pure extracellular fluid enhancer iomeprol-300 (300 mg I/ml). All agents were administered as rapid intravenous bolus injections. In an experiment in monkeys, spiral CT scans of the liver were performed before dosing and at 5 s, 2 min and 5 min after dosing, and then repeated at 10-min intervals up to 2 h after the dose (RUMMENY et al. 1999a). Peak enhancement of liver and spleen was highest after injection of BR23 (140±6 HU, and

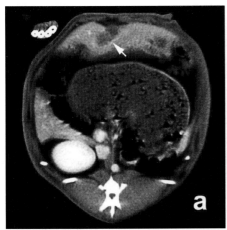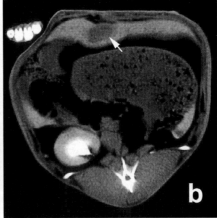

Fig. 46.2. CT in a rabbit following implantation of a VX2 tumor in a hepatic lobe. Note tumor (*arrow*) **a** 30 s and **b** 30 min after injection of BR23

143.5±5 HU, respectively). Compared with iomeprol-300, time ranges of sufficient (>50 HU) liver parenchyma radiodensity enhancement were significantly longer with both BR23 and BR24 (P<0.001). At 2 h after a dose, liver enhancement was still significantly more intense with both BR23 and BR24 (147 HU and 127 HU, respectively) than with iomeprol-300 (82 HU). Figure 46.2 illustrates the imaging capability of BR23 in a rabbit following earlier implantation of a VX2 carcinoma in the liver.

46.2.5
Blood Pool Radiopaque Agents

Contrast agents that specifically enhance and mark the blood pool would allow better and easier CT imaging of both the macrovasculature and the microvasculature by decreasing the diffusion and interstitial loss of contrast and by affording a longer temporal window for scanning.

Blood pool contrast media have to be either microparticulate or water-soluble polymers with a molecular weight that exceeds the renal excretion threshold. A diagnostically useful intravascular enhancer should selectively enhance the blood pool for at least 5 min, and must be inert and readily biodegradable to facilitate rapid elimination.

A number of blood pool markers have been synthesized and tested in animals, although none have yet been tested in humans. Ionic polymers of tri-iodinated moieties were explored, but were shown to be too viscous and toxic (SOVAK et al. 1994). Neither grafted polysaccharides nor peptides are suitable carriers, since they tend to be antigenic and the results of grafting are difficult to predict (SOVAK et al. 1994). Several polyacrylic iodine-containing copolymers have been synthesized and tested in animals, but have not shown adequate biological tolerance. Nanoparticles 200–400 nm in size have been made from the ethylester derivative of diatrizoic acid by milling in an aqueous solution containing a grinding medium and surfactants. In rabbits, these nanoparticles have been shown to produce superior enhancement of the blood pool, liver and spleen compared with the extracellular-fluid enhancer iohexol. Furthermore, the enhancement persisted for at least 30 min after injection (RUBIN et al. 1994). A surface-modified 10% chylomicron remnant-like lipid emulsion (ITG-PEG, University of Michigan and University of Wisconsin) has been developed and tested in animals (WEICHERT et al. 1998). ITG-PEG is similar to the purely hepatocyte-directed agent ITG, except

that polyethylene glycol (PEG)-modified phospholipids are embedded in the monolayer. It is speculated that by interfering in vivo with the apolipoprotein-E, a surface apoprotein necessary for receptor-site recognition in the liver, the PEG residues prevent liver sequestration of the remnant-like particle from the blood. A comparison of ITG and ITG-PEG in both normal and tumor-bearing rabbits has revealed that hepatic clearance from the blood is rapid with the standard ITG, and slower and less effective with ITG-PEG: by 60 min after injection 4.2% ITG and 56% ITG-PEG remained in the blood, with about 20 HU difference in blood pool density at the same time point.

Another approach is to make iodine-loaded liposomes that are not well recognized by the macrophages of the RES. Such liposomes take on "stealth" characteristics and are removed only very slowly from the circulation. A PEG-coated liposomal preparation of iopromide was developed as a potential blood-pool agent (SACHSE et al. 1997), the PEG coating giving the liposomes stealth characteristics. The suggested mechanism involves binding of the PEG-cholesterol part of the liposomes to the cell plasma membranes, thus inducing a decrease in surface hydrophobicity of the cell and consequently a marked decrease in the extent of phagocytic ingestion (VERTUT DOÏ et al. 1996).

Both the phospholipid composition and the size of the liposome play important parts in the circulation time and biodistribution, with the smallest particles tending to circulate longer than the larger ones (LITZINGER et al. 1994). Small stealth iomeprol-liposomes (BR22, Bracco) have recently been evaluated in monkeys and compared with iomeprol-300. Following rapid bolus injection, repeated thin spiral CT scans were performed before dosing and at 5 s, 2 min and 5 min after administration, and then repeated at 5-min intervals up to 20 min after administration (RUMMENY et al. 1999b). Images were analyzed quantitatively by measuring HU in the aorta, iliac artery and femoral artery. While no significant differences were seen between BR22 and iomeprol-300 in terms of peak enhancement in any of the vessels examined (aorta: 277±16 HU vs 273±15 HU, respectively), the time ranges for blood pool density enhancement over 60 HU were significantly longer with BR22 than with iopmepol-300 in all arteries. Radiodensity enhancement at 20 min in the femoral artery was 111±9 HU for BR22 and 66±8 HU for iomeprol-300. BR22 is finally taken up by the RES cells, permitting it to behave as a liver-specific agent on delayed acquisitions.

46.3
Conclusions

Though much has been achieved by pharmaceutical companies in terms of the development of safe and effective contrast media, there is still a reservoir of medical needs in several imaging areas that have not yet been met and which therefore represent a challenge for further advance. Surely one of the more challenging objectives for all companies involved in contrast media research and development is to improve the degree of accuracy in the detection and characterization of focal liver disease. This is particularly true for CT imaging, since CT is the "workhorse" for the investigation of any abdominal cancer, and of liver cancer in particular.

While a large number of new agents for CT of the liver have been synthesized and tested by many contrast medium drug discovery groups, only a few are still in development. The most promising agents are certainly the "dual" liver-specific and extracellular-fluid-specific agents and the blood pool markers. The dual agents may fulfill the full diagnostic potential of extracellular fluid agents while also improving the liver-lesion conspicuity afforded by purely liver-specific agents. The blood pool markers may further increase the potential of CT for the assessment of lesion hemodynamics, as well as prolonging the imaging window for the accurate detection of hypovascular lesions. Besides imaging of focal liver disease, blood pool agents might be useful for CT angiography procedures, venous imaging in particular, and vascular tagging.

Any decision to proceed with or stop a project is made on the basis of traditional minimal acceptable criteria, such as the demonstration of improved diagnostic accuracy or satisfactory safety, and after careful attention to acceptance and convenience on the part of the patient, the real utility in the daily clinical setting, and the cost-effectiveness of the contrast-enhanced procedure.

References

Aliiakparov MT, Rozenberg OA, Fomina EV, Loshakova LV, Gubareva AV (1981) Experimental hepatosplenography after the administration of liposomes with verografin (in Russian). Med Radiol (Mosk) 26:45–48

Anelli PL, Calabi L, de Haën C, Lattuada L, Lorusso V (1997) Hepatocyte-directed MRI agents: can we take advantage of bile acids? Acta Radiol 412: 125–133

Baron RL (1994) Understanding and optimizing use of contrast material for CT of the liver. AJR Am J Roentgenol 163:323–331

Behan M, O'Connell D, Mattrey RF, Carney DN (1993) Perfluorooctylbromide as a contrast agent for CT and sonography: preliminary clinical results. AJR Am J Roentgenol 160:399–405

Bergman A (1997) Hepatocyte-specific contrast media for CT. An experimental investigation. Acta Radiol Suppl 411:1–27

Bergman A, Sundin A, Magnusson A (1997) CT with different doses of the hepatocyte-specific contrast medium FP 736–03. Evaluation in a nude-rat model of experimental metastases. Acta Radiol 38:1003–1006

Bergman A, Magnusson A, Sundin A (1998) Detecting experimental liver metastases at CT with the hepatocyte-specific contrast medium FP 736–03. Acta Radiol 39:381–383

Bourin M, Jolliet P, Ballereau F (1997) An overview of the clinical pharmacokinetics of x-ray contrast media. Clin Pharmacokinet 32:180–193

Bruneton JN, Falewee MN, Francois E, Cambon P, Philip C, Riess JG, Balu-Maestro C, Rogopoulos A (1989) Liver, spleen and vessels: preliminary clinical results of CT with perfluorooctylbromide. Radiology 170:179–183

Cheng KT, Seltzer SE, Adams DF, Blau M (1987) The production and evaluation of contrast-carrying liposomes made with an automatic high-pressure system. Invest Radiol 22:47–55

Cohen Z, Seltzer SE, Davis MA, Hanson RN (1981) Iodinated starch particles: new contrast material for computed tomography of the liver. J Comput Assist Tomogr 5:843–846

Fouillet X, Tournier H, Khan H, Sabitha S, Burkhardt S, Terrier F, Schneider M (1995) Enhancement of computed tomography liver contrast using iomeprol-containing liposomes and detection of small liver tumors in rats. Acad Radiol 2:576–583

Havron A, Seltzer SE, Davis MA, Shulkin P (1981) Radiopaque liposomes: a promising new contrast material for computed tomography of the spleen. Radiology 140:507–511

Heiken JP, Weyman PJ, Lee JK, Balfe DM, Picus D, Brunt EM, Flye MW (1989) Detection of focal hepatic masses: prospective evaluation with CT, delayed CT, CT during arterial portography, and MR imaging. Radiology 171:47–51

Henze A, Freise J, Magerstedt P, Majewski A (1989) Radio-opaque liposomes for the improved visualisation of focal liver disease by computerized tomography. Comput Med Imaging Graphics 13:455–462

Ishikawa M, Munechika H (1987) Fundamental study of positive contrast media of hepatic CT by micro-barium sulphate particles. Nippon Igaku Hoshasen Gakkai Zasshi 47:1478–1488

Ivancev K, Lunderquist A, McCuskey R, McCuskey P, Wretlind A (1989) Experimental investigation of a new iodinated lipid emulsion for computed tomography of the liver. Acta Radiol 30:407–413

Jendrasiak GL, Frey GD, Heim RC Jr (1985) Liposomes as carriers of iodolipid radiocontrast agents for CT scanning of the liver. Invest Radiol 20:995–1002

Khanson KP, Rozenberg OA, Aliiakparov MT, Gubareva AV, Loshakova LV (1982) Use of liposome-bound x-ray contrast substances for the diagnosis of splenic lesions in generalized lymphoma in SJL/J mice. Vopr Onkol 28:35–39

Krause W, Leike J, Sachse A, Schuhmann-Giampieri G (1993)

Characterization of iopromide liposomes. Invest Radiol 28:1028–1032

Krause W, Sachse A, Wagner S, Kollenkirchen U, Rossling G (1991) Preclinical characterization of iopromide-carrying liposomes. Invest Radiol 26:S172-S174

Leander P (1996) A new liposomal contrast medium for CT of the liver. An imaging study in a rabbit tumour model. Acta Radiol 37:63–68

Leander P, Golman K, Strande P, Klaveness J, Besjakov J, Fält K (1993) A comparison between IEEC, a new biodegradable particulate contrast medium, and iohexol in a tumor model of computed tomography imaging of the liver. Invest Radiol 28:513–519

Leander P, Höglund P, Kloster Y, Børseth A (1998) New liposomal liver-specific contrast agent for CT. First human phase I clinical trial assessing efficacy and safety. Acad Radiol 5 [Suppl 1]:S6–8

Lee FT Jr, Sproat IA, Rappe AH, Kelcz F, Broghammer BG Jr, Chosy SG (1995) Lesion visualization by targeted computed tomography liver enhancement in dogs. Acad Radiol 2:484–491

Li C, Kan Z, Yang DJ, Kuang LR, Liu CW, Wright KC, Wallace S (1994) Preparation, characterization, and evaluation of ioxilan carbonate particles for computed tomography contrast enhancement of liver. Invest Radiol 29:1006–1013

Li C, McCuskey P, Yang DJ, Kan Z, Wallace S (1996a) Development of biodegradable ioxilan carbonate particles for contrast enhancement of the liver in computed tomography scanning: toxicity assessment. Acad Radiol 3 [Suppl 2]:S227–8

Li C, Yu D, Kan Z, Yang DJ, Tansey W, Kuang LR, Wallace S (1996b) Biodistribution of cyclic carbonate of ioxilan: a radiopaque particulate macrophage imaging agent. Acad Radiol 3:500–506

Litzinger DC, Buiting AM, van Rooijen N, Huang L (1994) Effect of liposome size on the circulation time and intraorgan distribution of amphipathic poly(ethylene glycol)-containing liposomes. Biochim Biophys Acta 1190:99–107

Long DM Jr, Lasser EC, Sharts CM, Multer FK, Nielsen M (1980) Experiments with radiopaque perfluorocarbon emulsions for selective opacification of organs and total body angiography. Invest Radiol 15:242–247

Longino MA, Bakan DA, Weichert JP, Counsell RE (1996) Formulation of polyiodinated triglyceride analogues in a chylomicron remnant-like liver-selective delivery vehicle. Pharm Res 13:875–879

Mackaness GB, Hou JP (1980) Contrast media containing liposomes as carriers. US Pat. 4,192,859

Magnusson A, Bergman A, Carneheim C, von Schèele L, Wessèn A (1998) Contrast enhancement of the liver in healthy male volunteers following intravenous administration of FP 736-04. Acad Radiol 5 [Suppl 1]:S9–12

Miller DL, Vermess M, Doppmann JL, Simon RM, Sugarbaker PH, O'Leary TJ, Grimes G, Chatterji DG, Willis M (1984) CT of the liver and spleen with EOE-13: review of 225 examinations. AJR Am J Roentgenol 143:235–243

Musu C, Felder E, Lamy B, Schneider M (1988) A liposomal contrast agent. Preliminary communication. Invest Radiol 23 [Suppl 1]:S126–129

Ranganathan RS, Arunachalam T, Song B, Mantha S, Ogan M, Wedeking F, Yost F, Jagoda E, Tweedle M (1998) Evaluation of N,N'-bis-dimethyldiatrizoic acid analogs as liver imaging agents. Acad Radiol 5 [Suppl 1]:S23-S27

Revel D, Corot C, Carrillon Y, Dandis G, Eloy R, Amiel M (1990) Ioxaglate-carrying liposomes. Computed tomographic study as hepatosplenic contrast agent in rabbits. Invest Radiol 25 [Suppl 1]:S95–97

Rozenberg OA, Hanson KP, Zherbin EA (1983) Re: Radiopaque liposomes for imaging of the spleen and liver [letter]. Radiology 149:877–878

Rubin DL, Desser TS, Qing F, Muller HH, Young SW, McIntire GL, Bacon E, Cooper E, Toner J (1994) Nanoparticulate contrast media: blood-pool and liver-spleen imaging. Invest Radiol 29:S280-S283

Rummeny EJ, Berning W, Fuest M, Fouillet X, Tournier H (1999a) Evaluation of a new blood pool agent for CT-angiography. Eur Radiol 9 [Suppl 1]:S24

Rummeny EJ, Berning W, Fuest M, Fouillet X, Tournier H, Bick U (1999b) New RES-specific contrast agents for computed tomography. Eur Radiol 9 [Suppl 1]:S269

Ryan PJ, Davis MA, DeGaeta LR, Woda B, Melchior DL (1984) Liposomes loaded with contrast material for image enhancement in computed tomography. Work in progress. Radiology 152:759–762

Sachse A, Leike JU, Rössling GL, Wagner SE, Krause W (1993) Preparation and evaluation of lyophilized iopromide-carrying liposomes for liver tumor detection. Invest Radiol 28:838–844

Sachse A, Leike JU, Schneider T, Wagner SE, Rössling GL, Krause W, Brandl M (1997) Biodistribution and computed tomography blood-pool imaging properties of polyethylene glycol-coated iopromide-carrying liposomes. Invest Radiol 32:44–50

Schmiedl UP, Krause W, Leike J, Nelson JA, Schuhmann-Giampieri G (1995) Liver contrast enhancement in primates using iopromide liposomes. Acad Radiol 2:967–972

Schumann-Giampieri G, Rupp K, Muschick P, Treher M, Krause W (1998) Dysprosium EOB DTPA: a new liver-specific contrast agent for computed tomography. Acad Radiol 5 [Suppl 1]:S90-S92

Seltzer SE (1988) Contrast-carrying liposomes. Current status. Invest Radiol 23 [Suppl 1]:S122–125

Seltzer SE, Gregoriadis G, Dick R (1988) Evaluation of the dehydration-rehydration method for production of contrast-carrying liposomes. Invest Radiol 23:131–138

Seltzer SE, Janoff AS, Blau M, Adams DF, Minchey SR, Boni LT (1991) Biodistribution and imaging characteristics of iotrolan-carrying interdigitation-fusion vesicles; Discussion. Invest Radiol [Suppl 1]:S169–171; S175–176

Small WC, Nelson RC, Bernardino ME, Brummer LT (1994) Contrast-enhanced spiral CT of the liver: effect of different amounts and injection rates of contrast material on early contrast enhancement [see comments]. AJR Am J Roentgenol 163:87–92

Sovak M, Douglass JG, Terry RC, Brown JW, Bakir F, Wasden TS (1994) Blood pool radiopaque polymers: design considerations. Invest Radiol 29:S271-S274

Spinazzi A, Ceriati S, Lorusso V, Pianezzola P, Zaccarini P, Fouillet X (1998) Safety and pharmacokinetics of BR21, a liver-specific CT agent, in healthy volunteers; Discussion. Acad Radiol [Suppl 1]:S20–22; S28–30

Trubetskoy VS, Gazelle GS, Wolf GL, Torchilin VP (1997) Block-copolymer of polyethylene glycol and polylysine as a carrier of organic iodine: design of long-circulating particulate contrast medium for X-ray computed tomography. J Drug Target 4:381–388

Vermess M (1984) Biodistribution study of intravenous lipoid contrast material – EOE13. Invest Radiol 19:S130-S134

Vertut Doï A, Ishiwata H, Miyajima K (1996) Binding and uptake of liposomes containing a poly(ethylene glycol) derivative of cholesterol (stealth liposomes) by the macrophage cell line J774: influence of PEG content and its molecular weight. Biochim Biophys Acta 1278:19–28

Violante MR, Dean PB, Fischer HW, Mahoney JA (1980a) Particulate contrast media for computed tomographic scanning of the liver. Invest Radiol 15: [Suppl] S171–175

Violante MR, Fischer HW, Mahoney JA (1980b) New media. Particulate contrast media. Invest Radiol 15: [Suppl] S329–334

Weichert JP, Longino MA, Bakan DA, Spigarelli MG, Schwendner SW, Francis IR, Counsell RE (1994) Targeted polyiodinated triglycerides for hepatic computed tomography. Invest Radiol 28:S284-S285

Weichert JP, Lee FT, Longino MA, Chosy SG, Counsell RE (1998) Lipid-based blood-pool CT imaging of the liver. Acad Radiol 5 [Suppl 1]:S16-S19

Zalutsky MR, Noska MA, Seltzer SE (1987) Characterization of liposomes containing iodine-125-labeled radiographic contrast agents. Invest Radiol 22:141–147

Zherbin EA, Davidenkova EF, Chanson KP, Gubareva AV, Zdanova NV, Alijakparov MT, Losakova LV, Fomina EV, Rozenberg OA (1983) A new procedure for contrast imaging of the liver and spleen using water-soluble contrast media in liposomes (in Russian). Radiol Diagn (Berl) 24:507–514

Zherbin EA, Davidenkova EF, Khanson KP, Shvarts EI, Zhdanova NV (1982) New approach to contrasting of liver and spleen using water-soluble roentgenocontrast media incorporated into liposomes (in Russian). Vestn Akad Med Nauk SSSR 4:84–89

47 Spiral CT Imaging Protocols for Abdominal Studies

G. Georgakopoulos, H.G. Khan, N. Howarth, M. Grossholz, F. Terrier

CONTENTS:

1	Abdomen and Pelvis – follow–up	532
2	Liver-hypovascular Lesion	532
3	Liver-hypervascular Lesion	533
4	Liver and Pancreas – Pancreatitis	533
5	Liver and Pancreas –Jaundice or Pancreatic Tumor	534
6	Liver-CT Angiography Before Liver Transplant	535
7	Pancreas with CT Angiogram	536
8	Pancreas – Endocrine Tumor	537
9	Suspected Mesenteric Infarction (Arterial or Venous)	538
10	Pelvis – Follow-up	539
11	Total-body Scan (Thorax-Abdomen-Pelvis)	539
12	Esophageal or Upper Digestive Tract Neoplasm	540
13	Liver-CT Portogram and CT Angiography	541
14	Abdominal Trauma	542
15	Abdominal Aorta	543
16	CT Cystogram After Renal or Pancreatic Transplant	543
17	Retroperitoneum-Retroperitoneal Hematoma	544
18	Renal Mass	544
19	Kidney and Excretory System: Calculus	545
20	Kidney-Acute Pyelonephritis	545
21	Urinary Excretory System-Tumor	546
22	Adrenal Glands	546

The spiral CT imgaging protocols that are presented are those that we use on a routine basis at the Geneva University Hospital for studies of the abdomen.

They have been designed for a fourth–generation, single–detector array scanner (PQ 5000 Picker International, Highland Heights, Ohio USA). This system has a scantime of 1 s per complete revolution and allows 70 revolutions with a pitch up to 2. The collimation can be as low as 1 mm.

The protocols described should be regarded as guidelines only and not be followed rigidly. They may differ from those utilized in other institutions, as can be seen in the relevant chapters of this book. For example, we use a constant amount of contrast medium without reference to body weight, whereas others calculate the amount of contrast medium according to the patient's body weight. Obviously, the imaging protocols should be adapted to the CT system and views of each institution.

G. Georgakopoulos, MD; Department of Radiology. Division de Radiodiagnostic et Radiologie Interventionnelle. Hôpital Cantonal, Rue Micheli–du–Crest 24. Ch-1211 Geneva 14, Switzerland

H.G. Khan, MD; Department of Radiology. Division de Radiodiagnostic et Radiologie Interventionnelle. Hôpital Cantonal, Rue Micheli–du–Crest 24. Ch-1211 Geneva 14, Switzerland

N. Howarth, MD; Department of Radiology. Division de Radiodiagnostic et Radiologie Interventionnelle. Hôpital Cantonal, Rue Micheli–du–Crest 24. Ch-1211 Geneva 14, Switzerland

M. Grossholz, MD; Department of Radiology. Division de Radiodiagnostic et Radiologie Interventionnelle. Hôpital Cantonal, Rue Micheli–du–Crest 24. Ch-1211 Geneva 14, Switzerland

F. Terrier, MD; Department of Radiology. Division de Radiodiagnostic et Radiologie Interventionnelle. Hôpital Cantonal, Rue Micheli–du–Crest 24. Ch-1211 Geneva 14, Switzerland

Protocol no. 1   Region of Interest: Abdomen and Pelvis – Follow–up

Oral contrast	1.0–1.5 positive contrast medium (e.g.: Gastrografin® 1:10 dilution), and 500–600 ml to be given on the table immediately before scanning.
Respiratory phase	Inspiration
Acquisition parameters	Slice collimation: 8 mm Reconstruction interval: 8 mm Pitch: 1.5–2.0
Scan range	Diaphragm to symphysis pubis
IV contrast	140 ml with 300 mg I/ml at 3 ml/s. Scan delay 60 s If necessary, acquire delayed slices on the bladder
Notes	1. In cases of hypervascular neoplasms (hepatocellular carcinoma, insulinoma, carcinoid, renal, thyroid or breast carcinoma, or sarcoma) use protocol no. 3.

Protocol no. 2   Region of Interest: Liver, Hypovascular Lesion

Oral contrast	1.0–1.5 positive contrast medium (e.g.: Gastrografin® 1: 10 dilution), and 500–600 ml to be given on the table immediately before scanning.
Respiratory phase	Inspiration
Acquisition parameters	Slice collimation: 5 mm Reconstruction interval: 5 mm Pitch: 1.5–2.0
Scan range	Diaphragm to iliac crest
IV contrast	140 ml with 300 mg I/ml at 3 ml/s Scan delay: 60 s
Notes	

Protocol no. 3   Region of Interest: Liver–Hypervascular Lesion

Oral contrast	600–900 ml positive contrast medium (e.g.: Gastrografin® 1:10 dilution), and 500–600 ml to be given on the table immediately before scanning.
Respiratory phase	Inspiration
Acquisition parameters	Collimation: 5mm Reconstruction interval: 5 mm Pitch: adjust (1.5–2.0) to fit one single spiral
Scan range	1st Spiral: From the inferior surface of the liver to the diaphragm 2nd Spiral: From the diaphragm to the inferior surface of the liver
IV contrast	150–180 ml of 300 mg I/ml at 5 ml/s 1st spiral: scan delay 20–25 s (arterial phase) 2nd spiral: scan delay 60 s (portal phase)
Notes	1. Hypervascular liver lesions: Hepatocellular carcinoma, insulinoma metastases, carcinoid metastases, kidney, thyroid, sarcoma, breast carcinoma metastases. 2. If no lesion is seen with the following tumors (kidney, carcinoid, insulinoma, breast carcinoma, thyroid, choriocarcinoma, leiomyosarcoma, or any other tumor likely to produce hypervascular metastases), acquire delayed slices (10 min after contrast injection).

Protocol no. 4   Region of Interest: Liver and Pancreas–Pancreatitis

Oral contrast	Water must be used as contrast medium to obtain negative contrast in the stomach and duodenum. 600–900 ml must be given 30 min before scanning, 600–900 ml on the table, immediately before. IV Buscopan® or Glucagon® may be administered to decrease intestinal peristalsis.
Respiratory phase	Inspiration
Acquisition parameters	1st Spiral: Slice collimation: 5 mm Reconstruction interval: 5 mm Pitch: 1.5–2.0 2nd Spiral: Slice collimation: 5 mm from 1 cm below the pancreas, scanning caudal to cephalad; 10 mm from below the pancreatic head to the symphysis Reconstruction interval: 5 mm from 1 cm below the pancreas, scanning caudal to cephalad; 10 mm from below the pancreatic head to the symphysis Pitch: 1.5–2.0
Scan range	1st spiral: Pancreas 2nd spiral: Starting 1 cm below the pancreas to the diaphragm (caudal to cephalad) and from below the pancreatic head to the symphysis pubis
IV contrast	1st spiral: None 2nd spiral: 140 ml of 300mg I/ml at 3 ml/s scan delay: 60 s
Notes	1. The purpose of the first spiral (unenhanced) is to localize the pancreas and exclude possible calcium-containing biliary stones.

Protocol no. 5   Region of Interest: Liver and Pancreas–Jaundice or Pancreatic Tumor

Oral contrast	Water must be used as contrast medium to obtain negative contrast in the stomach and duodenum: 600–900 ml must be given 30 min before scanning, 600–900 ml on the table, immediately before. IV Buscopan®, or Glucagon® may be administered to decrease intestinal peristalsis.

Respiratory phase   Inspiration

Acquisition Paramaeters

Unenhanced scan:
Slice collimation:	5 mm
Reconstruction interval:	5 mm
Pitch:	1.5–2.0
Enhanced scan:	Double–spiral CT:

1st spiral:
Slice collimation:	3–5 mm
Reconstruction interval:	3–5 mm
Pitch:	1.5–2.0

2nd spiral:
Slice collimation:	5–8 mm
Reconstruction interval:	5–8 mm
Pitch:	1.5–2.0

Scan Range

Unenhanced scan:	Superior abdomen
Enhanced scan:	
1st spiral:	Caudal to cephalad, starting 2 cm below the pancreas
2nd spiral:	Diaphragm to inferior surface of the liver

IV contrast

180 ml of 300 mg l/ml at 5 ml/s:
1st spiral:	Scan delay 25 s
2nd spiral:	Scan delay 60 s

Notes

1. The purpose of the unenhanced scan is to localize the pancreas and exclude possible biliary stones.
2. The first enhanced spiral is done with a 3–5 mm slice collimation, starting 2 cm below the pancreas, scanning caudal to cephalad, at the arterial phase (25 seconds after the beginning of contrast injection). The second enhanced spiral is acquired at the portal phase (60 seconds after the beginning of contrast injection).
3. If pancreatic surgery is being considered, see protocol no. 7 (CT–angio liver/pancreas).

Protocol no. 6   Region of Interest: Liver–CT Angiography (CTA) Before Liver Transplant

Oral contrast	Water must be used as contrast medium to obtain negative contrast in the stomach and duodenum. 600–900 ml must be given 30 min before scanning, 600–900 ml on the table, immediately before. Buscopan® or Glucagon® may be administered to decrease intestinal peristalsis.

Respiratory phase   Inspiration

Acquisition parameters

Unenhanced scan:
Slice collimation: 8 mm
Reconstruction interval: 8 mm
Pitch: 1.5–2.0
Enhanced scan: Double–spiral CT:

1st spiral (arterial phase):
Slice collimation: 3 mm
Reconstruction interval: 2 mm
Pitch: 1.5

2nd spiral: (portal phase):
Slice collimation: 3 mm
Reconstruction interval: 2 mm
Pitch: 1.5

Scan range

Unenhanced scan:	Diaphragm to 2–3 cm below the superior mesenteric artery
Enhanced scan:	
1st spiral:	Caudal to cephalad, starting 2 cm below the pancreas. Determine slice levels on the pre–contrast CT (see below).
2nd spiral:	Cephalad to caudal, diaphragm to 2 cm below the pancreas.

IV contrast

Double-spiral CT: Test-bolus: 20 ml at 5 ml/s. With 0 index at the level of the celiac trunk, program approximately 30 slices on the sequential program. Determine the peak enhancement in the aorta by measuring density.
– 180 ml of 300 mg I/ml at 5 ml/s:
– 1st spiral: Scan delay for the arterial phase = aortic peak enhancement (seconds) – 2 (seconds)
– 2nd spiral: scan delay 60 s (portal phase)

Notes

1. Unenhanced scan to localize the level of the vessels.
2. Angio CT with 3-mm collimation spiral. Beginning 2.5 cm below the superior mesenteric artery, caudal to cephalad. Start injection after calculating the peak enhancement with the test dose to obtain an arterial phase. The second spiral is for the portal phase.
3. Use a 2-mm reconstruction interval (for 3D reconstruction).
4. Postprocessing by Maximum Intensity Projection (MIP) and Surface Shade Display (SSD) for 3D reconstruction of the arteries and veins.
5. Measure the celiac trunk, common hepatic artery and portal vein diameters.

Protocol no. 7   Region of Interest: Pancreas with CT Angiogram (CTA)

Oral contrast	Water must be used as contrast medium to obtain negative contrast in the stomach and duodenum: 600–900 ml must be given 30 min before scanning, 600–900 ml on the table, immediately before. IV Buscopan® or Glucagon® may be administered to decrease intestinal peristalsis.

Respiratory phase   Inspiration

Acquisition parameters

Unenhanced scan:

Slice collimation: 8 mm
Reconstruction interval: 8 mm
Pitch: 1.5–2.0

Enhanced scan: Double–spiral CT:

1st spiral (arterial phase):
Slice collimation: 3 mm
Reconstruction interval: 2 mm
Pitch: 1.5

2nd spiral: (portal phase):
Slice collimation: 3 mm
Reconstruction interval: 2 mm
Pitch: 1.5

Scan range

Unenhanced scan: Diaphragm to 2–3 cm below the pancreas
Enhanced scan: 1st spiral: caudal to cephalad, starting 2 cm below the pancreas to the diaphragm.
2nd spiral: On the liver and pancreas, cephalad to caudal

IV contrast

Double–spiral enhanced CT: Test–bolus: 20 ml at 5 ml/s. With 0 index at the level of the celiac trunk, program approximately 30 slices on the sequential program. Determine the peak enhancement in the aorta by measuring density.

– 180 ml of 300 mg I/ml at 5 ml/s:
– 1st spiral: scan delay for the arterial phase = aortic peak enhancement (seconds) + 2 (seconds)
– 2nd spiral: scan delay 60 s (portal phase)

Notes

1. Unenhanced scan to localize the level of the vessels.
2. Double-spiral CT: CT angiogram with 3-mm collimation. Beginning 2.5 cm below the superior mesenteric artery, caudal to cephalad. Start injection after calculating the peak enhancement with the test dose to obtain an arterial phase. The second spiral is for the portal phase.
3. Use a 2-mm reconstruction interval for 3D reconstruction.

Protocol no. 8   Region of Interest: Pancreas, Endocrine Tumor

Oral contrast	Water must be used as contrast medium to obtain negative contrast in the stomach and duodenum. 600–900 ml must be given 30 min before scanning, 600–900 ml on the table, immediately before. IV Buscopan or Glucagon may be administered to decrease intestinal peristalsis.
Respiratory phase	Inspiration

Acquisition parameters

Unenhanced scan:
Slice collimation: 8 mm
Reconstruction interval: 8 mm
Pitch: 1.5–2.0
Enhanced scan: Double–spiral CT:

1st spiral (arterial phase):
Slice collimation: 3 mm
Reconstruction interval: 2 mm
Pitch: 1.5–2.0

2nd spiral: (portal phase):
Slice collimation: 5–8 mm
Reconstruction interval: 5–8 mm
Pitch: 1.5–2.0

Scan range

Unenhanced scan: Diaphragm to 2–3 cm below the pancreas
Enhanced scan:
1st spiral: On the liver and pancreas, caudal to cephalad, starting just below the pancreas. Try to cover the liver and pancreas with one single spiral.

2nd spiral: On the liver and pancreas, cephalad to caudal

IV contrast

Double-spiral CT: Test-bolus: 20 ml at 5 ml/s. With 0 index at the level of the celiac trunk, program approximately 30 slices on the sequential program. Determine the peak enhancement in the aorta by measuring density.
– 180 ml of 300 mg I/ml at 5 ml/s:
– 1st spiral: Scan delay for the arterial phase = aortic peak enhancement (seconds) + 2 (seconds)
– 2nd spiral: Scan delay 60 s (portal phase)

Notes

1. Unenhanced scan to localize the pancreas.
2. Double-spiral CT: Acquire the first enhanced scan with a 3 mm slice collimation. Begin slices just below the pancreas, caudal to cephalad. Start injection after calculating the peak enhancement with the test dose or the portal phase, after 60 s, cephalad to caudal.

Protocol no. 9   Region of Interest: Suspected Mesenteric Infarction (Arterial or Venous)

Oral contrast	Water must be used as contrast medium to obtain negative contrast in the stomach and duodenum: 600–900 ml must be given 30 min before scanning, 600–900 ml on the table, immediately before. IV Buscopan® or Glucagon® may be administered to decrease intestinal peristalsis.
Rectal Contrast	Water
Respiratory phase	Inspiration

Acquisition parameters

Unenhanced scan:
Slice collimation: 8 mm
Reconstruction interval: 8 mm
Pitch: 1.5–2.0
Enhanced scan:
Slice collimation: 5 mm
Reconstruction interval: 5 mm
Pitch: 1.5–2.0

Scan range	Diaphragm to symphysis pubis
IV contrast	150 ml of 300 mg l/ml at 3 ml/s Scan delay 60 s

Notes

1. Unenhanced slices are necessary to localize possible fresh, hyperdense thrombi.
2. Criteria for mesenteric infarction are:
   • Visualisation of the thrombus in the SMA or the SMV
   • Absence of bowel wall enhancement
   • Gas in the SMV or the portal vein
   • Intestinal pneumatosis
   • Bowel wall thickening (non–specific sign)
   • Infarction of a solid organ (non specific sign)

Protocol no. 10   Region of Interest: Pelvis–Follow–up

Oral contrast	Positive contrast medium (e.g. Gastrografin® 1:10 dilution), 600–900 ml 30 min before and 500–600 ml on the table immediately before scanning
	Rectal contrast medium (e.g. Telebrix Gastro®, 300 mg l/ml, 1:40 dilution)
	Vaginal tampon for women
Respiratory phase	Inspiration
Acquisition parameters	Slice collimation: 5 mm Reconstruction interval: 5 mm Pitch: 1.5–2.0
Scan range	Iliac crest to below the iliac branches
IV contrast	100 ml of 300 mg l/ml at 3 ml/s, Scan delay 90 seconds Consider delayed imaging with contrast medium filled bladder.
Notes	1. Venous opacification in the pelvis is maximal between 3 and 7 min after IV contrast medium injection (Teefey et al. Radiology 1990; 175:683–85)

Protocol no. 11   Region of Interest: Total Body Scan (thorax–abdomen–pelvis)

(Follow–up of Tumor for Patient with Known Malignancy)

Oral contrast	Positive contrast medium (eg: Gastrografin® 1:10 dilution), 600–900 ml 30 min before and 500–600ml on the table immediately before scanning Negative contrast medium (water) in case of gastric tumor If colon of pelvic tumor is a possibility: rectal contrast medium (eg: Telebrix Gastro® 300 mg l/ml, 1:40 dilution) Vaginal tampon for women
Respiratory phase	Inspiration
Acquisition parameters	Slice collimation: 8 mm Reconstruction interval: 8 mm Pitch: 1.5–2.0
Scan range	1st spiral: From the diaphragm to the lung apices 2nd spiral: From the diaphragm to the symphysis pubis
IV contrast	*Thorax–superior abdomen–inferior abdomen:* 140 ml of 300 mg l/ml at 3 ml/s 1st spiral: Scan delay 25 s, one single breathold 2nd spiral: Scan delay 60 s
Notes	1. Use a lung algorithm. 2. In case of strong suspicion of liver metastases, acquire slices with 5-mm collimation on the liver, with 140 ml of contrast at 3 ml/s.

Protocol no. 12   Region of Interest: Esophageal or Upper Digestive Tract Neoplasm

Oral contrast	Water must be used as contrast medium to obtain negative contrast in the stomach and duodenum. 600–900 ml must be given 30 min before scanning, 600–900 ml on the table, immediately before. IV Buscopan® or Glucagon® may be administered to decrease intestinal peristalsis and to obtain adequate duodenal distension.

Respiratory phase   Inspiration
Acquisition   Slice collimation: 5 mm
parameters   Reconstruction interval: 5 mm
                           Pitch: 1.5–2.0

Scan range   Superior or mid esophageal neoplasm:
                     Lung apex (see protocol 11) to iliac crest
                     Lower esophageal neoplasm:
                     Carina (see protocol 11) to iliac crest
                     Gastric or duodenal neoplasm: diaphragm to iliac crest

                     Direction: cephalad to caudal

IV contrast   140 ml of 300 mg I/ml at 3 ml/s
                     Start scanning 60 seconds after the beginning of the injection

Notes   1. Repositioning the patient may help to obtain better distension of the stomach (procline or left anterior oblique) or duodenum (right anterior oblique). Try these positions if the initial slices do not show adequate distension of the region under investigation.

                     2. Esophageal distension is always difficult to obtain. It may sometimes be necessary to ask the patient to swallow water just before scanning. This must be repeated before each additional slice. Giving esophageal paste may also be useful.

                     3. Always give more oral contrast medium before acquiring additional slices !

Protocol no. 13 Region of Interest: Liver, CT Portography (CTAP) and CT Angiography (CTA)

Oral contrast	Water must be used as contrast medium to obtain negative contrast.
Respiratory phase	Inspiration

Acquisition parameters

CTAP spiral:
Slice collimation: 5 mm
Reconstruction interval: 5 mm
Pitch: 1.5–2.0
CTA spiral:
Slice collimation: 5 mm
Reconstruction interval: 5 mm
Pitch: 1.5–2.0

Scan range

Diaphragm to lower surface of the liver

IV contrast

CT Portography: Done with the extremity of the catheter placed in the superior mesenteric artery or the splenic artery, 200 ml of 300 mg I/ml at 3 ml/s
Scan delay: 60 s
1 s per slice with 4–5 seconds delay between each slice (one breathold for each slice)

Hepatic CT Angiography: Extremity of the catheter placed in the hepatic artery. If one cannot opacify the left and right liver lobes simultaneously because of anatomical vascular variants, preference should be given to portography.
50 ml of 300 mg I/ml diluted with 150 ml of NaCl (total 200 ml) at 3–7 ml/s, (the injection flow must be determined by the angiographer: generally 5–7 ml/s in the hepatic artery)
For scan delay, see below.

Delayed Scan After IV contrast

After CTAP and CTA
Calculate how much contrast the patient has received during the Angiography and the CT. After the CT, inject more contrast medium for a total of 60 g of Iodine
Repeat the liver scan 4–6 hours later.

Notes

– CTAP spiral: delay 60 s. 5 mm collimation (use a 2.5 mm reconstruction interval if a small lesion is to be seen).
Spiral CT: delay = (contrast injection duration + 10 s) – (scanning time), thus
– CT ends 10 seconds after the end of the injection; 5-mm acquisition (2.5-mm reconstruction interval if a small lesion is to be visualized).

Protocol no. 14   Region of Interest: Abdominal Trauma (Superior Abdomen and Pelvis)

Oral contrast	If possible, positive contrast medium (Gastrografin® 1:10 dilution), 600–900 ml 30 min before (per os or through a naso–gastric tube), and 300 ml on the table immediately before scanning
Respiratory phase	Inspiration
Acquisition parameters	Slice collimation: 5–8 mm Reconstruction interval: 5–8 mm Pitch: 1.5–2.0
Scan range	Diaphragm to symphysis pubis (or lower if the thighs are to be examined)
IV contrast	140 ml of 300 mg l/ml at 3 ml/s, Scan delay 60 s Slice acquisition from the diaphragm to the symphysis pubis
CT Cystogram The filling of the bladder with contrast must be supervised by the radiologist	If necessary, must be performed before the abdomino–pelvic CT. 15 ml of 300 mg l/ml in 500 ml of sterile NaCl. Fill the bladder with 100 ml of contrast medium. Acquire 5–mm CT slices on the bladder to look for contrast medium leakage. Continue filling the bladder carefully up to a volume of 200–400 ml of contrast, even if extravasation is present. Acquire a spiral with 5– to 8–mm slice collimation for evaluation of intraperitoneal rupture. Unclamp the bladder catheter and continue with abdomino–pelvic CT.
Notes	1. In the patient is intubated and ventilated, ask the anesthesiologist for an apnea. 2. In case of severe injury to the spleen, liver or kidney, think of acquiring delayed slices to evaluate possible contrast medium extravasation (active bleeding).

Protocol no. 15 Region Interest: Abdominal Aorta

Oral contrast	Water must be used as contrast medium to obtain negative contrast in the stomach and duodenum. 600–900 ml must be given 30 min before scanning and 600–900 ml on the table, immediately before. IV Buscopan® or Glucagon® may be administered to decrease intestinal peristalsis.
Respiratory phase	Inspiration

Acquisition parameters

Unenhanced slices
Slice collimation: 10 mm
Reconstruction interval: 10 mm
Pitch: 1.5–2.0
Enhanced slices (covering the whole anevrismal region in one single breathold):
Slice collimation: 5–8 mm
Reconstruction interval: 5–8 mm
Pitch: 1.5–2.0

Scan Range

Unenhanced: diaphragm to symphysis pubis
Enhanced: use the unenhanced slices to determine the extension of the anevrism. Begin at least 3 cm above the celiac trunk and end at least 3 cm below the iliac bifurcation.

IV contrast

150 ml of 300 mg I/ml at 4 ml/s
Scan delay: 30 sec

Notes

1. 3 to 5 mm reconstruction interval for 3D reconstruction
2. If the patient is anesthesized, ask the anesthesiologist for a breathold.

Protocol no. 16 Region of Interest: CT Cystogram after Renal or Pancreatic Transplant

Oral contrast	Water
Respiratory phase	Breathold

Acquisition parameters

Slice collimation: 5 mm
Reconstruction interval: 5 mm
Pitch: 1.5–2.0

Scan range Iliac crest to symphysis pubis

IV contrast None

CT Cystogram

If necessary, must be performed before the abdomino–pelvic CT.

15 ml of 300 mg l/ml in 500 ml of sterile NaCl.

The filling of the bladder with contrast must be supervised by the radiologist

Fill the bladder with 100 ml of contrast medium. Acquire a spiral with 5-mm slice collimation on the bladder to look for extravasation. If extravasation is present, stop.

If negative or undetermined:
Continue filling the bladder carefully up to a volume of 200–400 ml of contrast.
Acquire a spiral with 5- to 8-mm slice collimation for evaluation of vesical rupture.

Protocol no. 17   Region of Interest: Retroperitoneum – Retroperitoneal Hematoma

Oral contrast	If possible, 600–900 ml positive contrast medium (e.g. Gastrografin 1:10 dilution), per os or through a naso gastric tube and 300ml on the table immediately before scanning
Respiratory phase	Inspiration
Acquisition parameters	Unenhanced slices Slice collimation: 10 mm Reconstruction interval: 10 mm Pitch: 1.5–2.0 Enhanced slices (if diagnosis is uncertain): Slice collimation: 5 mm Reconstruction interval: 5–mm Pitch: 1.5–2.0
Scan range	Diaphragm to symphysis pubis
IV contrast	IV contrast injection is necessary only if one wants to eliminate an arterial or parenchymal source of bleeding. 140 ml of 300 mg l/ml at 3 ml/s Scan delay 45 s
Notes	1. If a laceration of the femoral artery is suspected (after femoral artery catheterization, for example) additional slices on the thighs may be necessary.

Protocol no. 18   Region of Interest: Renal Mass

Oral contrast	1.0–1.5 l water, plus 500–600 ml on the table on the table immediately before scanning
Respiratory phase	Inspiration
Acquisition parameters	– Unenhanced: Collimation: 5 mm. If presence of fat is suspected within a lesion, repeat Slices on the lesion with 3-mm collimation Reconstruction interval: 5 mm Pitch: 1.5–2.0 – Enhanced: Collimation: 5 mm Reconstruction interval: 5 mm Pitch: 1.5–2.0
Scan range	Diaphragm to iliac crests
IV contrast	140 ml of 300 mg l/ml at 3 ml/s 2 spirals: 1. Scan delay: 90 s (nephrographic phase) 2. Scan delay: 180 s (excretory phase)
Notes	1. Always acquire unenhanced slices for evaluation of possible stones, of calcifications within the mass or of a retroperitoneal hematoma. Unenhanced slices are also useful to determine mass enhancement comparing pre- and postcontrast images. 2. If a very small lesion (less than 2 cm) is to be evaluated, it may be necessary to acquire thin (3 mm) slices of the mass to enable a precise evaluation of contrast uptake. 3. Unclamp the bladder catheter and acquire a cluster of 10-mm slices on the pelvis 4. A post-CT kidney urinary bladder film (KUB) must always be obtained.

Protocol no. 19   Region of Interest: Kidney and Excretory System – Calculus

Oral contrast	Neither oral nor rectal contrast medium
Respiratory phase	Inspiration
Acquisition parameters	Unenhanced

slice collimation: 5 mm
Reconstruction interval: 5 mm
Pitch: 1.5–2.0
Repeat the CT with IV contrast and identical parameters only if no calculus is visible.

Scan range	Top of kidneys to the bottom of the bladder
IV contrast	**Only if no calculus is visible.**

140 ml of 300 mg l/ml at 3 ml/s

2 scans:
1. Scan delay 90 s
2. Repeat slices on the kidneys 5 min after i.v. contrast injection to visualize the excretory system

Notes
1. A post CT Kidney – urinary bladder film (KUB) must always be obtained.
2. Reformat in coronal and sagital planes if necessary

Protocol no. 20   Region of Interest: Kidneys –Acute Pyelonephritis

Oral contrast	None
Respiratory phase	Breathold
Slice tickness, interval	Unenhanced scan:

Slice collimation: 10 mm
Reconstruction interval: 5 mm
Pitch: 1.5–2.0
Enhanced scan:
Slice collimation: 5 mm
Reconstruction interval: 10 mm
Pitch: 1.5–2.0

Scan range	Diaphragm to inferior pole of kidneys (bladder for the unenhanced scan)
IV contrast	120 ml of 300 mg l/ml

Scan delay: 45 s (parenchymal phase)
Scan delay: 180 s (excretory phase)

Notes
1. Kidney – urinary bladder film (KUB) at the end of the study
2. Reformat in coronal and sagital planes if necessary.

Protocol no. 21   Region of Interest: Urinary Excretory System – Tumor

Oral contrast	Water
Respiratory phase	Breathold

Acquisition parameters	Collimation:
	   3 mm on the region that is suspect on intravenous pyelography, 5 mm on the rest of the urinary system
	Reconstruction interval:
	   3 mm on region that is suspect on intravenous pyelography, 5 mm on the rest of the urinary system
	Pitch: 1.5–2.0

Scan range	Upper pole of kidneys to base of bladder
IV contrast	120 ml of 300 mg l/ml at 3 ml/s 2 scans: 1st scan delay: 90 seconds 2nd scan delay: 180 seconds
Notes	1. Kidney – urinary bladder film (KUB) at the end of the study. 2. Reformat in coronal and sagital planes if necessary.

Protocol no. 22   Region of Interest: Adrenal Glands

Oral contrast	Water must be used as contrast medium to obtain negative contrast in the stomach and duodenum. 600–900 ml must be given 30 min before scanning, 600–900 ml on the table, immediately before.
Respiratory phase	Breathold
Slice tickness interval	Collimation: 8 mm (to localize the adrenal glands) Reconstruction interval: 8mm Pitch: 1.5–2.0 If a mass is visualized, repeat slices with 3-mm collimation and 1–2.5-mm reconstruction interval on the mass. If no mass is seen and a pheochromocytoma is suspected, acquire slices with 5-mm collimation and 5-mm reconstruction interval down to the aortic bifurcation.
Scan range	Diaphragm to upper pole of kidneys (down to the aortic bifurcation if pheochromocytoma)
IV contrast	Only if the mass is infiltrating surrounding organs or vessels, to assess its relationship to these structures or to differentiate a tortuous splenic artery. 140 ml of 300 mg l/ml at 3 ml/s Scan delay: 60 s
Notes	1. An essential part of the study is the density measurement within the mass. 2. If an adrenal mass is seen during a routine contrast enhanced scan, then either a delayed scan (> 2 hours) can be obtained or ask the patient to return for an unenhanced scan.

Subject Index

A

abdominal
- abscess 486, 509
- aortic aneurysms (AAA) 420 pp.
- - inflammatory 423
- trauma 471 pp.
abscess
- abdominal 486, 509
- hepatic 141
- liver 507
- renal 357
acute
- cholecystitis 141
- pancreatic hemorrhage 237
- trauma 471
adenomatosis 107
adrenal
- cystic lesions 329
- hemorrhage 330
- infections 330
- metastases 327
adrenals 319 pp.
advanced 3D imaging 27 p.
ampullary carcinoma 178, 181
angiomyolipoma 297, 343, 351, 353, 362
aortic
- dissections 426
- hypoplasias 429
- stents 424, 431
aortitis 430
arterial phase (cortical phase) 261
arterio-portal shunting 135, 138
atypical liver hemangiomas 90

B

benign
- bile duct neoplasms 178
- postoperative bile strictures 183
biliary anastomoses 186
biopsy needle 492 pp.
blood pool contrast medium 526
bolus triggering 49
bowel tumors 377, 411
bright dot sign 91, 95
Budd-Chiari syndrome 136, 137

C

carcinoid tumors 380
cavernous transformation of the portal vein 135
celiac ganglion block 513

central stellate scar 100
cholangiocarcinomas 175, 178
- intrahepatic 178
cholangitis 182, 187
cholecystitis 508
choledocholithiasis 187, 188
colonic cancer 391
color imaging 16
color-coded doppler 443
common bile duct stones 191
complicated renal cysts 352
Conn's syndrome 322
contrast medium
- blood pool 526
- concentration 47, 197, 278
- dosis 47, 48, 169, 197, 277, 373, 483
- endoluminal 371, 372
- flow rate 47, 171, 373, 483
- liver-specific 521 pp.
- volume 48, 171, 197, 373, 483
contrast-induced nephropathy 276
cortical phase (arterial phase) 261
Couinaud's classification 69
Crohn's disease 374
CT (computed tomography)
- angiography (CTA) 198, 210, 266, 419, 451 pp., 465
- - evaluation 49
- arterial portography (CTAP) 61, 75, 77, 120
- cholangiopancreatoscopy 201
- entreocylis 369 pp.
- hepatic angiography (CTHA) 60, 75, 118
- semeiotics 375
- severity index (CTSI) 230
CT-guided interventions 312
curved multiplanar reformations 283
Cushing's syndrome 321, 324
cystic pancreatic tumor 174, 220 pp.

D

data/image processing 13 pp.
delayed contrast-enhanced CT 61
diffuse type of hepatocellular carcinoma 114
diseases (see syndromes)
double duct sign 205
dual-phase CT 60, 124, 157, 172, 218
dual-spiral CT 87
- CT arterial portography (CTAP) 75
- CT hepatic arteriography (CTHA) 75
dysplasic ectopic kidney 312

E

ectopic ureter 312
endoluminal contrast medium 371, 372
endometriosis 309
enteric fistulas 377
ERCP (endoscopic retrograde cholangio-pancreaticography) 234
excretory phase 262
expansive type of hepatocellular carcinoma 113

F

fatty morphosis 115
FEM (finite element modeling) 37
fibrolamellar hepatocellular carcinoma 124
filters 22, 24
finite element modeling (FEM) 37
focal
- nephritis 356
- nodular hyperplasia (FNH) 99 pp., 123

G

ganglioneuromas 333
gastrinoma 218
gastrointestinal injury 476
globular enhancement 88

H

hepatocellular carcinoma (HCC) 111 pp., 152, 499, 509
- diffuse type of 114
- expansive type of 113
- infiltrative type of 114
helical CT 105, 108
hemangiomas 499
hematoma 296
hemorrhage 497
- intra-abdominal 472
hepatic
- abscesses 141
- hemangioma 152
- vascular anatomy 143
- veno-occlusive disease 136, 137
hepatocarcinogenesis 112
hepatocellular adenoma 99, 104, 123
Hounsfield units 14
hydatid cysts 507
hypervascular hemangiomas 90

hypoattenuating hemangiomas 91
hypovascular hemangiomas 106

I
image
– noise 7
– reconstruction 45
image-based interventions 34
incidentalomas 325
infiltrative type of hepatocellular carcinoma 114
inflammatory aortic aneurysms 423
injury
– gastrointestinal 476
– liver 474
– renal 476
– splenic 473
insulinoma 217
interpolation 19
interventions 424, 430, 491 pp., 505
intestinal obstruction 410
intra-abdominal hemorrhage 472
intrahepatic cholangiocarcinoma 178
ischemic colitis 402
islet cell pancreatic tumor 174, 216

K
Klatskin's tumor 178, 180

L
leiomyomas 378
leiomyosarcomas 380
Leriche's syndrome 429
light model 31
lipiodol CT 61, 120
liver
– abscess 507
– cirrhosis 122
– hemangioma 85 pp., 103
– injury 474
– metastases 73 pp., 153
– segments 67
– transplantation 434
liver-specific contrast medium 521 pp.
living renal donors 437
look-up tables (LUTs) 14
lymph node metastases 288
lymphoma 296, 343, 381, 486, 500, 502

M
magnetic resonance cholangiopancreatography (MRCP) 252
malignant seeding 497
marching cubes (MCs) 29
maximum intensity projection (MIP) 32, 50, 199, 282, 425
MCs (marching cubes) 29
measurements 27
MEN (multiple endocrine neoplasia) 216
mesenteric
– ischemia 393 pp.
– – strangulation obsruction 401

– venous thrombosis 399
MIP (see maximum intensity projection) 32
morphological filtering 26
MR
– angiography 459 pp.
– cholangiography 192
– colonography 392
MRCP (magnetic resonance cholangiopancreatography) 252
MRI 251 pp.
multidetector-CT 209
multimodality imaging 37 pp.
multi-planar reconstruction 18, 20
multiple
– endocrine neoplasia (MEN) 216
– rows of detectors 10
multislice detectors 46
myeololipoma 327

N
navigation system 34
nephritis, focal 356
nephroblastoma 486
nephrographic phase 262
nephron-sparing surgery 261
neurolastomas 332
neurolysis 513

O
obstructive
– jaundice 187
– uropathy 275

P
PACS (picture archiving communication system) 38
paediatric abdomen 481 pp.
pancreatic
– adenocarcinomas 174, 197 pp., 203, 207, 245, 500
– cyst 224
– cystic tumors 245
– duct 206
– – calcification 234
– tumor 175, 200
pancreatitis 174, 175, 187, 227 pp., 243 p., 500, 508
PEI (percutaneous ethanol injection) 509
perfusion disorders 133 pp.
periaortic fibrosis 285
phaeochromocytoma 292, 320, 331, 332
picture archiving communication system (PACS) 38
pitch 5, 198
– factor 45
pneumothorax 497, 504
portal venous inflow obstruction 135
postoperative ureter 310
postradiation ureteritis 310
primary sclerosing cholangitis (PSC) 183

PSC (primary sclerosing cholangitis) 183
pseudo-color imaging 16, 18
pseudocysts 235
pyelonephritis 273, 357

R
radiation 482
– exposure 7 p.
ray paradigm 31
reconstruction
– interval 6
– techniques for CT angiography 41 pp.
registration 37
renal
– abscess 357
– adenocarcinoma 353, 362, 365, 339
– artery stenoses 434, 447, 452
– cell carcinoma 263, 339
– colic 264
– cystic tumors 339
– cysts 339, 349
– – complicated 352
– infarct 271
– injury 476
– metastases 355
– neoplasms 335 pp.
– transitional cell carcinoma 342, 366
– transplant 501
– tuberculosis 357
– tumors 349 pp., 359
– vein thrombosis 274
retrocaval ureter 312
retroperitoneal
– fibrosis 283, 286, 287
– tumors 291
rotation time 45

S
saline flush 48
satellite nodules 114
scan 60
sedation 482
segmentation 28
Seldinger technique 506
shaded surface renderings (SSR) 199
siphoning 140
slice
– collimation 43
– sensitivity profile (SSP) 5, 6
– thickness 5
smoothing 23
SPIO (see superparamagnetic iron oxide particles) 96
spiral CT 111, 157 pp., 247 pp.
– cholangiography 189, 192
splenic injury 473
SSD (see surface shaded displays) 51
SSP (slice sensitivity profile) 5, 6
SSR (shaded surface renderings) 199
start delay 48
superparamagnetic iron oxide particles (SPIO) 96, 162
surface shaded displays (SSD) 33, 51,

282, 425
surface visualization 30
syndromes / diseases (names only)
– *Budd-Chiari* syndrome 136, 137
– *Conn's* syndrome 322
– *Crohn's* disease 374
– *Cushing's* syndrome 321, 324
– *Leriche's* syndrome 429
– *Zollinger-Ellison* syndrome 216

T
test bolus injection 48
time to peak enhancement (TTP) 48,
    278
transjugular intrahepatic portosystemic
    shunt (TIPSS) 143

trocar technique 506
true-color imaging 17
tuberculosis 304
– renal 357

U
ultrasonography 151 pp.
ureteral tumors 300
ureteropelvic junction obstruction 437
urolithiasis 303

V
virtual
– colonoscopy 385 pp., 412
– reality 391

volume
– measurement 30
– rendering 283, 387
– – techniques (VRT) 32, 52, 425

W
windowing 14

Z
z-axis resolution 6
Zollinger-Ellison syndrome 216
zooming 19

List of Contributors

C. ALA EDINE, MD
Department of Radiology
Hôpital Huriez
Centre Hospitalier Regional
Universitaire de Lille
rue Michel Polonovski
F-59037 Lille Cedex, France

CARLO BARTOLOZZI, MD
Professor and Chairman
Division of Diagnostic and Interventional Radiology
Department of Oncology
University of Pisa
Via Roma 67
I-56125 Pisa, Italy

CHRISTOPH D. BECKER, MD
Department of Radiology
Division of Diagnostic
and Interventional Radiology
Geneva University Hospital
24, Rue Micheli-du-Crest
CH-1211 Geneva 14, Switzerland

MARIO BEZZI, MD
Department of Radiology
University of Rome "La Sapienza"
Policlinico Umberto I
Viale Regina Elena n. 324
I-00161 Rome, Italy

LUC BIDAUT, PhD
Division of Medical Informatics
Department of Radiology
University Hospitals of Geneva
24 rue Micheli-du-Crest
CH-1211 Geneva 14, Switzerland

ENNIO BISCALDI, MD
Assistant Chief of Radiology
Department of Radiology
Giannina Gaslini Children's Hospital
Largo Gaslini 5
I-16148 Genoa, Italy

DAVID A. BLUEMKE, MD, PhD
Assistant Professor
Department of Radiology
Clinical Director, MRI
Johns Hopkins Hospital
600 North Wolfe Street, MRI 143
Baltimore, MD 21287-6953, USA

VINCENT M. BONALDI, MD
Assistant-Chef de Clinique
Département d'Imagerie Médicale
Hôpital Universitaire de L'Archet II- (CHU de Nice)
BP 79-151, route de St. Antoine de Ginestière
F-06202 Nice Cedex 03, France

H.-J. BRAMBS, MD
Professor, Ärztlicher Direktor Abteilung Röntgendiagnostik
Radiologische Klinik und Poliklinik
Universitätsklinikum Ulm
Steinhövelstrasse 9
D-89075 Ulm, Germany

LAURA BROGLIA, MD
Department of Radiology
University of Rome "La Sapienza"
Policlinico Umberto I
Viale Regina Elena n. 324
I-00161 Rome, Italy

R. BROOKE JEFFREY, JR., MD
Professor of Radiology
Chief of Abdominal Imaging
Department of Radiology
Stanford University Medical Center
300 Pasteur Drive, H-1307
Stanford, CA 94305-5105, USA

JEAN MICHEL BRUEL, MD
Professeur, Imagerie Médicale
Hôpital Saint-Eloi
CHU de Montpellier
F-34295 Montpellier, France

CARLO CATALANO, MD
Istituto di Radiologia Cattedra II
Università Degli Studi di Roma "La Sapienza"
Policlinico Umberto I
Viale Regina Elena, 324
I-00161 Roma, Italy

OSMAN CAY, MD
Department of Radiology
Beth Israel Deaconess Medical Center
and Harvard Medical School
330 Brookline Avenue
Boston, MA 02215, USA

DANIA CIONI, MD
Division of Diagnostic
and Interventional Radiology
Department of Oncology
University of Pisa
Via Roma 67
I-56125 Pisa, Italy

LAURA CROCETTI, MD
Division of Diagnostic and Interventional Radiology
Department of Oncology
University of Pisa
Via Roma 67
I-56125 Pisa, Italy

JÖRG F. DEBATIN, MD
Zentralinstitut für Röntgendiagnostik
Universitätsklinikum Essen
Hufelandstrasse 55
D-45122 Essen, Germany

FRANCESCAMARIA DONATI, MD
Division of Diagnostic
and Interventional Radiology
Department of Oncology
University of Pisa
Via Roma 67
I-56125 Pisa, Italy

F. DUBRULLE, MD
Department of Radiology
Hôpital Huriez
Centre Hospitalier Regional
Universitaire de Lille
rue Michel Polonovski
F-59037 Lille Cedex, France

JEAN H.D. FASEL, MD
Division of Anatomy
Department of Morphology
University Medical Center
Rue Michel Servet 1
CH-1211 Geneva 4, Switzerland

XAVIER FOUILLET, PhD
Safety Asessment
Bracco Research SA
31, route de la Galaise
CH-1228 Plan-les-Ouates Geneva, Switzerland

FRANCESCO FRAIOLI, MD
Istituto di Radiologia Cattedra II
Università Degli Studi di Roma "La Sapienza"
Policlinico Umberto I
Viale Regina Elena, 324
I-00161 Roma, Italy

PATRICK C. FREENY, MD
Department of Radiology
Director, Abdominal Imaging
University of Washington School of Medicine
Box 357115
Seattle, WA 98195-7115, USA

BENOIT GALLIX, MD
Imagerie Médicale
Hôpital Saint-Eloi
CHU de Montpellier
F-34295 Montpellier, France

G. GEORGAKOPOULOS, MD
Department of Radiology
Division de Radiodiagnostie et
Radiologic Interventionnelle
Hôpital Cantonal
Rue Micheli-du-Crest 24
CH-1211 Genève 14, Switzerland

GIULIA GRANAI, MD
Division of Diagnostic and Interventional Radiology
Department of Oncology
University of Pisa
Via Roma 67
I-56125 Pisa, Italy

NICOLAS GRENIER, MD
Service de Radiologie
Centre Hospitalier Universitaire de Bordeaux
Groupe Hospitalier Pellegrin
Place Amélie Raba-Léon
F-33076 Bordeaux Cédex, France

MARIANNE GROSSHOLZ, MD
Hôpital de la Tour
CH-1217 Meyrin, Switzerland

BERND HAMM, MD
Professor, Head of Department of Radiology
Universitätsklinikum Charité
Medizinische Fakultät der Humboldt-Universität zu Berlin
Schumannstraße 20/21
D-10117 Berlin, Germany

PAUL R. HILFIKER, MD
Institute of Diagnostic Radiology
University Hospital Zurich
Rämistrasse 100
CH-8091 Zurich, Switzerland

H.-M. HOOGEWOUD, MD
Médecin-chef, Département de Radiologie
Hôpital Cantonal
CH-1708 Fribourg, Switzerland

NIGEL HOWARTH,
Department of Radiology
University Hospital of Geneva
CH-1211 Geneva 14, Switzerland

HEDVIG HRICAK, MD, PhD
Chief, Abdominal Imaging
Professor of Radiology, Urology, Radiation Oncology
and Obstetrics, Gynecology and Reproductive Sciences
Department of Radiology, Box 0628, L-308
505 Parnassus Avenue
San Francisco, CA 94143-0628, USA

W.A. KALENDER, PhD
Professor, Institut für medizinische Physik
Friedrich-Alexander-Universität Erlangen Nürnberg
Krankenhausstrasse 12
D-91054 Erlangen, Germany

HALEEM G. KHAN, MD
Department of Radiology
University Hospital of Geneva
24, Rue Micheli-du-Crest
CH-1211 Geneva 14, Switzerland

REINHARD KUBALE, MD
Institut für Radiologie und Nuclearmedizin,
Ringstr. 62–64
66953 Pirmasens, Germany

ANDREA LAGHI, MD
Istituto di Radiologia Cattedra II
Università Degli Studi di Roma "La Sapienza"
Policlinico Umberto I
Viale Regina Elena, 324
I-00161 Roma, Italy

MICHAEL J. LANE, MD
Clinical Instructor Radiology
Department of Radiology
Stanford University Medical Center
300 Pasteur Drive, H-1307
Stanford, CA 94305-5105, USA

L. LEMAÎTRE, MD
Professeur,
Chef de Service de Radiologie Ouest
Department of Radiology
Hôpital Huriez
Centre Hospitalier Regional
Universitaire de Lille
rue Michel Polonovski
F-59037 Lille Cedex, France

RICCARDO LENCIONI, MD
Division of Diagnostic
and Interventional Radiology
Department of Oncology
University of Pisa
Via Roma 67
I-56125 Pisa, Italy

GUY MARCHAL, MD
Professor, Department of Radiology
University Hospitals K.U.L.
Herestraat 49
B-3000 Leuven, Belgium

J. MARECEAUX, MD
Department of Radiology
Hôpital Huriez
Centre Hospitalier Regional
Universitaire de Lille
rue Michel Polonovski
F-59037 Lille Cedex, France

BORUT MARINCEK, MD
Professor and Chairman
Institute of Diagnostic Radiology
University Hospital Zurich
Rämistrasse 100
CH-8091 Zurich, Switzerland

L. MASQUILLIER, MD
Department of Radiology
Hôpital Huriez
Centre Hospitalier Regional
Universitaire de Lille
rue Michel Polonovski
F-59037 Lille Cedex, France

JEAN-YVES MEUWLY, MD
Department of Radiology
University Hospital
CHUV Lausanne
CH-1011 Lausanne, Switzerland

WILLIAM OKUNO, MD
Department of Radiology, Box 0628, L-308
505 Parnassus Avenue
San Francisco, CA 94143-0628, USA

JEAN PALUSSIÈRE, MD
Service de Radiologie
Institut Bergonié
F-33076 Bordeaux Cédex, France

VALERIA PANEBIANCO, MD
Istituto di Radiologia Cattedra II
Università Degli Studi di Roma "La Sapienza"
Policlinico Umberto I
Viale Regina Elena, 324
I-00161 Roma, Italy

ROBERTO PASSARIELLO, MD
Professor, Istituto di Radiologia Cattedra II
Università Degli Studi di Roma "La Sapienza"
Policlinico Umberto I
Viale Regina Elena, 324
I-00161 Roma, Italy

PAOLO PAVONE, MD
Professor
Department of Radiology
University of Parma
Via Antonio Gramsci, 14
43100 Parma, Italy

JEAN-PIERRE PELAGE, MD
Service de Radiologie Viscérale
Department of Radiology
Hôpital Lariboisière
2, rue Ambroise Paré
F-75745 Paris cedex 10, France

J.H. PRINGOT, MD
Department of Radiology
StLuc University Hospital
Avenue Hippocrate
B-1200 Brussels, Belgium

MATHIAS PROKOP, MD
Professor, Universitätsklinik für Radiodiagnostik
Allgemeines Krankenhaus der Stadt Wien
Abteilung Radiologie für konservative Fächer
A-1010 Wien, Austria

Vassilios Raptopoulos, MD
Department of Radiology
Beth Israel Deaconess Medical Center
and Harvard Medical School
330 Brookline Avenue
Boston, MA 02215, USA

Gian Andrea Rollandi, MD
Chairman of 2nd Service of Radiology
S.Martino Hospital
Universitarie Convenzionate
Largo R.Benzi, 10
I-16132 Genoa, Italy

Laura Rubbia-Brandt, MD
Department of Pathology
CMU University Hospital of Geneva
CH-1211 Geneva 4, Switzerland

Stefan G. Rühm, MD
Institute of Diagnostic Radiology
Zurich University Hospital
Rämistrasse 100
CH-8091 Zurich, Switzerland

Philippe Soyer, MD, PhD
Associate Professor
Department of Abdominal and Vascular Imaging
Hôpital Lariboisière
Université Paris VII
2, rue Ambroise Paré
F-75745 Paris cedex 10, France

Luc Spadola, MD
Department of Radiology
University Hospital of Geneva
CH-1211 Geneva 14, Switzerland

Alberto Spinazzi, MD
Bracco S.p.A.
Via Egidio Folli, 50
I-20134 Milano, Italy

Patrice Taourel, MD
Imagerie Médicale
Hôpital Saint-Eloi
CHU de Montpellier
F-34295 Montpellier, France

M. Taupitz, MD
Department of Radiology
Universitätsklinikum Charité
Medizinische Fakultät der Humboldt-Universität zu Berlin
Schumannstraße 20/21
D-10117 Berlin, Germany

François Terrier, MD
Professor, Division de radiodiagnostic et
radiologie interventionelle
Départment de radiologie
Hôpitaux Universitaires de Genève
Rue Micheli-du-Crest 24
CH-1211 Genève 14, Switzerland

Hervé Trillaud, MD, PhD
Service de Radiologie
Centre Hospitalier Universitaire de Bordeaux
Groupe Hospitalier Pellegrin
Place Amélie Raba-Léon
F-33076 Bordeaux Cédex, France

Heinz Tschäppeler, MD
Department of Diagnostic Radiology
Section of Pediatric Radiology
Inselspital
CH-3010 Bern, Switzerland

Dirk Vanbeckevoort, MD
Department of Radiology
University Hospital Gasthuisberg
Herestraat 49
B-3000 Leuven, Belgium

B.E. Van Beers, MD, PhD
Department of Radiology
St-Luc University Hospital
Av. Hippocrate 10
B-1200 Brussels, Belgium

Lieven Van Hoe, MD
Department of Radiology
University Hospital Gasthuisberg
Herestraat 49
B-3000 Leuven, Belgium

Geert Verswijvel, MD
Department of Radiology
University Hospital Gasthuisberg
Herestraat 49
B-3000 Leuven, Belgium

Valérie Vilgrain, MD
Department of Radiology
Hôpital Beaujon
100 bd du Général Leclerc
F-92118 Clichy Cedex, France

P. Vock, MD
Professor, Institut für Diagnostische Radiologie
der Universität Bern, Universitätsspital Bern
Inselspital
CH-3010 Bern, Switzerland

MEDICAL RADIOLOGY
Diagnostic Imaging and Radiation Oncology

Titles in the series already published

DIAGNOSTIC IMAGING

Innovations in Diagnostic Imaging
Edited by J. H. Anderson

Radiology of the Upper Urinary Tract
Edited by E. K. Lang

The Thymus – Diagnostic Imaging, Functions, and Pathologic Anatomy
Edited by E. Walter, E. Willich, and W. R. Webb

Interventional Neuroradiology
Edited by A. Valavanis

Radiology of the Pancreas
Edited by A. L. Baert, co-edited by G. Delorme

Radiology of the Lower Urinary Tract
Edited by E. K. Lang

Magnetic Resonance Angiography
Edited by I. P. Arlart, G. M. Bongartz, and G. Marchal

Contrast-Enhanced MRI of the Breast
S. Heywang-Köbrunner and R. Beck

Spiral CT of the Chest
Edited by M. Rémy-Jardin and J. Rémy

Radiological Diagnosis of Breast Diseases
Edited by M. Friedrich and E. A. Sickles

Radiology of the Trauma
Edited by M. Heller and A. Fink

Biliary Tract Radiology
Edited by P. Rossi

Radiological Imaging of Sports Injuries
Edited by C. Masciocchi

Modern Imaging of the Alimentary Tube
Edited by A. R. Margulis

Diagnosis and Therapy of Spinal Tumors
Edited by P. R. Algra, J. Valk, and J. J. Heimans

Interventional Magnetic Resonance Imaging
Edited by J. F. Debatin and G. Adam

Abdominal and Pelvic MRI
Edited by A. Heuck and M. Reiser

Orthopedic Imaging
Techniques and Applications
Edited by A. M. Davies and H. Pettersson

Radiology of the Female Pelvic Organs
Edited by E. K. Lang

Magnetic Resonance of the Heart and Great Vessels
Clinical Applications
Edited by J. Bogaert, A. J. Duerinckx, and F. E. Rademakers

Modern Head and Neck Imaging
Edited by S. K. Mukherji and J. A. Castelijns

Radiological Imaging of Endocrine Diseases
Edited by J. N. Bruneton
in collaboration with B. Padovani and M.-Y. Mourou

Trends in Contrast Media
Edited by H. S. Thomsen, R. N. Muller, and R. F. Mattrey

Functional MRI
Edited by C. T. W. Moonen and P. A. Bandettini

Radiology of the Pancreas
2nd Revised Edition
Edited by A. L. Baert
Co-edited by G. Delorme and L. Van Hoe

Radiology of Peripheral Vascular Diseases
Edited by E. Zeitler

Emergency Pediatric Radiology
Edited by H. Carty

Spiral CT of the Abdomen
Edited by F. Terrier, M. Grossholz, and C. D. Becker

Liver Malignancies
Diagnostic and Interventional Radiology
Edited by C. Bartolozzi and R. Lencioni

Medical Imaging of the Spleen
Edited by A. M. De Schepper and F. Vanhoenacker

Diagnostic Nuclear Medicine
Edited by C. Schiepers

Radiology of Blunt Trauma of the Chest
P. Schnyder and M. Wintermark

Portal Hypertension
Diagnostic Imaging-Guided Therapy
Edited by P. Rossi
Co-edited by P. Ricci and L. Broglia

Recent Advances in Diagnostic Neuroradiology
Edited by Ph. Demaerel

Virtual Endoscopy and Related 3D Techniques
Edited by P. Rogalla, J. Terwisscha Van Scheltinga, and B. Hamm

Multislice CT
Edited by M. F. Reiser, M. Takahashi, M. Modic, and R. Bruening

Pediatric Uroradiology
Edited by R. Fotter

Transfontanellar Doppler Imaging in Neonates
A. Couture and C. Veyrac

CT of the Peritoneum
Armando Rossi and Giorgio Rossi

Magnetic Resonance Angiography
2nd Revised Edition
Edited by I. P. Arlart, G. M. Bongratz, and G. Marchal

Pediatric Chest Imaging
Edited by Javier Lucaya and Janet L. Strife

Applications of Sonography in Head and Neck Pathology
Edited by J. N. Bruneton
in collaboration with C. Raffaelli and O. Dassonville

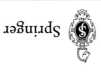

Springer

MEDICAL RADIOLOGY
Diagnostic Imaging and Radiation Oncology

Titles in the series already published

RADIATION ONCOLOGY

Lung Cancer
Edited by C. W. Scarantino

Innovations in Radiation Oncology
Edited by H. R. Withers
and L. J. Peters

**Radiation Therapy of Head
and Neck Cancer**
Edited by G. E. Laramore

Gastrointestinal Cancer – Radiation Therapy
Edited by R. R. Dobelbower, Jr.

**Radiation Exposure and
Occupational Risks**
Edited by E. Scherer, C. Streffer,
and K.-R. Trott

**Radiation Therapy of Benign
Diseases - A Clinical Guide**
S.E. Order and S.S. Donaldson

**Interventional Radiation Therapy
Techniques - Brachytherapy**
Edited by R. Sauer

Radiopathology of Organs and Tissues
Edited by E. Scherer,
C. Streffer, and K.-R. Trott

**Concomitant Continuous Infusion
Chemotherapy and Radiation**
Edited by M. Rotman
and C. J. Rosenthal

**Intraoperative Radiotherapy –
Clinical Experiences and Results**
Edited by F. A. Calvo,
M. Santos, and L. W. Brady

**Radiotherapy of Intraocular
and Orbital Tumors**
Edited by W. E. Alberti
and R. H. Sagerman

**Interstitial and Intracavitary
Thermoradiotherapy**
Edited by M. H. Seegenschmiedt
and R. Sauer

**Non-Disseminated Breast Cancer
Controversial Issues
in Management**
Edited by G. H. Fletcher
and S. H. Levitt

**Current Topics in Clinical Radiobiology
of Tumors**
Edited by H.-P. Beck-Bornholdt

**Practical Approaches to Cancer Invasion
and Metastases
A Compendium of Radiation
Oncologists' Responses to 40 Histories**
Edited by A. R. Kagan with the
Assistance of R. J. Steckel

Radiation Therapy in Pediatric Oncology
Edited by J. R. Cassady

Radiation Therapy Physics
Edited by A. R. Smith

Late Sequelae in Oncology
Edited by J. Dunst and R. Sauer

Mediastinal Tumors. Update 1995
Edited by D.E. Wood
and C.R. Thomas, Jr.

**Thermoradiotherapy
and Thermochemotherapy**

Volume 1:
Biology, Physiology, and Physics

Volume 2:
Clinical Applications
Edited by M. H. Seegenschmiedt,
P. Fessenden, and C. C. Vernon

Carcinoma of the Prostate
Innovations in Management
Edited by Z. Petrovich,
L. Baert, and L.W. Brady

**Radiation Oncology
of Gynecological Cancers**
Edited by H. W. Vahrson

Carcinoma of the Bladder
Innovations in Management
Edited by Z. Petrovich,
L. Baert, and L. W. Brady

**Blood Perfusion and Microenvironment
of Human Tumors**
Implications for Clinical
Radiooncology
Edited by M. Molls and P. Vaupel

**Radiation Therapy of Benign Diseases.
A Clinical Guide**
2nd Revised Edition
S. E. Order and S. S. Donaldson

**Carcinoma of the Kidney and Testis,
and Rare Urologic Malignancies**
Innovations in Management
Edited by Z. Petrovich,
L. Baert, and L. W. Brady

**Progress and Perspectives
in the Treatment of Lung Cancer**
Edited by P. Van Houtte, J. Klastersky,
and P. Rocmans

**Combined Modality Therapy of
Central Nervous System Tumors**
Edited by Z. Petrovich, L. W. Brady,
M. L. Apuzzo, and M. Bamberg

Age-Related Macular Degeneration
Current Treatment Concepts
Edited by W. A. Alberti, G. Richards,
and R. H. Sagerman

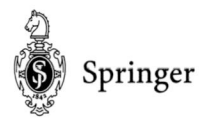 Springer